Carotenoids: Properties, Processing and Applications

Carotenoids: Properties, Processing and Applications

Edited by

Charis M. Galanakis
Research and Innovation Director, Galanakis Laboratories, Chania, Greece

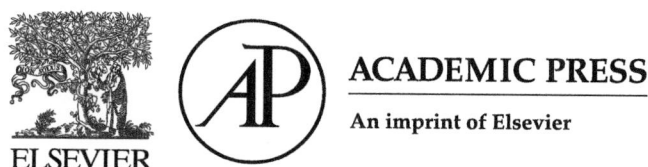

ELSEVIER

ACADEMIC PRESS

An imprint of Elsevier

Academic Press is an imprint of Elsevier
125 London Wall, London EC2Y 5AS, United Kingdom
525 B Street, Suite 1650, San Diego, CA 92101, United States
50 Hampshire Street, 5th Floor, Cambridge, MA 02139, United States
The Boulevard, Langford Lane, Kidlington, Oxford OX5 1GB, United Kingdom

Notices
Knowledge and best practice in this field are constantly changing. As new research and experience
broaden our understanding, changes in research methods, professional practices, or medical treatment
may become necessary.

Practitioners and researchers must always rely on their own experience and knowledge in evaluating
and using any information, methods, compounds, or experiments described herein. In using such
information or methods they should be mindful of their own safety and the safety of others, including
parties for whom they have a professional responsibility.

To the fullest extent of the law, neither the Publisher nor the authors, contributors, or editors, assume
any liability for any injury and/or damage to persons or property as a matter of products liability,
negligence or otherwise, or from any use or operation of any methods, products, instructions, or ideas
contained in the material herein.

Library of Congress Cataloging-in-Publication Data
A catalog record for this book is available from the Library of Congress

British Library Cataloguing-in-Publication Data
A catalogue record for this book is available from the British Library

ISBN: 978-0-12-817067-0

For information on all Academic Press publications
visit our website at https://www.elsevier.com/books-and-journals

Publisher: Charlotte Cockle
Acquisition Editor: Nina Bandeira
Editorial Project Manager: Redding Morse
Production Project Manager: James Selvam
Cover Designer: Christian J. Bilbow

Typeset by SPi Global, India

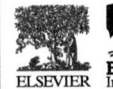

Working together
to grow libraries in
developing countries

www.elsevier.com • www.bookaid.org

Contents

Contributors

Margarita Aguilar-Espinosa Biochemistry and Molecular Biology of Plants, Yucatan Center for Scientific Research (CICY), A.C., Merida, Mexico

Ludmila Bogacz-Radomska Adaptive Food Systems Accelerator, Department of Biotechnology and Food Analysis, Wroclaw University of Economics, Wroclaw, Poland

Victor Manuel Carballo-Uicab Biochemistry and Molecular Biology of Plants, Yucatan Center for Scientific Research (CICY), A.C., Merida, Mexico

Yair Cárdenas-Conejo CONACYT -University of Colima, Colima, Mexico

A. Cepeda Department of Analytical Chemistry, Nutrition and Bromatology, Faculty of Veterinary Science, University of Santiago de Compostela, Lugo, Spain

Shi-Hui Cheng School of Biosciences, Faculty of Science, The University of Nottingham Malaysia Campus, Semenyih, Malaysia

I. Clemente School of Agriculture and Food Science, University College Dublin, Dublin 4, Ireland

María del Mar Contreras-Gámez Department of Chemical, Environmental and Materials Engineering, University of Jaén, Jaén, Spain

Cristina A. Fente Department of Analytical Chemistry, Nutrition and Bromatology, Faculty of Veterinary Science, University of Santiago de Compostela, Lugo, Spain

Carlos M. Franco Department of Analytical Chemistry, Nutrition and Bromatology, Faculty of Veterinary Science, University of Santiago de Compostela, Lugo, Spain

Charis M. Galanakis Research & Innovation Department, Galanakis Laboratories, Chania, Greece; Food Waste Recovery Group, ISEKI Food Association, Vienna, Austria

M. Garcia-Vaquero School of Veterinary Medicine, University College Dublin, Dublin 4, Ireland

Ana María Gómez-Caravaca Department of Analytical Chemistry, Faculty of Sciences, University of Granada, Granada, Spain

Sowmya Shree Gopal Department of Molecular Nutrition, CSIR-Central Food Technological Research Institute (CFTRI), Mysore, India

Joanna Harasym Adaptive Food Systems Accelerator, Department of Biotechnology and Food Analysis, Wroclaw University of Economics, Wroclaw, Poland

Hock Eng Khoo Department of Nutrition and Dietetics, Faculty of Medicine and Health Sciences, Universiti Putra Malaysia, Seri Kembangan, Malaysia

Kin Weng Kong Department of Molecular Medicine, Faculty of Medicine; Center for Natural Products Research and Drug Discovery, University of Malaya, Kuala Lumpur, Malaysia

T. Lafarga IRTA, XaRTA-Postharvest, Parc Científic i Tecnològic Agroalimentari de Lleida, Lleida, Spain

Rangaswamy Lakshminarayana Department of Biotechnology, Jnana Bharathi Campus, Bangalore University, Bengaluru, India

Alexandre Lamas Department of Analytical Chemistry, Nutrition and Bromatology, Faculty of Veterinary Science, University of Santiago de Compostela, Lugo, Spain

Aaron S.L. Lim School of Food and Nutritional Sciences, University College Cork; Food Chemistry & Technology Department, Teagasc Food Research Centre, Cork, Ireland

Wei Lu Food Chemistry & Technology Department, Teagasc Food Research Centre; School of Food and Nutritional Sciences, University College Cork, Cork, Ireland; School of Agriculture and Biology, Shanghai Jiao Tong University, Shanghai, China

Valentyn A. Maidannyk Food Chemistry & Technology Department, Teagasc Food Research Centre; School of Food and Nutritional Sciences, University College Cork, Cork, Ireland

Tehreem Maradgi Department of Molecular Nutrition, CSIR-Central Food Technological Research Institute (CFTRI), Mysore, India

Farah Ayuni Mohd Hatta International Institute for Halal Research and Training (INHART), Herbarium Unit, Department of Landscape Architecture, Kulliyyah of Architecture and Environmental Design, International Islamic University Malaysia, Kuala Lumpur, Malaysia

Rashidi Othman International Institute for Halal Research and Training (INHART), Herbarium Unit, Department of Landscape Architecture, Kulliyyah of Architecture and Environmental Design, International Islamic University Malaysia, Kuala Lumpur, Malaysia

Arkadiusz Piwowar Department of Management and Food Economy, Wroclaw University of Economics, Wroclaw, Poland

Ganesan Ponesakki Department of Molecular Nutrition, CSIR-Central Food Technological Research Institute (CFTRI), Mysore, India

Krishnamurthy Nagendra Prasad Chemical Engineering Discipline, School of Engineering, Monash University Malaysia, Bandar Sunway, Malaysia; World Pranic Healing Foundation India Research Centre, Mysore, India

Marisiddaiah Raju Department of Botany, St. Joseph's College Autonomous, Bengaluru, India

Patricia Regal Department of Analytical Chemistry, Nutrition and Bromatology, Faculty of Veterinary Science, University of Santiago de Compostela, Lugo, Spain

Renata Rivera-Madrid Biochemistry and Molecular Biology of Plants, Yucatan Center for Scientific Research (CICY), A.C., Merida, Mexico

Shivaprasad Shilpa Department of Biotechnology, Jnana Bharathi Campus, Bangalore University, Bengaluru, India

Hulikere Jagdish Shwetha Department of Biotechnology, Jnana Bharathi Campus, Bangalore University, Bengaluru, India

Ramamoorthy Siva Department of Biotechnology, School of Bio Sciences and Technology, Vellore Institute of Technology, Vellore, India

Preface

Carotenoids are a class of antioxidant compounds that occur widely in nature, especially in all colored fruits, vegetables, and flowers, and have diverse roles in photobiology, photochemistry, and medicine. These compounds have important health effects, for example, exert preventive activity against chronic diseases. The effectiveness of carotenoids depends on their metabolomics (e.g., bioactivity and bioavailability) as well as their functionality and stability during handling, extraction, and processing. Over the last years, researchers have investigated these issues, whereas the development of colorant and other food applications have attracted great interest due to the recent preference of consumers for natural compounds. Nevertheless, despite these demands, the industrial production of carotenoids is basically conducted chemically. This practice cannot be continued for a long time within the sustainability and bioeconomy frame of our times. In addition, modern food chemists, scientists, and technologists often face the development of new products and functional foods; thus a more integral point of view is required. To this line, there is a need for a new reference connecting properties, health effects, and metabolomics with extraction and processing techniques prior to exploring industrial applications that are affected by these aspects.

Over the last years, Food Waste Recovery Group (www.foodwasterecovery.group of ISEKI Food Association) has organized different training and development actions in the food science and technology field, for example, a basic theory ("The Universal Recovery Strategy"), a reference module, teaching activities (e-course, training workshops, and webinars), literature materials, e-course, an experts' database, several news channels (social media pages, videos, and blogs) for on-time dissemination of knowledge, and an open innovation network, aiming at bridging the gap between academia and food industry. In addition, the group has published books dealing with food waste recovery technologies, different food processing by-products' valorization (e.g., from olive, grape, cereals, coffee, meat, etc.), sustainable food systems, innovations in the food industry and traditional foods, nutraceuticals and nonthermal processing, as well as targeting functional compounds such as polyphenols, proteins, and dietary fiber.

Following these efforts, the current book aims to cover carotenoids' properties and health effects in view of the new trends in processing, sources (plant by-products, algae, microbial, etc.) and applications. The ultimate goal is to catalyze the development of new products and technologies to increase the competitiveness of the involved industries as well as to support the scientific community, professionals, and enterprises that aspire to develop industrial applications for carotenoids. In a broader perspective, the book aims to improve the knowledge of consumers about the importance of carotenoids in agro-food and their health benefits as well as to help public authorities refine nutritional advice to promote the health and well-being of consumers.

The book consists of 10 chapters. Chapter 1 provides an overview of carotenoids and their properties, for example, reactivity with singlet oxygen and free radicals that render them essential in dietary recommendations. Carotenoids have the particularity of acting to attenuate or prevent human chronic diseases (e.g., breast cancer, diabetes mellitus, eye illness, and cardiovascular ailments) and aging. In addition, mechanisms associated with the anti- and prooxidant behavior of carotenoids makes them essential elements for human health. Several studies, including cell cultures, animal studies, and epidemiological investigations have indicated the effect of dietary carotenoids in reducing the risk of chronic diseases such as cancer and coronary heart disease.

Chapter 2 discusses the factors affecting the bioaccessibility and bioefficacy of carotenoids. Due to lipophilic nature, and interfere with dietary and physical factors, the absorption of carotenoids at gastrointestinal level is very low. Bioaccessibility and bioefficacy of carotenoid are known to be influenced by various dietary (fat, fiber, the interaction between carotenoids and other phytomolecules/micronutrients, dosages, and location in the plant tissue) and physiological factors (genetic, gut health microflora, pH). Speciation and food processing methods are affecting bioaccessibility of carotenoids, too. The chemistry of these factors and their influence at various stages of absorption and metabolism of carotenoids are further discussed. In addition, the chapter highlights dietary approaches, as well as their merits and demerits in targeting enhancing bioaccessibility and bioefficacy of carotenoids in relation to nutrition-related health benefits.

Chapter 3 focuses on the antiobese molecular mechanisms of carotenoids particularly targeting adipocyte differentiation, thermogenesis, inflammation, and lipogenesis in view toward the management of obesity. Obesity is an abnormal condition in which excess fat is accumulated in adipose tissue. It has emerged as one of the biggest public-health concerns today as it is a major risk factor for developing type II diabetes, cardiovascular disease, hypertension, and certain types of cancer. Carotenoids play a key role in maintaining health and preventing diseases because of their remarkable structural and physical properties involving antioxidant, antiinflammatory and anticancer activities, which render them a remarkable position in the amelioration of various metabolic syndromes. Today, in vitro and in vivo as well as human interventional studies dealing with carotenoids shed light on the targets of major regulatory mechanisms of adipogenesis and pathophysiology concerning obesity and related metabolic disorders.

Chapter 4 discusses the occurrence of carotenoids in underutilized sources like agro-food by-products of vegetables, fruits, and cereals. Moreover, the impact of genetic and agronomical factors, pretreatment, extraction, and drying is revised, including examples of the potential use of carotenoids from agro-food by-products in foods. Today, carotenoids produced by chemical synthesis dominate the global market, but their obtaining from natural sources seems promising. This alternative can be useful to revalorize low-cost renewable resources, reduce industrial wastes and provide positive economic and environmental impacts. Besides, the importance of natural food additives is increasing as an alternative to synthetic additives in foods, cosmetics, and pharmaceuticals.

Chapter 5 deals with the production of carotenoids from microalgae. The latest is a rich source of high-value natural antioxidants, comprising an alternative to the chemically synthesized molecules currently dominating the global market. The chapter describes the recent advances of carotenoid production at multiple downstream processing stages like cultivation and harvesting (e.g., cultivation systems, conditions, and stresses), pretreatments (drying and cell disruption methods), extraction techniques (conventional and critical solvent extraction), purification, and storage conditions necessary to produce microalgal carotenoids. The challenges of the microalgal carotenoid industry like the advances in the chemical synthesis and the cost of production of microalgae are described in detail together with the recent developments in molecular approaches (metabolic and transcriptional engineering) to increase the synthesis of microalgal carotenoids.

Chapter 6 deals with the analysis of carotenoids. Liquid chromatography (LC) coupled to absorbance detectors (UV, Vis, PDA) and/or mass spectrometers (MS) are currently the most common instrumental methods for carotenoid and apocarotenoid analysis. Supercritical fluid chromatography (SFC) and comprehensive two-dimensional LC (LC×LC) are interesting alternatives to conventional LC separations, as they show extra capability to resolve complex mixtures of lipidic nature, including carotenoid isomers. On the the other hand, carotenoid analysis has recently moved from classical approaches to more modern and innovative solutions, as the high-throughput metabolomics.

In Chapter 7, the basic degradation process of carotenoids and the influence of encapsulation materials on the inhibition of carotenoids degradation are discussed with an attempt to facilitate the design of proper delivery systems for specific applications. Carotenoids show poor stability during storage, as they are labile to oxidation and degradation, which accordingly limit their potential as health-beneficial components. In addition, the extreme pH environment in the stomach can also result in the chemical instability of carotenoids. Hence, it is very important to maintain the stability of carotenoids during exposure to digestion tract environments after oral intake and inhibit the degradation of carotenoids during storage. Many encapsulation and delivery systems have been developed to improve the stability of carotenoids, and a correlation between the encapsulation materials and formulations with the stability and degradation velocity of encapsulated carotenoids has been observed.

Chapter 8 deals with the extraction techniques and recovery of carotenoids, as well as with their application in different fields. Owing to their multiple health prospects, carotenoids have gained significant interest in the pharmaceutical and food industries. The composition and bioavailability of the carotenoids in food are significantly influenced by the method of extraction used. Today, the application of "green" technologies in food processing has received great attention worldwide as they are environmentally friendly and considered safer for consumers. The chapter highlights also the use of greener solvents in the extraction of carotenoids as a new alternative approach. The advantages of applying such solvents (e.g., ionic liquids) over conventional ones are discussed in detail.

Carotenoids may pose as a good source of coloring agent that is capable of creating visuals that are appealing to consumers. They have also been acknowledged for positive bioactive compounds ability, including provitamin A and antioxidant properties that enhance human health. A perceptible visual aesthetics in terms of color is one of the most important aspects of product marketability and acceptability as the color itself is ubiquitous. It is capable of conveying the valuable message regarding the products effectively. Furthermore, colorants are added to products to replace the color that has vanished during product processing, while enhancing the existing color and ensuring minimal product dissimilarities within the same batch. Therefore, Chapter 9 focuses on the application of carotenoid as potential biocolorants, discussing a case study for the recovery of astaxanthin from shrimp waste.

Last but not least, Chapter 10 discusses the importance of carotenoids in different market sectors and revises current methods for commercial production and its regulation. In addition, it summarizes the most relevant patents and considers evidence supporting the health claims made by different industry sectors, focusing on the most commercially valuable carotenoids on the market (beta-carotene, lycopene, lutein, zeaxanthin, and astaxanthin). Although research has focused on the production of carotenoids in staple crops to improve nutritional welfare in developing countries, there is also an enormous market for carotenoids in the industrialized world (targeting pharmaceutical, nutraceutical, food/feed additive, cosmetics, and fine chemicals sectors), where they are produced both as commodities and luxury goods.

Conclusively, the book addresses food scientists, food technologists, and researchers working with food applications and processing as well as those who are interested in the development of innovative products and functional foods. It could be used by university libraries and institutes over the world as a textbook and ancillary reading in undergraduates and postgraduate level multidiscipline courses dealing with nutritional chemistry, food science and technology as well as bioresource technology.

Herein, I would like to thank all the authors for their fruitful collaboration in this book project. Accepting my invitation, editorial guidelines and timeline are highly appreciated. Indeed, I consider myself fortunate to have had the opportunity to collaborate with different experts around the world, for example, colleagues from India, Ireland, Malaysia, Mexico, Poland, and Spain. I would also like to thank the acquisition editor Nina Bandeira, the book manager Katerina Zaliva, and Elsevier's production team for their help during editing and publishing process. Finally, I have a message for every reader of this book. Those collaborative book projects of hundreds of thousands of words may always contain some errors or gaps. Therefore, instructive comments or even criticism are always welcome. So, please do not hesitate to contact me in order to discuss any issues of carotenoids properties, processing, and applications.

Charis M. Galanakis
Food Waste Recovery Group, ISEKI Food Association, Vienna, Austria
Research & Innovation Department, Galanakis Laboratories, Chania, Greece

Overview of carotenoids and beneficial effects on human health

Renata Rivera-Madrid*, Victor Manuel Carballo-Uicab*, Yair Cárdenas-Conejo†,
Margarita Aguilar-Espinosa*, Ramamoorthy Siva‡
*Biochemistry and Molecular Biology of Plants, Yucatan Center for Scientific Research
(CICY), A.C., Merida, Mexico, †CONACYT -University of Colima, Colima, Mexico,
‡Department of Biotechnology, School of Bio Sciences and Technology, Vellore Institute
of Technology, Vellore, India

Chapter outline

Introduction

Carotenoids are pigments synthesized by photosynthetic organisms and certain nonphotosynthetic bacteria and fungi. Carotenoid compounds are not synthesized by humans but are essential for several functions, so they need to be provided by the diet (Sun et al., 2018). The primary source of carotenoids are plants, mainly roots, flowers, fruits, and seeds (Águila & Rodríguez-Concepción, 2012). β-Carotene is also found in high contents (about 40 mg/g) in the red oil extracted from the African palm (*Elaeis guineensi*); this oil is also rich in α-carotenes (Fig. 1). Tomatoes are rich in lycopene

Carotenoids: Properties, Processing and Applications. https://doi.org/10.1016/B978-0-12-817067-0.00001-4

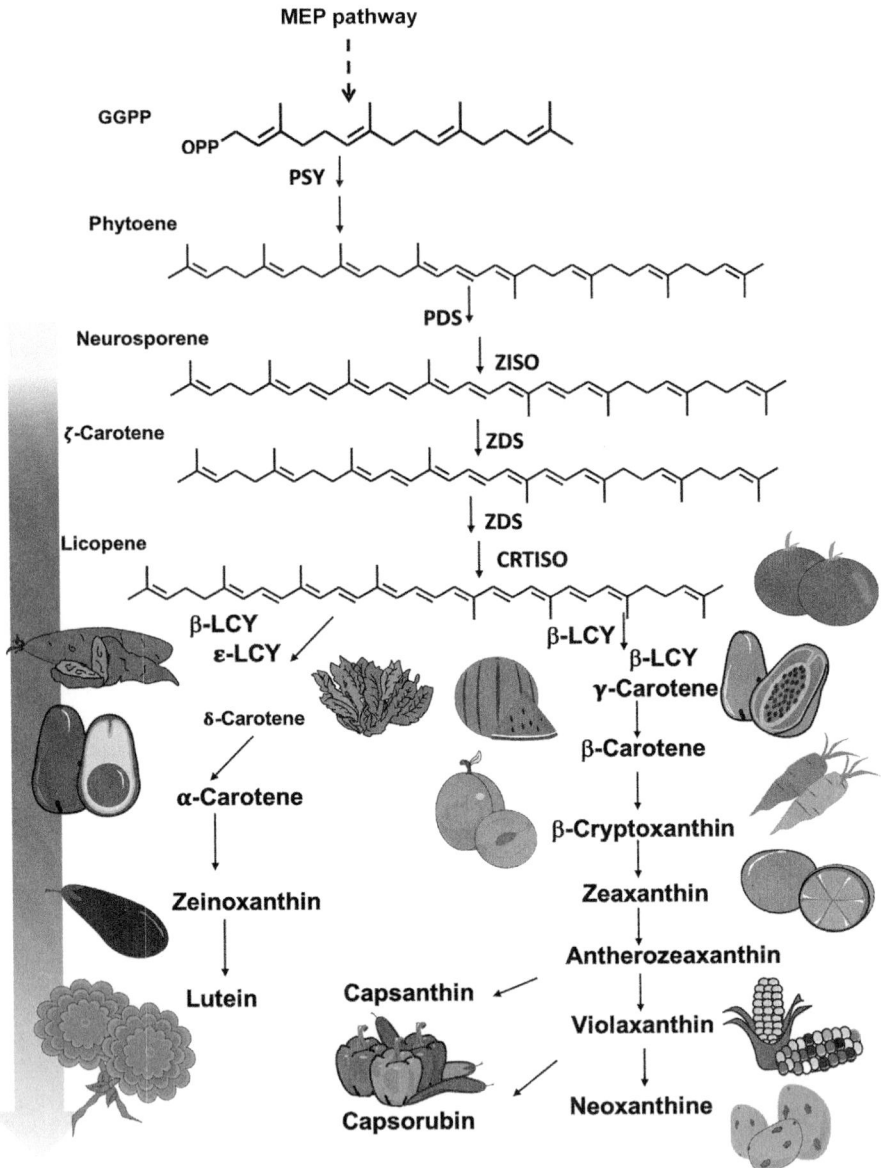

Fig. 1 Carotenoid pathway. Enzymatic conversions are represented by *arrows*, and the responsible enzymes are shown in *bold*. MEP pathway (glyceraldehyde 3-phosphate and pyruvate), *CRTISO*, carotene isomerase; *β-LCY*, lycopene beta-cyclase; *ε-LCY*, lycopene epsilon-cyclase; *PDS*, phytoene desaturase; *PSY*, phytoene synthase; *ZDS*, zeta-carotene desaturase. Fruits and vegetables have the main carotenoid from the pathway.

compound (around 100 µg/g when fresh) (Kavitha et al., 2013). Lutein is the most abundant carotenoid in plants. Marigold (*Tagetes erecta*) flowers are important sources.

Dietary carotenoids also provide provitamin A and have antioxidant properties which could help delay the onset of cardiovascular diseases (CVDs), cancers, and eye diseases as we age (Fiedor & Burda, 2014; Fraser & Bramley, 2004; Rao & Rao, 2007). Many natural carotenoids have been characterized, but only 40 are found in human diets. About 20 have been identified in blood and tissues (Rao & Rao, 2007). The mechanism of action of carotenoids includes antioxidant potential (Fiedor & Burda, 2014), anti-inflammatory activity, improving immune response, and preventing chronic diseases (Woodside, McGrath, Lyner, & McKinley, 2015). An impact of carotenoids on other functions related to aging has also been suggested, such as cognitive function and muscular strength (Woodside et al., 2015). Carotenoids concentration largely depends on the diet, tissue absorption, carotenoids release from tissues to blood and catabolism rate (Perera & Yen, 2007). Lutein, lycopene, zeaxanthin, β-cryptoxanthin, β-carotene, and α-carotene comprise 60%–70% of plasma carotenoid content (Khachik et al., 1992). These are found in all tissues, especially in adults' adipose tissue, liver, and plasma; β-carotene, lutein, lycopene, and canthaxanthin are found in the skin. About 90% of carotenoids are found in body tissues and 10% in plasma (Perera & Yen, 2007).

Dietary carotenoids, mainly from fruits and vegetables, have been associated with lower risk of chronic diseases, including type 2 diabetes, CVD, age-related macular degeneration, several types of cancers, antiinflammatory actions, and enhancement of the immune response. Some of these functions may result from the antioxidative properties of the carotenoids (Desmarchelier & Borel, 2017). However, stress, solar UV and IR radiation, alcohol abuse, and tobacco reduce carotenoids levels and promote aging (Lademann, Meinke, Sterry, & Darvin, 2011). The skin and the eyes are the only two organs of the human body exposed continuously to damage caused by the environment and require protection (Roberts et al., 2009).

Carotenoids and aging

Biologically, aging can be defined as the loss of cell, tissue, organ, and system functions occurring as the individual's chronological age increases, finally leading to death. It also involves gradual molecular changes that lead to homeostasis loss which predispose to chronic disease and to the distinctive fragility of the elderly, such as sarcopenia, osteoporosis, lipodystrophy, CVD, diabetes, cancer, and dementia (Kirkwood, 2005; Lees, Walters, & Cox, 2016).

The most noticeable characteristics of aging are a progressive decrease in physiological capabilities, reduced ability to respond adaptively to environmental stimuli, and greater susceptibility to disease (Farooqui & Farooqui, 2009). The biological mechanisms underlying aging are still uncertain. The central hypothesis of aging includes disturbances in proteins, DNA damage, less efficient DNA repair; inappropriate cross-linking of proteins, DNA, and other structural molecules; neuroendocrine secretion failure; increased oxidative stress mediated by free radicals; and changes in the order of gene expression (Farooqui & Farooqui, 2009).

In today's world, unhealthy eating habits and metabolic factors are among the primary causes of mortality risk (Eggersdorfer & Wyss, 2018). The most common causes of morbidity and premature death in developed countries are noncommunicable diseases such as heart disease, stroke, cancer, and diabetes mellitus (Eggersdorfer & Wyss, 2018).

It has been suggested that lifestyle factors, including diet, have an essential role in preventing chronic disease. Fruits and vegetables, through several mechanisms including the supply of antioxidants, dietary fiber, and micronutrients, such as carotenoids, flavonoids, vitamin C, and folic acid, may decrease oxidative damage and block carcinogens actions, helping reduce the risk of CVD and certain cancers (Eggersdorfer & Wyss, 2018; Woodside et al., 2015).

Skin aging

Just as the complete organism, the skin is subject to the unstoppable aging process. Skin aging is influenced by external factors, such as ultraviolet radiation or photoaging, one of the leading causes of skin aging (Kohl, Steinbauer, Landthaler, & Szeimies, 2011). The human skin is also under the constant influence of free radicals (FR), both from outside and inside the body. FR are produced continuously in the organism as a result of cellular metabolism, and they have an essential role in signaling between cells and destroying virus and bacteria. The human organism relies on antioxidants for protection against the action of FR (Lademann et al., 2011). Despite the antioxidant mechanisms—which deteriorate with age—cellular components of damage caused by reactive oxygen species (ROS) are abundant. Damage leads to further increase in ROS and to a reduction of antioxidant capacities, and finally, to cellular aging (Kohl et al., 2011) (Figs. 1 and 2).

Carotenoids are known to be potent antioxidant substances that have a crucial role in FR-neutralizing reactions. Carotenoid molecules in tissues are capable of neutralizing several FR attacks, especially by ROS (Darvin, Sterry, Lademann, & Vergou, 2011). Carotenoids such as α-, γ-, and β-carotenes, lutein, zeaxanthin, lycopene, and their isomers protect human skin against cell oxidation (Darvin et al., 2011).

Several studies have been conducted on the effect of carotenoids as human skin antioxidants (Lademann et al., 2011). Degradation of β-carotene and lycopene were measured in human skin after being exposed to UV irradiation, using the Raman spectrophotometer method. Researchers observed that β-carotene and lycopene do not decrease immediately after being exposed to UV and that the difference in time was caused by their capacity to react against FR (quenching). Lycopene response to radicals is better as compared to other carotenoids (Darvin et al., 2007).

An experiment was designed to evaluate the antioxidant protection of dietary supplements on healthy skin exposed to a moderate dose of UV. Several parameters were compared before and after 7 weeks of carotenoids, vitamin, and selenium (Se) supplements. Results demonstrated that oral ingestion of a complex of antioxidants significantly improved many of the parameters of epidermal defense against UV-induced damage (Césarini, Michel, Maurette, Adhoute, & Béjot, 2003); similar results have been reported recently with the increasing use of lutein and lycopene supplements as photoprotection agents (Marini, Jaenicke, Stahl, & Krutmann, 2017).

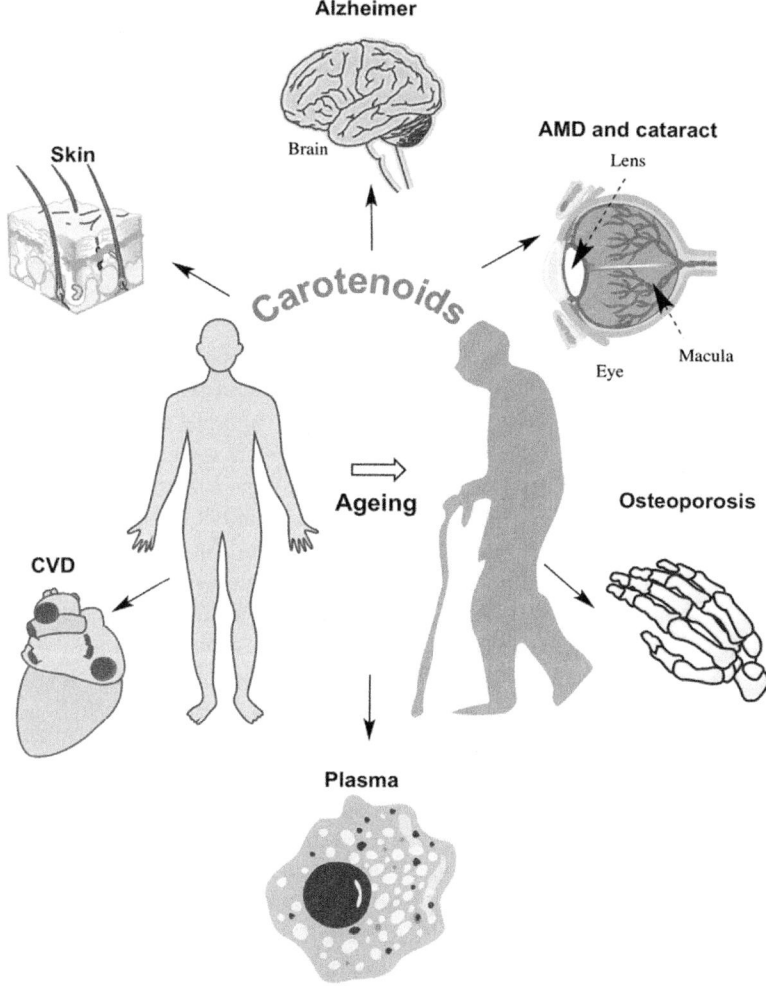

Fig. 2 Carotenoids are used against degenerative skin diseases, chronic cardiovascular diseases (CVDs), cataracts and age-related macular degeneration (AMD), Alzheimer's disease (AD), and osteoporosis.

Eye aging

Loss of vision or disease related to the eyes, such as cataracts and macular degeneration are the main disorders caused by aging in human eyes (Bernstein et al., 2016). Two carotenoids: lutein and zeaxanthin and the isomer meso-zeaxanthin are found in the human retina; they are responsible for screening light, acting as antioxidants against its iterative stress, and are known as macular pigments (Bernstein et al., 2016).

Low concentration of zeaxanthin and lutein lead to macular degeneration (age-related macular degeneration (AMD)) (Bernstein et al., 2016). AMD is the primary cause of blindness in people older than 65 years; besides age, the main factors of AMD are smoking, solar exposure, unhealthy eating, and genetics (Johnson, 2005). Several studies have confirmed the association between the quantity of lutein and zeaxanthin in the retina and macular degeneration by aging (Bernstein et al., 2001; Bone et al., 2001).

Most of the studies aiming to increase the levels of pigment in the retina are based on eating a diet rich in vegetables and fruits. However, it is necessary to consume large amounts (Bernstein et al., 2016).

The intake of supplements of vitamin C, E, β-carotene, and zinc against AMD were analyzed in persons between 55 and 80 years old. Results demonstrated that with the ingestion of these supplements, the progress of macular aging was 25% lower (Age-Related Eye Disease Study Research Group, 2001; Zhang, Jiang, Xie, Wu, & Zhang, 2015). After providingelderly people with or without AMD with supplements of lutein and zeaxanthin for6 months, mean serum levels of these compounds were significantly higher thanbaseline values, and so were their carotenoid metabolites. The serum levels of these carotenoidsgradually decline within 6 months of supplementation.(Khachik et al., 2006). However, lutein and zeaxanthin intake differ with age, sex, and ethnic group. In all the adult age groups, lutein intake is higher than that of zeaxanthin. Lower levels of zeaxanthin, as compared to lutein, have been reported in groups at risk of macular degeneration related to age (elderly and women) (Johnson, Maras, Rasmussen, & Tucker, 2010).

Age-related cataract (ARC) is a common disease of the eye affecting mainly women and old people. Its main feature is lens opacity, thus blocking the light from penetrating the eye; lens change is the consequence of aging, oxidative stress, and lack of defense against the oxidative damage (Karppi, Laukkanen, & Kurl, 2012; Zhang et al., 2015).

Lutein and zeaxanthin are the main antioxidants protecting the eye against the development of lens opacity and its severe form, cataracts (Hobbs & Bernstein, 2014; Mares, 2016). The relation of lutein and zeaxanthin concentrations in the elderly (61–80 years old) was evaluated to determine its association with ARC. The study found that high concentrations of lutein and zeaxanthin in plasma reduce the risk of suffering ARC (Karppi et al., 2012). AMD and cataracts are not independent processes. Oxidative stress is a common pathway in both diseases. Cataract is a self-defense reaction to reduce retinal damage (Wegner & Khoramnia, 2011).

Vascular aging

Old age is the stage of life with higher risk of suffering chronic CVD, such as myocardial infarction (Paneni, Diaz Cañestro, Libby, Lüscher, & Camici, 2017). Disturbances in the structure and function of arteries accompany the aging process and contribute to the increased risk of developing CVD (Camici, Savarese, Akhmedov, & Lüscher, 2015).

Two of the main characteristics of vascular changes during old age are endothelial dysfunction and rigidity of the central artery, which leads to a state of oxidative stress and inflammation of the arteries, causing CVD disease (Paneni et al., 2017).

Atherosclerosis is also one of the main manifestations of aging (Wolak & Paran, 2013). It is caused by an inflammatory process, leading to the formation of ROS, and reducing vascular nitric oxide (NO) (Celermajer et al., 1994). It has been demonstrated that lycopene and lutein are carotenoids that can reduce vascular aging in the arteries because of their antioxidative capacity, increasing the viability of NO. It has also been showed that tomato extracts (lycopene and β-carotene) decrease blood pressure and increase nitrate plasma levels (Paran, Novack, & Engelhard, 2009).

The level of lycopene in the blood may be significantly reduced during the aging process. Elderly persons show lower concentrations of lycopene in blood as compared to young people with similar diets and from the same ethnic group (Semba et al., 2010). However, the causes and mechanisms of lycopene deficiency in old age are not accurately known. DNA microarrays analyses revealed that the expression of lycopene supplements in mice prevents the activation of the genes involved in the aging process (Park et al., 2009).

Alzheimer

Among the aging-related diseases, neurodegenerative disease has received close attention because of their irreversibility and the lack of effective treatment (Hung, Chen, Hsieh, Chiou, & Kao, 2010). Oxidative stress, apoptosis, gene mutations, and neuroinflammation are associated with several chronic neurodegenerative diseases, such as Alzheimer's disease (AD) (Bao et al., 2014). AD is a neurodegenerative disorder caused by the accumulation of abnormal peptides β-amyloids and phosphorylation of Tau proteins in the brain, leading to memory loss, as well as loss of cognitive and behavioral functions, and has been associated with aging of the brain (Ademowo et al., 2017; Honarvar et al., 2017; Mariani, Polidori, Cherubini, & Mecocci, 2005; Swerdlow, 2011). Diet and carotenoid supplements have shown to have an essential role in several neurodegenerative diseases such as AD (Obulesu, Dowlathabad, & Bramhachari, 2011). The increase in dietary fruit and vegetable intake has been associated with the preservation of cognitive functions (Woodside et al., 2015). The Georgian Centenarian Study analyzed serum and demonstrated that lutein, zeaxanthin, and β-carotene are more closely associated with cognitive functions (Johnson, 2012). Lutein concentrations in the brain are lower in patients with slight cognitive impairment than in those with normal cognitive function (Johnson et al., 2013). On the other hand, lycopene has been showed to have antioxidant and antiinflammatory effects both in vivo and in vitro, it crosses the blood-brain barrier (Zhao et al., 2017) and contributes to reducing AD by decreasing the production of β-amyloid (Chen et al., 2015). Serum carotenoids, such as lycopene, lutein, and zeaxanthin reduce the risk of neurodegenerative disease (Min & Min, 2014; Zhao et al., 2017), while in patients with AD, vitamin A concentration and β-carotene in serum and plasma decrease (Molina et al., 1999); however, carotenoids concentration may increase after 6 months with dietary supplements (Ademowo et al., 2017). β-Carotene supplements also reduce β-amyloids concentration (Honarvar et al., 2017).

The association of lutein and zeaxanthin with brain functions was recently analyzed in 72-year-old patients who took lutein and zeaxanthin supplements for 1 year. Results indicated that lutein and zeaxanthin reduced cognitive impairment in tasks, such as verbal learning and seem to have benefits on the neurocognitive function, improving brain function even when consumed for a short period of time by elderly persons (Lindbergh et al., 2018).

Osteoporosis

Oxidative stress contributes to skeletal system disease (Rao & Rao, 2007). Bone is a dynamic tissue that preserves the size, shape, and structural integrity of the skeleton and regulates mineral homeostasis (Yamaguchi, 2012). Aging and numerous pathologic processes decrease bone formation and increase bone resorption which contributes to osteoporosis, a devastating skeletal disease (Weitzmann, Pacifici, Weitzmann, & Pacifici, 2006). Bone fractures associated with this disease affects one of every three women and one of every five men around the age of 50 years old. The primary test for the diagnosis of osteoporosis is bone mineral density (BMD) (Sacco, Horcajada, & Offord, 2013). Studies have shown that oxidative stress is associated with osteoporosis and that antioxidants can reduce this effect. Certain antioxidants, including vitamin C, E, and β-carotene can reduce the risk of osteoporosis (Holmberg, Wolk, Melhus, & Michae, 1999). Nutritional factors play an essential role in bone health during aging; a diet high in vegetables has demonstrated to be directly associated with BMD (McNaughton, Wattanapenpaiboon, Wark, & Nowson, 2011). On the other hand, carotenoids have direct in vitro effects on the bone, modulating osteoblastic, and osteoblastic activity (Maggio et al., 2006). A study conducted in 65 female patients with osteoporosis assessed the role of carotenoids on the disease; women with osteoporosis had a lower level of lutein, zeaxanthin, β-cryptoxanthin, lycopene, α-carotene, β-carotene, and retinol (Maggio et al., 2006). A positive relationship has been demonstrated between lycopene and total carotenoids levels in plasma with the bone mass and the risk of pelvic fracture among 75 years old men and women, which suggests that the intake of lycopene reduces the risk of bone fractures (Sahni et al., 2009). Carotenoids have many functions in human health and healthy aging. Nevertheless, elucidating the health benefits of each of the carotenoids is a challenge because the resources are similar and are highly correlated. Given the evidence of the role of specific carotenoids, particularly in the aging process, increasing their amount in the diet or taking them as supplements should be considered. However, ingestion of carotenoids in food products or as supplements in many population groups is low, particularly in the elderly.

Role of carotenoids against cancer

The highly antioxidant property displayed by carotenoids, scavenging ROS, suggest that these micronutrients have the ability to protect against chronic diseases, such as cancer, caused by ROS molecules. Recently, it has been suggested that a high intake of fruits and vegetables rich in carotenoids is related to a reduction in risk of cancer (Rodríguez-Concepción et al., 2018). The most abundant carotenoids in the human body are lycopene, β-carotene, α-carotene, β-cryptoxanthin, lutein, and zeaxanthin (Krinsky & Johnson, 2005); these carotenoids tend to be associated with specific tissues (Ahmed, Lott, & Marcus, 2005; Burri, La Frano, & Zhu, 2016; Jeon et al., 2017; Kaplan, Lau, & Stein, 1990), and probably provide protection to the tissue against cancer. For instance, lycopene showed high concentrations in the prostate compared to other tissues (Kaplan et al., 1990), and low lycopene concentrations in prostate have been associated with prostate cancer (Mariani et al., 2014). Many pieces of evidence have shown that carotenoids are implicated in the prevention of cancer in different tissues, such as lung, breast, prostate, liver, and leukemia (Nishino, Murakoshi, Tokuda, & Satomi, 2009) (Fig. 3).

The preventive anticancer activity of carotenoids has been associated mainly with the high antioxidant property that these micronutrients display; they are able to reduce the DNA damage induced by ROS molecules. However, the anticancer property of carotenoids also is linked to prooxidant activity and cellular mechanisms, inter alia, mechanism Nrf2 (NF-E2 related factor 2) mechanism NF-κB (nuclear factor kappa-light-chain-enhancer of activated B cells), intercellular communication via gap junctions (GJIC), and apoptosis, among others (Rao, Ray, & Rao, 2006; Rodriíguez-Concepción et al., 2018; Sharoni et al., 2012; van Breemen & Pajkovic, 2008).

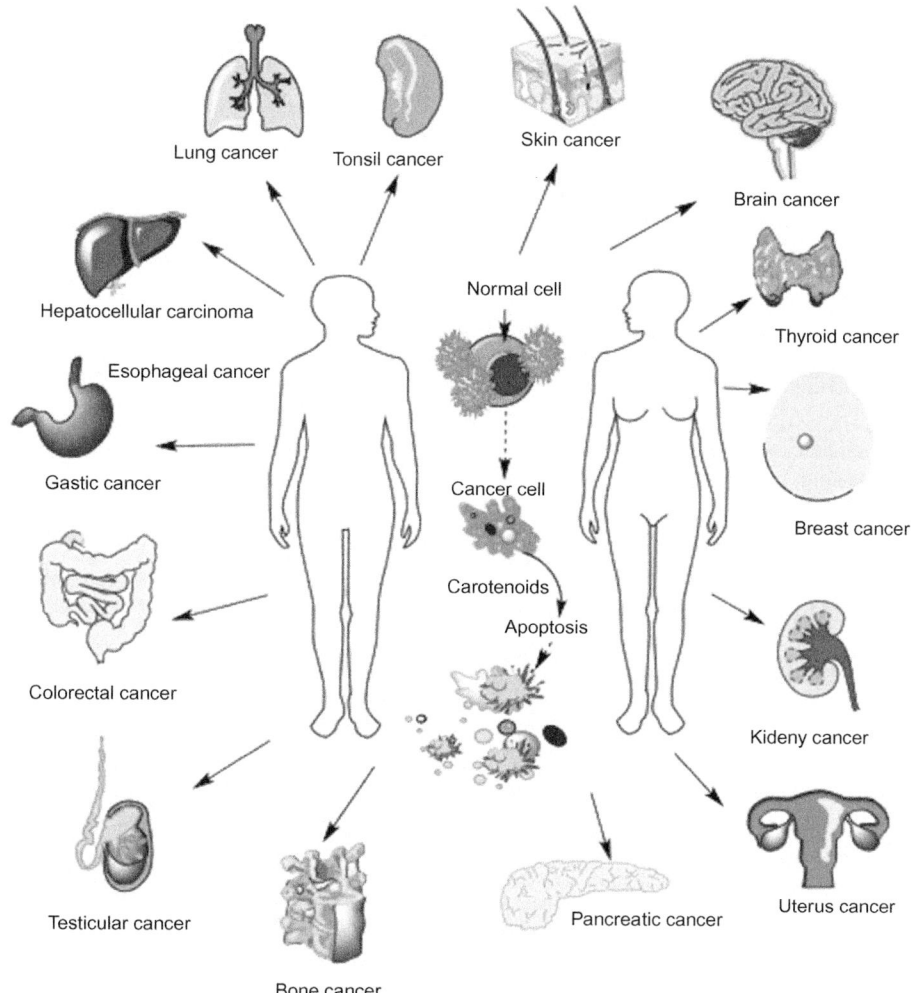

Fig. 3 Different kinds of human cancer. Suggested effect of carotenoids against cancer cells.

Antioxidant and prooxidant mechanism of carotenoids against cancer

Oxidative stress has important roles in human disease since they have the ability to damage cell macromolecules, such as proteins, lipids, and DNA (Martínez-Cayuela, 1995) by oxidation. ROS are generated within cells by aerobic metabolism including, singlet molecular oxygen ($^1O_2$), superoxide radicals (O_2^-), hydroxyl radicals, hydrogen peroxide (H_2O_2), peroxyl radicals, etc. Accumulation of ROS damage on DNA causes mutations and raises the possibility of starting the irregular cellular proliferation leading to cancer (Gill, Piskounova, & Morrison, 2016). Consistent with this idea, patients with high risk for breast, prostate, and lung cancer excrete higher levels of ROS generated by lipid peroxidation (Boyd & McGuire, 1991; Muindi, Scher, Rigas, Warrell, & Young, 1994). Additionally, tissues from lung, breast, colon, and ovary cancer have been associated with higher level of oxidized DNA adducts (Loft & Poulsen, 1996; Wang et al., 1996).

Antioxidants are compounds that provide protection against oxidative damage by inactivating ROS; therefore, it has been suggested that these compounds delay the onset of cancer (Gill et al., 2016). Enzymes within cells with antioxidant capacity include superoxide dismutases (SODs), glutathione peroxidase, glutathione reductase, and thioredoxin reductase (Gill et al., 2016). Additionally, cells produce metabolites acting as antioxidants, for instance, thioredoxin, glutathione, nicotinamide, and adenine dinucleotide phosphate (NADPH) (Gill et al., 2016). Some dietary compounds also help the cell to maintain ROS homeostasis. Carotenoids have been described as antioxidant molecules because having the ability to scavenge ROS molecules (Fiedor & Burda, 2014). The scavenging ability of carotenoids is given by a polyene backbone with a series of conjugated double-bonds which interact with $^1O_2$ and FR (Young & Lowe, 2018). The extended double-bonds system of carotenoids stabilizes unpaired electrons after radical quenching (Kaulmann & Bohn, 2014). Physical scavenging by carotenoids occurs via electron acceptance or donation, hydrogen transfer to free radical or radical adduct formation (Fiedor & Burda, 2014; Kaulmann & Bohn, 2014). The antioxidant capacity of carotenoid depends on the number of double-bonds in their backbone. Lycopene is the most efficient scavenger of $^1O_2$ and FR because is the carotenoid with more double-bonds (Britton, 1995; Ukai et al., 1994). In line with the anticancer activity via the antioxidant action of carotenoids, it has been shown that those that were treated with carotenoids reduce DNA damage in cancerous tissues in human patients, animal models, and cancerous cell lines (Bowen et al., 2002; Muzandu et al., 2005, 2006; Park, Hwang, & Moon, 2005) (Table 1).

Carotenoids can act as prooxidant agents under certain circumstances, such as high oxygen tension, high carotenoid concentration, and unbalanced intracellular redox status (Palozza, Serini, Di Nicuolo, Piccioni, & Calviello, 2003). For example, high oxygen tension transforms β-carotene into radical cation which is a reactive species with strong oxidizing properties (Burton & Ingold, 1984; Rao & Rao, 2007). The prooxidant activity has been observed mainly in β-carotene when it is administered without other antioxidants (Palozza, Serini, Di Nicuolo, et al., 2003). However, other carotenoids such as lycopene, lutein, and, zeaxanthin also display prooxidant activities

Table 1 Mechanism of carotenoid in cancer prevention.

Carotenoid	Mechanism	Cancer/model	Findings	References
Lycopene and β-carotene	Antioxidant	Chinese hamster lung fibroblasts cells (V79 cells)	Concentrations of both carotenoids ranging from 0.25 to 10 μM significantly inhibit DNA damage strand induced by ROS.	Muzandu et al. (2005)
Lycopene and β-carotene	Antioxidant	Chinese hamster lung fibroblasts	Concentrations of 0.31–10 μM of lycopene and β-carotene had protective effects on DNA damage due to their scavenging of ROS.	Muzandu et al. (2006)
Tomato sauce (lycopene)	Antioxidant	Prostate cancer/human	Patients supplemented with tomato sauce (30 mg of lycopene/day/3 weeks) had 28.3% lower prostate DNA 8-OH-deoxyguanosine/deoxyguanosine (predominant forms of free radical-induced oxidative lesions in DNA) in resected prostate compared with the control group ($P < .03$).	Bowen et al. (2002)
Lycopene	Antioxidant	Hepatic cancer/Hep3B cells	Hep3B cells growth was inhibited 20% at 0.2 μM lycopene and 40% at 50 μM lycopene after a 24-h incubation. Treated cells showed less DNA damage than did untreated cells.	Park et al. (2005)
Lutein	Prooxidant/apoptosis	Breast cancer/triple-negative breast cancer (TNBC) cells	Lutein treatment (2.0 μM for 3 h) significantly increases the intracellular ROS production in TNBC cells, but not in normal primary mammary epithelial cells (PmECs). Lutein treatment significantly increased levels of phosphorylated p53 and HSP60 protein in TNBC but not in PmECs.	Gong, Smith, Swanson, and Rubin (2018)
β-Carotene	Prooxidant	Leukemia and colon adenocarcinoma/HL-60, LS-174 and WiDr cells	Inhibition of HL-60 cell growth, LS-174 cells (and WiDr cells by significant increase of ROS ($P < .001$), ($P < .05$), and ($P < .05$), respectively. Prooxidant activity is associated with the regulation of NF-κB. If β-carotene is accompanied for antioxidant, the prooxidant activity is lost.	Palozza, Serini, Torsello, Di Nicuolo, Piccioni, et al. (2003b)

continued

Table 1 Continued

Carotenoid	Mechanism	Cancer/model	Findings	References
β-Carotene	Prooxidant	Lung cancer/lung carcinoma cell (A549)	A549 cells treated with β-carotene (5 μM) increased significantly (P < .05) the oxidative stress marker 8-oxo-dG.	van Helden et al. (2009)
Lycopene and lycopene oxidative products	Prooxidant/ apoptosis	Prostate cancer, breast cancer, and cervical cancer/PC-3 cells, MCF-7 cells and HeLa cells.	The cell viability decreased significantly (P < .05) when cancer cells were treated with 5 μM of lycopene. Interestingly, lycopene oxidative products showed lowest cell viability than lycopene in PC-3, HeLa and MCF-7 cells via apoptosis by ROS increased.	Arathi et al. (2016)
β-Carotene, zeaxanthin, lutein, and apocarotenal products of zeaxanthin and lutein.	Prooxidant	Liver cancer/Hep G2 cells	Hep G2 cells increased ROS when were treated with 2 μM of β-carotene, zeaxanthin or lutein. The apocarotenal products of zeaxanthin or lutein generated by oxidative cleavage β,β-carotene-9',10'-oxygenase dose-dependently increased (0.1–2.0 μM) ROS.	Amengual et al. (2011)
Lycopene (apo-10'-lycopenoic acid)	Activation of Nrf2 system	Human bronchial epithelial cell line (BEAS-2B)	Nuclear Nrf2 protein was increased by 50% in BEAS-2B cells treated with 10 μM of apo-10'-lycopenoic acid after 3 h. Apo-10'-lycopenoic acid also increased the expression of ARE genes and inhibit the endogenous generations of ROS.	Lian and Wang (2008)
Lycopene and β-carotene	Activation of the Nrf2 system	Breast cancer, liver cancer/MCF7, Hep G2	6 μmol/L of lycopene or breast cancer increase > twofold the mRNA levels of NQ01 and GCS genes in MCF7 and Hep G2 cells via the Nrf2 system.	Ben-Dor et al. (2005)
Lycopene	Activation of the Nrf2 system	Prostate cancer/LNCaP cells	Proteomic approaches displayed that lycopene alters the expression of the largest number of protein in LNCaP cells like epoxide hydrolase 1 (EPHX1), superoxide SOD-1, and catalase (CAT) via Nrf2.	Goo et al. (2007)

Carotenoid	Effect	Cell type	Description	References
Lycopene oxidative products	Inhibition of NF-κB	Prostate cancer/LNCaP cells	1 μmol/L of Lycopene or apo-10-lycopenal significantly reduced cell growth in LNCaP cells ($P<.05$) and relative quantities of NF-κB in the nucleus was significantive reduced cells ($P<.05$). Authors related the function of BCO2 with lycopene and NF-κB pathway.	Gong, Marisidddaiah, Zaripheh, Wiener, and Rubin (2016)
Lycopene oxidative products	Inhibition of NF-κB	Breast cancer/T47D human mammary cancer cells	10,100-Diapocarotene-10,100-dial and the derivative 6140 diapocar-otene-6140-dial inhibited 23% ± 0.03 of the basal NF-κB activation. Lycopene derivates interfere with thiol groups of both IKK and p65.	Linnewiel-Hermoni, Motro, Miller, Levy, and Sharoni (2014)
Lutein and β-carotene	Inhibition of NF-κB	Gastric cancer/AGS human gastric cancer cell	20 μmol/L of lutein or β-carotene significantly suppressed the NF-κB-DNA binding activity in AGS cells ($P<.05$).	Kim, Seo, and Kim (2011)
Lycopene	Inhibition of NF-κB	Liver cancer/SK-Hep-1 cells	Lycopene incorporation at a final concentration of 1–10 μmol significantly inhibited SK-Hep-1 invasion ($P<.05$) via inhibition of MMP-9 (matrix metalloproteinase, an important enzyme in cancer invasion) at the levels of enzyme activity ($r^2=0.94$, $P<.001$). Lycopene also significantly inhibited the binding abilities of NF-κB and Sp1 and decreased the expression of insulin-like growth factor-1 receptor (IGF-1R) and the ROS ($P<.05$)	Huang, Fan, Lin, and Hu (2007)
β-Carotene	activation of NF-κB	Leukemia and colon cancer/human leukemic cells (HL-60) and colon adenocarcinoma cells (LS-174 and WiDr)	β-Carotene significantly increased ROS levels ($P<.001$) and decreased cell growth ($P<.002$). β-Carotene-induced NF-κB DNA-binding activity at 20 μmol/L. β-Carotene inhibit cancer cell growth by increased production of ROS via activation of NF-κB.	Palozza, Serini, Torsello, Di Nicuolo, Piccioni, et al. (2003b)

continued

Table 1 Continued

Carotenoid	Mechanism	Cancer/model	Findings	References
Lycopene	GJIC enhanced	Oral cancer/KB-1 human oral tumor cells	Lycopene enhanced GJIC at 3–7 µmol/L, the enhanced of GJIC is accompanied by a significant increase of transcript levels ($P<.005$) and expression ($P<.05$) of connexin 43.	Livny et al. (2002)
β-Carotene (all-trans retinoic acid)	GJIC enhanced	Glial tumor/C6 rat glioma cells	The GJIC function of C6 glioma cells was significantly increased by all-trans retinoic acid at 1, 10, and 100 µmol/L. mRNA levels of connexin 43 connexin weren't increased by all-trans retinoic acid.	Zhang et al. (2002)
β-Carotene (all-trans retinoic acid)	GJIC enhanced	Embryo teratocarcinoma/teratocarcinoma stem cell line F9	0.1 µmol of all-trans retinoic acid increased the amount of connexin 43 protein and mRNA.	Clairmont, Tessmann, and Sies (1996)
β-Carotene, lycopene, canthaxanthin	GJIC enhanced	C3H10T1/2 cells	Seven days treatment with 10 µmol of tested carotenoids resulted in large increases in connexin 43 protein levels. Increased levels of connexin 43 were accompanied by increased in GJIC.	Zhang, Cooney, and Bertram (1992)
β-Carotene	Activation of apoptosis	Leukemia/HL-60 cells	β-Carotene treatment at the concentration of 10 µM for 24 h showed high percentage of apoptosis in HL-60 cells. Apoptosis was accompanied by caspase-3 activation in a dose-dependent manner. The activation of caspase-3 was carried out by both caspase-8 and caspase-9.	Palozza, Serini, Torsello, Di Nicuolo, Maggiano, et al. (2003a)
β-Carotene, lycopene, lutein, β-cryptoxanthin, and zeaxanthin	Activation of apoptosis	Leukemia/Jurkat E6.1 T-lymphoblast cells.	Carotenoids treatment at 20 µM induces apoptosis in Jurkat E6.1 cells after 24h. β-Carotene displayed the highest induction of apoptosis (56.5%). β-Carotene significantly induced chromatin condensation, nuclear fragmentation and DNA degradation at 50 mg/L via caspase 3 activation ($P<.01$).	Müller, Carpenter, Challis, Skepper, and Arends (2002)

β-Carotene	Activation of apoptosis	Gastric cancer/AGS cells	β-Carotene treatment at the concentration of 50 and 100μM for 30min significantly reduce AGS cells viability and enhanced DNA fragmentation via apoptosis ($P < .05$). Apoptosis is accompanied with increased levels of caspase 3, ROS, cytochrome c and Bax (proapoptotic effector molecules from Bcl-2 family).	Park, Choi, Lim, and Kim (2015)
Canthaxanthin- and β-carotene	Activation of apoptosis	Liver cancer/HepG2	1μM of β-carotene or canthaxanthin carotenoids significantly induced apoptosis in HepG2 cells ($P < .05$) by activation of caspase 3 via cytochrome c release.	Lobo, Isken, Hoff, Babino, and von Lintig (2012)
Lycopene	Activation of apoptosis	Prostate cancer/PC-3 and PCA cells	Cells incubated for 48h at 20μM of lycopene reduced 15% the PC-3 viability whereas decreased PCA viability at 1μM. In PCA cell, lycopene upregulated of Bax and CK18 genes.	Soares et al. (2013)
Lycopene	Activation of apoptosis	Breast cancer/ MDA-MB-468	Cells incubated for 72h at 20μM of lycopene induced growth decline in MDA-MB-468 cells via cell arrest and apoptosis. At 100μM of lycopene proapoptotic gene Bax was upregulated.	Takeshima et al. (2014)

(Amengual et al., 2011; Gong et al., 2018; Ribeiro, Freitas, Silva, Carvalho, & Fernandes, 2018). Prooxidant activity derived from carotenoids involve several mechanisms that increase ROS in the cells, such as processes of autoxidation of carotenoid and regulation of redox-sensitive genes and transcription factors (Palozza, Serini, Di Nicuolo, et al., 2003). Prooxidant activity of carotenoids could promote oxidative damage to DNA leading to cancer (Lowe, Booth, Young, & Bilton, 1999). The prooxidant activity of β-carotene increases lung cancer risk in hard cigarette smokers if β-carotene is supplemented without another antioxidant, such as vitamins C and E (Goralczyk, 2009). In this case, the prooxidant activity displayed by β-carotenes is possibly due to oxidized products generated by cigarette smoke which contains diverse carcinogens as well as oxidants such as NO (Centers for Disease Control and Prevention, 2010). Oxidants from cigarette smoke oxidize β-carotene into 4-nitro-β-carotene, β-apo-carotenal, and β-carotene epoxides (Baker, Krol, Jacobsen, & Liebler, 1999; Lowe et al., 2009), which probably alter the gene expression of *retinoic acid receptor* and *activator protein-1* genes enhancing lung tumorigenesis (Goralczyk, 2009; Wang et al., 1999).

While it is true that the prooxidant carotenoids can generate controversy because they could cause oxidative damage to normal cells, the prooxidant activity can also turn beneficial since several studies related to the toxicity of prooxidant carotenoids with inhibition of cancerous cell proliferation (Gong et al., 2018; Palozza, Serini, Di Nicuolo, et al., 2003; Ribeiro et al., 2018) (Table 1). The prooxidant activity of β-carotene has been associated with activity against adenocarcinoma cells, human leukemic (HL-60) cells, oral carcinoma cells, and HepG2 cells (Palozza, Serini, Di Nicuolo, et al., 2003). The toxicity caused on cancer cells by the prooxidant activity of β-carotene is due to the capacity of enhancing ROS production by autoxidation of β-carotene or through modulation of redox-sensitive genes mechanisms, such as SOD and glutathione-transferase, as well as regulating the activity of NF-κB transcription factor which induces the expression of pro-inflammatory genes (Palozza, Serini, Di Nicuolo, et al., 2003). The prooxidant effects of lycopene were first reported in normal human foreskin fibroblasts (Yeh & Hu, 2000). In cancer cells, lycopene oxidative products were able to increase ROS and induce apoptosis in human prostate (PC-3), breast (MCF-7) and cervical cancer cells (HeLa) (Arathi et al., 2016). Recently, lutein has shown a prooxidant activity in breast cancer cells. Lutein increased ROS and inhibited the growth of triple-negative breast cancer (TNBC) cells via cell cycle arrest and apoptosis (Gong et al., 2018). Interestingly, the prooxidant effect of lutein is selective for breast cancer cells, since normal primary mammary epithelial cells were not affected by lutein (Gong et al., 2018).

Prooxidant and antioxidant effects of carotenoids could be harmful as well as beneficial to fight against cancer. The antioxidant effect of carotenoids probably protects normal cells from oxidative damage caused by ROS while the same antioxidant activity increased the survival of cancerous cells because these kind of cells are more sensitive than normal cells to oxidative stress (Raj et al., 2011). On the other hand, prooxidant activity of carotenoids could produce oxidative damage and eventually cancer in normal cells, but in cancerous cells, the oxidative damage could inhibit cancer proliferation because oxidative stress limits cancer progression and metastasis. In fact, cancer cells use antioxidant proteins to overcome oxidative stress, such as Nrf2

(DeNicola et al., 2011; Wang et al., 2016) and SOD (DeNicola et al., 2011; Glasauer, Sena, Diebold, Mazar, & Chandel, 2014; Kamarajugadda et al., 2013). Both antioxidant and prooxidant effects displayed by carotenoids could be beneficial against cancer. In this sense, the antioxidant capacity of carotenoids should be used as cancer prophylaxis rather than treatment against cancer, while cancer should be treated with the prooxidant effect of carotenoids.

Modulation of Nrf2 and NF-κB pathways by carotenoids

In addition to the antioxidant activity via ROS scavenging, some carotenoids and apocarotenoids are able to interact and regulate the Nrf2 and NF-κB systems. The interaction with these systems allowed carotenoids to exert an indirect antioxidant action since Nrf2 and NF-κB systems are involved in the redox homeostasis in the cell.

Nrf2 is a transcription factor which activates a battery of antioxidant response genes, such as GSTA2 (glutathione S-transferase A2), NQO1 (NADPH: quinone oxidoreductase 1), and SODs, that protect cells from reactive oxygen species and other electrophilic molecules (Jaramillo & Zhang, 2013; Nguyen, Nioi, & Pickett, 2009). Genes activated by Nrf2 have a *cis*-acting element termed ARE (5'-RTGABNNNGCR-3') which is a DNA enhancer sequence (Jaramillo & Zhang, 2013). Nrf2 system defends cells against oxidative or electrophilic stress, promoting the survival of normal cells. In a few words, without oxidative stress condition, Nrf2 is located in the cytoplasm associated with Kelch-like ECH-associated protein 1 (Keap 1). Keap 1 induce the Nrf2 ubiquitination and subsequent degradation, this maintains Nrf2 at low levels. Oxidative stress or electrophilic stress causes a conformational change in Keap 1 that inhibits the Nrf2 ubiquitination and promotes Nrf2 accumulation and translocation at the nucleus of the cell. Within the nucleus, Nrf2 is associated with members of the masculoaponeurotic fibrosarcoma (Maf) protein family that facilitates the binding of Nrf2 to AREs of cell defense genes (reviewed from Jaramillo & Zhang, 2013).

Studies suggested that Nrf2 is able to protect the cell against tumor formation, Nrf2 knockout mice are more prone to developing neoplasia than wild-type mice (Jaramillo & Zhang, 2013). Carotenoids and their oxidative derivates have the ability to activate antioxidant response genes via the Nrf2 system (Rodríguez-Concepción et al., 2018). Therefore, they have been associated with antioxidant and anticancer functions (Table 1). Astaxantina, β-carotene, and lycopene are three carotenoids with the ability to activate the Nrf2 system (Ben-Dor et al., 2005; Goo et al., 2007; Inoue et al., 2017; Lian & Wang, 2008). Lycopene oxidative derivates (apo-100-lycopenoids) promote the nuclear accumulation of Nrf2 in BEAS-2B human bronchial epithelial cells activating ARE genes (Lian & Wang, 2008). It has been suggested that the aldehyde groups of apo-100-lycopenoids, rather than lycopene, have the ability to interrupting Keap1-mediated Nrf2 ubiquitination, allowing Nrf2 accumulation (Lian & Wang, 2008; Linnewiel et al., 2009). Although carotenoids promote the detoxification of normal cells via the Nrf2 system, their use in cancer patients needs to be studied thoroughly, because the Nrf2 system also promotes the survival of cancer cells. It has been shown that the accumulation of Nrf2 in cancer cell promotes their survival, protecting them against oxidative stress and cancer treatment as chemotherapy, and radiotherapy (Wang et al., 2008).

NF-κB is a transcription factor that modulates genes with canonical or noncanonical binding sites (Wong et al., 2011), which are related to innate immune response, embryogenesis, cell proliferation, and apoptosis (Serasanambati & Chilakapati, 2016). NF-κB also modulates the expression of antioxidant as well as prooxidant genes (Lingappan, 2018; Morgan & Liu, 2011). The NF-κB system works similarly to the Nrf2 system, briefly, in normal conditions transcription factor NF-κB is bound to cytoplasmatic inhibitory κB (IκB) protein family that arrests NF-κB in the cytoplasm, since IkB has nuclear export signals this pull off NF-κB proteins from the nucleus. In response to stress stimuli, such as cytokines, free radicals, bacterial antigens, viral antigens, etc., IkB kinases (IKK) induce phosphorylation of I-κB proteins promoting the ubiquitination and degradation of I-κB. This degradation allows NF-κB to be translocated and accumulated into the nucleus, leading to the activation of genes (reviewed from Lingappan, 2018; Morgan & Liu, 2011).

Constitutive activation of NF-κB transcription system could lead to inflammatory processes, producing cancer (Karin, 2009). Several lines of evidence suggest that carotenoids such as lycopene, β-carotene, lutein, and astaxanthin have the ability to modulate the NF-κB pathway, in some cases inhibiting cancer cell growth via NF-κB pathway (Cho, Kim, & Kim, 2018; Gong et al., 2016; Huang et al., 2007; Kim et al., 2008, 2011; Lee et al., 2003; Linnewiel-Hermoni et al., 2014; Palozza, Serini, Torsello, Di Nicuolo, Piccioni, et al., 2003b) (Table 1). In the case of lycopene, the electrophilic lycopene derivates, rather than lycopene itself, inhibit the NF-κB pathway (Linnewiel-Hermoni et al., 2014). Interestingly, in prostate cancer cells (LNCaP and DU145), which display low expression of the gen from β-carotene 9′,10′-oxygenase (BCO2) enzyme, lycopene was able to stop cancer cells proliferation and colony formation via inhibiting the NF-κB pathway only when the expression of bco2 gen was restored (Gong et al., 2016). The inhibiting mechanism of NF-κB pathway by electrophilic lycopene derivates is given by the interaction of lycopene derivates with thiol groups of p65 (member of NF-κB transcription factors family) and IKK kinase that leads to adducts formations that inhibit the protein activity, phosphorylation of IkB and DNA binding, respectively (Linnewiel-Hermoni et al., 2014).

Gap junctions enhanced by carotenoids

Gap junction intercellular communication term refers to groups of intercellular channels, formed by membrane proteins called connexins, that enable the diffusion of small molecules and ions between adjacent cells; this kind of communication is found in cells that form solid tissues (Goodenough & Paul, 2009). GJIC is considered crucial in tissue homeostasis, and alteration in this communication has been associated with cancer (Aasen, Mesnil, Naus, Lampe, & Laird, 2016). In fact, low levels of mRNA or proteins connexins are often found in human tumors (Cronier, Crespin, Strale, Defamie, & Mesnil, 2009). Restoration of GJIC and connexins levels have shown therapeutic advantages in early stages of cancer (Cronier et al., 2009). High mRNA expression of connexin in cancer tissues have been related with better prognosis; for example, high expression of connexin 43 is correlated with better prognosis in the prostate, pancreatic, breast, and colorectal cancers (Aasen et al., 2016).

Several lines of evidence have shown that carotenoids such as lycopene, β-carotene, α-carotene, lutein, and canthaxanthin have the ability to enhance GJIC (Aust et al., 2003; Krutovskikh et al., 1997; Livny et al., 2002; Novo, Azevedo, Minicucci, Zornoff, & SAR, 2013; Stahl et al., 1997; Zhang, Cooney, & Bertram, 1991, 1992; Zhang et al., 2002). The enhancement of GJIC is mainly due to the upregulation of the transcription of connexin 43 (Bertram, 1999; David Hieber et al., 2000; Livny et al., 2002; Zhang et al., 1992). It has also been described that enhanced GJIC is not related to the upregulation of connexin 43, but rather with mRNA stabilization of connexin 43 (Clairmont & Sies, 1997; Stahl, von Laar, Martin, Emmerich, & Sies, 2000). Studies in rats reveal that β-carotene is able to increase the content of total connexin 43 in animals (Krutovskikh et al., 1997; Novo et al., 2013). In cancer cells, carotenoids have shown the ability to upregulate connexin 43 gene and enhance GJIC (Clairmont et al., 1996; Livny et al., 2002; Zhang et al., 1992, 2002). Carotenoids have shown the ability to inhibit chemical-induced cancer in mouse fibroblast cell via GJIC (David Hieber et al., 2000) (Table 1).

Apoptosis induction in cancer cells by carotenoids

The anticancerogenic activity showed by carotenoids is also related to the ability to induce apoptosis selectively in cancer cells (Palozza, Serini, Di Nicuolo, & Calviello, 2004). Apoptosis is a cellular process that is essential for the correct development and for normal homeostasis and involves killing the cells (Nagata, 2018). Alterations of the apoptotic mechanism are considered to be a critical event for cancer initiation (Wong, 2011). Briefly, apoptosis is triggered mainly by a set of caspases that involved caspases 3 and 7 which are responsible for killing the cells. In mammalian systems, caspases 3 and 7 are activated by two pathways: intrinsic and extrinsic. Intrinsic pathway or mitochondrial pathway is controlled by proteins from Bcl-2 family, this pathway involved the cytochrome C released from the mitochondria to the cytoplasm. Cytochrome C forms a complex called apoptosome with Aoaf-1 protein which induced the caspases 3 and 7 via caspase 9. On the other hand, extrinsic apoptosis pathway is triggered by death factors from TNF family which are ligands for death receptors. The oligomerized formed by receptor and ligand propitiates the union of a complex called DISC (death-inducing signaling complex). DISC induce apoptosis via procaspase 8, member of DISC. Caspase 8 activate caspase 3 in cells type I or leading the cytochrome C released in cells type II, reviewed from Nagata (2018).

Several studies have suggested that carotenoids have proapoptotic capacity in cancer cells (Table 1) (Palozza et al., 2004), including cervical (Sowmya, Arathi, Vijay, Baskaran, & Lakshminarayana, 2015), prostate (Soares et al., 2013), breast (Sumantran, Zhang, Lee, & Wicha, 2000), colon (Palozza et al., 2010), leukemia (Müller et al., 2002), and gastric cancer (Park et al., 2015) cells. Carotenoids have shown selective proapoptotic activity for cancer cells, lutein, for example, selectively induced apoptosis in MCF-7 breast cancer cells but not in normal human mammary cells (Sumantran et al., 2000). Apoptosis induction carried out by carotenoids could be conducted by the activation of either, intrinsic or extrinsic pathway: β-carotene, for example, induces apoptosis by the activation of caspase-3 in human leukemia (HL-60) and colon adenocarcinoma (HT-29) via activation of caspase 8 and caspase 9 pathways (Palozza, Serini, Torsello, Di Nicuolo, Maggiano, et al., 2003a).

Cardiovascular diseases

According to the World Health Organization (Mendis, Puska, & Norrving, 2011), CVDs are the leading cause of death worldwide. The cardiovascular or circulatory system supplies the body with blood. It is comprised of the heart, arteries, veins, and capillaries. There are several types of CVD, but symptoms, treatment, and prevention often overlap. Currently, heart diseases are classified: as coronary heart disease (CHD) (myocardial infarction), rheumatic heart disease, congenital heart diseases, atherosclerosis heart disease, cerebrovascular disease (stroke), peripheral vascular disease, hypertension (high blood pressure), heart failure, and cardiomyopathies.

In 2012, 17.5 million people died from CVDs (30% of all deaths). A total of 7.4 million deaths were caused by coronary disease and 6.7 million by cerebrovascular accidents. Estimates for 2030 are 23.6 million deaths by CVD, mainly heart disease and cerebrovascular accidents (Mendis et al., 2011). The most common CVD deaths are CHDs, cerebrovascular disease, and peripheral vascular disease caused by atherosclerosis that affects blood vessels and results in heart attacks and strokes (Mendis et al., 2011).

Atherosclerosis is a condition in which a plaque made of cholesterol, fatty acids, calcium, fibrin, and cellular waste products builds up inside arterial wall and partially or totally blocks the blood flow through a vessel in the heart, brain, legs, or arms (Bergheanu, Bodde, & Jukema, 2017). The rupture of the atherosclerotic plaque triggers the formation of blood clots which are carried through the bloodstream and eventually cause a heart attack when they block a coronary artery or a stroke when they block a brain artery (Mendis et al., 2011). Although the actual causes of atherosclerosis and CVDs are not entirely known, the most accepted idea is that damage to the endothelium (inner layer) of the arterial wall initiates the plaque formation (Bergheanu et al., 2017). Experimental data that indicate the involvement of oxidative modification of low-density lipoproteins (LDL) components within the arterial wall support the "oxidant hypothesis of atherosclerosis" (Steinberg & Witztum, 2002). High-density lipoproteins (HDL) are strongly protective against atherosclerosis for they remove the excess of cholesterol from peripheral tissues. In addition, HDL inhibits LDL oxidation (Emanuelli, Augusti, & Roehrs, 2018).

Most CVDs could be prevented if the risk factors were addressed, that is, by consuming less alcohol and tobacco, reducing salt intake, avoiding sedentary lifestyles—particularly among children—and eating fresh fruits and vegetables (carrots, tomatoes, avocado, lettuce, oranges, and dark green vegetables). The latter contain carotenoids which are widespread in the vegetable kingdom and are also found in high concentrations in algae and microorganisms. Humans and other animals cannot synthesize them, so they must necessarily be ingested in food or via dietary supplements. Numerous epidemiological studies have demonstrated that eating rich-carotenoids diets (fruits and vegetables) is associated with lower incidence of CVDs mortality (Alissa & Ferns, 2017; Rissanen et al., 2003; Slavin & Lloyd, 2012; Tanaka et al., 2013; Woodside, Young, & McKinley, 2013; Zhan et al., 2015), reduced risk of stroke (He, Nowson, & MacGregor, 2006; Hjartåker, Knudsen, Tretli, & Weiderpass, 2015), and lower risk of CHD (Joshipura, Hu, & Manson, 2001; Shay et al., 2012).

Carotenoids are natural pigments found in plants, fungi, alga, and bacteria (Milani, Basirnejad, Shahbazi, & Bolhassani, 2017), and more than 650 different types exist in nature, including up to 100 that are present in the food chain and human diet (Milani et al., 2017). Carotenoids can be classified, according to their chemical structure, into carotenes (α-carotene, β-carotene, and lycopene) and xanthophylls, including lutein, fucoxanthin, canthaxanthin, zeaxanthin, beta-cryptoxanthin, capsorubin, and astaxanthin (Gammone, Riccioni, & D'Orazio, 2015).

The primary property of carotenoids is their antioxidant activity, which is considered the primary mechanism of their beneficial health effects (Seifried, Anderson, Fisher, & Milner, 2007). Because of their numerous conjugated double bonds (Krinsky, 1989), all carotenoids are effective antioxidants that protect the cellular system from a diversity of reactive oxygen (Rodrigues, Mariutti, Chisté, & Mercadante, 2012) and reactive nitrogen species (Chisté et al., 2011). They also help to prevent CVDs risk in humans (Müller, Caris-Veyrat, Lowe, & Böhm, 2016). It has been proposed that the antioxidant activity of carotenoids has a role in their protective effect against LDL cholesterol oxidation (Carpenter et al., 1997; Pashkow, Watumull, & Campbell, 2008). Some carotenoids have also been shown to reduce blood cholesterol levels (Fuhrman, Elis, & Aviram, 1997).

Carotenoids are also able to enhance gap junction communication by increasing the expression of connexin 43 (Polacek, Lal, Volin, & Davies, 1993). The role of the gap junctions is that of communication between vascular cells; this mechanism may also be involved in the cardiovascular protective effects of carotenoids (Zhang et al., 1991). Another biological activity of carotenoids is their ability to modulate the activated peroxisome proliferator receptors, thus modulating the expression of genes that control lipid and carbohydrate metabolism (Goto et al., 2012; Inoue et al., 2012; Jia et al., 2012; Kawada et al., 2000; Takahashi et al., 2009).

Numerous studies in humans involving dietary supplementation with β-carotene have shown the protective potential of β-carotene, lycopene, and astaxanthin. Other carotenoids, such as lutein, zeaxanthin and the annatto carotenoids (bixin and norbixin) have only been investigated in animals or in human epidemiological studies.

β-Carotene (major sources are carrots, spinach, and apricot) plays a crucial role in human health, being the major precursor of vitamin A (Burri, 1997). They also act as immune modulators, singlet oxygen quenchers and scavengers of peroxyl radicals (Wang & Russell, 1999). Another study showed that low serum β-carotene concentrations increased the risk of sudden cardiac death (Karppi, Laukkanen, Mäkikallio, Ronkainen, & Kurl, 2013). Studies on coronary artery disease found significantly lower β-carotene levels, in addition to elevated levels of the inflammatory marker IL-6; suggesting a potential protective effect of β-carotene on atherosclerosis due to inflammatory inhibition (Mužáková et al., 2010).

Lycopene is an acyclic isomer of β-carotene with no provitamin A activity (major sources are tomatoes) and it is the predominant carotenoid in human plasma (Clinton, 1998; Clinton et al., 1996). Lycopene is one of the most potent antioxidants, with a singlet-oxygen-quenching ability that is higher than that of β-carotene and α-tocopherol (Di Mascio, Kaiser, & Sies, 1989). It has also been associated with reduced CVD risk in epidemiological studies and human trials studying lycopene supplementation

(Riccioni, Mancini, Ilio, Bucciarelli, & Orazio, 2008). Another function of lycopene is to reduce the cholesterol synthesis and it is more effective than β-carotene (Riccioni et al., 2008). In addition, lycopene upregulates gap-junction communication in mouse embryonic fibroblast C3H710T1/2 cells (Zhang et al., 1992) and in human fetal skin fibroblasts junctions (Stahl et al., 2000).

Astaxanthin is a xanthophyll found in microalgae, fungi plants, seafood, and fla- mingos (Ambati, Moi, Ravi, & Aswathanarayana, 2014). Astaxanthin removes reactive oxygen and nitrogen species, is 11 and 550 times more efficient as a singlet oxygen scavenger than β-carotene and α-tocopherol, respectively (Krinsky, 1989; Shimidzu, Goto, & Miki, 1996). Its structure of carbon bonds and polar rings is able to remove FRs from the surface and inside the membrane (Pashkow et al., 2008). Astaxanthin protected hypercholesterolemic rabbits against oxidative stress in aortic tissue and serum, also preventing changes in the activities of thioredoxin reductase and paraoxo- nase; such protection could be useful in the treatment of CVDs (Augusti et al., 2012). There is no scientific information on astaxanthin in human with CVDs, but some clin- ical studies have investigated their effects in related events (Iwamoto et al., 2000).

Achiote (*Bixa orellana* L.) is a native plant of tropical America which accumu- lates several carotenoids derivatives (bixin and norbixin), terpenoids, tocotrienoles, and flavonoids in the seeds and the leaves. Annatto extract is a natural food color, which is obtained from the outer coatings of the seeds of the Annatto tree (Hagiwara et al., 2003). The most important pigment in annatto seeds is the carotenoid cis-bixin (up to 80% of the total pigment content), whereas norbixin (cis and trans) represent a minor portion of achiote seeds and have no provitamin A activity. Both carotenoids appeared in the plasma of subjects receiving 16 mg of bixin, but norbixin was found after bixin (Emanuelli et al., 2018; Levy, Regalado, Navarrete, & Watkins, 1997). Bixin has been earlier described as a biological singlet molecular oxygen quencher (Di Mascio, Devasagayam, Kaiser, & Sies, 1990) and norbixin has been shown to have higher antioxidant activity than lutein, β carotene, and lycopene against lipid oxida- tion in oil-in-water emulsion systems (Emanuelli et al., 2018; Kiokias & Oreopoulou, 2006). Additionally, norbixin was effective against DNA oxidative damage caused by methylmercury and UV radiation in rats and *Escherichia coli* cells, respectively (Barcelos et al., 2012; Junior Antonio et al., 2005). Although the antioxidant potential of annatto carotenoids has been described in several experimental models, little infor- mation is available on the potentially protective effect of these carotenoids in CVDs or related conditions. Only one study has evaluated the effects of annatto carotenoids in experimental atherosclerosis (Somacal et al., 2015). In this study, bixin showed an antiatherogenic effect by reducing the extent of atherosclerotic lesions in hypercho- lesterolemic rabbits. Such an effect was most likely mediated by antiinflammatory, antioxidant, and lipid-improving activities.

Lutein and zeaxanthin are oxygenated carotenoids found at a high concentration in the human retina. They are isomers obtained from supplements or from yellow corn, egg yolk, orange juice, and dark green vegetables, such as spinach and broccoli (Holden et al., 1999; Sommerburg, Keunen, Bird, & van Kuijk, 1998). However, their antioxidant and antiinflammatory capacity seem to be associated not only with eye health but also with decreasing CVD risk (Gammone et al., 2015). In addition, Adluri et al. (2013) reported the cardioprotective effect of a mix of carotenoids containing lutein (8.1%), zeaxanthin (1.23%), and 2% astaxanthin against myocardial ischemia-reperfusion injury in rats. However, zeaxanthin did not inhibit vascular smooth muscle cells migration, whereas its isomer, lutein, was able to exert such effect (Lo, Tsai, Du, Tsou, & Wu, 2012). The role of zeaxanthin and lutein in CVDs therapeutics has also been evaluated in human studies. Blood levels of lutein and zeaxanthin were inversely associated with the levels of soluble intercellular adhesion molecule 1 (sICAM-1) and with flow-mediated vasodilation (FMV) in serum samples from the general population (Van Herpen-Broekmans et al., 2004). This inverse association suggests that it is possible that the protective effect of carotenoids on atherosclerosis may occur through the modulation of inflammatory processes and endothelial function. Accordingly, Lidebjer, Leanderson, Ernerudh, and Jonasson (2007) demonstrated that lutein + zeaxanthin (and β-cryptoxanthin) were depleted in patients with coronary artery disease. In the Beijing atherosclerosis study, serum lutein was inversely associated with the intima-media thickness (IMT) of the common carotid artery, but no associations have been found for zeaxanthin or β-carotene (Zou et al., 2011). A study in Spain found no significant association between the risk of myocardial infarction and lutein + zeaxanthin blood levels measured within the first 24 h after the onset of the disease and 1 year later (Ruiz Rejón et al., 2002).

In conclusion, the human organism produces balanced FR and antioxidants, but when a disorder in their synthesis and degradation occurs, oxidative stress is unavoidable, increasing FR production which is associated with degenerative disease incidence. Nutrition plays a significant role in the prevention of many chronic diseases such as CVD, especially CHD and stroke. A diet high in fruit and vegetable is inversely associated with the risk of CVDs (Zhan et al., 2017). The effects of bixin and norbixin in human in an experimental model of CVDs still need to be investigated. The inconsistencies in the results of epidemiological studies involving lutein and zeaxanthin may be related to differences in xanthophyll intake and in the severity of the lesions and diseases in studied populations.

Uses

Many carotenoids, including annato seeds, have antifungal, antibacterial, antimalarial, and hypoglycemic preventive bioactivities. The apocarotenoid pigment bixin is known as a natural coloring agent in various products including dairy products, smoked fish, sausage, snack food, ice cream, cosmetics and body care products (Siva, Mathew, Venkat, & Dhawan, 2008; Zhan et al., 2017). Zsila, Molnár, Deli, and Lockwood (2005) reported that cis-bixin prevented lipid peroxidation and also interacts with human α1-acid glycoprotein. As β-carotene, prooxidant bixin quenches the singlet oxygen in liquid solution. Based on carcinogenesis, various toxicity and bioactivity studies were carried out using bixin (Dos Santos et al., 2012). Kovary et al. (2001) stated that bixin induced change in the xenobiotic metabolizing enzyme of different tissues, especially in carcinogenesis processes. In myeloma cancer, bixin induce apoptosis through the inhibition of thioredoxin and thioredoxin reductase activities. Bixin shows antitumor activity toward osteosarcoma, anaplastic thyroid, breast, colon, prostate, and papillary thyroid cancers. The cytotoxic potential of bixin and norbixin was due to the presence of a nonesterified carboxylic acid group and it also induced increased uptake of glucose by differentiated T3-L1 adipocytes in the presence of insulin.

The water soluble norbixin is a saponified product of bixin, which does not change the native structure of dairy proteins, such as casein and whey (Zhang, Dai, Zhang, Yang, & Liu, 2008). Norbixin protects plasmid DNA oxidative damage caused by H_2O_2 (Kovary et al., 2001). Various reports on the pharmacological activity of norbixin are available, yet its medicinal value remains unexplored.

Saffron stigma possesses a yellow-color pigment, crocin, which is utilized to enhance taste, color, and odor in multicuisine food preparations. Crocin is used in the treatment of many diseases for its antitumoral, antidepressant, cardioprotective, antitussive, genoprotective and neuroprotective (Amrita et al., 2015) properties. The therapeutic potential of crocin has been reported by many researchers conducting in vivo and clinical studies. Crocin showed a beneficial impact on several human organs, such as the gastrointestinal, immune, endocrine, and cardiovascular systems (Alavizadeh & Hosseinzadeh, 2014). It also prevented learning disorders and inhibited oxidative stress. Crocin acts as an anti-Alzheimer agent by inhibiting acetylcholinesterase activity and other pro-inflammatory activity triggered by the microglia. Crocetin is formed through hydrolyzation in the gastrointestinal system of orally administrated crocin. Kanakis, Tarantilis, Tajmir-Riahi, and Polissiou (2007) reported that in malignant cells, crocetin inhibits the synthesis of protein and nucleic acids and it also interacts with the Calf-Thymus DNA.

Carotenoids are the most abundant compounds among the secondary metabolites and are part of the terpenoids family (Barreiro & Barredo, 2018). Nearly 50 types of carotenoids have been detected in human blood and tissues, and all come from the diet, primarily fruits, and vegetables (Fiedor & Burda, 2014; Khachik, 2006). The positive effect on human health has been established by the association between the presence of carotenoids and good health condition. The positive effect of carotenoids on health is currently being investigated worldwide by many researchers. An association between their antiinflammatory activity and low incidence or decreased risk of suffering from chronic CVDs, some types of cancers, and eye disease and immune response enhancement has been reported (Coronado-Cáceres et al., 2014; Rivera-Madrid, Aguilar-Espinosa, Cárdenas-Conejo, & Garza-Caligaris, 2016). As mentioned above, part of the positive effects of carotenoids and human health results from the antioxidative properties of these compounds.

Besides natural food products, many carotenoids supplements are currently available, including β-carotene, xanthophylls, lycopene, and bixin. However, for carotenoids to be part of nutritional supplements or used as additives in processed food products they first have to be approved by the different health authorities, such as the FDA/HHS (Food and Drug Administration of the Department of Health and Human Services) in the United States, and the European Food Safety Authority (EFSA). Among the most important sources of carotenoids in the human diet are ß-carotene and norbixin (annatto), a yellow dye used to color dairy products. Primary sources of this pigments are the African palm and *B. orellana* (achiote) (Rivera-Madrid, Aguilar-Espinosa,

Cárdenas-Conejo, & Garza-Caligaris, 2016). Lycopene and canthaxanthin provide red dye for food and beverages; their primary source aretomatoes. Astaxanthin or canthaxanthin are added to animal feed in farmed salmons and trout, giving their meat the characteristics color of the species in nature (Higuera-Ciapara, Félix-Valenzuela, & Goycoolea, 2006). In the poultry industry, lutein, bixin, and capsanthin are used to give the typical yellow-red color to chicken skin and egg yolk; the natural sources of this pigment are marigold, achiote, and pepper, respectively (Tyckowski & Hamilton, 1986). Carotenoids such as astaxanthin and phytoene are used to produce makeup and dermatological treatments (Sandmann, 2014). The addition of carotenoids compounds used in the food and cosmetic industries preserves and improves human health.

Perspectives and conclusions

An association has been established between the absence or the reduction of chronic diseases in humans with the intake of carotenes and their presence in blood and tissues. The imbalance in ROS has adverse effects on health as it promotes several diseases and one of the crucial functions of carotenoids on human health is reducing the effects of oxidative stress. However, there is still much research to be done. A few carotenes have high demand in global trade owing to their use in industrialized products for human nutrition and feed for poultry and fish produced for human consumption. Industrial methods have been developed to increase the production of these natural compounds and reduce the use of synthetic carotenes. The two main challenges in the field of carotenoids research are, on one hand, the studies to increase our knowledge on the effects of carotenes on human health and, on the other hand, the development of technologies to increase their production at industrial level or genetically improve carotenoids-producing-crops to meet the growing global demand of this compounds.

Acknowledgments

This work was financially supported through grant from the Consejo Nacional de Ciencia y Tecnología (CONACYT) with Grant no. 220259. V. Carballo had CONACYT's PhD Grant No. 265369. FOMIX: YUC-2014-C17-247355.

References

Aasen, T., Mesnil, M., Naus, C. C., Lampe, P. D., & Laird, D. W. (2016). Gap junctions and cancer: communicating for 50 years. *Nature Reviews. Cancer*, *16*(12), 775–788. NIH Public Access. Available from: http://www.ncbi.nlm.nih.gov/pubmed/27782134.

Ademowo, O. S., Dias, H. K. I., Milic, I., Devitt, A., Moran, R., Mulcahy, R., et al. (2017). Phospholipid oxidation and carotenoid supplementation in Alzheimer's disease patients. *Free Radical Biology & Medicine*, *108*(September 2016), 77–85. Available from: https://linkinghub.elsevier.com/retrieve/pii/S0891584917301326.

Adluri, R. S., Thirunavukkarasu, M., Zhan, L., Maulik, N., Svennevig, K., Bagchi, M., et al. (2013). Cardioprotective efficacy of a novel antioxidant mix VitaePro against ex vivo myocardial ischemia-reperfusion injury. *Cell Biochemistry and Biophysics*, *67*(2), 281–286.

Age-Related Eye Disease Study Research Group. (2001). A randomized, placebo-controlled, clinical trial of high-dose supplementation with vitamins C and E, beta carotene, and zinc for age-related macular degeneration and vision loss: AREDS report no. 8. *Archives of Ophthalmology*, *119*(10), 1417.

Águila, R.-S.M., & Rodríguez-Concepción, M. (2012). Carotenoid biosynthesis in arabidopsis: a colorful pathway. In *The arabidopsis book* (pp. 2–28). The American Society of Plant Biologists.

Ahmed, S. S., Lott, M. N., & Marcus, D. M. (2005). The macular xanthophylls. *Survey of Ophthalmology*, *50*(2), 183–193.

Alavizadeh, S. H., & Hosseinzadeh, H. (2014). Bioactivity assessment and toxicity of crocin: a comprehensive review. *Food and Chemical Toxicology*, *64*, 65–80.

Alissa, E. M., & Ferns, G. A. (2017). Dietary fruits and vegetables and cardiovascular diseases risk. *Critical Reviews in Food Science and Nutrition*, *57*(9), 1950–1962. Taylor & Francis.

Ambati, R. R., Moi, P. S., Ravi, S., & Aswathanarayana, R. G. (2014). Astaxanthin: sources, extraction, stability, biological activities and its commercial applications—a review. *Marine Drugs*, *12*(1), 128–152.

Amengual, J., Lobo, G. P., Golczak, M., Li, H. N. M., Klimova, T., Hoppel, C. L., et al. (2011). A mitochondrial enzyme degrades carotenoids and protects against oxidative stress. *The FASEB Journal*, *25*(3), 948–959. The Federation of American Societies for Experimental Biology; Available from: http://www.ncbi.nlm.nih.gov/pubmed/21106934.

Amrita, A., Priya, R. R., Hridya, H., Akella, S., Subramanian, B., & Ramamoorthy, S. (2015). Studies on interaction of norbixin with DNA: multispectroscopic and in silico analysis. *Spectrochimica Acta Part A, Molecular and Biomolecular Spectroscopy*, *144*, 163–169.

Arathi, B. P., Sowmya, P. R. R., Kuriakose, G. C., Vijay, K., Baskaran, V., Jayabaskaran, C., et al. (2016). Enhanced cytotoxic and apoptosis inducing activity of lycopene oxidation products in different cancer cell lines. *Food and Chemical Toxicology*, *97*, 265–276. Elsevier Ltd. https://doi.org/10.1016/j.fct.2016.09.016.

Augusti, P. R., Quatrin, A., Somacal, S., Conterato, G. M., Sobieski, R., Ruviaro, A. R., et al. (2012). Astaxanthin prevents changes in the activities of thioredoxin reductase and paraoxonase in hypercholesterolemic rabbits. *Journal of Clinical Biochemistry and Nutrition*, *51*(1), 42–49.

Aust, O., Ale-Agha, N., Zhang, L., Wollersen, H., Sies, H., & Stahl, W. (2003). Lycopene oxidation product enhances gap junctional communication. *Food and Chemical Toxicology*, *41*(10), 1399–1407. Pergamon. Available from: https://www.sciencedirect.com/science/article/pii/S0278691503001480?via%3Dihub.

Baker, D. L., Krol, E. S., Jacobsen, N., & Liebler, D. C. (1999). Reactions of β-carotene with cigarette smoke oxidants. Identification of carotenoid oxidation products and evaluation of the prooxidant/antioxidant effect. *Chemical Research in Toxicology*, *12*(6), 535–543.

Bao, Q., Pan, J., Qi, H., Wang, L., Qian, H., Jiang, F., et al. (2014). Molecular and cellular endocrinology aging and age-related diseases—from endocrine therapy to target therapy. *Molecular and Cellular Endocrinology*, *394*, 115–118.

Barcelos, G. R. M., Grotto, D., Serpeloni, J. M., Aissa, A. F., Antunes, L. M. G., Knasmüller, S., et al. (2012). Bixin and norbixin protect against DNA-damage and alterations of redox status induced by methylmercury exposure in vivo. *Environmental and Molecular Mutagenesis*, *53*(7), 535–541.

Barreiro, C., & Barredo, J. L. (2018). Carotenoids production: a healthy and profitable industry. In C. Barreiro & J. L. Barredo (Eds.), *Microbial carotenoids Methods in molecular biology, Vol. 1852*. New York, NY: Humana Press.

Ben-Dor, A., Steiner, M., Gheber, L., Danilenko, M., Dubi, N., Linnewiel, K., et al. (2005). Carotenoids activate the antioxidant response element transcription system. *Molecular Cancer Therapeutics, 4*(1), 177–186. American Association for Cancer Research. Available from: http://www.ncbi.nlm.nih.gov/pubmed/15657364.

Bergheanu, S. C., Bodde, M. C., & Jukema, J. W. (2017). Pathophysiology and treatment of atherosclerosis: current view and future perspective on lipoprotein modification treatment. *Netherlands Heart Journal, 25*(4), 231–242.

Bernstein, P. S., Khachik, F., Carvalho, L. S., Muir, G. J., Zhao, D. Y., & Katz, N. B. (2001). Identification and quantitation of carotenoids and their metabolites in the tissues of the human eye. *Experimental Eye Research, 72*(3), 215–223.

Bernstein, P. S., Li, B., Vachali, P. P., Gorusupudi, A., Shyam, R., Henriksen, B. S., et al. (2016). Lutein, zeaxanthin, and meso-zeaxanthin: the basic and clinical science underlying carotenoid-based nutritional interventions against ocular disease. *Progress in Retinal and Eye Research, 50*, 34–66. Elsevier Ltd.

Bertram, J. S. (1999). Carotenoids and gene expression. *Nutrition, 57*(6), 182–191.

Bone, R. A., Landrum, J. T., Mayne, S. T., Gomez, C. M., Tibor, S. E., & Twaroska, E. E. (2001). Macular pigment in donor eyes with and without AMD: a case-control study. *Investigative Ophthalmology and Visual Science, 42*(1), 235–240.

Bowen, P., Chen, L., Stacewicz-Sapuntzakis, M., Duncan, C., Sharifi, R., Ghosh, L., et al. (2002). Tomato sauce supplementation and prostate cancer: lycopene accumulation and modulation of biomarkers of carcinogenesis. *Experimental Biology and Medicine (Maywood, N.J.), 227*(10), 886–893. Available from: http://www.ncbi.nlm.nih.gov/pubmed/12424330.

Boyd, N. F., & McGuire, V. (1991). The possible role of lipid peroxidation in breast cancer risk. *Free Radical Biology & Medicine, 10*(3–4), 185–190. Pergamon https://www.sciencedirect.com/science/article/pii/089158499190074D?via%3Dihub.

Britton, G. (1995). Structure and properties of carotenoids in relation to function. *The FASEB Journal, 9*(15), 1551–1558. Available from: http://www.ncbi.nlm.nih.gov/pubmed/8529834.

Burri, B. J. (1997). Beta-carotene and human health: a review of current research. *Nutrition Research, 17*(3), 547–580.

Burri, B. J., La Frano, M. R., & Zhu, C. (2016). Absorption, metabolism, and functions of β-cryptoxanthin. *Nutrition Reviews, 74*(2), 69–82.

Burton, G. W., & Ingold, K. U. (1984). beta-Carotene: an unusual type of lipid antioxidant. *Science, 224*(4649), 569–573. Available from: http://www.ncbi.nlm.nih.gov/pubmed/6710156.

Camici, G. G., Savarese, G., Akhmedov, A., & Lüscher, T. F. (2015). Molecular mechanism of endothelial and vascular aging: implications for cardiovascular disease. *European Heart Journal, 36*(48), 3392–3403.

Carpenter, K. L. H., Van Der Veen, C., Hird, R., Dennis, I. F., Ding, T., & Mitchinson, M. J. (1997). The carotenoids β-carotene, canthaxanthin and zeaxanthin inhibit macrophage-mediated LDL oxidation. *FEBS Letters, 401*(2–3), 262–266. Federation of European Biochemical Societies.

Celermajer, D. S., Sorensen, K. E., Spiegelhalter, D. J., Georgakopoulos, D., Robinson, J., & Deanfield, J. E. (1994). Aging is associated with endothelial dysfunction in healthy men years before the age-related decline in women. *Journal of the American College of Cardiology, 24*(2), 471–476. Elsevier Masson SAS.

Centers for Disease Control and Prevention. (2010). How tobacco smoke causes disease: the biology and behavioral basis for smoking-attributable disease: a report of the surgeon general.

Césarini, J. P., Michel, L., Maurette, J. M., Adhoute, H., & Béjot, M. (2003). Immediate effects of UV radiation on the skin: modification by an antioxidant complex containing carotenoids. *Photodermatology, Photoimmunology & Photomedicine*, *19*(4), 182–189.

Chen, W., Mao, L., Xing, H., Xu, L., Fu, X., Huang, L., et al. (2015). Lycopene attenuates Aβ1-42secretion and its toxicity in human cell and Caenorhabditis elegans models of Alzheimer disease. *Neuroscience Letters*, *608*, 28–33. Elsevier Ireland Ltd.

Chisté, R. C., Mercadante, A. Z., Gomes, A., Fernandes, E., da Costa Lima, J. L. F., & Bragagnolo, N. (2011). *In vitro* scavenging capacity of annatto seed extracts against reactive oxygen and nitrogen species. *Food Chemistry*, *127*(2), 419–426.

Cho, S. O., Kim, M.-H., & Kim, H. (2018). β-Carotene inhibits activation of NF-κB, activator protein-1, and STAT3 and regulates abnormal expression of some adipokines in 3T3-L1 adipocytes. *Journal of Cancer Prevention*, *23*(1), 37–43. Korean Society of Cancer Prevention. Available from: http://www.jcpjournal.org/journal/view.html?doi=10.15430/JCP.2018.23.1.37.

Clairmont, A., & Sies, H. (1997). Evidence for a posttranscriptional effect of retinoic acid on connexin43 gene expression via the 3′-untranslated region. *FEBS Letters*, *419*(2–3), 268–270. Wiley-Blackwell. Available from: http://doi.wiley.com/10.1016/S0014-5793%2897%2901468-3.

Clairmont, A., Tessmann, D., & Sies, H. (1996). Analysis of connexin43 gene expression induced by retinoic acid in F9 teratocarcinoma cells. *FEBS Letters*, *397*(1), 22–24. Wiley-Blackwell. Available from: http://doi.wiley.com/10.1016/S0014-5793%2896%2901129-5.

Clinton, S. K. (1998). Lycopene: chemistry, biology, and implications for human Health and disease. *Nutrition Reviews*, *1*, 35–51.

Clinton, S. K., Emenhiser, C., Schwartz, S. J., Bostwick, D. G., Williams, A. W., Moore, B. J., et al. (1996). Cis-trans lycopene isomers, carotenoids, and retinol in the human prostate. *Cancer Epidemiology, Biomarkers & Prevention*, *5*(10), 823–833.

Coronado-Cáceres, L. J., Lugo-Cervantes, E., Puebla-Pérez, A. M., Aguilar-Espinosa, M., Alcaraz-López, O. A., Mateos-Díaz, J. C., et al. (2014). *Actividad antitumoral y antioxidante de las proteínas de reserva de Bixa orellana L.* 1–10.

Cronier, L., Crespin, S., Strale, P.-O., Defamie, N., & Mesnil, M. (2009). Gap junctions and cancer: new functions for an old story. *Antioxidants & Redox Signaling*, *11*(2), 323–338. Mary Ann Liebert, Inc. 2 Madison Avenue Larchmont, NY 10538 USA. Available from: http://www.liebertpub.com/doi/10.1089/ars.2008.2153.

Darvin, M. E., Gersonde, I., Albrecht, H., Zastrow, L., Sterry, W., & Lademann, J. (2007). In vivo Raman spectroscopic analysis of the influence of IR radiation on the carotenoid antioxidant substances beta-carotene and lycopene in the human skin. Formation of free radicals. *Laser Physics Letters*, *4*(4), 318–321.

Darvin, M. E., Sterry, W., Lademann, J., & Vergou, T. (2011). The role of carotenoids in human skin. *Molecules*, *16*(12), 10491–10506.

David Hieber, A., King, T. J., Morioka, S., Fukushima, L. H., Franke, A. A., & Bertram, J. S. (2000). Comparative effects of all-trans β-carotene vs. 9-cis β-carotene on carcinogen-induced neoplastic transformation and connexin 43 expression in murine 10T1/2 cells and on the differentiation of human keratinocytes. *Nutrition and Cancer*, *37*(2), 234–244. Available from: http://www.tandfonline.com/doi/abs/10.1207/S15327914NC372_17.

DeNicola, G. M., Karreth, F. A., Humpton, T. J., Gopinathan, A., Wei, C., Frese, K., et al. (2011). Oncogene-induced Nrf2 transcription promotes ROS detoxification and tumorigenesis. *Nature*, *475*(7354), 106–109. Nature Publishing Group. Available from: http://www.nature.com/articles/nature10189.

Desmarchelier, C., & Borel, P. (2017). Overview of carotenoid bioavailability determinants: from dietary factors to host genetic variations. *Trends in Food Science and Technology*, *69*, 270–280. Elsevier Ltd https://doi.org/10.1016/j.tifs.2017.03.002.

Di Mascio, P., Devasagayam, T. P. A., Kaiser, S., & Sies, H. (1990). Carotenoids, tocopherols and thiols as biological singlet molecular oxygen quenchers. *Biochemical Society Transactions*, *18*(6), 1054–1056.

Di Mascio, P., Kaiser, S., & Sies, H. (1989). Lycopene as the most efficient biological carotenoid singlet oxygen quencher. *Archives of Biochemistry and Biophysics*, *274*(2), 532–538.

Dos Santos, G. C., Mendonça, L. M., Antonucci, G. A., dos Santos, A. C., Antunes, L. M. G., & de LP, B. M. (2012). Protective effect of bixin on cisplatin-induced genotoxicity in PC12 cells. *Food and Chemical Toxicology*, *50*(2), 335–340. Elsevier Ltd https://doi.org/10.1016/j.fct.2011.10.033.

Eggersdorfer, M., & Wyss, A. (2018). Carotenoids in human nutrition and health. *Archives of Biochemistry and Biophysics*, *652*(May), 18–26. Elsevier https://doi.org/10.1016/j.abb.2018.06.001.

Emanuelli, T., Augusti, P. R., & Roehrs, M. (2018). Protective effects of carotenoids in cardiovascular disease and diabetes. In *Fruit and vegetable phytochemicals: Chemistry and human health*. (pp. 347–382).

Farooqui, T., & Farooqui, A. A. (2009). Aging: an important factor for the pathogenesis of neurodegenerative diseases. *Mechanisms of Ageing and Development*, *130*, 203–215.

Fiedor, J., & Burda, K. (2014). Potential role of carotenoids as antioxidants in human health and disease. *Nutrients*, *6*(2), 466–488.

Fraser, P. D., & Bramley, P. M. (2004). The biosynthesis and nutritional uses of carotenoids. *Progress in Lipid Research*, *43*(3), 228–265.

Fuhrman, B., Elis, A., & Aviram, M. (1997). Hypocholesterolemic effect of lycopene and β-carotene is related to suppression of cholesterol synthesis and augmentation of LDL receptor activity in macrophages. *Biochemical and Biophysical Research Communications*, *233*(3), 658–662.

Gammone, M. A., Riccioni, G., & D'Orazio, N. (2015). Carotenoids: potential allies of cardiovascular health? *Food & Nutrition Research*, *59*(1), 26762.

Gill, J. G., Piskounova, E., & Morrison, S. J. (2016). Cancer, oxidative stress, and metastasis. *Cold Spring Harbor Symposia on Quantitative Biology* **LXXXI**. Cold Spring Harbor Laboratory Press.(pp. 163–175).

Glasauer, A., Sena, L. A., Diebold, L. P., Mazar, A. P., & Chandel, N. S. (2014). Targeting SOD1 reduces experimental non–small-cell lung cancer. *The Journal of Clinical Investigation*, *124*(1), 117–128. American Society for Clinical Investigation. Available from: http://www.ncbi.nlm.nih.gov/pubmed/24292713.

Gong, X., Marisiddaiah, R., Zaripheh, S., Wiener, D., & Rubin, L. P. (2016). Mitochondrial β-carotene 9',10' oxygenase modulates prostate cancer growth via NF-κB inhibition: a lycopene-independent function. *Molecular Cancer Research*, *14*(10), 966–975. American Association for Cancer Research.

Gong, X., Smith, J. R., Swanson, H. M., & Rubin, L. P. (2018). Carotenoid lutein selectively inhibits breast cancer cell growth and potentiates the effect of chemotherapeutic agents through ROS-mediated mechanisms. *Molecules*, *23*(4), 1–18.

Goo, Y. A., Li, Z., Pajkovic, N., Shaffer, S., Taylor, G., Chen, J., et al. (2007). Systematic investigation of lycopene effects in LNCaP cells by use of novel large-scale proteomic analysis software. *Proteomics Clinical Applications*, *1*(5), 513–523. NIH Public Access. Available from: http://www.ncbi.nlm.nih.gov/pubmed/20740054.

Goodenough, D. A., & Paul, D. L. (2009). Gap junctions. *Cold Spring Harbor Perspectives in Biology*, *1*(1), a002576. Cold Spring Harbor Laboratory Press. Available from: http://www.ncbi.nlm.nih.gov/pubmed/20066080.

Goralczyk, R. (2009). Beta-carotene and lung cancer in smokers: review of hypotheses and status of research. *Nutrition and Cancer*, *61*(6), 767–774.

Goto, T., Takahashi, N., Kato, S., Il, K. Y., Kusudo, T., Taimatsu, A., et al. (2012). Bixin activates PPARα and improves obesity-induced abnormalities of carbohydrate and lipid metabolism in mice. *Journal of Agricultural and Food Chemistry*, *60*(48), 11952–11958.

Hagiwara, A., Imai, N., Ichihara, T., Sano, M., Tamano, S., Aoki, H., et al. (2003). A thirteen-week oral toxicity study of annatto extract (norbixin), a natural food color extracted from the seed coat of annatto (*Bixa orellana* L.), in Sprague-Dawley rats. *Food and Chemical Toxicology*, *41*(8), 1157–1164.

He, F. J., Nowson, C. A., & MacGregor, G. A. (2006). Fruit and vegetable consumption and stroke: meta-analysis of cohort studies. *Lancet*, *367*(9507), 320–326.

Higuera-Ciapara, I., Félix-Valenzuela, L., & Goycoolea, F. M. (2006). Astaxanthin: a review of its chemistry and applications. *Critical Reviews in Food Science and Nutrition*, *46*(2), 185–196.

Hjartåker, A., Knudsen, M. D., Tretli, S., & Weiderpass, E. (2015). Consumption of berries, fruits and vegetables and mortality among 10,000 Norwegian men followed for four decades. *European Journal of Nutrition*, *54*(4), 599–608.

Hobbs, R. P., & Bernstein, P. S. (2014). Nutrient supplementation for age-related macular degeneration, cataract, and dry eye. *J Ophthalmic Vis Res*, *9*(4), 487–493.

Holden, J. M., Eldridge, A. L., Beecher, G. R., Marilyn Buzzard, I., Bhagwat, S., Davis, C. S., et al. (1999). Carotenoid content of U.S. foods: an update of the database. *Journal of Food Composition and Analysis*, *12*(3), 169–196.

Holmberg, L., Wolk, A., Melhus, H., & Michae, K. (1999). Smoking, antioxidant vitamins, and the risk of hip fracture. *Journal of Bone and Mineral Research*, *14*(1), 129–135.

Honarvar, N. M., Saedisomeolia, A., Abdolahi, M., Shayeganrad, A., Sangsari, G. T., Rad, B. H., et al. (2017). Molecular anti-inflammatory mechanisms of retinoids and carotenoids in Alzheimer's disease: a review of current evidence. *Journal of Molecular Neuroscience*, *61*(3), 289–304.

Huang, C.-S., Fan, Y.-E., Lin, C.-Y., & Hu, M.-L. (2007). Lycopene inhibits matrix metalloproteinase-9 expression and down-regulates the binding activity of nuclear factor-kappa B and stimulatory protein-1. *The Journal of Nutritional Biochemistry*, *18*(7), 449–456. Elsevier. Available from: https://www.sciencedirect.com/science/article/pii/S0955286306001914?via%3Dihub.

Hung, C. W., Chen, Y. C., Hsieh, W. L., Chiou, S. H., & Kao, C. L. (2010). Ageing and neurodegenerative diseases. *Ageing Research Reviews*, *9*(Suppl. 1), S36–S46. Elsevier B.V..

Inoue, Y., Shimazawa, M., Nagano, R., Kuse, Y., Takahashi, K., Tsuruma, K., et al. (2017). Astaxanthin analogs, adonixanthin and lycopene, activate Nrf2 to prevent light-induced photoreceptor degeneration. *Journal of Pharmacological Sciences*, *134*(3), 147–157. Elsevier; Available from: https://www.sciencedirect.com/science/article/pii/S1347861317300890?via%3Dihub.

Inoue, M., Tanabe, H., Matsumoto, A., Takagi, M., Umegaki, K., Amagaya, S., et al. (2012). Astaxanthin functions differently as a selective peroxisome proliferator-activated receptor γ modulator in adipocytes and macrophages. *Biochemical Pharmacology*, *84*(5), 692–700. Elsevier Inc.

Iwamoto, T., Hosoda, K., Hirano, R., Kurata, H., Matsumoto, A., Miki, W., et al. (2000). Inhibition of low-density lipoprotein oxidation by astaxanthin. *Journal of Atherosclerosis and Thrombosis*, *7*(4), 216–222.

Jaramillo, M., & Zhang, D. (2013). The emerging role of the Nrf2–Keap1 signaling pathway in cancer. *Genes & Development*, *27*, 2179–2191. Available from: http://genesdev.cshlp.org/content/27/20/2179.short.

Jeon, S., Neuringer, M., Johnson, E. E., Kuchan, M. J., Pereira, S. L., Johnson, E. J., et al. (2017). Effect of carotenoid supplemented formula on carotenoid bioaccumulation in tissues of infant rhesus macaques: a pilot study focused on lutein. *Nutrients*, *9*(1), 1–15.

Jia, Y., Kim, J. Y., Jun, H. J., Kim, S. J., Lee, J. H., Hoang, M. H., et al. (2012). The natural carotenoid astaxanthin, a PPAR-agonist agonist antagonist, agonist and PPAR-antagonist, reduces hepatic lipid accumulation by rewiring the transcriptome in lipid-loaded hepatocytes. *Molecular Nutrition & Food Research*, *56*(6), 878–888.

Johnson, E. J. (2005). Obesity, lutein metabolism, and age-related macular degeneration: a web of connections. *Nutrition Reviews*, *63*(1), 9–15.

Johnson, E. J. (2012). A possible role for lutein and zeaxanthin in cognitive function in the elderly. *The American Journal of Clinical Nutrition*, *96*(5), 1161S–1165S.

Johnson, E. J., Maras, J. E., Rasmussen, H. M., & Tucker, K. L. (2010). Intake of lutein and zeaxanthin differ with age, sex, and ethnicity. *Journal of the American Dietetic Association*, *110*(9), 1357–1362. Elsevier Inc.

Johnson, E. J., Vishwanathan, R., Johnson, M. A., Hausman, D. B., Davey, A., Scott, T. M., et al. (2013). Relationship between serum and brain carotenoids α-tocopherol, and retinol concentrations and cognitive performance in the oldest old from the Georgia Centenarian Study. *Journal of Aging Research*, *2013*, [Mci].

Joshipura, K. J., Hu, F. B., & Manson, J. E. (2001). The effect of fruit and vegetable intake on risk for coronary heart disease. *Annals of Internal Medicine*, *9*(3), 483–496.

Junior Antonio, C. T. S., Asad, L.M.B.O., De Oliveira, E. B., Kovary, K., Asad, N. R., & Felzenszwalb, I. (2005). Antigenotoxic and antimutagenic potential of an annatto pigment (norbixin) against oxidative stress. *Genetics and Molecular Research*, *4*(1), 94–99.

Kamarajugadda, S., Cai, Q., Chen, H., Nayak, S., Zhu, J., He, M., et al. (2013). Manganese superoxide dismutase promotes anoikis resistance and tumor metastasis. *Cell Death & Disease*, *4*(2), e504. Nature Publishing Group. Available from: http://www.ncbi.nlm.nih.gov/pubmed/23429290.

Kanakis, C. D., Tarantilis, P. A., Tajmir-Riahi, H. A., & Polissiou, M. G. (2007). Interaction of tRNA with safranal, crocetin, and dimethylcrocetin. *Journal of Biomolecular Structure & Dynamics*, *24*(6), 537–545.

Kaplan, L., Lau, J., & Stein, E. (1990). Carotenoid composition, concentrations, and relationships in various human organs. *Clinical Physiology and Biochemistry*, *8*(1), 1–10.

Karin, M. (2009). NF-kappaB as a critical link between inflammation and cancer. *Cold Spring Harbor Perspectives in Biology*, *1*(5), a000141. Cold Spring Harbor Laboratory Press. Available from: http://www.ncbi.nlm.nih.gov/pubmed/20066113.

Karppi, J., Laukkanen, J. A., & Kurl, S. (2012). Plasma lutein and zeaxanthin and the risk of age-related nuclear cataract among the elderly Finnish population. *The British Journal of Nutrition*, *108*(1), 148–154.

Karppi, J., Laukkanen, J. A., Mäkikallio, T. H., Ronkainen, K., & Kurl, S. (2013). Serum β-carotene and the risk of sudden cardiac death in men: a population-based follow-up study. *Atherosclerosis*, *226*(1), 172–177. Elsevier Ltd.

Kaulmann, A., & Bohn, T. (2014). Carotenoids, inflammation, and oxidative stress-implications of cellular signaling pathways and relation to chronic disease prevention. *Nutrition Research*, *34*(11), 907–929. Elsevier Inc. https://doi.org/10.1016/j.nutres.2014.07.010.

Kavitha, P., Shivashankara, K., Rao, V. K., Avverahally, T. S., Ravishankar, K., & Gonchigar, J. S. (2013). Genotypic variability for antioxidant and quality parameters among tomato cultivars, hybrids, cherry tomatoes and wild species. *Journal of the Science of Food and Agriculture* *94*(5), 993–999.

Kawada, T., Kamei, Y., Fujita, A., Hida, Y., Takahashi, N., Sugimoto, E., et al. (2000). Carotenoids and retinoids as suppressors on adipocyte differentiation via nuclear receptors. *BioFactors*, *13*(1–4), 103–109.

Khachik, F. (2006). Distribution and metabolism of dietary carotenoids in humans as a criterion for development of nutritional supplements. *Pure and Applied Chemistry*, *78*(8), 1551–1557. Available from: https://www.degruyter.com/view/j/pac.2006.78.issue-8/pac200678081551/pac200678081551.xml.

Khachik, F., Beecher, G. R., Goli, M. B., Lusby, W. R., Smith, J. C., Beecher, G. R., et al. (1992). Separation and identification of carotenoids and their oxidation products in the extracts of human plasma. *Analytical Chemistry*, *64*(18), 2111–2122.

Khachik, F., De Moura, F. F., Chew, E. Y., Douglass, L. W., Ferris, F. L., Kim, J., et al. (2006). The effect of lutein and zeaxanthin supplementation on metabolites of these carotenoids in the serum of persons aged 60 or older. *Investigative Ophthalmology and Visual Science*, *47*(12), 5234–5242.

Kim, J.-H., Na, H.-J., Kim, C.-K., Kim, J.-Y., Ha, K.-S., Lee, H., et al. (2008). The non-provitamin A carotenoid, lutein, inhibits NF-κB-dependent gene expression through redox-based regulation of the phosphatidylinositol 3-kinase/PTEN/Akt and NF-κB-inducing kinase pathways: role of H2O2 in NF-κB activation. *Free Radical Biology & Medicine*, *45*(6), 885–896. Pergamon.

Kim, Y., Seo, J. H., & Kim, H. (2011). β-Carotene and lutein inhibit hydrogen peroxide-induced activation of NF-κB and IL-8 expression in gastric epithelial AGS cells. *Journal of Nutritional Science and Vitaminology (Tokyo)*, *57*(3), 216–223. Center for Academic Publications Japan. Available from: http://joi.jlc.jst.go.jp/JST.JSTAGE/jnsv/57.216?from=CrossRef.

Kiokias, S., & Oreopoulou, V. (2006). Antioxidant properties of natural carotenoid extracts against the AAPH-initiated oxidation of food emulsions. *Innovative Food Science and Emerging Technologies*, *7*(1–2), 132–139.

Kirkwood, T. B. L. (2005). Understanding the odd science of aging. *Cell*, *120*(4), 437–447.

Kohl, E., Steinbauer, J., Landthaler, M., & Szeimies, R. (2011). Skin ageing. *Journal of the European Academy of Dermatology and Venereology*, *25*(8), 873–884.

Kovary, K., Louvain, T. S., Silva, M., Albano, F., Pires, B. B. M., Laranja, G. A. T., et al. (2001). Biochemical behaviour of norbixin during in vitro DNA damage induced by reactive oxygen species. *The British Journal of Nutrition*, *85*(4), 431–440.

Krinsky, N. I. (1989). Antioxidant functions of carotenoids. *Free Radical Biology & Medicine*, *7*, 617–635.

Krinsky, N. I., & Johnson, E. J. (2005). Carotenoid actions and their relation to health and disease. *Molecular Aspects of Medicine*, *26*(6), 459–516.

Krutovskikh, V., Asamoto, M., Takasuka, N., Murakoshi, M., Nishino, H., & Tsuda, H. (1997). Differential dose-dependent effects of alpha-, beta-carotenes and lycopene on gap-junctional intercellular communication in rat liver in vivo. *Japanese Journal of Cancer Research*, *88*(12), 1121–1124. Wiley-Blackwell. Available from: http://www.ncbi.nlm.nih.gov/pubmed/9473727.

Lademann, J., Meinke, M. C., Sterry, W., & Darvin, M. E. (2011). Carotenoids in human skin. *Experimental Dermatology*, *20*(5), 377–382.

Lee, S.-J., Bai, S.-K., Lee, K.-S., Namkoong, S., Na, H.-J., Ha, K.-S., et al. (2003). Astaxanthin inhibits nitric oxide production and inflammatory gene expression by suppressing IkB kinase-dependent NF-kB activation. *Molecules and Cells*, *16*(1), 97–105. The Korean Society for Molecular and Cellular Biology. Available from: http://www.molcells.org/journal/view.html?year=2003&volume=16&number=1&spage=97.

Lees, H., Walters, H., & Cox, L. S. (2016). Animal and human models to understand ageing. *Maturitas*, *93*, 18–27. Elsevier Ireland Ltd.

Levy, L. W., Regalado, E., Navarrete, S., & Watkins, R. H. (1997). Bixin and norbixin in human plasma: determination and study of the absorption of a single-dose of annatto food color. *The Analyst*, *122*(9), 977–980.

Lian, F., & Wang, X. (2008). Enzymatic metabolites of lycopene induce Nrf2-mediated expression of phase II detoxifying/antioxidant enzymes in human bronchial epithelial cells. *International Journal of Cancer*, *123*(6), 1262–1268. Wiley-Blackwell. Available from: http://doi.wiley.com/10.1002/ijc.23696.

Lidebjer, C., Leanderson, P., Ernerudh, J., & Jonasson, L. (2007). Low plasma levels of oxygenated carotenoids in patients with coronary artery disease. *Nutrition, Metabolism, and Cardiovascular Diseases*, *17*(6), 448–456.

Lindbergh, C. A., Renzi-Hammond, L. M., Hammond, B. R., Terry, D. P., Mewborn, C. M., Puente, A. N., et al. (2018). Lutein and zeaxanthin influence brain function in older adults: a randomized controlled trial. *Journal of the International Neuropsychological Society*, *24*(1), 77–90.

Lingappan, K. (2018). NF-κB in oxidative stress. *Current Opinion in Toxicology*, *7*, 81–86. Elsevier.

Linnewiel, K., Ernst, H., Caris-Veyrat, C., Ben-Dor, A., Kampf, A., Salman, H., et al. (2009). Structure activity relationship of carotenoid derivatives in activation of the electrophile/antioxidant response element transcription system. *Free Radical Biology & Medicine*, *47*(5), 659–667. Pergamon. Available from: https://www.sciencedirect.com/science/article/pii/S0891584909003438?via%3Dihub.

Linnewiel-Hermoni, K., Motro, Y., Miller, Y., Levy, J., & Sharoni, Y. (2014). Carotenoid derivatives inhibit nuclear factor kappa B activity in bone and cancer cells by targeting key thiol groups. *Free Radical Biology & Medicine*, *75*, 105–120. Pergamon. Available from: https://www.sciencedirect.com/science/article/pii/S0891584914003414?via%3Dihub.

Livny, O., Kaplan, I., Reifen, R., Polak-Charcon, S., Madar, Z., & Schwartz, B. (2002). Lycopene inhibits proliferation and enhances gap-junction communication of KB-1 human Oral tumor cells. *The Journal of Nutrition*, *132*(12), 3754–3759. Oxford University Press. Available from: https://academic.oup.com/jn/article/132/12/3754/4712113.

Lo, H. M., Tsai, Y. J., Du, W. Y., Tsou, C. J., & Wu, W. B. (2012). A naturally occurring carotenoid, lutein, reduces PDGF and H2O2 signaling and compromised migration in cultured vascular smooth muscle cells. *Journal of Biomedical Science*, *19*(1), 1–10.

Lobo, G. P., Isken, A., Hoff, S., Babino, D., & von Lintig, J. (2012). BCDO2 acts as a carotenoid scavenger and gatekeeper for the mitochondrial apoptotic pathway. *Development*, *139*(16), 2966–2977. Available from: http://dev.biologists.org/cgi/doi/10.1242/dev.079632.

Loft, S., & Poulsen, H. E. (1996). Cancer risk and oxidative DNA damage in man. *Journal of Molecular Medicine*, *74*(6), 297–312.

Lowe, G. M., Booth, L. A., Young, A. J., & Bilton, R. F. (1999). Lycopene and beta-carotene protect against oxidative damage in HT29 cells at low concentrations but rapidly lose this capacity at higher doses. *Free Radical Research*, *30*(2), 141–151. Available from: http://www.ncbi.nlm.nih.gov/pubmed/10193582.

Lowe, G. M., Vlismas, K., Graham, D. L., Carail, M., Caris-Veyrat, C., & Young, A. J. (2009). The degradation of (all-E)-β-carotene by cigarette smoke. *Free Radical Research*, *43*(3), 280–286.

Maggio, D., Polidori, M. C., Barabani, M., Tufi, A., Ruggiero, C., Cecchetti, R., et al. (2006). Low levels of carotenoids and retinol in involutional osteoporosis. *Bone*, *38*, 244–248.

Mares, J. (2016). Lutein and zeaxanthin isomers in eye health and disease. *Annual Review of Nutrition*, *36*, 571–602.

Mariani, S., Lionetto, L., Cavallari, M., Tubaro, A., Rasio, D., De Nunzio, C., et al. (2014). Low prostate concentration of lycopene is associated with development of prostate cancer in patients with high-grade prostatic intraepithelial neoplasia. *International Journal of Molecular Sciences*, *15*(1), 1433–1440.

Mariani, E., Polidori, M. C., Cherubini, A., & Mecocci, P. (2005). Oxidative stress in brain aging, neurodegenerative and vascular diseases: an overview. *Journal of Chromatography B, Analytical Technologies in the Biomedical and Life Sciences*, *827*(1), 65–75.

Marini, A., Jaenicke, T., Stahl, W., & Krutmann, J. (2017). Molecular evidence that oral supplementation with lycopene or lutein protects human skin against ultraviolet radiation: results from a double-blinded, placebo-controlled, crossover study. *The British Journal of Dermatology*, 231–240.

Martínez-Cayuela, M. (1995). Oxygen free radicals and human disease. *Biochimie*, *77*(3), 147–161.

McNaughton, S. A., Wattanapenpaiboon, N., Wark, J. D., & Nowson, C. A. (2011). An energy-dense, nutrient-poor dietary pattern is inversely associated with bone health in women. *The Journal of Nutrition*, *141*(8), 1516–1523.

Mendis, S., Puska, P., & Norrving, B. (2011). *Global atlas on cardiovascular disease prevention and control*. WHO.2–13.

Milani, A., Basirnejad, M., Shahbazi, S., & Bolhassani, A. (2017). Carotenoids: biochemistry, pharmacology and treatment. *British Journal of Pharmacology*, *174*(11), 1290–1324.

Min, J. Y., & Min, K. B. (2014). Serum lycopene, lutein and zeaxanthin, and the risk of Alzheimer's disease mortality in older adults. *Dementia and Geriatric Cognitive Disorders*, *37*(3–4), 246–256.

Molina, J. A., De Bustos, F., Jiménez-Jiménez, F. J., Esteban, J., Guerrero-Sola, A., Zurdo, M., et al. (1999). Serum levels of beta-carotene, alpha-carotene, and vitamin A in patients with amyotrophic lateral sclerosis. *Acta Neurologica Scandinavica*, 315–317.

Morgan, M. J., & Liu, Z. (2011). Crosstalk of reactive oxygen species and NF-κB signaling. *Cell Research*, *21*(1), 103–115. Nature Publishing Group.

Muindi, J. F., Scher, H. I., Rigas, J. R., Warrell, R. P. J., & Young, C. W. (1994). Elevated plasma lipid peroxide content correlates with rapid plasma clearance of all-trans-retinoic acid in patients with advanced cancer. *Cancer Research*, *54*(8), 2125–2128.

Müller, L., Caris-Veyrat, C., Lowe, G., & Böhm, V. (2016). Lycopene and its antioxidant role in the prevention of cardiovascular diseases—a critical review. *Critical Reviews in Food Science and Nutrition*, *56*(11), 1868–1879.

Müller, K., Carpenter, K. L. H., Challis, I. R., Skepper, J. N., & Arends, M. J. (2002). Carotenoids induce apoptosis in the T-lymphoblast cell line Jurkat E6.1. *Free Radical Research*, *36*(7), 791–802. Taylor & Francis. Available from: http://www.tandfonline.com/doi/full/10.1080/10715760290032539.

Mužáková, V., Kand'ár, R., Meloun, M., Skalický, J., Královec, K., Žáková, P., et al. (2010). Inverse correlation between plasma β-carotene and interleukin-6 in patients with advanced coronary artery disease. *International Journal for Vitamin and Nutrition Research*, *80*(6), 369–377.

Muzandu, K., El Bohi, K., Shaban, Z., Ishizuka, M., Kazusaka, A., & Fujita, S. (2005). Lycopene and beta-carotene ameliorate catechol estrogen-mediated DNA damage. *The Japanese Journal of Veterinary Research*, *52*(4), 173–184. Available from: http://www.ncbi.nlm.nih.gov/pubmed/15822859.

Muzandu, K., Ishizuka, M., Sakamoto, K. Q., Shaban, Z., El Bohi, K., Kazusaka, A., et al. (2006). Effect of lycopene and β-carotene on peroxynitrite-mediated cellular modifications. *Toxicology and Applied Pharmacology, 215*(3), 330–340.

Nagata, S. (2018). Apoptosis and clearance of apoptotic cells. *Annual Review of Immunology, 36*(1), 489–517. Available from: http://www.annualreviews.org/doi/10.1146/annurev-immunol-042617-053010.

Nguyen, T., Nioi, P., & Pickett, C. B. (2009). The Nrf2-antioxidant response element signaling pathway and its activation by oxidative stress. *The Journal of Biological Chemistry, 284*(20), 13291–13295.

Nishino, H., Murakoshi, M., Tokuda, H., & Satomi, Y. (2009). Cancer prevention by carotenoids. *Archives of Biochemistry and Biophysics, 483*(2), 165–168. Elsevier Inc. https://doi.org/10.1016/j.abb.2008.09.011.

Novo, R., Azevedo, P. S., Minicucci, M. F., Zornoff, L. A. M., & SAR, P. (2013). Effect of beta-carotene on oxidative stress and expression of cardiac connexin 43. *Arquivos Brasileiros de Cardiologia, 101*(3), 233–239. Available from: http://www.ncbi.nlm.nih.gov/pubmed/23917457.

Obulesu, M., Dowlathabad, M. R., & Bramhachari, P. V. (2011). Carotenoids and Alzheimer's disease: an insight into therapeutic role of retinoids in animal models. *Neurochemistry International, 59*(5), 535–541. Elsevier B.V.

Palozza, P., Colangelo, M., Simone, R., Catalano, A., Boninsegna, A., Lanza, P., et al. (2010). Lycopene induces cell growth inhibition by altering mevalonate pathway and Ras signaling in cancer cell lines. *Carcinogenesis, 31*(10), 1813–1821.

Palozza, P., Serini, S., Di Nicuolo, F., & Calviello, G. (2004). Modulation of apoptotic signalling by carotenoids in cancer cells. *Archives of Biochemistry and Biophysics, 430*(1), 104–109. Academic Press. Available from: https://www.sciencedirect.com/science/article/pii/S0003986104001225?via%3Dihub#BIB1.

Palozza, P., Serini, S., Di Nicuolo, F., Piccioni, E., & Calviello, G. (2003). Prooxidant effects of β-carotene in cultured cells. *Molecular Aspects of Medicine, 24*(6), 353–362.

Palozza, P., Serini, S., Torsello, A., Di Nicuolo, F., Maggiano, N., Ranelletti, F. O., et al. (2003a). Mechanism of activation of caspase cascade during $β$-carotene-induced apoptosis in human tumor cells. *Nutrition and Cancer, 47*(1), 76–87. Available from: http://www.ncbi.nlm.nih.gov/pubmed/14769541.

Palozza, P., Serini, S., Torsello, A., Di Nicuolo, F., Piccioni, E., Ubaldi, V., et al. (2003b). β-Carotene regulates NF-κB DNA-binding activity by a redox mechanism in human leukemia and colon adenocarcinoma cells. *The Journal of Nutrition, 133*(2), 381–388. Oxford University Press.

Paneni, F., Diaz Cañestro, C., Libby, P., Lüscher, T. F., & Camici, G. G. (2017). The aging cardiovascular system: understanding it at the cellular and clinical levels. *Journal of the American College of Cardiology, 69*(15), 1952–1967.

Paran, E., Novack, V., & Engelhard, Y. N. (2009). The effects of natural antioxidants from tomato extract in treated but uncontrolled hypertensive patients. *Cardiovascular Drugs and Therapy, 23*(2), 145–151.

Park, Y., Choi, J., Lim, J. W., & Kim, H. (2015). β-Carotene-induced apoptosis is mediated with loss of Ku proteins in gastric cancer AGS cells. *Genes & Nutrition, 10*(4), 467. BioMed Central.

Park, Y. O., Hwang, E.-S., & Moon, T. W. (2005). The effect of lycopene on cell growth and oxidative DNA damage of Hep3B human hepatoma cells. *Biofactors, 23*(3), 129–139. Available from: http://www.ncbi.nlm.nih.gov/pubmed/16410635.

Park, S. K., Kim, K., Page, G. P., Allison, D. B., Weindruch, R., & Prolla, T. A. (2009). Gene expression profiling of aging in multiple mouse strains: identification of aging biomarkers and impact of dietary antioxidants. *Aging Cell*, *8*(4), 484–495.

Pashkow, F. J., Watumull, D. G., & Campbell, C. L. (2008). Astaxanthin: a novel potential treatment for oxidative stress and inflammation in cardiovascular disease. *The American Journal of Cardiology*, *101*(10), S58–S68.

Perera, C. O., & Yen, G. M. (2007). Functional properties of carotenoids in human health. *International Journal of Food Properties*, *10*(2), 201–230.

Polacek, D., Lal, R., Volin, M. V., & Davies, P. F. (1993). Gap junctional communication between vascular cells: induction of connexin43 messenger RNA in macrophage foam cells of atherosclerotic lesions. *The American Journal of Pathology*, *142*(2), 593–606.

Raj, L., Ide, T., Gurkar, A. U., Foley, M., Schenone, M., Li, X., et al. (2011). Selective killing of cancer cells by a small molecule targeting the stress response to ROS. *Nature*, *475*(7355), 231–234. Nature Publishing Group. Available from: http://www.nature.com/doifinder/10.1038/nature10167.

Rao, A. V., & Rao, L. G. (2007). Carotenoids and human health. *Pharmacological Research*, *55*, 207–216.

Rao, A. V., Ray, M. R., & Rao, L. G. (2006). Lycopene. *Advances in Food and Nutrition Research*, *51*(06), 99–164.

Ribeiro, D., Freitas, M., Silva, A. M. S., Carvalho, F., & Fernandes, E. (2018). Antioxidant and pro-oxidant activities of carotenoids and their oxidation products. *Food and Chemical Toxicology*, *120*(August), 681–699. Elsevier. https://doi.org/10.1016/j.fct.2018.07.060.

Riccioni, G., Mancini, B., Ilio, E. D. I., Bucciarelli, T., & Orazio, N. D. (2008). Protective effect of lycopene in cardiovascular disease. *European Review for Medical and Pharmacological Sciences*, *12*(November 2007), 183–190.

Rissanen, T. H., Voutilainen, S., Virtanen, J. K., Venho, B., Vanharanta, M., Mursu, J., et al. (2003). Low intake of fruits, berries and vegetables is associated with excess mortality in men: the Kuopio Ischaemic Heart Disease Risk Factor (KIHD) Study. *The Journal of Nutrition*, *133*(1), 199–204.

Rivera-Madrid, R., Aguilar-Espinosa, M., Cárdenas-Conejo, Y., & Garza-Caligaris, L. E. (2016). Carotenoid derivates in achiote (*Bixa orellana*) seeds: synthesis and health promoting properties. *Frontiers in Plant Science*, *7*(September), 1–7. Available from: http://journal.frontiersin.org/Article/10.3389/fpls.2016.01406/abstract.

Roberts, R. L., Green, J., Lewis, B., Health, K., Avenue, E. C., Suite, A., et al. (2009). Lutein and zeaxanthin in eye and skin health. *Clinics in Dermatology*, *27*(2), 195–201. Elsevier Inc. https://doi.org/10.1016/j.clindermatol.2008.01.011.

Rodrigues, E., Mariutti, L. R. B., Chisté, R. C., & Mercadante, A. Z. (2012). Development of a novel micro-assay for evaluation of peroxyl radical scavenger capacity: application to carotenoids and structure-activity relationship. *Food Chemistry*, *135*(3), 2103–2111. Elsevier Ltd.

Rodríguez-Concepción, M., Avalos, J., Bonet, M. L., Boronat, A., Gómez-Gómez, L., Hornero-Mendez, D., et al. (2018). A global perspective on carotenoids: metabolism, biotechnology, and benefits for nutrition and health. *Progress in Lipid Research*, *70*(February), 62–93.

Ruiz Rejón, F., Martín-Peña, G., Granado, F., Ruiz-Galiana, J., Blanco, I., & Olmedilla, B. (2002). Plasma status of retinol, α- and γ-tocopherols, and main carotenoids to first myocardial infarction: case control and follow-up study. *Nutrition*, *18*(1), 26–31.

Sacco, S. M., Horcajada, M., & Offord, E. (2013). Phytonutrients for bone health during ageing. *British Journal of Clinical Pharmacology*, *75*(3), 697–707.

Sahni, S., Hannan, M. T., Gagnon, D., Blumberg, J., Cupples, L. A., Kiel, D. P., et al. (2009). Protective effect of total and supplemental vitamin C intake on the risk of hip fracture-a 17-year follow-up from the Framingham Osteoporosis Study. *Osteoporosis International*, *20*(11), 1853–1861.

Sandmann, G. (2014). Carotenoids of biotechnological importance. In T. Scheper (Ed.), *Biotechnology of isoprenoids. Springer-V* (pp. 450–463). Germany: Springer.

Seifried, H. E., Anderson, D. E., Fisher, E. I., & Milner, J. A. (2007). A review of the interaction among dietary antioxidants and reactive oxygen species. *The Journal of Nutritional Biochemistry*, *18*(9), 567–579.

Semba, R. D., Patel, K. V., Ferrucci, L., Sun, K., Roy, C. N., Guralnik, J. M., et al. (2010). Serum antioxidants and inflammation predict red cell distribution width in older women: the Women's Health and Aging Study I. *Clinical Nutrition*, *29*(5), 600–604. Elsevier Ltd.

Serasanambati, M., & Chilakapati, S. R. (2016). Function of nuclear factor kappa B (NF-kB) in human diseases—a review. *South Indian Journal of Biosocial Science*, *2*(4), 368. Available from: http://www.sijbsojms.com/index.php/SIJBS/article/view/103443.

Sharoni, Y., Linnewiel-Hermoni, K., Khanin, M., Salman, H., Veprik, A., Danilenko, M., et al. (2012). Carotenoids and apocarotenoids in cellular signaling related to cancer: a review. *Molecular Nutrition & Food Research*, *56*(2), 259–269.

Shay, C. M., Stamler, J., Dyer, A. R., Brown, I. J., Chan, Q., Elliott, P., et al. (2012). Nutrient and food intakes of middle-aged adults at low risk of cardiovascular disease: the international study of macro-/micronutrients and blood pressure (INTERMAP). *European Journal of Nutrition*, *51*(8), 917–926.

Shimidzu, N., Goto, M., & Miki, W. (1996). Carotenoids as singlet oxygen quenchers in marine organisms. *Fisheries Science*, *62*(1), 134–137. Available from: https://www.jstage.jst.go.jp/article/fishsci1994/62/1/62_1_134/_article.

Siva, R., Mathew, G. J., Venkat, A., & Dhawan, C. (2008). An alternative tracking dye for gel electrophoresis. *Current Science*, *94*(6), 765–767.

Slavin, J. L., & Lloyd, B. (2012). Health benefits of fruits and vegetables. *Advances in Nutrition*, *3*(4), 506–516.

Soares, N., Teodoro, A. J., Oliveira, F. L., Santos, C. A., Takiya, C. M., Junior, O. S., et al. (2013). Influence of lycopene on cell viability, cell cycle, and apoptosis of human prostate cancer and benign hyperplastic cells. *Nutrition and Cancer*, *65*(7), 1076–1085. Taylor & Francis Group. Available from: http://www.tandfonline.com/doi/abs/10.1080/01635581.2013.812225.

Somacal, S., Figueiredo, C. G., Quatrin, A., Ruviaro, A. R., Conte, L., Augusti, P. R., et al. (2015). The antiatherogenic effect of bixin in hypercholesterolemic rabbits is associated to the improvement of lipid profile and to its antioxidant and anti-inflammatory effects. *Molecular and Cellular Biochemistry*, *403*(1–2), 243–253.

Sommerburg, O., Keunen, J. E., Bird, A. C., & van Kuijk, F. J. (1998). Fruits and vegetables that are sources for lutein and zeaxanthin: the macular pigment in human eyes. *The British Journal of Ophthalmology*, *82*(8), 907–910.

Sowmya, P.R.-R., Arathi, B. P., Vijay, K., Baskaran, V., & Lakshminarayana, R. (2015). Role of different vehicles in carotenoids delivery and their influence on cell viability, cell cycle progression, and induction of apoptosis in HeLa cells. *Molecular and Cellular Biochemistry*, *406*(1–2), 245–253. Springer US. Available from: http://link.springer.com/10.1007/s11010-015-2442-y.

Stahl, W., Nicolai, S., Briviba, K., Hanusch, M., Broszeit, G., Peters, M., et al. (1997). Biological activities of natural and synthetic carotenoids: induction of gap junctional communication and singlet oxygen quenching. *Carcinogenesis*, *18*(1), 89–92.

Stahl, W., von Laar, J., Martin, H.-D., Emmerich, T., & Sies, H. (2000). Stimulation of gap junctional communication: comparison of acyclo-retinoic acid and lycopene. *Archives of Biochemistry and Biophysics*, *373*(1), 271–274. Academic Press.

Steinberg, D., & Witztum, J. L. (2002). Is the oxidative modification hypothesis relevant to human atherosclerosis? Do the antioxidant trials conducted to date refute the hypothesis? *Circulation*, *105*(17), 2107–2111.

Sumantran, V. N., Zhang, R., Lee, D. S., & Wicha, M. S. (2000). Differential regulation of apoptosis in normal versus transformed mammary epithelium by lutein and retinoic acid. *Cancer Epidemiology, Biomarkers & Prevention*, *9*(3), 257–263.

Sun, T., Yuan, H., Cao, H., Yazdani, M., Tadmor, Y., & Li, L. (2018). Carotenoid metabolism in plants: the role of plastids. *Molecular Plant*, *11*(1), 58–74.

Swerdlow, R. H. (2011). Brain aging, Alzheimer's disease, and mitochondria. *Biochimica et Biophysica Acta, Molecular Basis of Disease*, *1812*(12), 1630–1639. Elsevier B.V.

Takahashi, N., Goto, T., Taimatsu, A., Egawa, K., Katoh, S., Kusudo, T., et al. (2009). Bixin regulates mRNA expression involved in adipogenesis and enhances insulin sensitivity in 3T3-L1 adipocytes through PPARγ activation. *Biochemical and Biophysical Research Communications*, *390*(4), 1372–1376. Elsevier Inc.

Takeshima, M., Ono, M., Higuchi, T., Chen, C., Hara, T., & Nakano, S. (2014). Anti-proliferative and apoptosis-inducing activity of lycopene against three subtypes of human breast cancer cell lines. *Cancer Science*, *105*(3), 252–257. Wiley/Blackwell (10.1111). Available from: http://doi.wiley.com/10.1111/cas.12349.

Tanaka, S., Yoshimura, Y., Kamada, C., Tanaka, S., Horikawa, C., Okumura, R., et al. (2013). Intakes of dietary fiber, vegetables, and fruits and incidence of cardiovascular disease in Japanese patients with type 2 diabetes. *Diabetes Care*, *36*(12), 3916–3922.

Tyckowski, J. K., & Hamilton, P. B. (1986). Absorption, transport, and deposition in chickens of lutein diester, a carotenoid extracted from marigold (*Tagetes erecta*) petals. *Poultry Science*, *65*(8), 1526–1531.

Ukai, N., Lu, Y., Etoh, H., Yagi, A., Ina, K., Oshima, S., et al. (1994). Photosensitized oxygenation of lycopene. *Bioscience, Biotechnology, and Biochemistry*, *58*(9), 1718–1719. Taylor & Francis.

van Breemen, R. B., & Pajkovic, N. (2008). Multitargeted therapy of cancer by lycopene. *Cancer Letters*, *269*(2), 339–351.

van Helden, Y. G. J., Keijer, J., Heil, S. G., Pico, C., Palou, A., Oliver, P., et al. (2009). Beta-carotene affects oxidative stress-related DNA damage in lung epithelial cells and in ferret lung. *Carcinogenesis*, *30*(12), 2070–2076. Oxford University Press. Available from: https://academic.oup.com/carcin/article-lookup/doi/10.1093/carcin/bgp186.

Van Herpen-Broekmans, W., Klöpping-Ketelaars, I., Michiel, B., Cornelis, K., Hans, P., Hendriks, F. J., et al. (2004). Serum carotenoids and vitamins in relation to markers of endothelial. *European Journal of Epidemiology*, *19*(10), 915–921.

Wang, M., Dhingra, K., Hittelman, W. N., Liehr, J. G., de Andrade, M., & Li, D. (1996). Lipid peroxidation-induced putative malondialdehyde-DNA adducts in human breast tissues. *Cancer Epidemiology, Biomarkers & Prevention*, *5*(September), 705–710.

Wang, X. D., Liu, C., Bronson, R. T., Smith, D. E., Krinsky, N. I., & Russell, M. (1999). Retinoid signaling and activator protein-1 expression in ferrets given beta-carotene supplements and exposed to tobacco smoke. *Journal of the National Cancer Institute*, *91*(1), 60–66. Available from: http://www.ncbi.nlm.nih.gov/pubmed/9890171.

Wang, H., Liu, X., Long, M., Huang, Y., Zhang, L., Zhang, R., et al. (2016). NRF2 activation by antioxidant antidiabetic agents accelerates tumor metastasis. *Science Translational Medicine*, *8*(334), 334ra51. Available from: http://www.ncbi.nlm.nih.gov/pubmed/27075625.

Wang, X., & Russell, R. M. (1999). Procarcinogenic and anticarcinogenic effects of β-carotene. *Nutrition Reviews*, *57*(9), 263–272.

Wang, X.-J., Sun, Z., Villeneuve, N. F., Zhang, S., Zhao, F., Li, Y., et al. (2008). Nrf2 enhances resistance of cancer cells to chemotherapeutic drugs, the dark side of Nrf2. *Carcinogenesis*, *29*(6), 1235–1243. Oxford University Press. Available from: http://www.ncbi.nlm.nih.gov/pubmed/18413364.

Wegner, A., & Khoramnia, R. (2011). Cataract is a self-defence reaction to protect the retina from oxidative damage. *Medical Hypotheses*, *76*(5), 741–744. Elsevier Ltd. https://doi.org/10.1016/j.mehy.2011.02.013.

Weitzmann, M. N., Pacifici, R., Weitzmann, M. N., & Pacifici, R. (2006). Estrogen deficiency and bone loss: an inflammatory tale. *The Journal of Clinical Investigation*, *116*(5), 1186–1194.

Wolak, T., & Paran, E. (2013). *Can carotenoids attenuate vascular aging?* (59). Elsevier Inc..63–66.

Wong, R. S. Y. (2011). Apoptosis in cancer: from pathogenesis to treatment. *Journal of Experimental & Clinical Cancer Research*, *30*(1), 87. BioMed Central. Available from: http://www.ncbi.nlm.nih.gov/pubmed/21943236.

Wong, D., Teixeira, A., Oikonomopoulos, S., Humburg, P., Lone, I. N., Saliba, D., et al. (2011). Extensive characterization of NF-κB binding uncovers non-canonical motifs and advances the interpretation of genetic functional traits. *Genome Biology*, *12*(7), R70. BioMed Central; Available from: http://www.ncbi.nlm.nih.gov/pubmed/21801342.

Woodside, J. V., McGrath, A. J., Lyner, N., & McKinley, M. C. (2015). Carotenoids and health in older people. *Maturitas*, *80*(1), 63–68. Elsevier Ireland Ltd. https://doi.org/10.1016/j.maturitas.2014.10.012.

Woodside, J. V., Young, I. S., & McKinley, M. C. (2013). Fruit and vegetable intake and risk of cardiovascular disease. *The Proceedings of the Nutrition Society*, *72*(4), 399–406.

Yamaguchi, M. (2012). Role of carotenoid β-cryptoxanthin in bone homeostasis. *Journal of Biomedical Science*, *19*(1), 1–14.

Yeh, S.-L., & Hu, M.-L. (2000). Antioxidant and pro-oxidant effects of lycopene in comparison with β-carotene on oxidant-induced damage in Hs68 cells. *The Journal of Nutritional Biochemistry*, *11*(11–12), 548–554. Elsevier.

Young, A., & Lowe, G. (2018). Carotenoids—antioxidant properties. *Antioxidants*, *7*(2), 28. Available from: http://www.mdpi.com/2076-3921/7/2/28.

Zhan, J., Liu, Y.-J., Cai, L.-B., Xu, F.-R., Xie, T., & He, Q.-Q. (2015). Fruit and vegetable consumption and risk of cardiovascular disease: a meta-analysis of prospective cohort studies. *Critical Reviews in Food Science and Nutrition*, *57*(8), 1650–1663.

Zhan, J., Liu, Y.-J., Cai, L.-B., Xu, F.-R., Xie, T., & He, Q.-Q. (2017). Fruit and vegetable consumption and risk of COPD: a prospective cohort study of men. *Thorax*, *72*(6), 500–509.

Zhang, L. X., Cooney, R. V., & Bertram, J. S. (1991). Carotenoids enhance gap junctional communication and inhibit lipid peroxidation in C3H/10T1/2 cells: relationship to their cancer chemopreventive action. *Carcinogenesis*, *12*(11), 2109–2114. Available from: http://www.ncbi.nlm.nih.gov/pubmed/1934296.

Zhang, L. X., Cooney, R. V., & Bertram, J. S. (1992). Carotenoids up-regulate connexin43 gene expression independent of their provitamin A or antioxidant properties. *Cancer Research*, *52*(20), 5707–5712.

Zhang, Y. Z., Dai, J., Zhang, X. P., Yang, X., & Liu, Y. (2008). Studies of the interaction between Sudan I and bovine serum albumin by spectroscopic methods. *Journal of Molecular Structure*, *888*, 152–159.

Zhang, Y., Jiang, W., Xie, Z., Wu, W., & Zhang, D. (2015). Review article vitamin E and risk of age-related cataract: a meta-analysis. *Public Health Nutrition*, *18*(May 2014), 2804–2814.

Zhang, X., Ren, Z., Zuo, J., Su, C., Wang, R., Chang, Y., et al. (2002). The effect of all-trans retinoic acid on gap junctional intercellular communication and connexin 43 gene expression in glioma cells. *Chinese Medical Sciences Journal = Chung-kuo i hsueh k'o hsueh tsa chih*, *17*(1), 22–26. Available from: http://www.ncbi.nlm.nih.gov/pubmed/12894880.

Zhao, B., Ren, B., Guo, R., Zhang, W., Ma, S., Yao, Y., et al. (2017). Supplementation of lycopene attenuates oxidative stress induced neuroinflammation and cognitive impairment via Nrf2/NF-κB transcriptional pathway. *Food and Chemical Toxicology*, *109*(April), 505–516. Elsevier.

Zou, Z., Xu, X., Huang, Y., Xiao, X., Ma, L., Sun, T., et al. (2011). High serum level of lutein may be protective against early atherosclerosis: the Beijing atherosclerosis study. *Atherosclerosis*, *219*(2), 789–793.

Zsila, F., Molnár, P., Deli, J., & Lockwood, S. F. (2005). Circular dichroism and absorption spectroscopic data reveal binding of the natural cis-carotenoid bixin to human α1-acid glycoprotein. *Bioorganic Chemistry*, *33*(4), 298–309.

Further reading

Siva, R., Doss, F. P., Kundu, K., Satyanarayana, V. S. V., & Kumar, V. (2010). Molecular characterization of bixin—an important industrial product. *Industrial Crops and Products*, *32*(1), 48–53.

Factors affecting bioaccessibility and bio-efficacy of carotenoids

Shivaprasad Shilpa*, Hulikere Jagdish Shwetha*, Marisiddaiah Raju†,
Rangaswamy Lakshminarayana*
*Department of Biotechnology, Jnana Bharathi Campus, Bangalore University,
Bengaluru, India., †Department of Botany, St. Joseph's College Autonomous,
Bengaluru, India.

Chapter outline

Carotenoids: Properties, Processing and Applications. https://doi.org/10.1016/B978-0-12-817067-0.00002-6

Introduction

Carotenoids are nonpolar compounds which impart yellow, orange, and red hues to a number of commonly consumed fruits and vegetables. They are synthesized by plants and other photosynthetic organisms including certain bacteria, fungi, and yeasts (Liaaen-Jensen, 2004). To date, more than 750 carotenoids have been identified in various natural sources (Britton, Liaaen-Jensen, & Pfander, 2004). In general, carotenoids are classified into two primary types: hydrocarbon carotenoids such as β-carotene and lycopene, which are composed entirely of hydrogen and carbon, and xanthophylls (lutein, zeaxanthin, canthaxanthin, astaxanthin, fucoxanthin) contain oxygen in addition to carbon and hydrogen. Some carotenoids, like β-carotene, α-carotene, and β-cryptoxanthin serve as an important source of provitamin A in the human diet. Consumption of the carotenoid lycopene has been associated with a reduced risk of developing cardiovascular disease and cancer. Xanthophyll carotenoids like lutein and zeaxanthin have been shown to provide potential beneficial effects on human eye health particularly in delaying progression of age-related macular degeneration (AMD) (Lakshminarayana et al., 2008; Maiani, Periago Caston, Catasta, et al., 2009; Tang, Qin, Dolnikowski, Russell, & Grusak, 2009). Recently, astaxanthin (keto-carotenoids) and fucoxanthin (epoxy-carotenoids) are recognized as promising marine carotenoids with an anticipated role against diabetes, obesity, angiogenesis, and cancers (Arathi, Sowmya, Vijay, Baskaran, & Lakshminarayana, 2016).

Apart from these diverse structures of carotenoids showed certain common properties such as antioxidant activity, cell signaling, immunomodulation, and inhibit on cancer growth (Arathi et al., 2016). Dietary ingestion is the only source to obtain them, since humans cannot synthesize. Epidemiological studies correlated that consumption of dietary carotenoids decreased risk of VAD, cancer, atherosclerosis, and AMD. These vital health benefits of carotenoid led to an increasing interest on their bioavailability and bioefficacy. Though carotenoids are important nutraceuticals, their intestinal absorption and transport process at cellular (enterocyte) level addressed recently (Tyssandier et al., 2003). Since carotenoids are lipids soluble, its bioavailability is extremely low, further it may interfere with various dietary and physiological factors (During & Harrison, 2006; Van het Hof, West, Weststrate, & Hautvast, 2000). In this regard, several studies have revealed the bioavailability of dietary carotenoids based on their postprandial levels in plasma/serum of humans and rodents. However, the assessment of astaxanthin (crustaceans) and fucoxanthin (seaweeds) bioavailability from respective edible source or its nutraceuticals supplements is still not much available though the exploration of marine source is one of the major concerns of food industry (Suleria, Osborne, Masci, & Gobe, 2015). Focus to bioavailability, direct gavages of carotenoids is limited due to poor solubility, chemical instability, and sensitive to oxidative modifications during gastrointestinal transit.

Interest in the metabolism of carotenoids has increased because of the inverse association between chronic diseases and dietary intake of these molecules or their blood or tissue concentrations. In addition, clinical studies have systematically observed that a huge variability in blood or tissue response of food derived carotenoids. Therefore, understanding the absorption, metabolism, and bioefficacy of these compounds is considered to be very important for making or ensure adequate carotenoids recommendation to combat vitamin A status and reduce the risk of developing specific diseases. Nutritional biochemist believes that food-based strategies are the best and promising approach to combat VAD and other health-related problems worldwide (Arathi et al., 2016; Drammeh et al., 2002; Tang, Serfaty-Lacrosniere, Camilo, & Russell, 1996). With this context, this chapter highlights the critical factor (dietary or nondietary) involved in solubilization, processing and formation of carotenoid-rich mixed micelles, and their influence on bioaccessibility/bioavailability and bioefficacy of carotenoids. Further, influence of each factor and its regulation on biochemical and molecular mechanism of carotenoids absorption and transport processes are systematically illustrated.

Carotenoids bioaccessibility and bioavailability

Since, carotenoids are lipophilic in nature, they get processed in a similar manner as other fat-soluble compounds are absorbed in the gastrointestinal transit. Major dietary provitamin and nonprovitamin A carotenoids have different biological activities and efficacy, depending on their food content, dietary intake, bioavailability, and bioconversion (Maiani et al., 2009). To understand the metabolism of carotenoids and the influence of their rich foods, three important terms have been commonly used: bioaccessibility, bioavailability, and bioefficacy. "Bioaccessibility" is a digestive process to release carotenoids from the food matrix and consider being most crucial step to support carotenoids bioavailability at enterocyte levels. Bioavailability is defined as "the fraction of an ingested nutrient that is available for utilization in normal physiological functions or for storage". Bioefficacy is the efficiency of ingested carotenoids that are made available as such or converted to active form of metabolite for executing desired function in the body (Van Lieshout, West, & Van Breemen, 2003). All these terms are pertaining only to the provitamin A carotenoids as they give the end product, retinol by the enzyme β-carotene 15,15′-oxygenase-1 (BCO1) through their metabolism. Other carotenoid cleavage enzyme β-carotene 9,10′-oxygenase-2 (BCO2) is presumed to be acting on the lycopene or other xanthophyll carotenoids metabolism or it may be having broad substrate specificity on different carotenoids. However, the metabolites or other carotenoids and the substrate specificity of different metabolizing enzymes are yet to be determined. Published information on the carotenoids bioavailability of is based on the measurement of their levels in serum or plasma. Dietary matrix or components interferes the rate of each of the absorption steps that affect the bioavailability of the ingested carotenoids are shown in Fig. 1.

Intestinal absorption and distribution of carotenoids

The process of carotenoid absorption requires movement of the digested food components into the mucosal cells of the intestinal wall. Uptake occurs when the carotenoids or its metabolites diffuse through the mucosal cells into the portal or lymphatic system (Fig. 1). Generally, intestinal absorption of carotenoids involves few major steps:

(1) release from the food matrix,
(2) solubilization into mixed lipid micelles in the lumen,
(3) cellular uptake by intestinal mucosal cells,

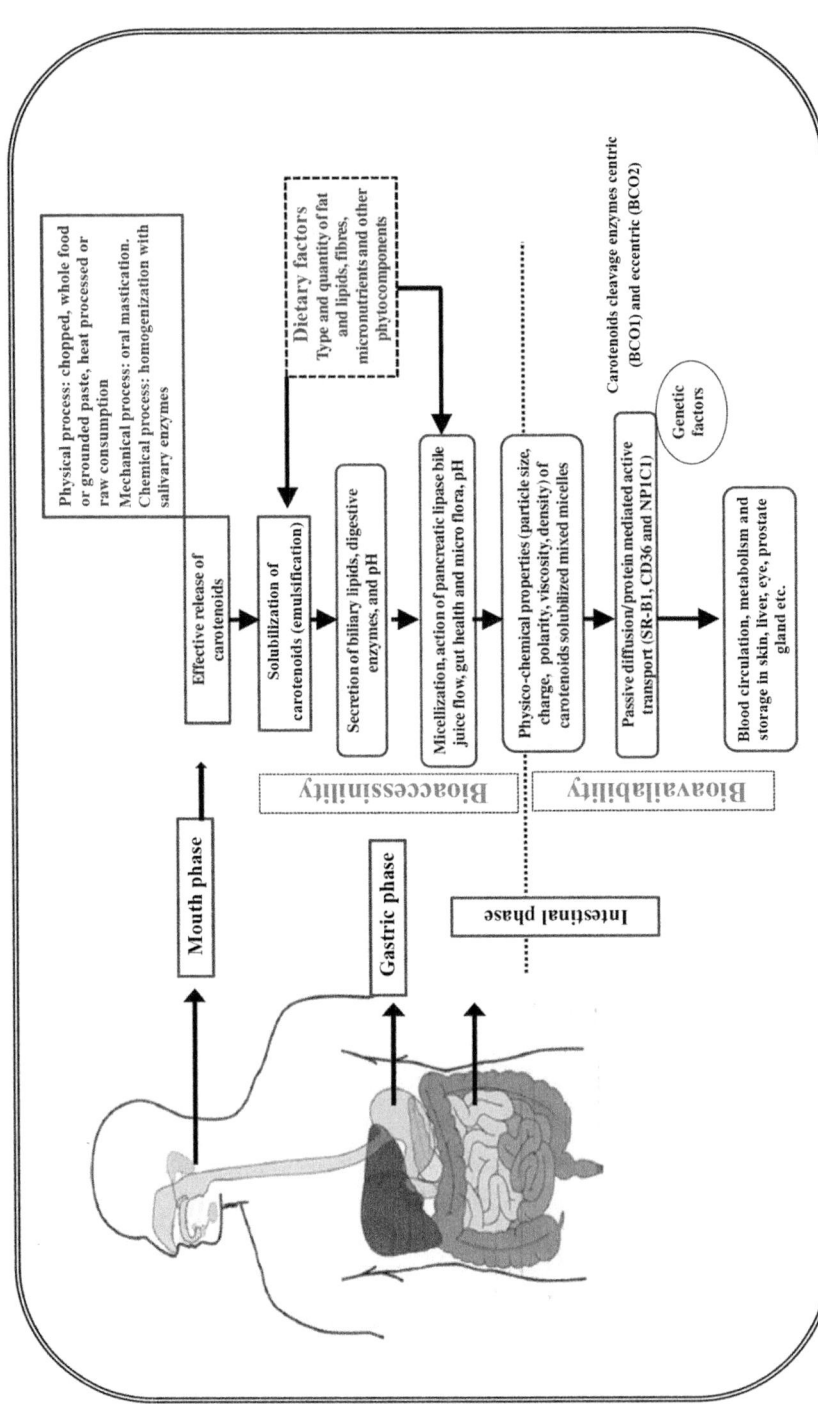

Fig. 1 Schematic demonstration of intestinal absorption of carotenoids.

(**4**) incorporation into chylomicrons, and.

(**5**) secretion into the lymph (Erdman, Bierer, & Gugger, 1993; Furr & Clark, 1997; van Vliet, 1996; Yeum & Russell, 2002).

Carotenoids are released from the food matrix by heat, physical and mechanical food processing, and in the mouth by mastication and the action of salivary enzymes. Carotenoids are lipophilic compounds and must undergo solubilization from the food matrix, followed by micellization. This refers to their incorporation into micelles, which are molecular aggregates that transport fat-soluble material, and making it accessible by the intestinal epithelium. Digestion begins in the oral cavity by mechanical action and lubrication with saliva before entering the stomach. Hydrochloric acid, pepsin, and gastric lipase are secreted into the gastric lumen and mixed with the ingested foods, resulting in partial release of the carotenoids from the food matrix into the emulsified oil droplets. Then, the mixed micelles are formed due to biliary secretion and diffuse across the unstirred water layer and deliver carotenoids, and other fat-soluble compounds through the apical surface of the mucosal epithelium. Nonpolar carotenoids such as β-carotene/lycopene reside in the core of lipid droplets, whereas polar carotenoids, lutein/zeaxanthin are preferentially distributed at the surface (Borel et al., 1996). The transfer of carotenoids from micelles to the apical surface of epithelial cell, lining of the small intestine, suggested that the absorption of carotenoid is saturable (Diwadkar-Navsariwala et al., 2003; Furr & Clark, 1997; Parker, 1996). These observations suggest that like cholesterol and fatty acids, carotenoids may be transported across the brush border membrane by a partially facilitated process (Davis et al., 2004; Schaffer, 2002). Once taken into the enterocyte, portion of the carotenoids may be converted into their metabolites. For example, β-carotene can be converted to retinol by the action of β-carotene cleavage enzymes. Retinal formed from β-carotene is reduced to retinol by retinal reductase.

The uptake of carotenoids from the intestinal lumen takes place partially by simple diffusion through the brush border membrane into the cytoplasm of the enterocytes. However, reports have suggested that the carotenoid transport is also mediated by receptor-binding protein. The hairpin-like external domain forms a hydrophobic channel that may facilitate the uptake of carotenoids by the enterocytes, without energy expenditure (Yonekura & Nagao, 2007). In this regard, several receptors such as, scavenger receptor-binding protein I (SR-BI), cluster of differentiation 36 (CD36), and Niemann-Pick C1-Like 1 protein (NPC1L1) were eventually identified as facilitators of the absorption of cholesterol and carotenoids (van Bennekum et al., 2005). A protein facilitated lipid uptake mechanism is also consistent with the observation of a pronounced interindividual variability in cholesterol absorption efficiency in both animals and humans that have been attributed to genetic factors at the enterocytes level (Wang, Chuang, & Hsu, 2008). It is noteworthy that there is also interindividual variability in the response to dietary β-carotene (Borek et al., 1998). The cellular uptake and efflux of carotenoids, likely involve more than one transporter. During, Dawson, and Horrison (2005) have shown that the carotenoids transport decreased with an increased polarity of carotenoids. Similarly, Reboul et al. (2005) examined carotenoids transport processes in cultured intestinal cells. Purified lutein mixed with phospholipids, lysophospholipid, cholesterol, mono-olein, oleic acid, and taurocholate to obtain carotenoid-rich mixed micelles, which are mimicked those found under physiological conditions. Co-incubation of β-carotene, but not lycopene decreased the lutein absorption significantly. Further they demonstrated that lutein absorption is at least partly protein-mediated.

Studies indicate that the carotenoids reaches peak concentration in chylomicron fraction at approximately 2 h, detected a peak in serum at about 16 h of postingestion (Kostic, White, & Olson, 1995; O'Neill & Thurnham, 1998). Absorption of carotenoid from purified crystalline supplements is almost twice than that from spinach or other vegetable sources (Castenmiller, West, Linssen, Van het Hof, & Voragen, 1999). Carotenoids released, and retinyl esters synthesized after cleavage of provitamin A carotenoids are incorporated into nascent chylomicrons in the Golgi of enterocytes (Parker, 1996). Conversion of chylomicrons to remnants is associated with uptake of the particles by liver, where the carotenoids may be utilized, stored or resecreted into plasma associated with very low-density lipoproteins (VLDLs) and high-density lipoproteins (HDLs).

It is hypothesized that xanthophylls are surface oriented (Britton, 1995; Deming & Erdman, 1999). The chylomicrons are eventually set free into the bloodstream, where they lose triglycerides content and shrink in size by the action of lipoprotein lipase. Carotenoids remain in the liver or enter into the blood stream back with the help of VLDLs, are then transferred by either low-density lipoproteins (LDLs) or HDLs to target sites. Where, lutein or oxygenated carotenoids binds equally with LDL and HDLs in human blood, in contrast to the hydrocarbon carotenoids (BC and lycopene), which are preferentially found in LDL fractions (Erdman et al., 1993; Parker. 1996). HDL is the primary transporter of lutein. Recently, Wang et al. (2007) have reported that the lutein and zeaxanthin are transported primarily by lipoprotein in normal and AMD patients. They observed that that transport of these carotenoids are not significantly different from the AMD and control groups. Non-dietary factors such as age, body composition, gender, malabsorption of fat, alcohol consumption, smoking, and liver or kidney diseases also affects the bioavailability (Albanes et al., 1997; Alberg, 2002; Brady, Mares-Perlman, Bowen, & Stacewicz-Sapuntzakis, 1996; Williams, Boileau, & Erdman, 1998). The detailed process of carotenoids metabolism is shown in Fig. 2.

Bioefficacy of carotenoids with provitamin A activity

Carotenoids should have some structural requirements for conversion into vitamin A. Carotenoid those with at least one β-ionone ring, without oxygenated functional groups, along with polyene chain containing at least 11 carbon atoms are potential precursors of vitamin A. Among natural carotenoids described only 10% have shown provitamin A activity. The most important ones, as much for their high activity level as for their availability are α- and β-carotene, and including xanthophyll carotenoid, β-cryptoxanthin, and apocarotenoids (Hornero-Mendez & Minguenz-Mosquera, 2000). Of these, β-carotene has the greatest provitamin A activity since each molecule of pigment produces two of retinal, which is then reduced to vitamin A (retinol).

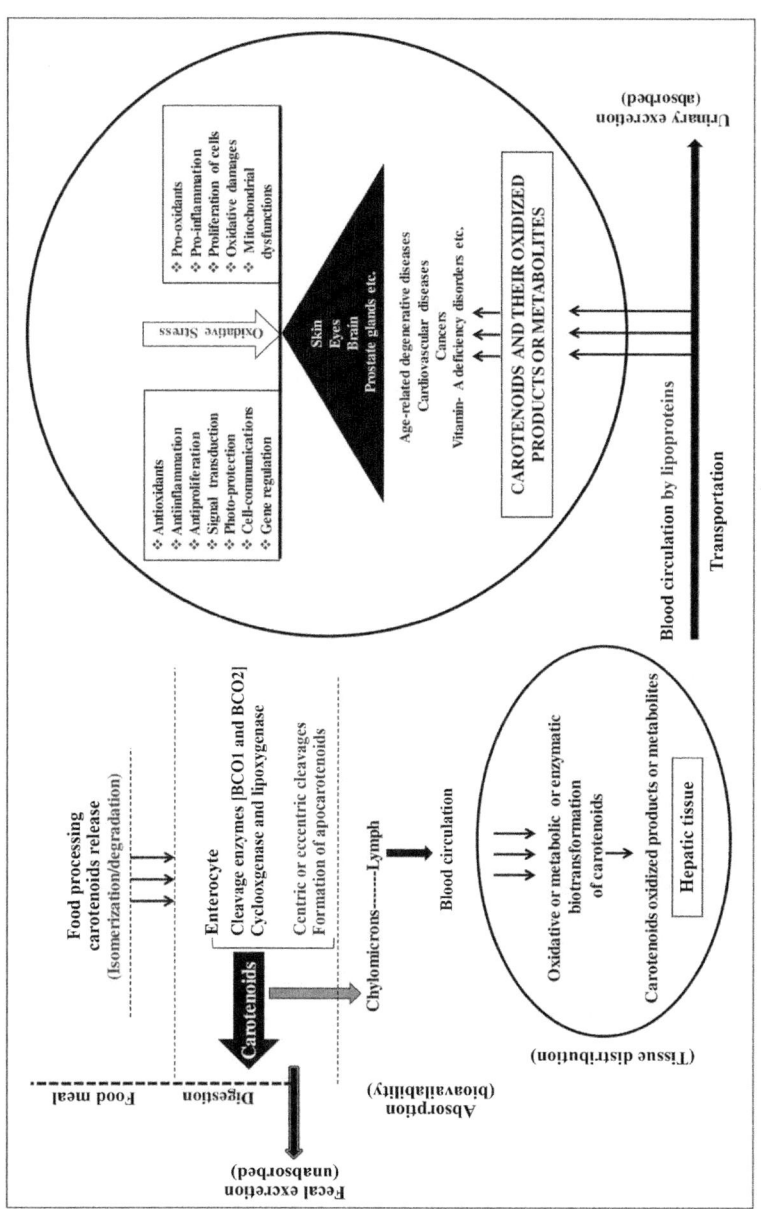

Fig. 2 Overview of bioavailability and bioefficacy of carotenoids.

In 1967, the World Health Organization (WHO) defined the term bioefficiency as "the fraction of ingested carotenoids with provitamin A activity that is absorbed and converted to its active form retinol." Estimating the bioefficacy of carotenoids from a diet is one-third of that of retinol and recognizing that the equivalence between β-carotene and retinol is 2:1, a ratio value of 6 was introduced to calculate the efficacy of β-carotene and 12 for other carotenoids with retinol equivalence. However, it was recognized that these ratios could overestimate or underestimate the bioavailability when considering other factors that alter the bioavailability efficiency, such as carotenoid content in the food, type of food, degree of processing, and so on. Van het Hof, Tiijburg, Pietrzik, and Weststrate (1999) conducted the study with stable isotopes and confirmed the fact behind overestimation of bioavailability efficiency, which is a more crucial factor than the conversion to retinol. Further, they demonstrated that the efficiency of dietary β-carotene absorption corresponding to β-carotene administration in oil. The Institute of Medicine of the National Academy of Sciences (USA) report from 2001 reduced the ratios to 12 for β-carotene and 24 for other carotenoids with retinol equivalence (Scott & Rodriguez-Amaya, 2000). The abovementioned change in ratios between β-carotene and carotenoids with provitamin A activity obtained from the consumption of fruits and vegetables prompted by bioavailability studies. These dietary trials indicate that the amount of intake of food that is required to meet the daily vitamin A requirement is higher than established previously (Thurnham, 2007).

Assessment of carotenoid bioavailability by isotopes labeling

Approaches using stable isotopes, coupled with mass spectral analysis of the carotenoid and its metabolites isolated from the postprandial triglyceride-rich lipoprotein plasma fraction are the most promising method in terms of accurate measurement of carotenoid absorption (Lin, Dueker, Burri, Neidlinger, & Clifford, 2000; Novotny, Dueker, Zech, & Clifford, 1995; Tang, Qin, Doinikowski, & Russell, 2000; Yao, Liang, Trahanovsky, Serfass, & White, 2000). Though such methods are great promising in assessing carotenoid bioavailability and bioefficacy from different food sources in humans (Van Lieshout et al., 2003), but they do not provide mechanistic information about the carotenoid absorption process itself. De Moura, Ho, Getachew, Hickenbottom, and Clifford (2005) reveal that the highest lutein level labeled with ^{14}C appeared in 1 h after dosing of ^{14}C-lutein (125 nmol, 36 nCi ^{14}C) in adult woman. Further, they documented that 45% and 10% of the ^{14}C was eliminated in feces and urine in the first 2 d after dosing, respectively. Lienau et al. (2003) determined relative bioavailability of lutein from food in humans by stable isotope method. The study subjects were administered a dose of deuterium-labeled carotenoids from intrinsically labeled spinach or collard green. The serum level of labeled lutein was measured at various time points and calculated its enrichment. Furthermore, they also predicted the subjects yielded serum lutein responses of dietary supplements, following an acute dose of spinach. These techniques show the efficacy of carotenoids bioavailability from different foods of diverse composition and following various methods of food preparation procedures.

Effect of dietary and nondietary factors affecting bioaccessibility, bioavailability, and bioefficacy of carotenoids

As mentioned earlier, carotenoid is an important molecule obtained from dietary consumption since de novo not synthesized it (Van het Hof et al., 2000). Carotenoids concentration in human plasma and tissue depends on their dietary intake and bioavailability. It has been assumed that the lipophilic micronutrients such as fat-soluble vitamins, carotenoids, phytosterols, and other phytochemicals have the same metabolic process in the human's upper gastrointestinal tract and they follow the similar pathway as lipids (Tyssandier et al., 2003). Carotenoid bioaccessibility is limited and conditioned by different factors, mainly the degree of food processing and matrix composition (Deming & Erdman, 1999). The type and quantity of fat is a relevant factor that is required in minimum quantities to ensure bioaccessibility (Jalal, Nesheim, Agus, Sanjur, & Habicht, 1998; Van het Hof et al., 2000). The factors influencing carotenoid bioaccessibility and bioavailability can be categorized to carotenoid-related and unrelated groups. The carotenoid related includes dosage, chemical structure (isomeric forms), and interactions between different carotenoids, and the unrelated includes cooking, nutrient composition of co-consumed foods, particle size of digested foods, biometric of consumers, efficiency of micellarization, and transport from the enterocytes to the lymph system (Colle, Lemmens, Knockaert, Van Loey, & Hendrickx, 2016; de Pee et al., 1998; Donhowe & Kong, 2014; Lemmens et al., 2014; Reboul, 2013). Bioavailability depends on several dietary and non-dietary factors including the level and origin of dietary fat, the amount and type or mixture of carotenoids, the digestibility of food, the presence of antioxidants or fibers, as well as vitamin A status (Erdman et al., 1993). The factors that influence the bioavailability of carotenoids are often summarized in the mnemonic 'SLAMENGHI,' which means 'S'pecies of carotenoid, molecular 'L'inkage, 'A'mount consumed in a meal, 'M'atrix in which the carotenoid is incorporated, 'E'ffectors of absorption and bioconversion, 'N'utrient status of the host, 'G'enetic factors, 'H'ost-related factors, and 'I'nteractions (Borel, 2003; Castenmiller & West, 1998; de Pee & West, 1996; Van den Berg et al., 2000). The mechanism of intestinal absorption of carotenoids from emulsion lipid droplets to mixed micelles is governed by the carotenoid type, their hydrophobicity, pH of emulsion, and bile lipid concentration (Borel et al., 1996; Tyssandier, Lyan, & Borel, 2001). Also absorption of dietary carotenoids is influenced by the amount ingested, the physicochemical properties of the carotenoid, its subcellular location in the plant tissue that constitutes the food, the method of food preparation, and the chemical composition of the meal may affect bioavailability.

Garrett, Failla, and Sarama (1999) studied the bioavailability of dietary β-carotene, lutein, lycopene, and their aqueous fraction of digesta and determined the quantity of carotenoids transferred from the food to micellar fractions. They found that micellization of lutein was higher than that of β-carotene and lycopene. Although lutein and β-carotene share a common lipophilic characteristic, their structural variation affects the process of absorption (Borel et al., 1996; Gartner, Stahl, & Sies, 1996). In the three main stages of carotenoid absorption (release from the food matrix, incorporation into mixed micelles, and intestinal uptake by mucosa), the higher polarity of lutein seems to have advantage in the mass transfer processes. The main reason is that polar carotenoids are distributed at the surface of emulsions, whereas carotenes are located in the hydrophobic core. Thus, the former can transfer directly from emulsions to mixed micelles. Van het Hof et al. (1999) and Erdman (1999) reported that the bioavailability of β-carotene and lutein vary substantially among vegetables, and found relative bioavailability of lutein from vegetables is higher than that of β-carotene. Riso, Brusamolino, Ciappellano, and Porrini (2016) observed that the ingestion of spinach or broccoli increased the levels of lutein in serum. Van den Berg and van Vliet (1998) revealed that lutein negatively affected the β-carotene absorption when given simultaneously, but lycopene had no effect. The bioavailability of carotenoids from food sources was reported to be different, and it is dependent on its nature (whole food or supplement), state of the food (raw, cooked or processed), and extent of destruction of the cellular matrix via mastication and digestive enzymes. Therefore, food processing is the most important facilitator of carotenoid bioavailability. Food processing (e.g., cooking in the presence of oil) has been reported to affect the bioavailability of carotenoids for absorption. While Rodriguez-Amaya and Kimura (2004) reported that different cooking processes lowered the lutein content dramatically, which decreased its bioavailability. Carotenoids absorption from a green vegetable varies with different degrees of processing, and the absorption of lutein is lower from chopped spinach than from whole-leaf spinach. Increased carotenoids absorption correlated to slower gastrointestinal transit for the whole-leaf meal (Faulks, Hart, Brett, Dainty, & Southon, 2004). Castenmiller et al. (1999) showed that enzymatic disruption of cell wall structure of spinach enhanced the plasma β-carotene level, but the level of lutein was not affected in vitro. Mechanical homogenization or heat treatment resulted in higher plasma response for lutein from chopped versus whole-leaf spinach (van het Hof et al. 1999). Heat treatment of carotenoid-containing foods converts some of the dominant *all-trans* carotenoids to a *cis*-form. Although *cis*-isomers are apparently better incorporated into the mixed micelles than the *all-trans* form, there is no evidence of higher absorption of *cis*-isomers in rodents (Levin & Mokady, 1994). Tanumihardjo, Li, and Dosti (2005) reported that lutein is absorbed faster when supplemented with vitamin C than E.

Lutein was absorbed more efficiently than β-carotene when administered in oil to human subjects (Castenmiller et al., 1999; Van het Hof et al., 1999). β-Carotene bioavailability has been reported to be influenced by the food matrix (Castenmiller et al., 1999; Micozzi et al., 1992). These observations suggest that carotenoid bioavailability is affected by both chemical speciation and food matrix. However, interpretation is confounded by a lack of information about the extent of β-carotene conversion, potential interactions between carotenoids during digestion and uptake and transport across the mucosal epithelium, and the rates of plasma clearance for individual carotenoids. Moderate cooking, mashing, and juicing destroys plant tissue structure thereby increasing surface area and interactions of hydrolytic enzymes and emulsifiers with food particles in gastric and small intestinal region during digestion (Edwards et al., 2002; Livny et al., 2003). Processing may also induce conversion of all-*trans* isomers of some carotenoids to *cis*-isomers.

Dietary fat and carotenoids bioavailability

Dietary fat increases carotenoid bioavailability by providing a depot for hydrophobic compounds released from the food matrix, stimulating the secretion of bile salts and pancreatic lipases required for micelle formation, and inducing chylomicron synthesis (Borel, 2003). Approximately 5–10 g fat in a meal is required for efficient absorption of carotenoids. A greater amount of fat is required when the dietary source is lutein ester instead of free lutein (Roodenberg, Leenen, Van het Hof, Weststrate, & Tijburg, 2000). The type of fat may also affect carotenoid absorption. For example, absorption of carotenoids (lycopene and astaxanthin) was more efficient when administered to rats with olive oil than in corn oil (Clark, Yao, & Furr, 2000). Among various dietary factors, fat is an important factor facilitate the solubilization and transfer of carotenoids from food matrix to tissues. In particular, fatty acids influence the formation of carotenoid-rich mixed micelles and also influence its physiochemical properties. The fatty acid composition of emulsion droplets and their structure may influence the lipolysis and enhance the bioaccessibility of carotenoids at enterocyte level (Tyssandier et al., 2001). Similarly, the presence of unsaturated fatty acids, particularly oleic acid, modulates β-carotene absorption from the perfused rat intestine (Hollander & Ruble, 1978). Hu, Jandacek, and White (2000) reported that the efficiency of β-carotene absorption by human subjects increased when the meal was rich in sunflower oil compared with beef tallow. Raju, Lakshminarayana, Krishnakantha, and Baskaran (2006) reported the type of fatty acids in mixed micelles modulated the β-carotene uptake and its cleavage into retinol in rats. Dietary triacylglycerols with long-chain rather than medium-chain fatty acids enhanced the absorption of β-carotene and retinyl palmitate (Borel, Tyssandier, et al., 1998). The potential of phospholipids to affect carotenoid bioavailability is supported by the observation demonstrated that lysophosphatidylcholine stimulated carotenoid absorption in mice (Baskaran, Sugawara, & Nagao, 2003).

As mentioned elsewhere, normal absorption of carotenoids with "very low-fat" diet is due to the presence of endogenous lipid and cholesterol from biliary sources (Furr & Clark, 1997). Sugawara et al. (2001) and including our previous reports (Lakshminarayana, Raju, Krishnakantha, & Baskaran, 2006; Raju et al., 2006) have showed that specific phospholipids and fatty acids in the mixed micelles positively influence the intestinal absorption of carotenoids and its cleavage in human intestinal cells and rat models. Further, dietary study revealed that supplementation of green leafy vegetables with olive oil might enhance the intestinal accessibility of lutein, which is reflected in higher levels of lutein and zeaxanthin in plasma and eye samples of aged lutein deficient rats. The mechanism by which dietary olive oil influences the intestinal uptake of lutein is may be due to its oleic acid content, which facilitates the incorporation and formation of lutein solubilized mixed micelles (Lakshminarayana, Raju, Keshava Prakash, & Baskaran, 2009). Chemical composition and properties of vegetable oils may act differently at various stages of absorption and metabolism of carotenoids. Also, we have shown that higher levels of dietary unsaturated fat as carrier for lutein may be avoided if oxidative stress is a critical issue in nutrition-related degenerative diseases. The relative bioavailability of lutein could be improved either by single, repeated, and dietary feeding with oleic acid micelles or dispersed in olive oil that in turn may help in modulating the activity of antioxidant molecules when compared to linoleic acid micelles or dispersed in sunflower oil (Lakshminarayana et al., 2009).

Brown et al. (2004) reveals that the level of carotenoids in chylomicrons increased with the ingestion of salads dressing with fat as compared to salads without fat. Deming, Boileau, Lee, and Erdman (2000) observed the effects of dietary fat level and fiber type on β-carotene bioavailability. Further, they suggested that an increasing dietary fat resulted higher vitamin A level and lower accumulation of β-carotene in the liver. Dietary lutein and zeaxanthin are esterified with fatty acids either before or after absorption. Esterification decreases their polarity in comparison with that of the corresponding free form. Thus, the distribution of xanthophyll esters in lipid emulsions normally concentrated in the core, not at the surface, which impairs their diffusion into micelles or binding with lipoproteins, increasing the requirements of bile salts and intestinal enzymes to digest the triacylglycerol bulk (Hollander & Ruble, 1978). Moreover, as no carotene esters have been detected in plasma and peripheral tissues, they must be hydrolyzed, implying a new stage before absorption. Khachik et al. (1992) reported that the xanthophyll esters would be hydrolyzed in the gut before absorption. Experimental data on the absorption of esters in humans were reported by Wingerath, Stahl, and Sies (1995) and Herbst et al. (1997). Thus, they assumed that the esters were equally absorbed like free lutein and suggested that hydrolysis of esters is essential. This could be rectified with an adequate intake of dietary fat that has been established as a factor affects the intestinal absorption of carotenoids (Baskaran et al., 2003). Apart from these, other also indicated that addition of scraped coconut milk significantly improved the β-carotene bioaccessibility from carrot. Also, Noakes et al. (2002) demonstrated that spreading of sterol or stanol esters with high-carotenoid vegetable or fruit maintains carotenoids concentrations while reducing LDL-cholesterol concentration in plasma. Roodenberg et al. (2000) compared the absorption of lutein esters with a low-fat and high-fat spreads. The response was significantly higher in the case of high-fat spread, with an increase in lutein levels than the low-fat spread, but the increase with respect to the control subjects was lower. Contrarily, Bowen, Herbst-Espinosa, Hussain, and Stacewicz-Sapuntzakis (2002) have shown that bioavailability of the lutein ester supplement was higher than that of free lutein. In case of xanthophyll esters, they decrease the polarity and accumulated on the core rather than the surface, thus limiting their transfer into bile salt micelles (Perez-Galvez, Marti, Sies, & Stahl, 2003). Breithaupt and Bamedi (2002) reported that xanthophyll esters as substrates for typical lipases from human pancreas. Chitchumroonchokchai and Failla (2005) suggested that dietary zeaxanthin esters are hydrolyzed to free form of zeaxanthin in the small intestine by carboxyl ester lipase and intestinal epithelial cells preferentially absorb free zeaxanthin. The above studies suggest that dietary carotenoids esters are hydrolyzed during intestinal phase of digestion and absorption. This selective absorption could be established in some pathway of enzymatic hydrolysis or based on physicochemical properties of the interface of mixed micelles.

Though implication of dietary fat on bioaccessibility of carotenoid is demonstrated from the last three decades, nevertheless the quantity and type of the dietary fat required for optimal bioavailability of carotenoids is still under standardization.

Castenmiller and West (1998) suggested that essentially a minimum quantity of fat (~5 g/day) is required for optimum carotenoid absorption. Ribaya-Mercado, Solon, and Solon (2000) revealed that the serum retinol or β-carotene response vs. carotenes supplements with different amounts of fat. Further, they suggested that minimal quantity of fat, 5 g in a meal rich with carotenoids diet is recommended for maximum absorption from the supplements. Drammeh et al. (2002) results support the use of dietary supplementation with dried mangoes and a source of fat as one of several concurrent strategies that can be used to help maintain vitamin A status of children in developing countries where there is a severe seasonal shortage of carotenoid-rich foods. Mutsokoti et al. (2017) investigated by a kinetic approach of release of free fatty acids and monoacylglycerides from triacylglyceride proceeded faster than their incorporation into micelles. Salvia-Trujillo and McClements (2016) study highlights the potential of using nanoemulsions to modulate lipid digestion which indicates possible interactions between food components and lipid digestion products during the formation of mixed micelles and its implications on the bioaccessibility of lipophilic bioactives such as carotenoids. Various fats and oils and long-chain triacylglycerols enhanced the bioaccessibility of β-carotene present in spinach, but not of lutein and α-tocopherol, which are less hydrophobic than β-carotene. Free fatty acid, monoacylglycerol, and diacylglycerol also enhanced the bioaccessibility of β-carotene present in spinach (Nagao, Kotake-Nara, & Hase, 2013). Excipient emulsions containing mainly medium-chain triacylglycerols and coconut oils had faster initial lipid digestion rates, higher overall digestibility, smaller mixed micelle sizes, and higher lutein bioaccessibilities than those containing mainly long-chain triacylglycerols (corn, olive, and fish oils) (Yuan, Liu, McClements, Cao, & Xiao, 2018). Zhang et al. (2016) also concluded that excipient emulsions are highly effective at increasing carotenoid bioaccessibility from carrots, which can be attributed to the ability of the small lipid droplets to rapidly solubilize the carotenoids. Liu, Shao, Zhang, & Wang, 2015 results facilitated the rational design of excipient emulsions that boost the bioavailability of phytochemicals in fruits and vegetables. The influence of oil type (medium-chain triglycerides, MCT; long chain triglycerides, LCT; and, indigestible orange oil, OO) on microstructural changes, particle properties, lipid digestibility, and carotenoid bioaccessibility was investigated. Oil type had a major impact, with carotenoid bioaccessibility decreasing in the following order: LCT > MCT > OO > control (no oil). Conversely, thermal treatment (raw versus boiled) had little influence on carotenoid bioaccessibility.

Interaction of carotenoids

The interaction between carotenoids is likely to occur at various stages of the absorption process, that is, during micellar incorporation, transport to different organs, or within tissues after absorption. Competition between carotenoids for micellar incorporation in the gastrointestinal tract has been possibly occurs at higher dose. Food containing mixture of carotenoids affects their intestinal absorption depending on the type and the level of each carotenoid. Micozzi et al. (1992) observed that lowered serum response of lutein after a 6-week period of β-carotene supplementation.

In another study with human subjects, lutein impaired β-carotene absorption, but did not affect the secretion of retinyl esters in chylomicrons (Van den Berg & van Vliet, 1998).

Also, they studied the interaction between carotenoids and compared their retinyl palmitate response in triglycerol-rich lipoprotein fraction of men given a single dose of β-carotene (15 mg) with that of 15 mg β-carotene plus 15 mg lycopene or 15 mg lutein. Data on the intestinal absorption of carotenoids other than β-carotene are limited, it seems that polar carotenoids especially xanthophylls are absorbed better than carotenes. To support the hypothesis, Kostic et al. (1995) reported that an interaction between lutein and β-carotene on intestinal absorption and serum clearance after oral administration of single equimolar doses of lutein and/or β-carotene with oil in adult human subjects. Further, they reported that the plasma response of lutein was double as compare to β-carotene. Gartner et al. (1996) suggested that the lutein and zeaxanthin were increased in chylomicron compared to that of β-carotene after ingestion of a carotenoid mixture. Raju and Baskaran (2009) reported that lutein did not affect the intestinal uptake of β-carotene in rats. In addition, the relative bioavailability of lutein from vegetables was reported to be five times higher than that of β-carotene (Van het Hof et al., 1999), but in the same study the plasma response of lutein was substantially lower than that of β-carotene after simultaneous ingestion of pure lutein and β-carotene. Tyssandier et al. (2003) reported that the absorption of β-carotene, lutein and lycopene from a single vegetable was greater when the food was administered alone than when it was co-administered with either a second carotenoid-rich vegetable or the purified carotenoid from the second vegetable. Van den Berg (1999) demonstrated the possibility of preabsorptive interactions between carotenoids include their competition for incorporation into micelles, uptake by intestinal cells, competitive binding to β-carotene 15,15′-monooxygenase, and incorporation into chylomicrons.

Dietary fiber and carotenoids bioavailability

The water soluble fibers such as pectin, guar gum, and alginate decrease the absorption of carotenoids (Riedl, Linseisen, & Hoffmann, 1999). Possible mechanism responsible for the fiber-mediated decrease in carotenoid bioavailability include decreased micellarization due to binding of bile acids and phospholipids, inhibition of lipase activity, increased viscosity and volume of luminal contents, and increased rate of transit of enterocytes (Riedl et al., 1999). Pasquier et al. (1996) have reported that soluble dietary fibers could alter the process of intra-gastric lipid emulsification and subsequent triacylglycerol lipolysis. It has been reported that the concentration of viscous fibers increases the size of the emulsified droplets. Further Serrano, Isabel, and Saura-Calixto (2005) demonstrated that the droplet size and its surface area were strongly correlated the viscosity of medium containing lignin and enzymatic release of carotenoids. Rock and Swendseid (1992) reported that dietary pectin had a negative effect on plasma β-carotene response after a single dose of purified β-carotene administered with a meal. Viscous polysaccharides, such as pectin reported to delay gastric emptying and interfere with micelle formation, whereas gastric emptying is delayed in human subjects by the addition of 15 g pectin to a meal (Di Lorenzo, Williams, Hajnal, & Valenzuela, 1988). Rock and Swendseid (1992) noted that presence of pectin reduced plasma β-carotene concentration by 42% as compared to control group in humans. Further, they hypothesized and explained the two possible mechanisms, such as one effect occurs due to soluble fibers diminishing formation micelles by increasing fecal excretion of bile acids. Other role is due to interfere the contact between micelle and intestinal mucosal cells by enhancing viscosity of the gastrointestinal fluids (Van den Berg et al., 2000). Unlu, Bohn, Clinton, and Schwartz (2005) demonstrated that inhibitory effect of dietary fiber on the absorption of carotenoids, since avocado consists of good source of dietary fiber (6.8 g fiber/100 g edible portion), and comprises with 72% of insoluble fibers such as cellulose, pectin, and hemicelluloses. In contrast to these studies, Castenmiller et al. (1999) reported that there was no inhibition of carotenoid absorption when dietary fiber added to liquefied spinach. Apart from these, Mamatha and Baskaran (2011) reported that ingestion of lutein with pectin and β-carotene suppresses lutein absorption. Further, they suggested that diet containing appropriate fat like soya bean oil and phospholipid with less dietary fiber and β-carotene moderately monitor the lutein level in lutein deficient aged rats.

Dosage of carotenoids

To improve bioefficacy of food product or nutrient requires appropriate dosage. Determination of bioaccessibility and bioavailability of carotenoids/nutrients provide basic platform to select required dosage and source of food matrices to ensure nutritional efficacy. Also, adequate measurements of biofunctionality in vitro and in vivo models support health benefits of carotenoids may be accomplished with their bioaccessibility, to its nutritional significance. Food matrix determines intestinal absorption availability of carotenoids and effects bioaccessibility. Huo, Ferruzzi, Schwartz, and Failla (2007) reported that transfer of α-carotene, β-carotene, and lycopene from chyme to mixed micelles requires 0.5%–1% of lipid content in the meal, and is affected by type of fatty acids. Serum β-carotene concentration depends on the amount of β-carotene in the meal. Generally, less absorption was noted with the administration of higher doses (Castenmiller & West, 1998). Prince and Frisoli (1993) revealed that administration of β-carotene in three divided dietary doses/day raised the β-carotene in serum concentration threefold as compared with the same doses administered once a day. Further, they opinion that the prediction of an optimal dose of β-carotene is difficult. Van het Hof et al. (1999) observed that that there is a marked difference in the bioavailability of β-carotene and lutein vs. different leafy vegetables supplementation. Spinach contains higher fold of β-carotene as compared to other green vegetables (broccoli or green peas). However, dietary study confirms that plasma β-carotene levels were comparatively lower in spinach fed group than that of other green leafy vegetables supplementation. The reason may be due to difference in the phytochemical contents and their composition of natural source. Similarly, carotenoid content of fruits or vegetables is higher; the transferring of carotenoids into the micelles becomes lower. Spinach which had the highest content of lutein had the lowest (18.9%). O'Connell, Ryan, and O'Brien (2007) demonstrated that the highest content of lutein in spinach shown lowest bioaccessibility. Dimitrov et al. (1988) observed that the degree of increase of plasma β-carotene levels is extensively interindividual variation. Koch, Wilson, and Hill (2016) reported the importance of dosage fixation to elucidate the limited vs surplus carotenoids levels intake. Johnson, Qin, Krinsky, and Russell (1997) suggested that ingestion of a combined dose of β-carotene and lycopene has little effect on the absorption of β-carotene, but improves lycopene in men.

Influence of other phytoconstituents on carotenoid bioaccessibility, bioavailability, and bioefficacy

Co-consumption of other dietary phytoconstituents such as flavonoids, alkaloids, polyphenols, vitamins, and spice principles may also alter physicochemical properties of micelles, and affect carotenoid bioaccessibility, bioavailability, and bioefficacy. Nagao, Maeda, Lim, Kobayashi, and Terao (2000) have demonstrated the influence of dietary antioxidants and flavonoids on BCMO activity in pig intestinal homogenate. Butylated hydroxytoluene strongly inhibited the BCMO activity, whereas butylated hydroxyanisole, nordihydroguaiaretic acid, n-propyl gallate, and curcumin were moderately inhibited the conversion of retinol in intestinal cells. Flavonoids such as luteolin, quercetin, rhamnetin, and phloretin remarkably inhibited the BCMO activity noncompetitively. Further, they believed that some dietary flavonoids derived from food sources modulate conversion of β-carotene to vitamin A in intestinal cells. Claudie, Bertrand, Franck, and Marie-Josephe (2013) positively attributed that bioactivities of carotenoids depend on their bioavailability that could be enhanced by the presence of certain dietary constituents like polyphenols and vitamin C. Further, they suggested that hesperidin in the presence of iron restored the bioavailability as compared to only supplemented with iron. Others have also revealed that influence of four common food acidulants amchur, lime, tamarind, and kokum on increased bioaccessibility of β-carotene from the vegetable sources in rats (Veda, Platel, & Srinivasan, 2008). Likewise, they also reported that dietary spices alters ultrastructure and permeability characteristics of intestines in-turn enhanced carotenoids absorption in rats fed with dietary spices such as black pepper, red pepper, ginger, piperine, and capsaicin. Whereas, they found that the bioconversion of β-carotene to vitamin A, the activity of intestinal and hepatic β-carotene cleavage enzymes remain unaffected in spice treatments (Veda & Srinivasan, 2009, 2011).

Particle size

Several studies have been demonstrated that mechanical and chemical disruptions are important to improve bioaccessibility of carotenoids by decreasing particle size and increasing surface area available for the digestive enzymes to act efficiently, and release carotenoids from food matrix (Furr & Clark, 1997; Gartner et al., 1996; Hedren, Diaz, & Svanberg, 2002; Torronen, Lehmusaho, Hakkinen, Hanninen, & Mykkanen, 1996). Castenmiller et al. (1999) carried out the experiments and showed that higher bioavailability of β-carotene from liquefied spinach than that of the whole leaf or minced spinach consumption.

Moelants et al. (2012) predicted the carotenoid bioaccessibility in carrot and tomato derived purees. Further, they indicated that carotenoid bioaccessibility determined by the cell wall integrity (related with particle size). Gence, Servent, Poucheret, Hiol, and Dhuique-Mayer (2018) reported that pectin structure and particle size modify carotenoid bioaccessibility from citrus juices vs. concentration. Zhang et al. (2016) demonstrated that influence of particle size of digestible lipid droplets on carotenoid bioaccessibility from carrots using excipient emulsions. In addition, they also discussed positive implications of designing excipient foods, such as dressings, dips, creams, and sauces.

Physiological factors: Gut health

The absorption of dietary carotenoids is also modulated by phenotypic characteristics of the host that affect processes associated with digestive and absorptive events. Typically composition and activity of luminal fluids, morphological and functional integrity of the absorptive epithelium also affects the bioavailability of carotenoid. Plasma response to a single dose of β-carotene was significantly lower in subjects administered omeprazole to increase gastric pH to the neutral range as compared with gastric pH acidic (Tang et al., 1996). Also, cholestasis, pancreatic inefficiency, biliary cirrhosis, cystic fibrosis, and other syndromes may be responsible for fat malabsorption which in turn decrease carotenoid bioavailability and induce VAD, especially in children (Olson, 1999). Apart from these, intestinal parasites can impair carotenoid metabolism, absorption, and utilization of β-carotene enhanced after de-worming in children infected with *Ascaris lumbricoides* (Jalal et al., 1998). In contrast, plasma retinol concentrations in helminth-infected preschool children fed a stew with dark green cassava and kapok supplemented with fat and β-carotene was not further elevated by administration of antihelminthics (Takyi, 1999).

Goni, Serrano, and Saura-Calixto (2006) revealed that during complete digestion process, 91% of α-carotene, lutein, and lycopene were bioaccessible from the dietary fruits and vegetables. Bioaccessibility of carotenoids may vary between small intestine and large intestine with respect to enzymatic digestion and colonic fermentation. Henceforth, in case of small intestine, bioaccessibility of lutein > lycopene > α-carotene found to be 79%, 40%, and 29%, whereas in large intestine, similar amount of lycopene and α-carotene (57%) and 17% of lutein were released from food matrix, respectively.

Nutritional status

Nutritional status of the host can affect the bioavailability of carotenoids. The plasma vitamin A response following the administration of β-carotene in protein deficient rats found to be decreased as compared to control rats (Parvin & Sivakumar, 2000). Further, they suggested that this suppression is due to a decline in the activity of β-carotene 15,15'-monooxygenase. Because of the central role of retinoic acid in cellular differentiation, VAD compromises the integrity of epithelial barriers. Mild

VAD reduced the number of duodenal goblet cells per villus and luminal mucus and decreased cellular division in the crypts of intestinal villi (McCullough, Northrop-Clewes, & Thurnham, 1999). Gastrointestinal integrity, assessed by the dual-sugar gastrointestinal permeability test, was markedly improved when retinol-deficient children in Gambian and India ingested β-carotene-rich mango and received vitamin A supplementation, respectively (Thurnham, Northrop-Clewes, McCullough, Das, & Lunn, 2000). Studies have reported a decreased uptake of micellar β-carotene by brush border membrane vesicles isolated from retinol deficient Mongolian gerbils and rats compared with membrane preparations from animals fed vitamin A adequate diet (Boileau, Lee, & Erdman, 2000; Moore, Gugger, & Erdman, 1996). It is unknown if the differences were due to immaturity of plasma membranes from donor cells or due to other biochemical alterations associated with dietary inadequacy. Decreased uptake of micellar β-carotene across the brush border membrane may offset the greater activity of β-carotene 15,15′-monooxygenase associated with VAD. Also, activity of this enzyme in the soluble fraction of homogenized intestinal mucosa was positively correlated with the iron content of the tissue prepared from rats fed diets with different quantities of the trace metal (During, Fields, Lewis, & Smith, 2000). Kana-Sop et al. (2015) evaluated the influence of zinc, iron, and their combination on bioavailability of provitamin A carotenoid in humans. Zinc and iron + zinc supplements monitored the optimal intact appearance of α-carotene, β-carotene, and β-cryptoxanthin. However, supplementation of iron showed greatest bioavailability of provitamin A carotenoids from papaya and its conversion to retinol. Further, Dijkhuizen, Wieringa, and West (2004) revealed that zinc plus β-carotene supplementation improves the vitamin A status as compared with the only β-carotene supplementation in mother and infants. Whereas, Corte-Real et al. (2018) investigated that magnesium reduce the carotenoid bioaccessibility by forming insoluble complexes with bile salt/fatty acids and inhibiting micelles formation.

Karin et al. (1999) investigated the disruption of the vegetable matrix would enhance the bioavailability and bioefficacy of micronutrients. Bioavailability of β-carotene and lutein vary substantially among different vegetables. Whereas, bioavailability of lutein, folate, and vitamin C from spinach improved by disruption of the vegetable matrix.

Genotype

Recent studies with tracer isotope techniques have confirmed emarked variability in the absorption of β-carotene by human subjects (Hickenbottom et al., 2002; Lin et al., 2000). Moreover, plasma β-carotene and retinol were not predictive for the absorption or conversion of β-carotene. These differences in absorption efficiency originally resulted in the classification of individuals as "responders," "low responders," and "nonresponders." Explanations for the observed variation among healthy subjects tested under well-controlled conditions have included differences in the rate of cleavage of β-carotene to retinal, the efficiency of incorporation of the carotenoid into chylomicrons and the rate and extent of clearance from circulation

(Borel, 2003). Lin et al. (2000) also suggested that differences in the ability to transfer the carotenoid from a complex matrix to the absorptive cell might be the basis for the reported variability, because all individuals were "responders" when administered high doses of β-carotene in oil (Borel, Grolier, et al., 1998). Genetic factors are also likely to affect the efficiency of carotenoid absorption and conversion. Polymorphisms in genes whose products are required for the many reactions affecting the transfer of carotenoids from food matrix to micelles during digestion, assembly and secretion of chylomicrons and the kinetics of postabsorptive delivery of carotenoids and retinoids to tissues may contribute to the observed variations in the absorption and conversion efficiency of provitamin A carotenoids by individuals.

Chemical speciation, food matrix, and location of carotenoids in the plant tissue

Absorption of dietary carotenoids is influenced by numerous factors in addition to the amount ingested. The physicochemical properties of the carotenoid of interest, its subcellular location in the plant tissue that constitutes the food, the method of food preparation, and the chemical composition of the meal may affect its bioavailability. Lutein was absorbed more efficiently than β-carotene when administered in oil to human subjects (Castenmiller et al., 1999; Van het Hof et al., 1999). β-Carotene bioavailability has been reported to be influenced by the food matrix, with absorption from carrots > broccoli > spinach (Castenmiller et al., 1999; Micozzi et al., 1992). These observations suggest that carotenoid bioavailability is affected by both chemical speciation and food matrix. However, interpretation is confounded by a lack of information about the extent of β-carotene conversion, potential interactions between carotenoids during digestion and uptake and transport across the mucosal epithelium and the rates of plasma clearance for individual carotenoids. Food processing methods like, moderate cooking, mashing, and juicing destroys plant tissue structure thereby increasing surface area and interactions of hydrolytic enzymes and emulsifiers with food particles during the gastric and small intestinal phases of digestion, which increases the carotenoid bioavailability (Edwards et al., 2002; Livny et al., 2003). Carotenoids occur in natural sources that exist in various forms within cell. They are located in chromoplasts, and that they either dissolved in oil droplets (e.g., pumpkin) or crystalline form (e.g., carrot and tomato). In this case, carotenoids can be more bioaccessible from fruits or vegetables as compared to green leafy vegetables, where they are complexes with proteins and chloroplast (Castenmiller & West, 1998; de Pee, West, Hautvast, & Karyadi, 1995). The population study suggested that an additional daily intake of dark-green leafy vegetables found no improvement in vitamin A status. However, a similar quantity of β-carotene from a simpler matrix showed the improvement of vitamin A status. Also, others have revealed the lutein bioavailability in healthy men administered with lutein supplement, lutein ester supplement (lutein equivalent), and spinach with lutein-enriched egg supplement separately. The results indicated that serum lutein level was significantly increased with the consumption of egg than that of lutein supplements. This difference is due to the presence of digestible lipid matrix consists of cholesterol, triglycerides, and phospholipids in the egg yolk (Chung, Rasmussen, & Johnson, 2004). O'Connell et al. (2007) suggested that transferring of xanthophylls to the micelles and their intestinal uptake from fruits was greater than green leafy vegetables.

Carotenoids speciation and isomeric form

Carotenoid-type species

Carotenoids transfer from emulsified lipid droplets to micelles is dependent on lipophilicity. Polar carotenoids (xanthophylls) are more easily absorbed than less polar carotenoids (lycopene and β-carotene) as they are incorporated into the outer surface of the lipid droplets. As a result, polar carotenoids easily transfer into mixed micelles (Borel et al., 1996; Tyssandier et al., 2001, 2002). Chitchumroonchokchai, Schwartz, and Failla (2004) in an in vitro study showed that micellarization of lutein and zeaxanthin in Caco-2 human intestinal cells exceeded that of β-carotene. Khachik et al. (1992) have shown that epoxy carotenoids (neoxanthin, violaxanthin, lutein epoxide, and carotenol fatty acid esters) are missing in the nonpolar solvent extractions from human plasma even their concentrations are high in the supplemented diets. Further, they presumed that absorption and metabolism of epoxy carotenoids are different from the other hydroxyl and hydrocarbon carotenoids. The parent compounds of carotenoid esters have been found in the plasma and prediction was made that they undergo enzymatic hydrolysis. Asai, Terasaki, and Nagao (2004) characterized the conversion of stereoisomers (R/S) of neochrome from the dietary neoxanthin by intragastric acidity before absorption. The bioavailability of hydroxyl carotenoid lutein is 5 times greater than that of β-carotene (Van het Hof et al., 1999).

Isomeric form

The plasma response all-*trans*-β-carotene was shown to be absorbed preferentially with a higher amount incorporated into chylomicrons compared to 9-*cis*-β-carotene (Gaziano et al., 1995; Stahl, Schwarz, von Laar, & Sies, 1995). Nevertheless, lycopene from tomato juice showed *cis*-isomers was better absorbed than all-*trans* form (Stahl & Sies, 1992). The promising reason may be due to higher solubility of cis-isomers from lycopene (Boileau, Boileau, & Erdman, 2002). In plant foods, ~90% of lycopene occurs as all-trans isomer form; however, research evidences demonstrated that cis-isomers are the major type in human tissue. Deming, Baker, and Erdman (2002) concluded that the value of isomeric form of β-carotene such as 9-*cis* and 13-*cis* isomeric forms have lower vitamin A biopotencies than all-*trans*-β-carotene. Furthermore, they discussed the lower value could be due to destruction or slower absorption in the intestine.

Overview of bioaccessibility and bioavailability of carotenoids from carotenoid-rich fruits and vegetables

The ranking of food sources may be decided based on enrichment of vital nutri-ents/phytochemicals and their relative bioavailability. The bioaccessibility and bioavailability of carotenoids from each dietary source are considered to be very important to monitor adequate level of nutrient. Carotenoid-rich sources, majorly fruits and green vegetables comprise the phytocomponents, including nutrition and anti-nutrition factors. The profiling of these phytocomponents in respective diet and their accurate assessment gives more precise information on the determination of carotenoids bioavailability. Further, mode of consumption as either raw or pro-cessed food or chopped or whole leaf/grains/fruits also plays a role on extent of carotenoids/nutrients absorption at intestinal levels (Carbonell-Capella, Buniowska, Barba, Esteve, & Frigola, 2014; Palafox Carlos, Ayala Zavala, & Gonzalez Aguilar, 2011). Since, bioavailability of carotenoids from green vegetables is generally very low, due to the interference of food matrices including complexes with protein and lipids, dietary fibers and cellulose. Therefore, the bioavailability of carotenoids from fruits and their forms of consumption is adequate to improve their level in tissue. Further, overcoming with these possibilities necessitates the understanding of the native food matrix and its effect on digestibility and phytochemical (carotenoids) intestinal accessibility.

Studies have demonstrated that plasma carotenoids are biomarkers of intake of fruits and vegetables and associated with lower risk of CVD, cancer and age-related eye diseases (Al-Delaimy et al., 2005; Moeller et al., 2008; Sommerburg, Keunen, Bird, & van Kuijk, 1998). The chemistry of food matrix, dietary fats, or oils or carotenoids esters may greatly exert absorption and metabolism of carotenoids. Bioavailability of vitamins and other food components from fruits and green veg-etables has significantly increased interest for different reasons, like existence of malnourished populations worldwide with micronutrient deficiencies. Also the ep-idemiological and clinical trials positively correlate the health beneficial aspects of carotenoids supplementation on the reduction of chronic diseases. Development of such carotenoids-rich traits is necessary to address the potential impact on pub-lic health nutritional status. Generally, green leafy vegetables and fruits consists of lycopene, β-carotene, β-cryptoxanthin, zeaxanthin, lutein, violaxanthin, and neoxanthin, whereas, fruits contains xanthophyll's ester. In certain fruits such as mango, papaya, orange, etc., carotenoids are found in oil droplets in the chloroplast and esterified with fatty acids that make them liberated easily during digestion. In addition, intestinal absorption of carotenoids is also affected due to competition among co-consumed carotenoids, food matrix, cooking, and processing methods (Lemke et al., 2003). Stahl and Sies (1992) demonstrated that dietary intake of heated tomato juice increases lycopene level in serum as compared to consump-tion of same quantity without heated samples. de Pee et al. (1998) demonstrated that higher bioavailability β-carotene when diet with high fruits than vegetable-supplemented groups in vitamin A deficient population. This difference may be due to carotenoids in dark green leafy vegetables that are bound with chloroplasts to protein and fiber, whereas in fruit, carotenoids are accumulated in chromoplasts dissolved in oil droplets. Similarly, Ornelas-Paz, Yahia, and Gardea-Bejar (2007) compared the in vitro bioaccessibility of carotene and xanthophyll carotenoids in different fruits and vegetables and reported better transfer of carotenoids to the micelles from fruits, In addition, they have shown highly bioaccessible lutein, zeaxanthin, and β-cryptoxanthin from fruits, (50%–100%) compared to dark green vegetables (19%–38%), respectively.

The differences in bioaccessibility between the fruits and vegetables indicate that certain carotenoids are potentially more available from fruit for absorption. Edwards et al. (2003) shown consumption of water melon juice and canned tomato fruit juice increases plasma concentrations of lycopene and β-carotene in humans. Further, they observed that fresh-frozen watermelon juice favors the intestinal uptake of lycopene than from canned tomato juice. Unlu et al. (2005) suggested that carotenoid bioavailability from salad and salsa by humans was enhanced by the inclusion of avocado fruit or avocado oil in humans (Fernandez-Garcia et al., 2012). Therefore, formulation of fruit carotenoids in an oily matrix expected to enhance the higher bioaccessibility of carotenoids. An interesting study on carotenoid bioaccessibility was demonstrated using carotenoid-rich fruits and vegetables. These sources of carotenoids have a different chromoplast morphology, and may influence the release of carotenoids from the food matrix. In fruits like mango and papaya, xanthophylls and their esters accumulate as liquid crystalline and lipid dissolved state in globular-tubular substructures of the chromoplasts. Carotenes (β-carotene and lycopene) are localized in crystalloid structures in chromoplasts of carrots, tomato, and papaya. Recently, Aschoff et al. (2015) studied and compared the effect of differently processed oranges (freshly squeezed, flash-pasteurized, and pasteurized juices) and orange juices on bioaccessibility in vitro.

During intestinal uptake, xanthophyll esters are hydrolyzed by carboxyl ester lipase before entering into enterocytes, this process resulting in an enhanced cellular uptake of xanthophyll's than from dark leafy vegetables and other vegetables. Administration of paprika oleoresin rich in xanthophylls esters in healthy volunteers was significantly increase the zeaxanthin, β-cryptoxanthin, and β-carotene levels in the chylomicrons fraction of plasma. However, none of them identified esterified form, even if administered with carotenoid-rich esters oleoresin (Perez-Galvez et al., 2003). The bioavailability of zeaxanthin di-palmitate from wolfberry increased plasma zeaxanthin concentration in a human supplementation trial (Cheng, Chung, Szeto, & Benzie, 2005). The increase in plasma concentration after supplementation with this fruits is important since zeaxanthin bioavailability from spinach or corn is low (Bone, Landrum, Dixon, Chen, & Llerena, 2000; Mozaffarieh, Sacu, & Wedrich, 2003). Chitchumroonchokchai and Failla (2006) and Granado-Lorencio et al. (2007) have reported that the addition of the enzyme cholesterol esterase may also be considered as necessary requirement for the hydrolysis of xanthophyll esters present in fruits. Overall bioavailability studies detailed that fruits are suitable source to enhance carotenoid bioavailability.

Conclusion

Carotenoids released from the food matrix are sequential, produced primarily by mastication, then by digestive enzymes, followed by emulsification and enzymatic activity at intestinal microbiota. The efficient release of carotenoids from food only occurs when the plant cell ruptured during food processing. Although certain nutrient in a food is potentially bioaccessible, however absorption of lipophilic carotenoids is very low and highly variable depends upon various dietary and physiological factors, and may be interindividual variation. The bioaccessibility of a nutrient is monitored by the physical properties of the food matrix, which primarily affect the efficiency of the physical and chemical digestion processes, though dietary fat, heat treatment, and reduced particle size shown the positive support. In contrast to these, interactions between carotenoids and dietary fiber have negative effect on bioaccessibility and bio-efficacy of carotenoids. Polarity and structural properties of carotenoids is crucial in the rate of transferring of carotenoids from emulsified lipid to micelles in gastrointestinal transit. Knowledge on carotenoids interaction with other dietary phytochemicals (flavonoids, phenolics, alkaloids, etc.), cleavage enzyme, and their regulatory mechanism during digestion process is yet to be explored in detail and understood. The modulation of intestinal uptake of carotenoids by specific dietary factors and understanding their metabolism could enable to formulate food-based approaches to combat with VAD, age, and other chronic diseases.

Acknowledgments

Authors acknowledge Indian council of medical research, Govt. of India, Grant reference number GIA/54/2014-DHR, Dt.29.12.2014. Authors also acknowledge the support of Department of Biotechnology, Jnana Bharathi Campus, Bangalore University.

References

Albanes, D., Virtamo, J., Talo, P. R., Rautalahti, M., Pietinen, P., & Heinonen, O. P. (1997). Effects of supplemental β-carotene, cigarette smoking and alcohol consumption on serum carotenoids in the α-tocopherol, β-carotene cancer prevention study. *The American Journal of Clinical Nutrition, 66*, 366–372.

Alberg, A. (2002). The influence of cigarette smoking on circulating concentrations of antioxidant micronutrients. *Toxicology, 180*, 121–137.

Al-Delaimy, W. K., Slimani, N., Ferrari, P., Key, T., Spencer, E., Johansson, I., et al. (2005). Plasma carotenoids as biomarkers of intake of fruits and vegetables: Ecological-level correlations in the European Prospective Investigation into Cancer and Nutrition (EPIC). *European Journal of Clinical Nutrition, 59*, 1397–1408.

Arathi, B. P., Sowmya, P. R., Vijay, K., Baskaran, V., & Lakshminarayana, R. (2016). Enhanced cytotoxic and apoptosis inducing activity of lycopene oxidation products in different cancer cell lines. *Food and Chemical Toxicology, 97*, 265–276.

Asai, A., Terasaki, M., & Nagao, A. (2004). An epoxide-furanoid rearrangement of spinach neoxanthin occurs in the gastrointestinal tract of mice and in vitro: Formation and cytostatic activity of neochrome stereoisomers. *The Journal of Nutrition*, *134*, 2237–2243.

Aschoff, J. K., Kaufmann, S., Kalkan, O., Neidhart, S., Carle, R., & Schweiggert, R. M. (2015). In vitro bioaccessibility of carotenoids, flavonoids, and vitamin C from differently processed oranges and orange juices [*Citrus sinensis* (L.) Osbeck]. *Journal of Agricultural and Food Chemistry*, *63*, 578–587.

Baskaran, V., Sugawara, T., & Nagao, A. (2003). Phospholipids affect the intestinal absorption of carotenoids in mice. *Lipids*, *38*, 705–711.

Boileau, A. C., Lee, C. M., & Erdman, J. W. (2000). Vitamin A deficiency reduces uptake of β-carotene by brush border membrane vesicles but does not alter intestinal retinyl ester hydrolase activity in the rat. *The Journal of Nutritional Biochemistry*, *11*, 436–442.

Boileau, T. W. M., Boileau, A. C., & Erdman, J. W. (2002). Bioavailability of all-trans and cis–Isomers of lycopene. *Experimental Biology and Medicine*, *227*, 914–919.

Bone, R. A., Landrum, J. T., Dixon, Z., Chen, Y., & Llerena, C. M. (2000). Lutein and zeaxanthin in the eyes, serum and diet of human subjects. *Experimental Eye Research*, *71*, 239–245.

Borek, P., Grolier, P., Mekki, N., Boiric, Y., Rochette, Y., Le Roy, B., et al. (1998). Low and high responders to pharmacological doses of β-carotene: Proportion in the population, mechanisms involved and consequences on β-carotene metabolism. *Journal of Lipid Research*, *39*, 2250–2260.

Borel, P. (2003). Factors affecting intestinal absorption of highly lipophilic food microconstituents (fat-soluble vitamins, carotenoids and phytosterols). *Clinical Chemistry and Laboratory Medicine*, *41*, 979–994.

Borel, P., Grolier, P., Armand, M., Partier, A., Lafont, H., Lairon, D., et al. (1996). Carotenoids in biological emulsions: Solubility, surface-to-core distribution and release from lipid droplets. *Journal of Lipid Research*, *37*, 250–261.

Borel, P., Grolier, P., Mekki, N., Boirie, Y., et al. (1998). Low and high responders to pharmacological doses of β-carotene: Proportion in the population, mechanisms involved and consequences on beta-carotene metabolism. *Journal of Lipid Research*, *39*, 2250–2260.

Borel, P., Tyssandier, V., Mekki, N., Grolier, P., Rochette, Y., Alexandre-Gouabau, M. C., et al. (1998). Chylomicron β-carotene and retinyl palmitate responses are dramatically diminished when men ingest β-carotene with medium chain rather than long chain triglycerides. *The Journal of Nutrition*, *128*, 1361–1367.

Bowen, P. E., Herbst-Espinosa, S. M., Hussain, E. A., & Stacewicz-Sapuntzakis, M. (2002). Esterification does not impair lutein bioavailability in humans. *The Journal of Nutrition*, *132*, 3668–3673.

Brady, W. E., Mares-Perlman, J. A., Bowen, P., & Stacewicz-Sapuntzakis, M. (1996). Human serum concentrations are related to physiologic and life style factors. *The Journal of Nutrition*, *126*, 129–137.

Breithaupt, D. E., & Bamedi, A. (2002). Carotenoids and carotenoid esters in potatoes (*Solanum tuberosum* L.): New insights into an ancient vegetable. *Journal of Agricultural and Food Chemistry*, *50*, 7175–7181.

Britton, G. (1995). Structure and properties of carotenoids in relation to function. *The FASEB Journal*, *9*, 1551–1558.

Britton, G., Liaaen-Jensen, S., & Pfander, H. (2004). Carotenoids Handbook. *Photosynthetica*: *42* (p. 186). Basel, Switzerland: Birkhauser.

Brown, M. J., Ferruzzi, M. G., Nguyen, M. L., Cooper, D. A., Eldridge, A. L., Schwartz, S. J., et al. (2004). Carotenoid bioavailability is higher from salads ingested with full-fat than with fat-reduced salad dressings as measured with electrochemical detection. *The American Journal of Clinical Nutrition*, *80*, 396–403.

Carbonell-Capella, J. M., Buniowska, M., Barba, F. J., Esteve, M. J., & Frigola, A. (2014). Analytical methods for determining bioavailability and bioaccessibility of bioactive compounds from fruits and vegetables: A review. *Comprehensive Reviews in Food Science and Food Safety, 13*, 155–171.

Castenmiller, J. J. M., & West, C. E. (1998). Bioavailability and bioconversion of carotenoids. *Annual Review of Nutrition, 18*, 19–38.

Castenmiller, J. J. M., West, C. E., Linssen, J. H., Van het Hof, K. H., & Voragen, A. G. J. (1999). The food matrix of spinach is a limiting factor in determining the bioavailability of β-carotene and to a lesser extent of lutein in humans. *The Journal of Nutrition, 129*, 349–355.

Cheng, C. Y., Chung, W. Y., Szeto, Y. T., & Benzie, I. F. (2005). Fasting plasma zeaxanthin response to *Fructus barbarum* L. (wolfberry; Kei Tze) in a food-based human supplementation trial. *The British Journal of Nutrition, 93*, 123–130.

Chitchumroonchokchai, C., & Failla, M. L. (2005). Bioavailability of zeaxanthin esters: Investigations using in vitro digestion and Caco-2 human intestinal cells. *The FASEB Journal, 19*, A1457.

Chitchumroonchokchai, C., & Failla, M. L. (2006). Hydrolysis of zeaxanthin esters by carboxyl ester lipase during digestion facilitates micellarization and uptake of the xanthophyll by Caco-2 human intestinal cells. *The Journal of Nutrition, 136*, 588–594.

Chitchumroonchokchai, C., Schwartz, S. J., & Failla, M. L. (2004). Assessment of lutein bioavailability from meals and a supplement using simulated digestion and Caco-2 human intestinal cells. *The Journal of Nutrition, 134*, 2280–2286.

Chung, H. Y., Rasmussen, H. M., & Johnson, E. J. (2004). Lutein bioavailability is higher from lutein-enriched eggs than from supplements and spinach in men. *The Journal of Nutrition, 134*, 1887–1893.

Clark, R. M., Yao, L., & Furr, H. C. (2000). A comparison of lycopene and astaxanthin absorption from corn oil and olive oil emulsions. *Lipids, 37*, 803–806.

Claudie, D. M., Bertrand, C., Franck, T., & Marie-Josephe, A. (2013). Citrus flavanones enhance carotenoid uptake by intestinal Caco-2 cells. *Food & Function, 4*, 1625–1631.

Colle, I. J. P., Lemmens, L., Knockaert, G., Van Loey, A., & Hendrickx, M. (2016). Carotene degradation and isomerization during thermal processing: A review on the kinetic aspects. *Critical Reviews in Food Science and Nutrition, 56*, 1844–1855.

Corte-Real, J., Desmarchelier, C., Borel, P., Richling, E., Hoffmann, L., & Bohn, T. (2018). Magnesium affects spinach carotenoid bioaccessibility in vitro depending on intestinal bile and pancreatic enzyme concentrations. *Food Chemistry, 239*, 751–759.

Davis, H. R., Zhu, L. J., Hoos, L. M., Tetzloff, G., Maguire, M., Liu, J., et al. (2004). Niemann-Pick C1 Like 1 (NPC1L1) is the intestinal phytosterol and cholesterol transporter and a key modulator of whole-body cholesterol homeostasis. *The Journal of Biological Chemistry, 279*, 33586–33592.

De Moura, F. F., Ho, C. C., Getachew, G., Hickenbottom, S., & Clifford, A. J. (2005). Kinetics of ^{14}C distribution after tracer dose of ^{14}C-lutein in an adult woman. *Lipids, 40*, 1069–1073.

de Pee, S., Bloen, M. W., Gorstein, J., Sari, M., Satoto Yip, R., & Muhilal, S. R. (1998). Reappraisal of the role of vegetables in the vitamin A status of mothers in Central Java, Indonesia. *The American Journal of Clinical Nutrition, 68*, 1068–1074.

de Pee, S., & West, C. E. (1996). Dietary carotenoids and their role in combating vitamin A deficiency: A review of the literature. *European Journal of Clinical Nutrition, 50*, S38–S53.

de Pee, S., West, C. E., Hautvast, J. G., & Karyadi, D. (1995). Lack of improvement in vitamin A status with increased consumption of dark-green leafy vegetables. *Lancet, 346*, 75–81.

Deming, D. M., Baker, D. H., & Erdman, J. W. (2002). The relative vitamin A value of 9-cis β-carotene is less and that of 13-cis β-carotene may be greater than the accepted 50% that of all-trans β-carotene in gerbils. *The Journal of Nutrition, 132*, 2709–2712.

Deming, D. M., Boileau, A. C., Lee, C. M., & Erdman, J. W. (2000). Amount of dietary fat and type of soluble fiber independently modulate post absorptive conversion of β-carotene to vitamin A in Mongolian gerbils. *The Journal of Nutrition, 130*, 2789–2796.

Deming, D. M., & Erdman, J. W. (1999). Mammalian carotenoids absorption and metabolism. *Pure and Applied Chemistry, 71*, 2213–2223.

Di Lorenzo, C., Williams, C. M., Hajnal, F., & Valenzuela, J. E. (1988). Pectin delays gastric emptying and increases satiety in obese subjects. *Gastroenterology, 95*, 1211–1215.

Dijkhuizen, M. A., Wieringa, F. T., & West, C. E. (2004). Zinc plus β-carotene supplementation of pregnant women is superior to β-carotene supplementation alone in improving vitamin A status in both mothers and infants. *The American Journal of Clinical Nutrition, 80*, 1299–1307.

Dimitrov, N. V., Meyer, C., Ullrey, D. E., Chenoweth, W., Michelakis, A., Malone, W., et al. (1988). Bioavailability of beta-carotene in humans. *The American Journal of Clinical Nutrition, 48*, 298–304.

Diwadkar-Navsariwala, V., Novotny, J. A., Gustin, D. M., Sosman, J. A., Redvold, K. A., Crowell, J. A., et al. (2003). A physiological pharmacokinetic model describing the disposition of lycopene in healthy men. *Journal of Lipid Research, 44*, 1927–1939.

Donhowe, E. G., & Kong, F. (2014). Beta-carotene: Digestion, microencapsulation, and in vitro bioavailability. *Food Bioprocess Technology, 7*, 338–354.

Drammeh, B. S., et al. (2002). A randomized, 4-month mango and fat supplementation trial improved vitamin A status among young Gambian children. *The Journal of Nutrition, 132*, 3693–3699.

During, A., Dawson, H. D., & Horrison, E. H. (2005). Carotenoid transport is decreased and expression of the lipid transporters SR-BI, NPC1L1 and ABCA1 is down regulated in Caco-2 cells treated with estimable. *The Journal of Nutrition, 135*, 2305–2312.

During, A., Fields, M., Lewis, C. G., & Smith, J. C. (2000). Intestinal β-carotene 15,15′-dioxygenase activity is markedly enhanced in copper deficient rats fed on high-iron diets and fructose. *The British Journal of Nutrition, 84*, 117–124.

During, A., & Harrison, E. H. (2006). Digestion and intestinal absorption of dietary carotenoids and vitamin A. In *Vol. 2. Physiology of the Gastrointestinal Tract* (4th ed., pp. 1735–1752). New York: Academic Press.

Edwards, A. J., Nguyen, C. H., You, C. S., Swanson, J. E., Emenhiser, C., & Parker, R. S. (2002). α- and β-carotene from a commercial carrot puree are more bioavailable to humans than from boiled-mashed carrots, as determined using an extrinsic stable isotope reference method. *The Journal of Nutrition, 132*, 159–167.

Edwards, A. J., Vinyard, B. T., Wiley, E. R., Brown, E. D., Collins, J. K., Perkins-Veazie, P., et al. (2003). Consumption of watermelon juice increases plasma concentrations of lycopene and β-carotene in humans. *The Journal of Nutrition, 133*, 1043–1050.

Erdman, J. W. (1999). Variable bioavailability of carotenoids from vegetables. *The American Journal of Clinical Nutrition, 70*, 179–180.

Erdman, J. W., Bierer, T. L., & Gugger, E. T. (1993). Absorption and transport of carotenoids. *Annals of the New York Academy of Sciences, 691*, 76–85.

Faulks, R. M., Hart, D. J., Brett, G. M., Dainty, J. R., & Southon, S. (2004). Kinetics of gastrointestinal transit and carotenoid absorption and disposal in ileostomy volunteers fed spinach meals. *European Journal of Nutrition, 43*, 15–22.

Fernandez-Garcia, E., Carvajal-Lerida, I., Jaren-Galan, M., Garrido-Fernandez, J., Perez-Galvez, A., & Hornero-Mendez, D. (2012). Carotenoids bioavailability from foods: From plant pigments to efficient biological activities. *Food Research International, 46*, 438–450.

Furr, H. C., & Clark, R. M. (1997). Intestinal absorption and tissue distribution of carotenoids. *The Journal of Nutritional Biochemistry, 8*, 364–377.

Garrett, D. A., Failla, M. L., & Sarama, R. J. (1999). Development of an *in vitro* digestion method to assess carotenoid bioavailability from meals. *Journal of Agricultural and Food Chemistry, 47*, 4301–4309.

Gartner, C., Stahl, W., & Sies, H. (1996). Preferential increase in chylomicron levels of the xanthophylls lutein and zeaxanthin compared to beta-carotene in the human. *International Journal for Vitamin and Nutrition Research, 66*, 119–125.

Gaziano, J. M., Johnson, E. J., Russell, R. M., Krinsky, N. I., Frei, B., Ridker, P., et al. (1995). Discrimination in absorption of transport of β-carotene isomers following oral supplementation with either all-trans or 9-cis β-carotene. *The American Journal of Clinical Nutrition, 61*, 1248–1254.

Gence, L., Servent, A., Poucheret, P., Hiol, A., & Dhuique-Mayer, C. (2018). Pectins structure and particle size modify the carotenoid bioaccessibility and uptake by caco-2 cells in citrus juices vs. concentrates. *Food & Function, 9*, 3523–3531.

Goni, I., Serrano, J., & Saura-Calixto, F. (2006). Bioaccessibility of β-carotene, lutein, and lycopene from fruits and vegetables. *Journal of Agricultural and Food Chemistry, 54*, 5382–5387.

Granado-Lorencio, F., Olmedilla-Alonso, B., Herrero-Barbudo, C., Perez-Sacristan, B., Blanco-Navarro, I., & Blazquez-Garcia, S. (2007). Comparative in vitro bioaccessibility of carotenoids from relevant contributors to carotenoid intake. *Journal of Agricultural and Food Chemistry, 55*, 6387–6394.

Hedren, E., Diaz, V., & Svanberg, U. (2002). Estimation of carotenoid accessibility from carrots determined by an in vitro digestion method. *European Journal of Clinical Nutrition, 56*, 425–430.

Herbst, S., Bowen, P., Hussain, E., Stecewicz-Sapuntzakis, M., Damayanti, B., & Burns, J. (1997). Evaluation of the bioavailability of lutein (L) and lutein diesters (LD) in humans. *The FASEB Journal, 11*, A447.

Hickenbottom, S. J., Lemke, S. L., Dueker, S. R., Lin, Y., Follett, J. R., Carkeet, C., et al. (2002). Dual isotope test for assessing β-carotene cleavage to vitamin A in humans. *European Journal of Nutrition, 41*, 141–147.

Hollander, D., & Ruble, P. E. (1978). β-Carotene intestinal absorption: Bile, fatty acid, pH and flow rate effects on transport. *American Journal of Physiology, 235*, E686–E692.

Hornero-Mendez, D., & Minguenz-Mosquera, M. I. (2000). Xanthophyll esterification accompanying carotenoid overaccumulation in chromoplast of *Capsicum annuum* ripening fruits is a constitutive process and useful for ripeness index. *Journal of Agricultural and Food Chemistry, 48*, 1617–1622.

Hu, X., Jandacek, R. J., & White, W. S. (2000). Intestinal absorption of β-carotene ingested with a meal rich in sunflower oil or beef tallow: Postprandial appearance in triacylglycerol-rich lipoproteins in women. *The American Journal of Clinical Nutrition, 71*, 1170–1180.

Huo, T., Ferruzzi, M. G., Schwartz, S. J., & Failla, M. L. (2007). Impact of fatty acyl composition and quantity of triglycerides on bioaccessibility of dietary carotenoids. *Journal of Agricultural and Food Chemistry, 55*, 8950–8957.

Jalal, F., Nesheim, M. C., Agus, Z., Sanjur, D., & Habicht, J. P. (1998). Serum retinol concentrations in children are affected by food sources of β-carotene, fat intake, and anthelmintic drug treatment. *The American Journal of Clinical Nutrition, 68*, 623–629.

Johnson, E. J., Qin, J., Krinsky, N. I., & Russell, R. M. (1997). Ingestion by men of a combined dose of β-carotene and lycopene does not affect the absorption of β-carotene but improves that of lycopene. *The Journal of Nutrition, 127*, 1833–1837.

Kana-Sop, M. M., Gouado, I., Achu, M. B., Van Camp, J., Zollo, P. H. A., Schweiger, F. J., et al. (2015). The influence of iron and zinc supplementation on the bioavailability of provitamin A carotenoids from papaya following consumption of a vitamin A-deficient diet. *Journal of Nutritional Science and Vitaminology, 61*, 205–214.

Karin, H., van het Hof, K. H., Lilian, B. M., Tijburg, L. B., Pietrzik, K., & Weststrate, J. A. (1999). Influence of feeding different vegetables on plasma levels of carotenoids, folate and vitamin C. Effect of disruption of the vegetable matrix. *The British Journal of Nutrition, 82*, 203–212.

Khachik, F., Goli, M. B., Beecher, G. R., Holden, J., Lusby, W. R., Tenorio, M. D., et al. (1992). Effect of food preparation on qualitative and quantitative distribution of major carotenoid constituents of tomatoes and several green vegetables. *Journal of Agricultural and Food Chemistry, 40*, 390–398.

Koch, R. E., Wilson, A. E., & Hill, G. E. (2016). The importance of carotenoid dose in supplementation studies with songbirds. *Physiological and Biochemical Zoology, 89*, 61–71.

Kostic, D., White, W. S., & Olson, J. A. (1995). Intestinal absorption, serum clearance and interactions between lutein and β-carotene when administered to human adults in separate or combined oral doses. *The American Journal of Clinical Nutrition, 62*, 604–610.

Lakshminarayana, R., Aruna, G., Sangeetha, R. K., Bhaskar, N., Divakar, S., & Baskaran, V. (2008). Possible degradation/biotransformation of lutein *in vitro* and *in vivo*: Isolation and structural elucidation of lutein metabolites by HPLC and LC-MS (atmospheric pressure chemical ionization). *Free Radical Biology & Medicine, 45*, 982–993.

Lakshminarayana, R., Raju, M., Keshava Prakash, M. N., & Baskaran, V. (2009). Phospholipids, oleic acid micelles and dietary olive oil influence the lutein absorption and activity of antioxidant enzymes in rats. *Lipids, 44*, 799–806.

Lakshminarayana, R., Raju, M., Krishnakantha, T. P., & Baskaran, V. (2006). Enhanced lutein bioavailability by lyso-phosphatidylcholine in rats. *Molecular and Cellular Biochemistry, 281*, 103–110.

Lemke, S. L., Dueker, S. R., Follett, J. R., Lin, Y., Carkee, C., Buchholz, B. A., et al. (2003). Absorption and retinol equivalence of β-carotene in humans is influenced by dietary vitamin A intake. *Journal of Lipid Research, 44*, 1591–1600.

Lemmens, L., Colle, I., Van Buggenhout, S., Palmero, P., Van Loey, A., & Hendrickx, M. (2014). Carotenoid bioaccessibility in fruit-and vegetable-based food products as affected by product (micro)structural characteristics and the presence of lipids: A review. *Trends in Food Science & Technology, 38*, 125–135.

Levin, G., & Mokady, S. (1994). Antioxidant activity of 9-cis compared to all-trans β-carotene in vitro. *Free Radical Biology & Medicine, 17*, 77–82.

Liaaen-Jensen, S. (2004). Basic carotenoid chemistry. In *Vol. 13. Oxidative stress and disease* (pp. 1–30): Marcel Dekker.

Lienau, A., Glaser, T., Tang, G., Dolnikowski, G. G., Grusak, M. A., & Albert, K. (2003). Bioavailability of lutein in humans from intrinsically labelled vegetables determined by LC-APCI-MS1. *The Journal of Nutritional Biochemistry, 14*, 663–670.

Lin, Y., Dueker, S. R., Burri, B. J., Neidlinger, T. R., & Clifford, A. J. (2000). Variability of the conversion of β-carotene to vitamin A in women measured by using a double-tracer study design. *The American Journal of Clinical Nutrition, 71*, 1545–1554.

Liu, L., Shao, Z., Zhang, M., & Wang, Q. (2015). Regulation of carotenoid metabolism in tomato. *Molecular Plant, 8*, 28–39.

Livny, O., Reifen, R., Levy, I., Madar, Z., Faulks, R., Southon, S., et al. (2003). β-Carotene bioavailability from differently processed carrot meals in human ileostomy volunteers. *European Journal of Nutrition, 42*, 338–345.

Maiani, G., Periago Caston, M. J., Catasta, G., et al. (2009). Carotenoids: Actual knowledge on food sources, intakes, stability and bioavailability and their protective role in humans. *Molecular Nutrition & Food Research, 53*, S194–S218.

Mamatha, B. S., & Baskaran, V. (2011). Effect of micellar lipids, dietary fiber and β-carotene on lutein bioavailability in aged rats with lutein deficiency. *Nutrition, 27*, 960–966.

McCullough, F. S., Northrop-Clewes, C. A., & Thurnham, D. I. (1999). The effect of vitamin A on epithelial integrity. *Proceedings of the Nutrition Society, 58*, 289–293.

Micozzi, M. S., Brown, E. D., Edwards, B. K., Bieri, J. G., Taylor, P. R., Khachik, F., et al. (1992). Plasma carotenoid response to chronic intake of selected foods and beta-carotene supplements in men. *The American Journal of Clinical Nutrition, 55*, 1120–1125.

Moelants, K. R., Lemmens, L., Vandebroeck, M., Van Buggenhout, S., Van Loey, A. M., & Hendrickx, M. E. (2012). Relation between particle size and carotenoid bioaccessibility in carrot-and tomato-derived suspensions. *Journal of Agricultural and Food Chemistry, 60*, 11995–12003.

Moeller, S. M., Voland, R., Tinker, L., Blodi, B. A., Klein, M. L., Gehrs, K. M., et al. (2008). Associations between age-related nuclear cataract and lutein and zeaxanthin in the diet and serum in the carotenoids in the age-related eye disease study (CAREDS), an ancillary study of the women's health initiative. *Archives of Ophthalmology, 126*, 354–364.

Moore, A. C., Gugger, E. T., & Erdman, J. W. (1996). Brush border membrane vesicles from rats and gerbils can be used to study uptake of all-trans and 9-cis β-carotene. *The Journal of Nutrition, 126*, 2904–2912.

Mozaffarieh, M., Sacu, S., & Wedrich, A. (2003). The role of the carotenoids, lutein and zeaxanthin, in protecting against age-related macular degeneration: A review based on controversial evidence. *The Journal of Nutrition, 2*, 1–8.

Mutsokoti, L., Panozzo, A., Pallares, A. P., Jaiswal, S., Van Loey, A., Grauwet, T., et al. (2017). Carotenoid bioaccessibility and the relation to lipid digestion: A kinetic study. *Journal of Food Chemistry, 232*, 124–134.

Nagao, A., Kotake-Nara, E., & Hase, M. (2013). Effects of fats and oils on the bioaccessibility of carotenoids and vitamin E in vegetables. *Bioscience, Biotechnology, and Biochemistry, 77*, 1055–1060.

Nagao, A., Maeda, M., Lim, B. P., Kobayashi, H., & Terao, J. (2000). Inhibition of β-carotene-15, 15′-dioxygenase activity by dietary flavonoids. *The Journal of Nutritional Biochemistry, 11*, 348–355.

Noakes, M., Clifton, P., Ntanios, F., Shrapnel, W., Record, I., & McInerney, J. (2002). An increase in dietary carotenoids when consuming plant sterols or stanols is effective in maintaining plasma carotenoid concentrations. *The American Journal of Clinical Nutrition, 75*, 79–86.

Novotny, J. A., Dueker, S. R., Zech, L. A., & Clifford, A. J. (1995). Compartmental analysis of the dynamics of beta-carotene metabolism in an adult volunteer. *Journal of Lipid Research, 36*, 1825–1838.

Olson, J. A. (1999). Carotenoids and human health. *Archivos Latinoamericanos de Nutrición, 49*, 7S–11S.

O'Neill, M. E., & Thurnham, D. I. (1998). Intestinal absorption of β-carotene, lycopene and lutein in men and women following a standard meal: Response curves in the triglycerol-rich lipoprotein fraction. *The British Journal of Nutrition, 79*, 149–159.

O'Connell, O. F., Ryan, L., & O'Brien, N. M. (2007). Xanthophyll carotenoids are more bioaccessible from fruits than dark green vegetables. *Nutrition Research, 27*, 258–264.

Ornelas-Paz, J. D. J., Yahia, E. M., & Gardea-Bejar, A. (2007). Identification and quantification of xanthophyll esters, carotenes, and tocopherols in the fruit of seven mexican mango cultivars by liquid chromatography–atmospheric pressure chemical ionization–time-of-flight mass spectrometry [LC-(APCI+)-MS]. *Journal of Agricultural and Food Chemistry, 55*, 6628–6635.

Palafox Carlos, H., Ayala Zavala, J. F., & Gonzalez Aguilar, G. A. (2011). The role of dietary fiber in the bioaccessibility and bioavailability of fruit and vegetable antioxidants. *Journal of Food Science, 76*, R6–R15.

Parker, R. S. (1996). Absorption, metabolism and transport of carotenoids. *The FASEB Journal, 10*, 542–551.

Parvin, S. G., & Sivakumar, B. (2000). Nutritional status affects intestinal carotene cleavage activity and carotene conversion to vitamin A in rats. *The Journal of Nutrition, 130*, 573–577.

Pasquier, B., Armand, M., Guillon, F., Castelain, C., Borel, P., Lafont, H., et al. (1996). Emulsification and lipolysis of triacylglycerols are altered by viscous soluble dietary fibres in acidic gastric medium in vitro. *The Biochemical Journal, 314*, 269–275.

Perez-Galvez, A., Marti, H. D., Sies, H., & Stahl, W. (2003). Incorporation of carotenoids from paprika oleoresin into human chylomicrons. *The British Journal of Nutrition, 89*, 787–793.

Prince, M. R., & Frisoli, J. K. (1993). Beta-carotene accumulation in serum and skin. *The American Journal of Clinical Nutrition, 57*, 175–181.

Raju, M., & Baskaran, V. (2009). Bioefficacy of β-carotene is improved in rats after solubilized as equimolar dose of β-carotene and lutein in phospholipid-mixed micelles. *Nutrition Research, 29*, 588–595.

Raju, M., Lakshminarayana, R., Krishnakantha, T. P., & Baskaran, V. (2006). Micellar oleic and eicosapentaenoic acid but not linoleic acid influences the β-carotene uptake and its cleavage into retinol in rats. *Molecular and Cellular Biochemistry, 288*, 7–15.

Reboul, E. (2013). Absorption of vitamin a and carotenoids by the enterocyte: Focus on transport proteins. *Nutrients, 5*, 3563–3581.

Reboul, E., Aboul, L., Mikail, C., Ghiringhelli, O., Andre, M., Portugal, H., et al. (2005). Lutein transport by Caco-2, TC-7 cells occurs partly by a facilitated process involving the scavenger receptor class B type 1 (SR-B1). *The Biochemical Journal, 387*, 455–461.

Ribaya-Mercado, J. D., Solon, F. S., & Solon, M. A. (2000). Bioconversion of plant carotenoids to vitamin A in Filipino school-aged children varies inversely with vitamin A status. *The American Journal of Clinical Nutrition, 72*, 455–465.

Riedl, J., Linseisen, J., & Hoffmann, J. (1999). Wolfram. Some dietary fibers reduce the absorption of carotenoids in women. *The Journal of Nutrition, 129*, 2170–2176.

Riso, P., Brusamolino, A., Ciappellano, S., & Porrini, M. (2016). Comparison of lutein bioavailability from vegetables and supplement. *International Journal for Vitamin and Nutrition Research, 73*, 201–205.

Rock, C. L., & Swendseid, M. E. (1992). Plasma β-carotene response in human after meals supplemented with dietary pectin. *The American Journal of Clinical Nutrition, 55*, 96–99.

Rodriguez-Amaya, D. B., & Kimura, M. (2004). *HarvestPlus: Handbook for carotenoid analysis*.

Roodenberg, A. J., Leenen, R., Van het Hof, K. H., Weststrate, J. A., & Tijburg, L. B. (2000). Amount of fat in the diet affects bioavailability of lutein esters but not of α-carotene, β-carotene and vitamin E in humans. *The American Journal of Clinical Nutrition, 71*, 1187–1193.

Salvia-Trujillo, L., & McClements, D. J. (2016). Improvement of β-carotene bioaccessibility from dietary supplements using excipient nanoemulsions. *Journal of Agricultural and Food Chemistry, 64,* 4639–4647.

Schaffer, J. E. (2002). Fatty acid transport: The roads taken. *American Journal of Physiology, 282,* E239–E246.

Scott, K. J., & Rodriguez-Amaya, D. (2000). Pro-vitamin A carotenoid conversion factors: Retinol equivalents. Fact or fiction? *Food Chemistry, 69,* 125–127.

Serrano, J., Isabel, G., & Saura-Calixto, F. (2005). Determination of β-carotene and lutein available from green leafy vegetables by an in vitro digestion and colonic fermentation method. *Journal of Agricultural and Food Chemistry, 53,* 2936–2940.

Sommerburg, O., Keunen, J. E., Bird, A. C., & van Kuijk, F. J. (1998). Fruits and vegetables that are sources for lutein and zeaxanthin: The macular pigment in human eyes. *The British Journal of Ophthalmology, 82,* 907–910.

Stahl, W., Schwarz, W., von Laar, J., & Sies, H. (1995). All-trans β-carotene preferentially accumulates in human chylomicrons and very low density lipoproteins compared with the 9-cis geometrical isomer. *The Journal of Nutrition, 125,* 2128–2133.

Stahl, W., & Sies, H. (1992). Uptake of lycopene and its geometrical isomers is greater from heat-processed than from unprocessed tomato juice in humans. *The Journal of Nutrition, 122,* 2161–2166.

Sugawara, T., Kushiro, M., Zhang, H., Nara, E., Ono, H., & Nagao, A. (2001). Lysophosphatidylcholine enhances carotenoid uptake from mixed micelles by Caco-2 human intestinal cells. *The Journal of Nutrition, 131,* 2921–2927.

Suleria, H. A. R., Osborne, S., Masci, P., & Gobe, G. (2015). Marine-based nutraceuticals: An innovative trend in the food and supplement industries. *Marine Drugs, 13,* 6336–6351.

Takyi, E. E. K. (1999). Children's consumption of dark green, leafy vegetables with added fat enhances serum retinol. *The Journal of Nutrition, 129,* 1549–1554.

Tang, G., Qin, J., Doinikowski, G. G., & Russell, R. M. (2000). Vitamin A equivalence of β-carotene in women as determined by a stable isotope reference method. *European Journal of Nutrition, 39,* 7–11.

Tang, G., Qin, J., Dolnikowski, G. G., Russell, R. M., & Grusak, M. A. (2009). Golden rice is an effective source of vitamin A. *The American Journal of Clinical Nutrition, 89,* 1776–1783.

Tang, G., Serfaty-Lacrosniere, C., Camilo, M. E., & Russell, R. (1996). Gastric acidity influences the blood response to a β-carotene dose in humans. *The American Journal of Clinical Nutrition, 64,* 622–626.

Tanumihardjo, S. A., Li, J., & Dosti, M. P. (2005). Lutein absorption is facilitated with cosupplementation of ascorbic acid in young adults. *Journal of the American Dietetic Association, 105,* 114–118.

Thurnham, D. I. (2007). Bioequivalence of β-carotene and retinol. *Journal of the Science of Food and Agriculture, 87,* 13–39.

Thurnham, D. I., Northrop-Clewes, C. A., McCullough, F. S., Das, B. S., & Lunn, P. G. (2000). Innate immunity, gut integrity and vitamin A in Gambian and Indian infants. *The Journal of Infectious Diseases, 182,* S23–S28.

Torronen, R., Lehmusaho, M., Hakkinen, S., Hanninen, O., & Mykkanen, H. (1996). Serum β-carotene response to supplementation with raw carrots, carrot juice or purified β-carotene in healthy non-smoking women. *Nutrition Research, 16,* 565–575.

Tyssandier, V., Cardinault, N., Caris-Veyrat, C., Amiot, M. J., Grolier, P., Bouteloup, C., et al. (2002). Vegetable-borne lutein, lycopene, and β-carotene compete for incorporation into chylomicrons, with no adverse effect on the medium-term (3-wk) plasma status of carotenoids in humans. *The American Journal of Clinical Nutrition, 75,* 526–534.

Tyssandier, V., Lyan, B., & Borel, P. (2001). Main factors governing the transfer of carotenoids from emulsion lipid droplets to micelles. *Biochimica et Biophysica Acta - Molecular and Cell Biology of Lipids, 1533*, 285–292.

Tyssandier, V., Reboul, E., Dumas, J. F., Bouteloup-Demange, C., Armand, M., Marcand, J., et al. (2003). Processing of vegetable-borne carotenoids in the human stomach and duodenum. *American Journal of Physiology. Gastrointestinal and Liver Physiology, 284*, G913–G923.

Unlu, N. Z., Bohn, T., Clinton, S. K., & Schwartz, S. J. (2005). Carotenoid absorption from salad and salsa by humans is enhanced by the addition of avocado or avocado oil. *The Journal of Nutrition, 135*, 431–436.

van Bennekum, A., Werder, M., Thuahnai, S. T., Han, C. H., Duong, P., Williams, D. L., et al. (2005). Class B scavenger receptor-mediated intestinal absorption of dietary β-carotene and cholesterol. *Biochemistry, 44*, 4517–4525.

Van den Berg, H. (1999). Carotenoid interactions. *Nutrition Reviews, 57*, 1–10.

Van den Berg, H., Faulks, R., Granado, H. F., Hirschberg, J., Olmedilla, B., Sandmann, G., et al. (2000). The potential for the improvement of carotenoid levels in foods and the likely systemic effects. *Journal of the Science of Food and Agriculture, 80*, 880–912.

Van den Berg, H., & van Vliet, T. (1998). Effect of simultaneous, single oral doses of b-carotene with lutein or lycopene on the b-carotene and retinyl ester responses in the triacylglycerol-rich lipoprotein fraction of men. *The American Journal of Clinical Nutrition, 68*, 82–89.

Van het Hof, K. H., Tiijburg, L. B. M., Pietrzik, K., & Weststrate, J. A. (1999). Influence of feeding different vegetables on plasma levels of carotenoids, folate and vitamin C. Effect of disruption of the vegetable matrix. *The British Journal of Nutrition, 82*, 203–212.

Van het Hof, K. H., West, C. E., Weststrate, J. A., & Hautvast, J. G. (2000). Dietary factors that affect the bioavailability of carotenoids. *The Journal of Nutrition, 130*, 503–506.

Van Lieshout, M., West, C. E., & Van Breemen, R. B. (2003). Isotopic tracer techniques for studying the bioavailability and bioefficacy of dietary carotenoids, particularly β-carotene, in humans: A review. *The American Journal of Clinical Nutrition, 77*, 12–28.

van Vliet, T. (1996). Absorption of β-carotene and other carotenoids in humans and animal models. *European Journal of Clinical Nutrition, 50*, 32–37.

Veda, S., Platel, K., & Srinivasan, K. (2008). Influence of food acidulants and antioxidant spices on the bioaccessibility of β-carotene from selected vegetables. *Journal of Agricultural and Food Chemistry, 56*, 8714–8719.

Veda, S., & Srinivasan, K. (2009). Influence of dietary spices—black pepper, red pepper and ginger on the uptake of β-carotene by rat intestines. *Journal of Functional Foods, 1*, 394–398.

Veda, S., & Srinivasan, K. (2011). Influence of dietary spices on the in vivo absorption of ingested β-carotene in experimental rats. *The British Journal of Nutrition, 105*, 1429–1438.

Wang, Y., Chuang, Y., & Hsu, H. (2008). The flavonoid, carotenoid and pectin content in peels of citrus cultivated in Taiwan. *Food Chemistry, 106*, 277–284.

Wang, W., Connor, S. L., Johnson, E. J., Klein, M. L., Hughes, S., & Connor, W. E. (2007). Effect of dietary lutein and zeaxanthin on plasma carotenoids and their transport in lipoproteins in age-related macular degeneration. *The American Journal of Clinical Nutrition, 85*, 762–769.

Williams, A. W., Boileau, T. W., & Erdman, J. W. (1998). Factors influencing the uptake and absorption of carotenoids. *Proceedings of the Society for Experimental Biology and Medicine, 218*, 106–108.

Wingerath, T., Stahl, W., & Sies, H. (1995). β-Cryptoxanthin selectively increases in human chylomicrons upon ingestion of tangerine concentrate rich in β-cryptoxanthin esters. *Archives of Biochemistry and Biophysics, 324*, 385–390.

Yao, L., Liang, Y., Trahanovsky, W. S., Serfass, R. E., & White, W. S. (2000). Use of a ^{13}C tracer to quantify the plasma appearance of a physiological dose of lutein in humans. *Lipids*, *35*, 339–348.

Yeum, K. J., & Russell, R. M. (2002). Carotenoid bioavailability and bioconversion. *Annual Review of Nutrition*, *22*, 483–504.

Yonekura, L., & Nagao, A. (2007). Intestinal absorption of dietary carotenoids. *Molecular Nutrition & Food Research*, *51*, 107–115.

Yuan, X., Liu, X., McClements, D. J., Cao, Y., & Xiao, H. (2018). Enhancement of phytochemical bioaccessibility from plant-based foods using excipient emulsions: Impact of lipid type on carotenoid solubilization from spinach. *Food & Function*, *9*, 4352–4365.

Zhang, R., Zhang, Z., Zou, L., Xiao, H., Zhang, G., Decker, E. A., et al. (2016). Enhancement of carotenoid bioaccessibility from carrots using excipient emulsions: Influence of particle size of digestible lipid droplets. *Food & Function*, *7*, 93–103.

Further reading

Reboul, E., Richelle, M., Perrot, E., Desmoulins-Malezet, C., Pirisi, V., & Borel, P. (2006). Bioaccessibility of carotenoids and vitamin E from their main dietary sources. *Journal of Agricultural and Food Chemistry*, *54*, 8749–8755.

Rodriguez-Amaya, D. B., & Kimura, M. (2004). *HarvestPlus handbook for carotenoid analysis*. *Vol. 2*. Washington, DC: International Food Policy Research Institute (IFPRI).

Antiobese properties of carotenoids: An overview of underlying molecular mechanisms

Sowmya Shree Gopal, Tehreem Maradgi, Ganesan Ponesakki
Department of Molecular Nutrition, CSIR-Central Food Technological Research Institute (CFTRI), Mysore, India

Chapter Outline

Introduction

Obesity is defined as one of the phenotypic manifestations characterized by excessive deposition of fat (hyperplasia) and increased in fat cell mass (hypertrophy). It is a multifactorial metabolic syndrome, is associated with an increased risk of major secondary complications like cardiovascular diseases, diabetes, hypertension, and cancer (Cascio, Schiera, & Di Liegro, 2012). The prevalence of obesity has increased rapidly at an alarming rate worldwide during the past three decades. According to the WHO (2016), more than 39% (1.9 billion) of the world's adult population were overweight, out of which over 13% (650 million) were obese. Notably, the prevalence of overweight and obesity among children and adolescents aged 5–19 years has risen dramatically from 4% to 18% since 1975–2016. It was reported that, there are about 44% of diabetes cases worldwide, and 23% of ischemic heart diseases and 7%–41% certain cancer patients are attributed to overweight and obesity (Mathieu, Lemieux, & Després, 2010). The strong association between obesity and other chronic diseases such as diabetes and cardiovascular disorders generates economic instability in health sector, creating greatest challenge for the underdeveloped and developing countries. Studies carried out across the different countries state that obese individuals spent 25% more in health care than healthy individuals (Withrow & Alter, 2011).

From an etiological point of view, genetic and environmental interactions cause dysfunction of adipose tissue by initiating a sequence of adipocyte hypertrophy, hypoxia, several stresses, and inflammatory processes. As a consequence, impaired adipose tissue function contributes to a pro-inflammatory, atherogenic, and diabetogenic state, which in turn mechanistically linked to the development of obesity-associated disorders. Studies on genetic disposition on obesity reports, heredity as major contributor for obesity. Hereditary components in obesity were studied in twins, family and adoptions with an outcome of 60%–90% of genetic influence (Grundy, 2012). Obesity increases apparently in childhood with a greater impact in adulthood. Research reports highlight that parental obesity is the highest risk factor for childhood obesity (Hebebrand & Hinney, 2009). Intrauterine environment and the dietary practice during gestation are found to have a direct influence on childhood obesity (Mamun et al., 2010). Large-scale epidemiological studies noticed that polygenic variant might be a major causative factor contributing to obesogenic. However, some individuals carrying these variants may not develop obesity due to other gene-gene interaction or gene-environment interaction (Stöger, 2008). Genetic factors are considered to contribute much lesser extent to obesity as they are modified by environment and/or dietary component.

The adipose tissue is typically attributed toward storage of lipids and release of fatty acids during energy requirement. Thus, it plays an essential role in maintaining the balance between energy intake and energy expenditure. It is an inert tissue comprised of brown adipose tissue (BAT) and white adipose tissue (WAT), both of which possess different morphology, cellular distribution, gene expression, and function. WAT contributes the major component of adipose tissue in the body and is dispersed in varied anatomic body site majorly deposited as subcutaneous fat, visceral fat, and intramuscular fat (Gesta, Tseng, & Kahn, 2007). The cellular composition of adipose tissue includes adipocytes and stromal vascular fractions, the latter comprises of blood cells, endothelial cells, pericytes, and adipose precursor cells (Ahima & Flier, 2000; Bernlohr, Jenkins, & Bennaars, 2002; Fonseca-Alaniz, Takada, Alonso-Vale, & Lima, 2007; Saely, Geiger, & Drexel, 2012).

Adipose tissue is capable of expanding by accommodating the increased number of lipids droplets through a combinatorial mechanism of hypertrophy and hyperplasia via initiating differentiation of preadipocytes to mature adipocytes (Coelho, Oliveira, & Fernandes, 2013). The adipose tissue also serves as a crucial integrator of glucose homeostasis, inflammatory processes, insulin sensitivity, redox mechanism, and immune pathways (Trayhurn & Beattie, 2001). The sequential process of buffering the daily influx of dietary fat and secretion of adipokines has rendered adipose tissue as a highly active metabolic and endocrine organ. Adipose tissue dysfunction plays a central mechanism leading to obesity and obesity-related disorders such as coronary heart disease, type 2 diabetes, hypertension, and certain types of cancers.

Enlarged adipocytes due to excessive accumulation of fat in the adipose tissue with reduced buffering capacity for lipid storage exposes the adjacent tissues to an excessive influx of lipids leading to ectopic fat deposition and insulin resistance. Under this circumstance, an increased energy intake exceeds energy expenditure favoring excessive fat storage in nonadipose tissues, which induces hypoxic condition in adipose tissue. This adipose tissue hypoperfusion induced hypoxic condition further results in altered adipokine secretion and increased macrophage infiltration. The established hypoxic condition further induces disturbances in the blood flow, which affects the lipid-handling capacity and ectopic fat deposition in adipose tissue. Impaired blood flows are also associated with insulin sensitivity (Goossens, 2008). The altered haemostasis elicits cellular stress which consequently activates the inflammatory processes in metabolically active sites such as WAT, liver, and immune cells. This chronic inflammatory condition is associated with the development of obesity-related inflammatory diseases (Balistreri, Caruso, & Candore, 2010). Apparently, uncontrolled adipose tissue remodeling is one of the histological features of chronic inflammation, where the adipocyte cell death favors macrophage recruitment, causing insulin resistance and chronic inflammation (Lee, Wu, & Fried, 2010). In contrast, BAT predominantly known as the thermogenic tissue is broadly identified as the site of uncoupling protein 1 (UCP1) (Nicholls & Rial, 1999). Several studies have elucidated the mechanisms underlying the activity of UCP1 in the uncoupling mitochondrial oxidative phosphorylation to produce heat without producing adenosine triphosphate (ATP). In this way, BAT can partition excess energy intake toward oxidation, and thus reduce storage of body fat. Epidemiological studies indicate that obese individuals are associated with reduced energy expenditure (Braitman, Adlin, & Stanton Jr, 1985).

For the past few decades, an enormous amount of progress has been made toward understanding the molecular mechanisms of adipose tissue dysfunction and the pathogenesis of obesity. Most of the research findings suggest the importance of primary intervention in obesity. Although the prevention strategies of obesity through education and changes to the obesogenic environment are long-term goals, treatment plan is necessary for those who are already obese. However, the preventive/treatment options are scarce or very limited. The mechanisms of action by which those antiobesity drugs play their role include appetite suppression, increased rate of metabolism, reducing the capacity of the body to absorb certain food nutrients like lipids, and triggering the process of thermogenesis and enhancing lysis of lipids (Chopra, Kaur, & Lalit, 2014). Orlistat and sibutramine are prescribed in case of patients with the body mass index (BMI) above $28 \, kg/m^2$ (Wirth, Wabitsch, & Hauner, 2014). Orlistat, a pancreatic lipase inhibitor reduces the absorption of dietary fat and is found to be effective both in short- and long-term preventive measures. Sibutramine is a centrally acting serotonin-norepinephrine reuptake inhibitor that increase satiety and promote energy expenditure. Various studies demonstrated the positive outcome of sibutramine on triglyceride, high-density lipoprotein cholesterol, and glycemic control. The other pharmacological approaches include using cholecystokinin as a satiety signal moiety, anticonvulsant medications such as topiramate and zonisamide, and cannabinoid receptor antagonist, and some drugs that target peptide neurotransmitters (Lawlor & Chaturvedi, 2006). Few studies say that changes in the lifestyle which include dieting and/or exercise does not generally produce sustainable weight loss (Dansinger, Gleason, Griffith, Selker, & Schaefer, 2005; LeBlanc, O'connor, Whitlock, Patnode, & Kapka, 2011), while few of the effective physiological therapies like cognitive behavioral therapy do reduce obesity, but they may not be accessed in a larger scale due to the disappointing long-term results (Wing, Tate, Gorin, Raynor, & Fava, 2006).

Bariatric surgery (weight loss surgery) is another alternative in case of long-term obesity that reduces stomach volume and bowel length resulting in satiety and less uptake of food (O'Brien, MacDonald, Anderson, Brennan, & Brown, 2013). Liposuction or liposculpture suction and lipectomy are the new curative strategies gaining a concern now-a-days, and a cosmetic surgical for fat removal from different parts of the body also reported to possess various side effects. The major investigation resulted with a reduction of gastric pouch using two procedures are, laparoscopic gastric banding and gastric bypass. Both those procedures are focused on reducing the volume of stomach. Laparoscopic gastric banding includes an operation which decrease food intake with a small gastric pouch and limited outlet. On the other hand, gastric bypass involves modification of digestion and uptake process by excluding the food from stomach. These are the two procedures which are majorly practiced surgeries around the world (Pories, 2008). Besides, few other effective strategies like bariatric surgery, such as Roux-en-Y bypass or gastric banding, which is even more effective in terms of weight loss, reduced comorbidity, and enhanced survival (Kral & Näslund, 2007; Sjöström et al., 2007). But, due to the associated complications such as perioperative mortality, surgical complications, and frequent need of reoperation, these procedures are advisable only for the morbidly obese individuals (Field, Chaudhri, & Bloom, 2009; Melnikova & Wages, 2006). An alternative strategy to surgery is to develop therapeutic agents that can reduce body weight by decreasing the consumption or absorption of food, and/or by increasing energy expenditure (Cooke & Bloom, 2006; Sargent & Moore, 2009). Unfortunately, although avidly pursued for more than half a century, this strategy has thus far only shown limited success. Many new agents that were heralded as the answer to the obesity problem were hastily withdrawn owing to an unacceptable burden of side effects. Indeed, a recent review rather pessimistically concluded that "the history of antiobesity drug development is far from glorious, with transient magic bullets and only a handful of agents currently licensed for clinical use" (Rodgers, Holch, & Tallett, 2010). Therefore, new treatments for obesity that are both better tolerated and more efficacious are urgently needed (Halford, Boyland, Blundell, Kirkham, & Harrold, 2010; Kennett & Clifton, 2010; Rodgers et al., 2010; Vickers & Cheetham, 2007). In this context, major recent advances in our understanding of the basic neurobiology of appetite and energy homeostasis have identified numerous targets for potential antiobesity drug development (Halford et al., 2010; Heal, Gosden, & Smith, 2009; Wilding, 2007).

Ayurveda, also known as the "Science of Life," is a comprehensive, holistic traditional health care system that originated in the ancient Vedic period of India. Ayurveda mainly focuses on promotion of health by prevention and curation of diseases. A novel mechanistic approach toward understanding and management of these disorders is available from the comprehensive, holistic health care system known as Ayurveda. The complex set of disorders (Prameha) in Ayurveda correlates in many ways with obesity, metabolic syndrome, and diabetes mellitus (Sharma & Chandola, 2011). Ayurveda utilizes the theoretical background and comprehensive set of strategies to manage Prameha in treating these disorders in an efficacious and cost-effective manner. Ayurveda utilizes the botany and the medicinal properties of some of the currently popular medicinal herbs that are documented in Charaka Samhitha. Ayurvedic herbs such as Dashamula, Triphala, Cyavananprasa, and Guggula are some of the ancient oral plant-derived, multicomponent drugs in popular use and are available commercially. Many of the spices and substances used in domestic cooking (e.g., pepper, ginger, circumin, and garlic) are used extensively. Plant and tree gum resins, called gugullu (e.g., *Commiphora mukul* and *Boswellia serrata*), have been used since times immemorial to treat numerous ailments, especially arthritis and obesity (Chopra & Doiphode, 2002).

Pharmacological management of obesity involves various US Food and Drug Administration (FDA) approved antiobesity drugs viz., orlistat, sibutramine, and diethylpropion. These drugs exert their effect through various molecular mechanisms against obesity. However, they are found to cause chronic side effects viz., nausea, insomnia, dry mouth, dizziness, nervousness, hand tremor, palpitation, and elevation in blood pressure and pulse rate. The extended side effects and contracted therapeutic index of the drugs have paved the way for the search of plant-based substances that have been used to treat/prevent diseases and maintain health for centuries.

Phytonutrients, the substantial constituents of plants are known for their intense role in the maintenance of good health, and also, are an immense preventive tool for various diseases/disorders. Phytochemicals or active ingredients of plants, comprising of carotenoids, flavonoids, glucosinolates (isothiocyanates and indoles), phenolic acids, phytates, and phytoestrogens (isoflavones and lignans) are capable of efficiently combating metabolic diseases due to their novel antiinflammatory, antiobesity, and antidiabetic properties. Regular consumption of fruits and vegetables provides a rich amount of these phytonutrients. Antiinflammatory properties contribute to counteract the obesogenic state (Williams et al., 2013). Phytochemicals target key components of pathways related to obesity (Holubková, Penesová, Šturdík, Mošovská, & Mikušová, 2012). Dietary phytochemicals act on various stages of life cycle of adipocytes. Some probable mechanisms of action of these plants derived products are reduction in adipose tissue mass by inhibition of precursor cell proliferation, enhancing apoptosis of fat cells, and hindering the absorption of triglyceride by reducing formation of pancreatic lipase. They are inhibitors of preadipocyte differentiation and stimulators of lipolysis (Williams et al., 2013). Antiobesity mechanism of plant-derived supplements is attributed to several effects they elicit; these are reduced lipid absorption, decreased intake of energy, more expenditure of energy, and reduced lipogenesis (Chandrasekaran et al., 2012). Carotenoids are one of the classes of phytonutrients, and are natural fat-soluble pigments known for their structural and functional diversity.

Carotenoids are a ubiquitous group of isoprenoid pigments. They are formed by the tail-to-tail linkage of two C20 moieties [geranyl-geranyl pyrophosphate (GGPP)] resulting in the formation of the linear hydrocarbon backbone. These C40 tetraterpenoids contain a rigid backbone that is susceptible to structural modifications (Fig. 1). Carotenoids are essential components of all photosynthetic organisms including plants, algae, and microorganisms, and also few nonphotosynthetic bacteria, yeasts, and molds (Cazzonelli, 2011; Dufosse et al., 2005; Mata-Gómez, Montañez, Méndez-Zavala, & Aguilar, 2014). It was documented that in the year of 1907, Willstatter chemically characterized and classified carotenoids into two major groups, namely oxygen-containing xanthophylls and oxygen-devoid carotenes depending on the presence or the absence of oxygen in their structure (Eugster, 1995). The simple carotenoids belonging to a type of carotene, lycopene from which α and β carotenes are derived by cyclization of end chain (Faure et al., 1999). On the other hand, xanthophyll carotenoids like lutein and zeaxanthin are synthesized by hydroxylation of carotenes, and the oxidative reactions of these xanthophyll carotenoids cause the formation of their subsequent epoxides like antheraxanthin (Jackson, Braun, & Ernst, 2008; Kovary et al., 2001). Currently, around 750 carotenoids are identified from the natural sources (Takaichi, 2011). Decades of research on carotenoids have accumulated more knowledge on the important roles of these omnipresent pigments. They play a

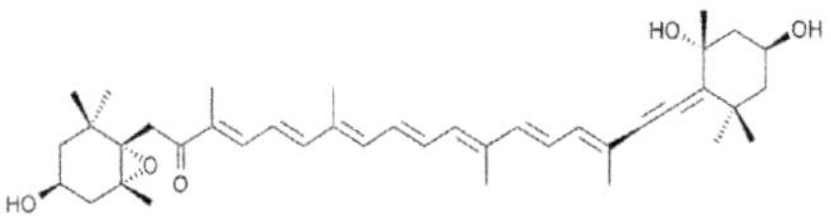

Fucoxanthinol

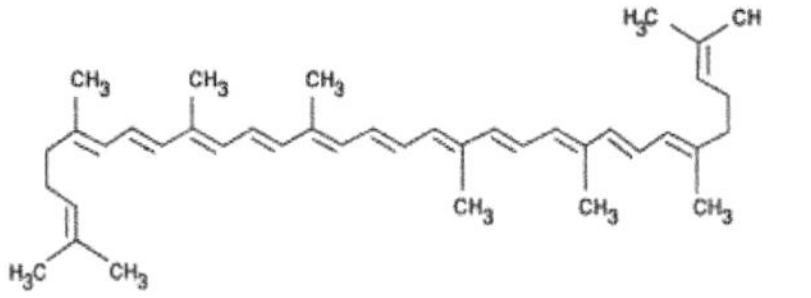

Lycopene

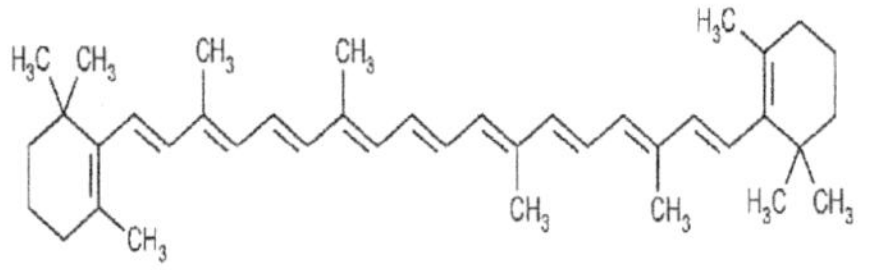

β - carotene

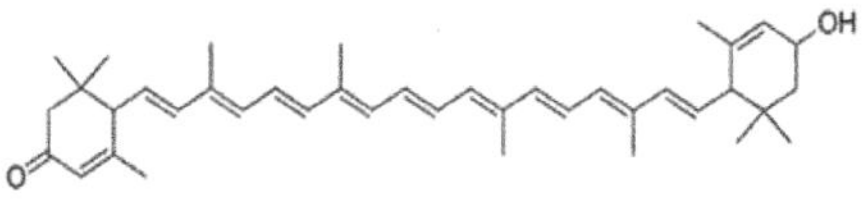

3′-hydroxy-ε,ε-caroten-3-one

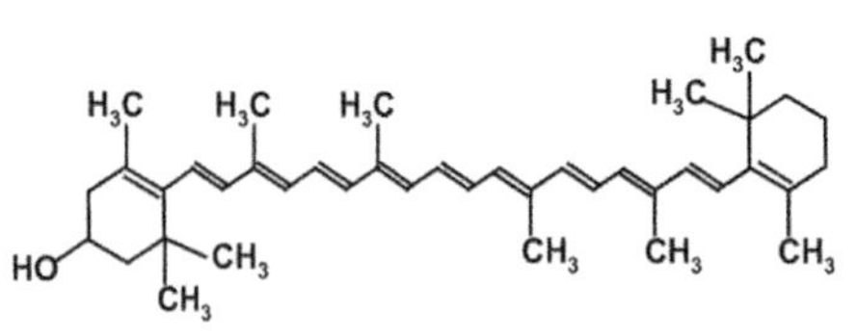

β - cryptoxanthin

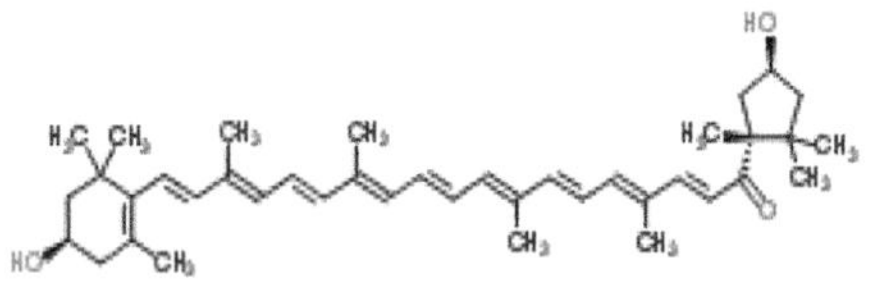

Capsanthin

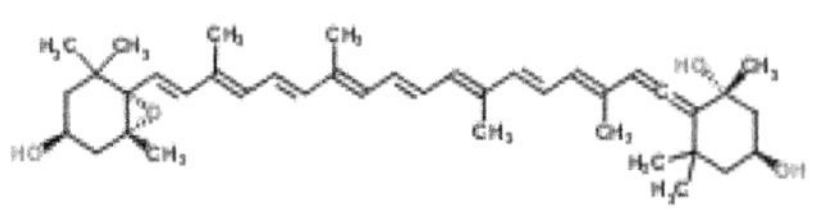

Neoxanthin

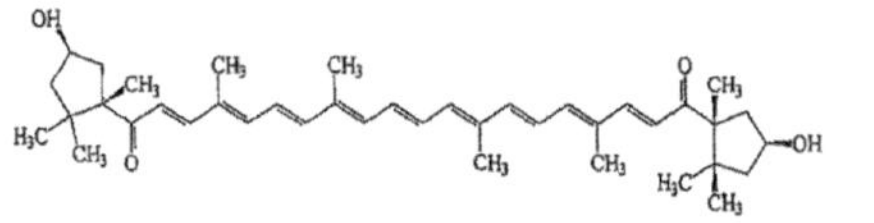

Casporubin

Fig. 1 Chemical structure of carotenoids which possess antiobese properties.

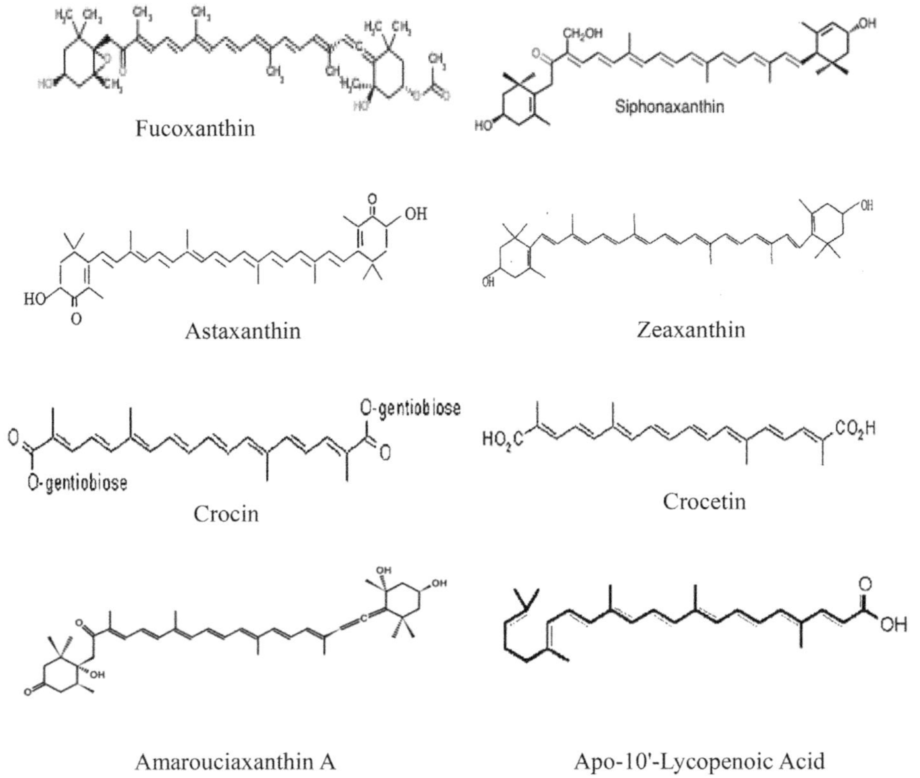

Fucoxanthin

Siphonaxanthin

Astaxanthin

Zeaxanthin

Crocin

Crocetin

Amarouciaxanthin A

Apo-10'-Lycopenoic Acid

Fig. 1 Cont'd

prominent role in plant kingdom during photosynthesis and also as natural colorants in food. The scientific evidence on the carotenoid biosynthetic pathway potentiates the diverse roles of carotenoids in photobiology, photochemistry, and also photomedicine (Pryor, Stahl, & Rock, 2000). Among the total 750 carotenoids identified, only 50 possess vitamin A activity. There are around 40 carotenoids form the constituents of human diet, whereas only 14 and some of their metabolic intermediates are detected in the human blood and tissues (Akoh & Min, 1997).

The unique antioxidant properties of carotenoids have uplifted their protective roles against chronic diseases such as cardiovascular diseases, cancers, cataracts, age-related macula degeneration, aging, and obesity (Bermudez, Ribaya-Mercado, Talegawkar, & Tucker, 2005; Bowen, Stacewicz-Sapuntzakis, & Diwadkar-Navsariwala, 2015; Pantavos et al., 2015; Rao & Rao, 2007). Although humans and animals cannot synthesize carotenoids de novo, their metabolism takes place in a characteristic manner (Kiokias, Proestos, & Varzakas, 2016). Dietary intake of carotenoids results in the absorption and transportation into blood circulation through sequential mechanisms (Erdman, Bierer, & Gugger, 1993). Cellular uptake of carotenoids by intestinal mucosa cells facilitates their transportation to the circulatory system (Berni, Chitchumroonchokchai, Canniatti-Brazaca, De Moura, & Failla, 2015). The carotenoids absorbed via passive diffusion follow the metabolism of chylomicron. The lipoprotein carrying carotenoids are taken up by the liver and are then released to the bloodstream (Faure et al., 1999). Carotenoids are found to accumulate in various human tissues like cervix, lung, skin, eye, liver, and adipose tissue (Li et al., 2014). Adipose tissue and liver are the main storage sites of carotenoids while adrenal glands, kidney, and testes are found to contain minor proportions. The serum concentration of carotenoids mainly depends on dietary intake, age, sex, geographic origin, seasonal variations, smoking, and drinking habits (Olmedilla, Granado, Blanco, & Rojas-Hidalgo, 1994).

Numerous epidemiological studies asserted that antioxidants like carotenoids could be used as an inexpensive means of preventing metabolic disorders (Riccioni, Gammone, & D'Orazio, 2015). According to the prudent individual daily intake (PIDI), the daily total carotenoid intake has been assumed to be 9.0–18.0 mg (Concepcion et al., 2018). The most common carotenoids found in the human diet are α/β-carotene, lycopene, lutein, zeaxanthin, β-cryptoxanthin, and astaxanthin. Epidemiological studies depict a positive link between the dietary intake and serum/tissue concentrations of carotenoids, which is associated with lower risk of chronic diseases (Agarwal & Rao, 2000; Gerster, 1997; Johnson, 2002). The consumption of the most common carotenoids such as β-carotene and lycopene is inversely related to the risk of cardiovascular diseases and certain cancers, while lutein and zeaxanthin are found to curtail eye-related disorders. Apart from the antioxidant nature of carotenoids, recent reports suggest that the biological roles of carotenoids also associated with dysregulated cell growth and gap junction communication, and modulated gene expression, immune response, and phase-I and II drug metabolizing enzymes (Astorg, 1997; Bertram, 1999; Jewell & O'Brien, 1999; Paiva & Russell, 1999). The multiple mechanistic approaches of carotenoids have uplifted the potentiality of these molecules in preventing chronic diseases. The antidiabetic, antiobesity (Maeda et al., 2006), cardio protective, and antiinflammatory properties (Di Pietro, Di Tomo, & Pandolfi, 2016) of carotenoids have paved the way for a positive approach to manage various metabolic diseases. The emerging scientific interest in exploring the innovative strategies of utilizing carotenoids against human diseases highlights the common etiological and molecular mechanistic approaches of the diseases. This chapter focuses on the promising role of carotenoids in the management/prevention of obesity and its related abnormalities. The possible molecular mechanisms of action of carotenoids in combating obesity are highlighted.

Molecular mechanisms of obesity

The accuracy and precision in maintaining the energy balance in the body are crucial as even a small error can create detrimental effect overtime (Goran, 2000). The process of metabolism plays a preferential role in maintaining the homeostatic equilibria, which entail physiological response to changing environmental condition. The metabolism of macronutrients is critical for channelizing the energy contained in food to usable cellular energy. The balance between energy intake and energy expenditure or the balance between energy fuels flow to the cells and release as cellular work determines the body size. The adipose tissue, an important site for lipid storage which actively participate in regulating energy homeostasis by synchronizing complex communications with other physiological systems and also within the tissue. The highly specialized adipocytes respond to hormonal and nutritional inputs for the storage of excess nutrients as intracellular lipids or it mobilizes the stored fat for utilization (Siersbæk et al., 2012). However, the role of adipocytes is not only confined to produce free fatty acids but also to secrete a large array of hormones, cytokines, chemokines, and growth factors. Synchronized regulation of metabolic pathways that balance the uptake, esterification, and hydrolysis of lipid is accomplished through the involvement of various protein kinases and nuclear receptors (Pol, Gross, & Parton, 2014). Metabolic regulation of adipocytes encompasses differentiation, biogenesis, and remodeling of adipocytes.

Obesity is associated with impaired or dysregulated adipose tissue that predisposes to metabolic dysfunction. Changes in the adipose tissue function and its secretion due to excess adipose tissue are linked to low-grade inflammation, developing insulin resistance, dyslipidemia, type 2 diabetes, and metabolic syndrome. Thus, adipose dysfunction is favored through the activation of the inflammatory pathway through the activation of inflammatory pathway, down-regulation of lipid turnover, and excess accumulation of fat in ectopic locations (Sam & Mazzone, 2014). Adipogenesis involves differentiation of mesenchymal stem cells into unipotent fibroblast-like preadipocytes, which then undergo marked changes in their gene expression and morphology to form mature lipid-rich adipocytes. The terminal differentiation of preadipocytes to mature adipocytes is mainly dependent on the transcription factors, peroxisome proliferator-activated receptor (PPAR)-γ, C/enhancer-binding protein (EBP)-α, FOXO-1, and other factors such as PCG-1α, sterol regulatory element-binding protein 1 (SREBP-1), and mTOR (Rosen & MacDougald, 2006). The mature adipocytes acquire insulin sensitivity, and express the fatty acid-binding protein (FABP/aP2), lipoprotein lipase (LPL), and glucose transporter 4 (GLUT4) on the cell surface that control the overall metabolic health (Stephens, 2012). Adipose tissue enlarges by hypertrophy (increased adipocyte size) and hyperplasia (increased adipocyte number) or both. Hypertrophy is associated with cell death and infiltration of inflammatory macrophages into adipose tissue (Cinti et al., 2005). As the mature adipocytes reach the diffusional limit of oxygen, hypoxia acts as the primary determinant for healthy expansion. Therefore, proper expansion requires especially coordinated responses among different cell types like endothelial cells and immune cells, and preadipocytes promoting adipose tissue remodeling (Sun, Kusminski, & Scherer, 2011). But, dysregulated hypertrophy- and hyperplasia-mediated adipocyte expansion leads to a myriad of effects including hypoxia, apoptosis, elevated chemokine secretion, and impaired free fatty acid refluxes (Sun & Scherer, 2010). Besides, insulin resistance due to adipose hypertrophy affects the glucose metabolism which is a principle switch between lipolysis/fatty acid oxidation. Chronic elevated threshold of insulin resistance plays a key role in the pathophysiology of obesity (Shi, Ansari, McGuinness, Wasserman, & Johnson, 2013). Hypertrophic obesity is associated with an infiltration of macrophage into the adipose tissue which in turn promotes the induction of pro-inflammatory factors such as interleukin (IL)-6, monocyte chemotactic protein 1 (MCP-1), IL-8, and tumor necrosis factor α (TNF-α) (Weisberg et al., 2003).

The elevated levels of pro-inflammatory cytokines also contribute to insulin resistance by inhibiting insulin-dependent glucose uptake which is also a prime factor of obesity (Xu et al., 2003).

Epidemiological studies authenticate that carotenoids and their derivatives act as nutritional regulators of adipose tissue homeostasis (Bonet, Canas, Ribot, & Palou, 2015). Extensively studied carotenoids in this context are fucoxanthin (Maeda et al., 2006), fucoxanthinol (Maeda, Kanno, Kodate, Hosokawa, & Miyashita, 2015), β-carotene (Kameji, Mochizuki, Miyoshi, & Goda, 2010), cryptoxanthin (Shirakura, Takayanagi, Mukai, Tanabe, & Inoue, 2011), astaxanthin (Ikeuchi, Koyama, Takahashi, & Yazawa, 2007), neoxanthin (Okada et al., 2008), capsanthin (Jo et al., 2017), lycopene (Zeng, He, Jia, & Hao, 2017), siphonoxanthin, zeaxanthin (Liu et al., 2018), and together with 3′-hydroxy-ε,ε-carotene-3-one (Kotake-Nara, Hase, Kobayashi, & Nagao, 2016). Recently, researchers are most interested to explore the potential roles of these compounds on the essential aspects of adipose tissue biology by focusing adipocyte differentiation, adipocyte metabolism, oxidative stress and adipose tissue-derived regulatory signals, and inflammation. Reports demonstrate that carotenoids and their derivatives negatively regulate adipogenesis and adipocyte hypertrophy by increasing fatty acid oxidation in brown and white adipocytes (Bonet et al., 2015). Studies on assessment of the daily intake, blood levels, and adipocyte content of carotenoids report a negative impact on the intensity of obesity. Although sparse, specifically designed human intervention studies indicate that carotenoid supplementation is beneficial in ameliorating abdominal adiposity (Bonet et al., 2015).

Antiobese properties of carotenoids

Effect on adipocyte differentiation

Adipocyte differentiation or adipogenesis is a multistep process characterized by the formation of adipocytes from the precursor cells (White & Stephens, 2010). The process of adipogenesis is attributed by an increased insulin sensitivity, and altered cell morphology and secretory capacity of the cells. Differentiation of preadipocytes is initiated when the committed preadipocytes withdraw from cell cycle before the adipose conversion. Upon hormonal induction, the growth-arrested proliferative preadipocytes reenter the cell cycle and undergo mitotic clonal expansion leading to terminal differentiation (Fajas, 2003). At this stage, the cells acquire characteristics of mature adipocyte where they attain specialized machinery required for lipid transport and synthesis, insulin action, and the secretion of adipocyte-specific proteins. Adipocyte differentiation is controlled by a cascade of transactivation factors and cell cycle regulatory proteins (Lefterova & Lazar, 2009). The molecular regulation of adipogenesis occurs primarily at the transcriptional level. Several transcription factors mainly the PPAR-γ and CCAAT/EBP-α (C/EBP-α) coordinate the expression of genes that create and maintain the adipocyte phenotype (Zhao, Gregoire, & Sul, 2000). In the initial stage of adipocyte differentiation, there is a rapid induction in the expression of C/EBP-α, C/EBP-β, and C/EBP-δ, the key regulators of adipogenesis. The targets of C/EBP-β and C/EBP-δ are the genes that encode key adipogenic transcription factors, PPAR-γ and C/EBP-α, and the regulators of the lipogenic gene, SREBP-1. PPAR-γ activates the promoter of the gene that encodes C/EBP-α and vice versa. During the terminal phase of differentiation, activation of the transcriptional cascade of PPAR-γ and C/EBP-α regulates the expression of the genes involved in insulin sensitivity, lipogenesis, and lipolysis, including GLUT4, FABP4 (aP2), LPL, *sn*-1-acylglycerol-3-phosphate acyltransferase 2 (AGPAT2), perilipin, and the secreted factors adiponectin and leptin resulting in the development of mature adipocytes (Payne et al., 2010; Rosen & MacDougald, 2006; White & Stephens, 2010).

Despite the presence of carotenoids in serum and tissues, with the recent bioavailability reports, it is evident that adipose tissue is a major storage site for carotenoids (El-Sohemy et al., 2002). The antiobesity actions of carotenoids have recently been received considerable attention as high serum carotenoid is found to associate with lower risk of metabolic syndrome (Sugiura et al., 2006). Carotenoids and their metabolites are shown to exert vivid health beneficial properties including antiadipogenic effect (Kotake-Nara et al., 2016). Carotenoids such as fucoxanthin, siphonaxanthin, neoxanthin, β-carotene, and β-cryptoxanthin have been reported to inhibit adipocyte differentiation and thereby reduce the cellular triacylglycerol (TAG) levels (Lobo et al., 2010; Maeda et al., 2006; Shirakura et al., 2011).

In this aspect, 3′-hydroxy-ε,ε-caroten-3-one, a metabolite of lutein inhibited adipocyte differentiation in 3T3-L1 adipocyte cells, and reduced triglyceride (TG) production (Kotake-Nara et al., 2016). Zeaxanthin, a major xanthophyll carotenoid exists abundantly in eggs, yellow corn, orange pepper, and paprika showed an efficient antiobesity effect by significantly decreasing the intracellular lipid accumulation in adipocytes. Upon zeaxanthin treatment, the progression of obesity was found to be attenuated in high-fat diet (HFD) fed animals, and improved dyslipidemia. Zeaxanthin treatment enhanced the phosphorylation of adenosine monophosphate-activated protein kinase (AMPK) in differentiated 3T3-L1 cells as well as in epididymal adipose tissues of HFD-fed mice (Liu et al., 2018).

β-Cryptoxanthin, a carotenoid found in mango, papaya, and persimmon was found to reduce the level of intracellular lipids in 3T3-L1 adipocyte cells (Shirakura et al., 2011). The study demonstrated that β-cryptoxanthin activates the members of retinoic acid receptor (RAR) family and subsequently down-regulates the mRNA expression of PPAR-γ during adipocyte differentiation. Neoxanthin is an intermediate carotenoid in the synthesis of abscisic acid from violaxanthin (Kim et al., 2011). Neoxanthin is present in *Undaria pinnatifida*, *Amaranthus viridis*, *Gynandrophi spentaphylla*, and *Phyllanthus niruri*. Adipocytes treated with neoxanthin exhibited an effective reduction in lipid accumulation and glycerol-6-phosphate dehydrogenase (GPDH) activity. Furthermore, neoxanthin treatment reduced the mRNA expressions of the major transcription factors C/EBP-α and PPAR-γ (Okada et al., 2008). The authors hypothesize that the presence of allele bond and an additional hydroxyl group on the side chain may be contributed to the suppressive effect on adipocyte differentiation in 3T3-L1 cells.

Crocin is an active carotenoid present in *Crocus sativus* L. (saffron) showed enhanced inhibition of adipocyte differentiation. Crocin affected the energy homeostasis by significantly increasing AMPK protein expression, a key regulator of energy homeostasis (Kianbakht & Hashem Dabaghian, 2015). Obese Wistar rats treated with saffron extract significantly reduced body weight, food intake and leptin levels, and increased insulin sensitivity. Crocin treatment significantly down-regulates the expression of PPAR-γ (Gul, Balkhi, & Haq, 2017).

Siphonaxanthin, a xanthophyll carotenoid, is found in green algae such as *Codium fragile, Caulerpa lentillifera*, and *Umbraulva japonica* (Takaichi, 2011). Studies emphasize that the presence of an additional hydroxyl group in its C19 may contribute to its potential health beneficial effects including its potential role in adipogenesis (Ganesan et al., 2011; Sugawara, Ganesan, Li, Manabe, & Hirata, 2014). Siphonaxanthin significantly inhibited the cytosolic lipid accumulation in differentiated preadipocyte (3T3-L1) cells (Li et al., 2014). They found that the effect of siphonaxanthin was largely limited to the early stages of adipocyte differentiation. The study further demonstrated that it significantly inhibited the expressions of key adipogenic genes, including C/EBP-α, PPAR-γ, FABP4, and stearoyl-CoA desaturase 1 (SCD1). Further, oral administration of siphonaxanthin to KK-Ay mice significantly decreased the total weight of WAT, especially the mesenteric WAT. Daily administration of siphonaxanthin for 6 weeks inhibited lipogenesis and increased fatty acid oxidation in adipose tissue. Two to threefold higher accumulation of siphonaxanthin was observed in mesenteric WAT than in epididymal and perirenal WAT (Li et al., 2014). Inhibitory potential of carotenoids on adipocyte differentiation is illustrated in Fig. 2.

Fucoxanthinol, a metabolite of a common and major carotenoid, fucoxanthin is shown to exert its inhibitory activity on the differentiation of 3T3-L1 preadipocytes. The antiadipogenic activity of fucoxanthinol was found to be stronger than fucoxanthin. Fucoxanthinol exhibited suppressive effects on lipid accumulation and GPDH activity. Also, adipocyte cells treated with fucoxanthin and fucoxanthinol, down-regulated PPAR-α in a dose-dependent manner. These results demonstrate that fucoxanthin and fucoxanthinol potently inhibit adipogenesis through down-regulation of PPAR-α (Maeda et al., 2015). Astaxanthin, an oxygenated carotenoid was found to consider as a novel selective modulator of PPAR (PPAR-γ). Astaxanthin antagonized the process of adipocyte

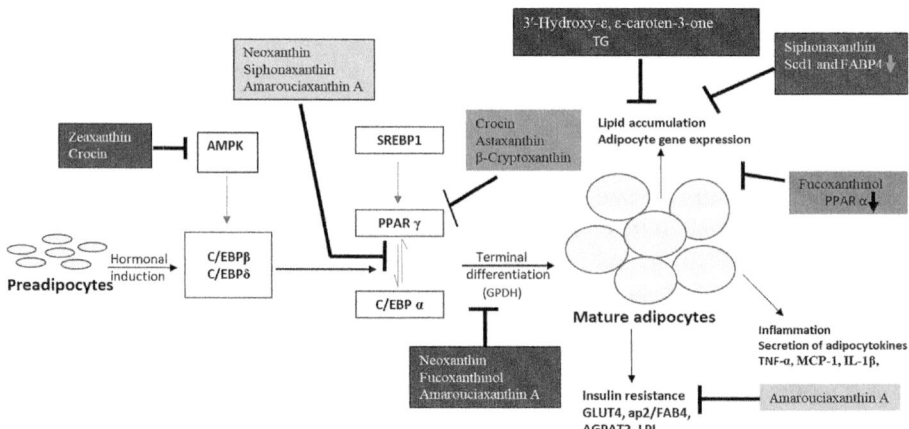

Fig. 2 Effect of carotenoids on adipocyte differentiation.

differentiation, lipid accumulation, and the transcriptional activation induced by PPAR-γ agonist rosiglitazone (RGZ) by suppressing ap2 and LPL mRNA. The molecular interaction studies between PPAR-γ and co-activators CREB-binding protein (CBP), SRC-1, TIF-2, and PGC-1 showed that astaxanthin increased the interactions of PPAR-γ with TIF-2 and SRC-1 but not with CBP which showed that expression of CBP is essential for the activation of PPAR-γ and adipocyte differentiation (Inoue et al., 2012).

Amarouciaxanthin A, a dominant metabolite of fucoxanthin has reported having a strong suppressive effect on adipocytes differentiation in comparison to other derivatives of fucoxanthin like isofucoxanthinol, fucoxanthinol, and amarouciaxanthin B. It has shown the suppressive effect on adipocyte differentiation by down-regulating two key adipogenic transcriptional factors, PPAR-γ and C/EBP-α. Amarouciaxanthin A treatment resulted in a significant reduction in GPDH activity, an indicator of adipocyte differentiation. Further, it down-regulated FABP (aP2), LPL, and GLUT4 in 3T3-L1 adipocytes cells (Yim et al., 2011) (Table 1).

Table 1 Effect of carotenoids on the molecular mechanism underlying adipocyte differentiation

Carotenoids	Experiment-al model	Molecular mechanism	References
Lutein	3T3-L1	• Reduce TG level	Kotake-Nara et al. (2016)
Zeaxanthin	3T3-L1	• Inhibit AMPK phosphorylation • Reduce intracellular lipid accumulation • Improved dyslipidemia	Daval, Foufelle, and Ferré (2006) Liu et al. (2018)
β-Cryptoxanthin	3T3-L1	• Down-regulate mRNA expression of PPARγ	Shirakura et al. (2011)
Neoxanthin	3T3-L1	• Reduce mRNA expression of CEBP-α and PPARγ • Reduce glycerol-6-phosphate dehydrogenase (GPDH) activity • Decrease lipid accumulation	Okada et al. (2008)
Siphonaxanthin	3T3-L1; KK-Ay mice	• Inhibit c/EBPα, PPARγ, FABP4 and scd1 • Retard cytosolic lipid accumulation • In vivo, reduce WAT by decreasing lipogenesis and enhance fatty acid oxidation	Li et al. (2014)

Continued

Table 1   Continued

Carotenoids	Experiment-al model	Molecular mechanism	References
Fucoxanthin/ fucoxanthinol	3T3-L1	• Decrease GPDH activity • Down-regulate PPARγ expression • Suppress lipid accumulation	Maeda et al. (2015)
Astaxanthin	3T3-L1	• Modulates PPARγ expression • Suppress mRNA expression of aP2 and LPL • Increase PPARγ interaction with TIF2 and SRC • Antagonize adipocyte differentiation • Prevent lipid accumulation	Inoue et al. (2012)
Crocin	3T3-L1; obese wistar rats	• Maintain energy homeostasis by upregulating AMPK expression • Inhibit adipocyte differentiation • In vivo, down-regulate PPARγ expression • Increase insulin sensitivity	Kianbakht and Hashem Dabaghian (2015)
Amarociaxanthin A	3T3-L1	• Down-regulated PPARγ and C/EBPα expression • Reduce GDPH activity • Down-regulated aP2, LPL and GLUT 4	Yim et al. (2011)

Effect on inflammation-mediated obesity

Since obesity is an over nutritive condition, it impairs the systemic metabolic homeostasis through adipocyte hypertrophy, hypoxia, and stress in the adipose tissue, which obviously leads to an elevated inflammatory response in adipose tissue. Obesity and inflammation are a highly coordinated process in the pathogenesis of insulin resistance, diabetes, atherosclerosis, and nonalcoholic fatty liver diseases (NAFLD) (Blüher, 2009). An inflammatory process up-regulated in the metabolically active sites like WAT, liver, and immune cells determine the circulating levels of pro-inflammatory cytokines (Lago, Dieguez, Gómez-Reino, & Gualillo, 2007; Lago, Gómez, Gómez-Reino, Dieguez, & Gualillo, 2009; Wozniak, Gee, Wachtel, & Frezza, 2009). Macrophage infiltration, the prime factor that links obesity with increased BMI and adipocyte hypertrophy (Cancello & Clement, 2006; Harman-Boehm et al., 2007). Excessive secretion of MCP-1 and colony-stimulating factors 1 and 3 by mature adipocyte attract monocytes from the blood circulation. Increased levels of TNF-α, IL-6, IL-1β, and resistin by the activated macrophages, and up-regulation of NF-κB pathway contribute to insulin resistance in the adipose depots. This inflammatory condition in the expanded adipose tissue mass is responsible for altered adipokines and obesity-related insulin resistance (Tomas et al., 2002).

Modulatory effects of carotenoids on inflammation associated markers of obesity is shown in Fig. 3. Lycopene, the major carotenoid in tomatoes, watermelons, red grape fruits, and guava was evaluated for its antiobesity property, and the results showed that this carotenoid improves glucose tolerance in HFD-fed mice. Lycopene notably prevented HFD-induced IL-1β, TNF-α, and C-reactive protein (CRP) levels in mice fed with HFD (Zeng et al., 2017). Beta-carotene is one of the most abundant carotenoids in green leafy vegetables has a potent antioxidant property which renders its role in preventing metabolic diseases. Beta-carotene treatment at 10 μM reduced the expression of genes related to insulin sensitivity in 3T3-L1 adipocyte cells. The cellular accumulation of β-carotene eliminated reactive oxygen species (ROS) induced by TNF-α thereby reducing the gene expression of adiponectin, adipocyte lipid-binding protein (ALBP), GLUT4 and their transcriptional factor, PPAR-γ in insulin resistant adipocytes. These results showed that β-carotene accumulation restores ROS levels and promotes the expression of genes related to insulin sensitivity (Kameji et al., 2010).

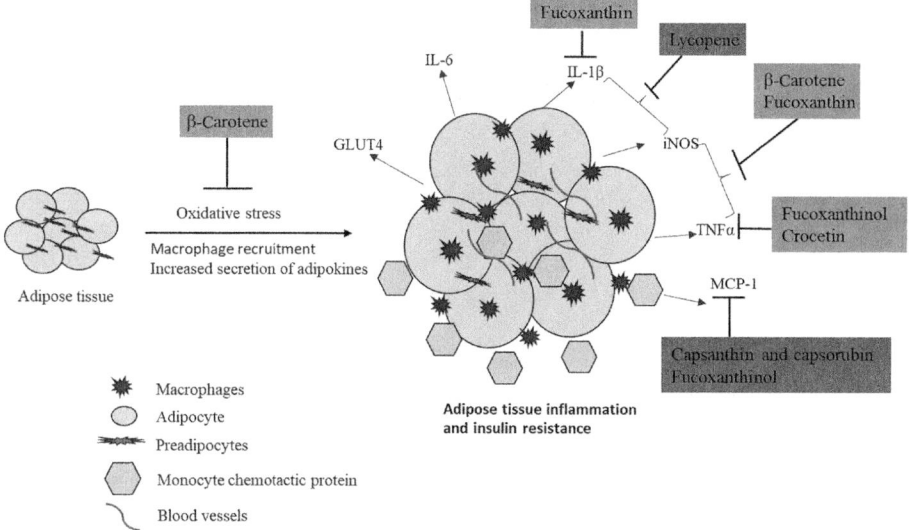

Fig. 3 Effect of carotenoids on inflammation-associated obesity.

Capsanthin and capsorubin, the major carotenoids of paprika were evaluated for their effects on adipocytokines secretion, and the data showed a suppressive effect on chronic inflammation in 3T3-L1 adipocyte cells. Paprika pigments treatment was shown to recover the insulin resistance by promoting differentiation, and up-regulating adiponectin mRNA expression and secretion in 3T3-L1 cells. Capsanthin and capsorubin attenuated inflammatory changes when the adipocytes were co-cultured with macrophage by suppressing the mRNA expression of IL-6, TNF-α, MCP-1, and resistin. From these results, it is apparent that capsanthin and capsorubin ameliorated inflammatory changes in 3T3-L1 adipocyte cells induced by macrophage migration (Maeda, Saito, Nakamura, & Maoka, 2013). Crocetin, a derivative of saffron was found to improve the impaired insulin sensitivity and dysregulated expression of TNF-α and adiponectin induced by palmitate in rat adipocyte (Xi, Qian, Xu, Zhou, & Sun, 2007).

Fucoxanthin, a marine carotenoid significantly inhibited obesity-induced up-regulation of IL-1β, TNF-α, iNOS, and COX-2 in HFD-fed mice. It further suppressed maleic dialdehyde (MDA) and infiltration of polymorpho nuclear cells (PMNs) which depicts that supplementation of fucoxanthin might be a favoring strategy for blocking macrophage-mediated inflammation and inflammation-induced obesity (Tan & Hou, 2014). Fucoxanthinol found to suppress low-grade chronic inflammation by down-regulating the mRNA and protein levels TNF-α and MCP-1 in a coculture system of adipocytes and macrophages cells (Maeda et al., 2015) (Table 2).

Effect on thermogenesis

Energy balance is often referred to the result of an equilibrium between energy intake and energy expenditure. When energy intake exceeds expenditure, the excess energy is stored as body tissue, which is the major driver of weight gain. Although adipocytes possess the capacity of storing surplus energy in the form of lipids, they also can transform chemical energy into heat. The BAT is a specialized tissue that contains an increased number of mitochondria which dissipate energy in the form of heat by the nonshivering thermogenesis. The elevated expression of UCP1 in the inner mitochondrial membrane of BAT is the critical player that dissipate the pH-gradient generated by oxidative phosphorylation through releasing chemical energy as heat (Ntambi & Young-Cheul, 2000). In addition to UCP-1, brown adipocytes differ from WAT at the molecular level by expressing high levels of type 2 iodothyronine deiodinase (DIO2), transcription co-regulators, PRDM16 and PGC-1α, and the regulators of lipolysis (Gesta et al., 2007). BAT being highly vascularized and densely innervated by the sympathetic nervous system, it is activated by cold exposure and increased caloric intake. The sympathetic activation of BAT results in increased expression of thermogenic genes, and recruitment of enzymes required for uptake, mobilization, and oxidation of lipids (Townsend & Tseng, 2014).

UCP-1 gene expression is stimulated by various factors like β3-agonists, adrenergic stimulation, and thyroid hormones, whose dysfunction results in weight gain, a significant co-factor for the development of obesity (Ntambi & Young-Cheul, 2000). UCP-1, the long-chain fatty acid-activated protein which catalyzes the proton leak

Table 2 Effect of carotenoids on inflammation-associated obesity

Carotenoids	Experimental model	Molecular mechanism	References
Lycopene	High fat diet (HFD) fed mice	• Down-regulate IL-1β, TNFα and CRP level • Increase glucose tolerance	Zeng et al. (2017)
β-Carotene	3T3-L1	• Down-regulate adiponectin, adipocyte lipid binding protein, GLUT4 and PPARγ	Kameji et al. (2010)
Capsaxanthin/ casporubin	Coculture of 3T3-L1 and RAW246.7	• Attenuate I-L6, TNFα, MCP1 and resistin mRNA expression • Improved insulin resistance	Maeda et al. (2013)
Fucoxanthin	HFD fed mice	• Inhibits IL 1β, TNFα, iNOS and COX2 • Suppress MDA and PMNs • Block macrophage-mediated inflammation-induced obesity	Tan and Hou (2014)
Fucoxanthinol	Coculture of 3T3-L1 and RAW246.7	• Down-regulate mRNA expression of TNF α and MCP 1 • Suppress low-grade chronic inflammation	Maeda et al. (2015)
Crocetin	Rat model	• Improve insulin sensitivity • Reduced adiponectin and disordered TNF-α	Xi et al. (2007)

across the inner membrane of mitochondria dissipating the electrochemical gradient that has been generated via electron transport chain (ETC) (Bartelt et al., 2011; Fedorenko, Lishko, & Kirichok, 2012; Krauss, Zhang, & Lowell, 2005). Cells lacking UCP1 dissipate this proton gradient only through the formation of ATP via complex V (ATP synthase) in the ETC. Under physiological stimuli, chronic cold exposure, hormonal stimuli such as irisin and pharmacological treatment with PPAR-γ agonist or β-adrenergic stimuli, a brown fat-like gene expression program is activated in WAT. This process is known as browning where WAT takes up the characteristics of BAT including increased expression of UCP1, multilocular lipid droplets, and mitochondria numbers. Indeed, browning of WAT has been shown to have antiobesity and antidiabetic effects in rodents (Wu, Cohen, & Spiegelman, 2013).

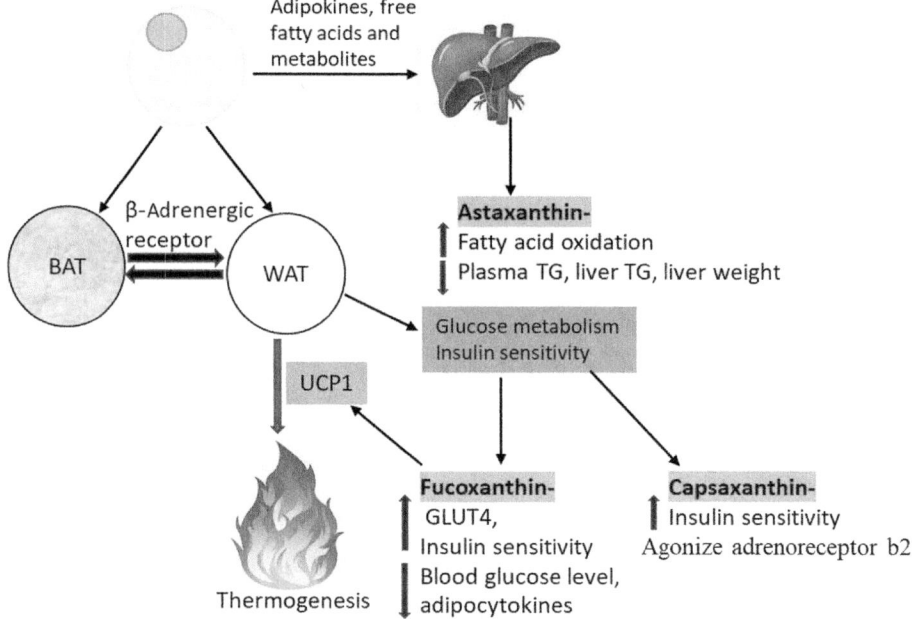

Fig. 4 Effect of carotenoids on thermogenesis in obesity.

Effect of carotenoids on thermogenesis is outlined in Fig. 4. In vitro and in vivo studies indicate that carotenoids and carotenoid derivatives have a greater impact on fatty acid oxidation and thermogenesis (Bonet et al., 2015). Capsanthin, a major carotenoid present in *Capsicum annuum* L. effectively inhibited adipogenesis in the 3T3-L1 cell model. The pharmacological activity of capsanthin on adipogenesis was found to be mainly due to its adrenoceptor-b2-agonistic activity. Capsanthin treatment enhanced the production of ATP through its adrenoceptor b2-agonistic activity in HFD-fed mice. It also improves insulin sensitivity by activating AMPK which is a key regulator of energy homeostasis (Jo et al., 2017).

The nutrigenomics studies reveal that fucoxanthin, a characteristic carotenoid belongs to the group of xanthophylls containing an allenic bond and two hydroxyl groups, favors up-regulation of UCP1 in abdominal WAT mitochondria. It increases the amount of energy, which is generated as heat in fat tissue, thus stimulating thermogenesis and fatty acid oxidation (Kozak & Anunciado-Koza, 2009). Fucoxanthin also improved insulin resistance and decreased blood glucose levels through the down-regulation of adipocytokines and up-regulated GLUT4 in skeletal muscle (Maeda et al., 2015).

Astaxanthin, a major carotenoid present in shrimp, exerts its antiobesity effect by decreasing body weight and adipose tissue weight caused by a HFD. Also, astaxanthin reduced liver weight, liver triglyceride, plasma triglyceride, and total cholesterol in HFD-fed mice. Besides that, this carotenoid increased fatty acid oxidation and stimulated thermogenesis, but the exact mechanism has to be delineated (Ikeuchi et al., 2007) (Table 3).

Table 3 Effect of carotenoids on thermogenesis linked with obesity

Carotenoids	Cell line model	Molecular mechanism	References
Fucoxanthin	Skeletal muscle cell	• Up-regulate UCP1 and stimulate fatty acid oxidation • Increase GLUT4 expression • Down-regulate adipocytokines • Stimulate thermogenesis and improve insulin resistance	Maeda et al. (2015) and Kozak and Anunciado-Koza (2009)
Capsaxanthin	3T3-L1; HFD fed mice	• Adrenoreceptor-b2 activity • Phosphorylates AMPK and improves insulin sensitivity • Accelerates oxidation of fatty acid	Jo et al. (2017)
Astaxanthin	HFD fed mice	• Increase fatty acid oxidation and thermogenesis	Ikeuchi et al. (2007)

Effect on lipogenesis

Excessive accumulation of fat is determined by the imbalance between fat synthesis (lipogenesis) and fat breakdown (lipolysis/fatty acid oxidation). Lipogenesis takes place both in the liver and adipose tissue, which comprises the process of fatty acid synthesis and subsequent triglyceride synthesis (Rosen & Spiegelman, 2000). Diet rich in carbohydrate stimulates lipogenesis leading to increased postprandial plasma TG levels, whereas unsaturated fatty acids suppress lipogenesis by inhibiting enzymes that are involved in fatty acid synthesis (Jump, Clarke, Thelen, & Liimatta, 1994). Fasting reduces lipogenesis in adipose tissue, but it increases lipolysis leading to net loss of TGs in adipocytes. In liver, TG synthesis is increased due to increased fatty acid arrival from adipocytes. Lipogenesis is positively regulated by insulin, recruitment of GLUTs, and the activation of lipogenic and glycolytic enzymes (Assimacopoulos-Jeannet, Brichard, Rencurel, Cusin, & Jeanrenaud, 1995).

The conversion of glucose to fatty acids is nutritionally regulated by glucose and insulin signaling pathways. Insulin and glucose trigger the activation of few major intracellular kinases [protein kinase B (AKT), protein kinase C (PKC), mammalian target of rapamycin (mTOR) ½] and phosphatases (PP1 and PP2) which control the activation of transcription factors such as SREBP, liver X receptors (LXRs), and carbohydrate-responsive element-binding protein (ChREBP). These transcription factors induce genes that encode lipogenic enzymes such as acetyl-CoA carboxylase 1

(ACC1), fatty acid synthase (FAS), and SCD1 (Wang, Viscarra, Kim, & Sul, 2015). Nuclear receptor, LXRα is activated by ligands like endogenous oxysterols forming a heterodimer with retinoid X receptor (RXR), which is activated by 9 *cis*-retinoic acid. LXRα activation in turn induces the expression of target genes including nuclear transcription factor, SREBP-1c. Several reports described as an enhanced expression of LXRα, SREBP, and ChREBP in fatty liver diseases (Higuchi et al., 2008).

Inhibitory effects of carotenoids on lipid biosynthetic pathway is shown in Fig. 5. Lycopene, a lipophilic nonprovitamin A carotenoid reported to display antiinflammatory activity in adipose tissue (Gouranton et al., 2011; Marcotorchino et al., 2012) and liver (Ip et al., 2013; Luvizotto et al., 2013; Wang, Ausman, Greenberg, Russell, & Wang, 2010) was evaluated for its inhibitory effect on hepatosteatosis and lipid metabolism in liver of HFD-fed animals. Lycopene found to regulate hepatosteatosis and lipid metabolism by effectively down-regulating the expression of transcription factor SREBP-1c. Lycopene supplementation reduced the expression of key genes of fatty acid synthesis and lipid metabolism such as FAS and acetyl-CoA carboxylase, aP2, Cd36, and LPL. Lycopene treatment also increased the expression of genes involved in fatty acid β-oxidation such as Cpt-1 and Acox and PPAR-α (Fenni et al., 2017). Further, lycopene administration was found to prevent expression and phosphorylation of STAT3 in the liver (Zeng et al., 2017).

In a recent demonstration, a biologically active metabolite of lycopene, apo-10′-lycopenoic acid (ALA) was analyzed for its effect on steatosis induced by a liquid HFD in male *ob/ob* mice. ALA supplementation markedly decreased steatosis by increasing the mRNA and protein levels of SIRT1, a NAD+-dependent protein deacetylase which is a key regulator of lipid homeostasis. The increased SIRT1 activity was associated with lower levels of acetylated forkhead box class O1 (FOXO1) protein levels. Also, ALA down-regulated the mRNA levels of ACC1.

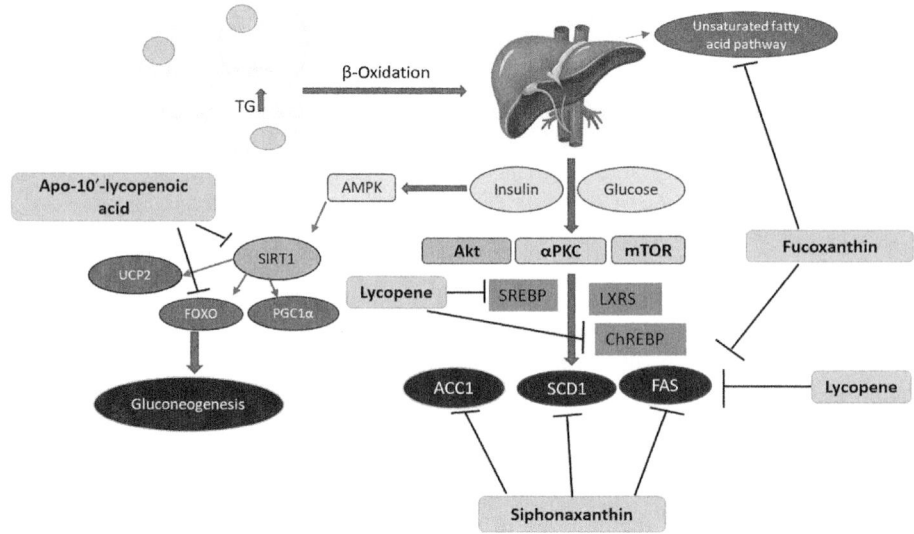

Fig. 5 Effect of carotenoid on lipogenesis.

These results together suggest that the lycopene metabolite, ALA protects from the development of steatosis in ob/ob mice by up-regulating SIRT1 gene expression and activity (Chung et al., 2012).

Studies using HEPG2 cells treated with siphonaxanthin exhibited a strong inhibitory effect on aggravated hepatic lipogenesis. Siphonaxanthin significantly suppressed the excess accumulation of triacylglycerol induced by LXR (LXRα) agonist. Further, it down-regulated the expression of a nuclear transcription factor, SREBP-1c and lipogenic enzymes, FAS, SCD1, and ACC1. Siphonaxanthin also down-regulated the expression of fatty acid translocase (CD36) and FABP1, which are responsible for uptake and transportation of fatty acids. Further, it blocked LXRα activation. From these results, it was assumed that the siphonaxanthin might be a promising candidate as an antagonist of LXRα in NAFLD (Zheng et al., 2018).

Fucoxanthin-treated HFD-fed C57BL/6N mice showed increased fatty acid oxidation and decreased hepatic lipid contents with inhibited hepatic lipogenic enzymes such as glucose-6-phosphate dehydrogenase, malic enzymes, FAS, and phosphatide phosphohydrolase (Woo et al., 2010). Also, fucoxanthin treatment reduced the hepatic glycogen content by significantly up-regulating glycolytic enzymes such as glucokinase in the liver, which further increased the ratio of hepatic glucokinase/ glucose 6 phosphatase and glycogen content (Park, Lee, Park, Shin, & Choi, 2011). Male Wistar rats and female KK-Ay mice supplemented with *Undaria pinnatifida,* a rich source of fucoxanthin, enhanced the content of docosahexanoic acid only in the liver but not in the intestine. Also, fucoxanthin-fed mice showed an increase in arachidonic acid content in liver indicates that fucoxanthin might modify the metabolic pathways of ω-3 and ω-6 unsaturated fatty acids (Airanthi et al., 2011; Tsukui et al., 2007) (Table 4).

Table 4   Effect of carotenoids on lipogenesis

Carotenoids	Experimental model	Molecular mechanism	References
Siphonaxanthin	HepG2	• Down-regulate SREBP-1c • Reduce FAS, ACC-1 and SCD1 expression • Down-regulate CD36 and FABP1 expression • Block LXRα activation	Zheng et al. (2018)
Fucoxanthin	HFD C57BL/6N Male Wistar rats/ female KK-Ay mice	• Enhance DHA and AA • Modify metabolic ω 6 and ω 3 pathway	Tsukui et al. (2007) and Airanthi et al. (2011)

Continued

Table 4   Continued

Carotenoids	Experimental model	Molecular mechanism	References
Lycopene	HFD fed mice	• Down-regulate SREBP1c expression • Reduce FAS, aP2, Cd36 and LPL • Suppress SREBP-1c, FAS and ACC-1 expression • Prevent phosphorylation of STAT3	Luvizotto et al. (2013), Wang et al. (2010), Ip et al. (2013), Fenni et al. (2017), and Zeng et al. (2017)
Apo-10′-lycopenoic acid (ALA)	HFD fed ob/ob male mice	• Decrease steatosis by up-regulation of SIRTI • Down-regulate FOXO1 and ACOX expression	Chung et al., 2012

Conclusions

Humans do no biosynthesize carotenoids, but they exert a vital role in human health and disease prevention. The emerging scientific interest in exploring the novel functions of carotenoids against metabolic diseases underlines the common etiological and molecular mechanistic approaches of the diseases. This chapter summarizes the antiobese properties of carotenoids with a special focus on the molecular mechanisms of adipocyte differentiation, inflammation, thermogenesis, and lipogenesis. Data collected from the available literature emphasize that carotenoids have vast potency in ameliorating obesity and related dysfunctions. More interestingly, the derivatives of carotenoid attributed more potent antiobese activity than the parent molecule. The antiobese capacity of carotenoids shown in epidemiological and human intervention studies might be through the reported molecular mechanisms by which carotenoids exert their effect. Apart from having various disease preventive roles of carotenoids, from a powerful antioxidant to anticarcinogenic molecule, this chapter highlights the preventive role of carotenoids against obesity, which propose a strategy to utilize these bioactive molecules for nutraceutical applications toward the management of obesity.

Acknowledgments

The authors acknowledge the award of Junior Research Fellowship by the University Grants Commission (UGC), and the Department of Biotechnology (DBT), New Delhi, India. Sowmya Shree G and Tehreem M thank the Academy of Scientific and Innovative Research (AcSIR), New Delhi. The authors acknowledge the Director, CSIR-CFTRI for the constant support to carry out this work.

References

Agarwal, S., & Rao, A.V. (2000). Carotenoids and chronic diseases. *Drug Metabolism and Drug Interactions, 17*(1–4), 189–210.

Ahima, R. S., & Flier, J. S. (2000). Adipose tissue as an endocrine organ. *Trends in Endocrinology and Metabolism, 11*(8), 327–332.

Airanthi, M. W. A., Sasaki, N., Iwasaki, S., Baba, N., Abe, M., Hosokawa, M., et al. (2011). Effect of brown seaweed lipids on fatty acid composition and lipid hydroperoxide levels of mouse liver. *Journal of Agricultural and Food Chemistry, 59*(8), 4156–4163.

Akoh, C. C., & Min, B. D. (1997). *Food lipid chemistry, nutrition and biotechnology.* New York: Marcel Dekker.

Assimacopoulos-Jeannet, F., Brichard, S., Rencurel, F., Cusin, I., & Jeanrenaud, B. (1995). In vivo effects of hyperinsulinemia on lipogenic enzymes and glucose transporter expression in rat liver and adipose tissues. *Metabolism, 44*(2), 228–233.

Astorg, P. (1997). Food carotenoids and cancer prevention: An overview of current research. *Trends in Food Science & Technology, 8*(12), 406–413.

Balistreri, C. R., Caruso, C., & Candore, G. (2010). The role of adipose tissue and adipokines in obesity-related inflammatory diseases. *Mediators of Inflammation, 2010*, 1–19.

Bartelt, A., Bruns, O. T., Reimer, R., Hohenberg, H., Ittrich, H., Peldschus, K., et al. (2011). Brown adipose tissue activity controls triglyceride clearance. *Nature Medicine, 17*(2), 200.

Bermudez, O. I., Ribaya-Mercado, J. D., Talegawkar, S. A., & Tucker, K. L. (2005). Hispanic and non-Hispanic white elders from Massachusetts have different patterns of carotenoid intake and plasma concentrations. *Journal of Nutrition, 135*(6), 1496–1502.

Berni, P., Chitchumroonchokchai, C., Canniatti-Brazaca, S. G., De Moura, F. F., & Failla, M. L. (2015). Comparison of content and in vitro bioaccessibility of provitamin A carotenoids in home cooked and commercially processed orange fleshed sweet potato (*Ipomea batatas* Lam). *Plant Foods for Human Nutrition, 70*(1), 1–8.

Bernlohr, D. A., Jenkins, A. E., & Bennaars, A. A. (2002). Adipose tissue and lipid metabolism. In J. E. Vence & D. Vence (Eds.), *Biochemistry of lipids, lipoproteins and membranes.* (4th ed., pp. 263–289). Amsterdam: Elsevier Science.

Bertram, J. S. (1999). Carotenoids and gene regulation. *Nutrition Reviews, 57*(6), 182–191.

Blüher, M. (2009). Adipose tissue dysfunction in obesity. *Experimental and Clinical Endocrinology & Diabetes, 117*(06), 241–250.

Bonet, M. L., Canas, J. A., Ribot, J., & Palou, A. (2015). Carotenoids and their conversion products in the control of adipocyte function, adiposity and obesity. *Archives of Biochemistry and Biophysics, 572*, 112–125.

Bowen, P. E., Stacewicz-Sapuntzakis, M., & Diwadkar-Navsariwala, V. (2015). *Carotenoids in human nutrition.* In *Pigments in fruits and vegetables.* (pp. 31–67). New York, NY: Springer.

Braitman, L. E., Adlin, E. V., Stanton, J. L., Jr. (1985). Obesity and caloric intake: The National Health and nutrition examination survey of 1971–1975 (HANES I). *Journal of Chronic Diseases, 38*(9), 727–732.

Cancello, R., & Clement, K. (2006). Is obesity an inflammatory illness? Role of low-grade inflammation and macrophage infiltration in human white adipose tissue. *BJOG: An International Journal of Obstetrics & Gynaecology, 113*(10), 1141–1147.

Cascio, G., Schiera, G., & Di Liegro, I. (2012). Dietary fatty acids in metabolic syndrome, diabetes and cardiovascular diseases. *Current Diabetes Reviews, 8*(1), 2–17.

Cazzonelli, C. I. (2011). Carotenoids in nature: Insights from plants and beyond. *Functional Plant Biology, 38*(11), 833–847.

Chandrasekaran, C. V., Vijayalakshmi, M. A., Prakash, K., Bansal, V. S., Meenakshi, J., & Amit, A. (2012). Herbal approach for obesity management. *American Journal of Plant Sciences*, *3*(07), 1003.

Chopra, A., & Doiphode, V. V. (2002). Ayurvedic medicine: Core concept, therapeutic principles, and current relevance. *Medical Clinics*, *86*(1), 75–89.

Chopra, A., Kaur, N., Lalit. (2014). Herbal drugs—A promising approach to obesity management. *Journal of Pharmaceutical Sciences and Research*, *2*, 1–5.

Chung, J., Koo, K., Lian, F., Hu, K. Q., Ernst, H., & Wang, X. D. (2012). Apo-10′-lycopenoic acid, a lycopene metabolite, increases Sirtuin 1 mRNA and protein levels and decreases hepatic fat accumulation in ob/ob mice-3. *Journal of Nutrition*, *142*(3), 405–410.

Cinti, S., Mitchell, G., Barbatelli, G., Murano, I., Ceresi, E., Faloia, E., et al. (2005). Adipocyte death defines macrophage localization and function in adipose tissue of obese mice and humans. *Journal of Lipid Research*, *46*(11), 2347–2355.

Coelho, M., Oliveira, T., & Fernandes, R. (2013). Biochemistry of adipose tissue: An endocrine organ (State of the art paper). *Archives of Medical Science*, *9*(2), 191–200.

Concepcion, M. R., Avalos, J., Bonet, M. L., Boronat, A., Gomez-Gomez, L., Hornero-Mendez, D., et al. (2018). A global perspective on carotenoids: Metabolism, biotechnology, and benefits for nutrition and health. *Progress in Lipid Research*, *70*, 62–93.

Cooke, D., & Bloom, S. (2006). The obesity pipeline: Current strategies in the development of anti-obesity drugs. *Nature Reviews Drug Discovery*, *5*(11), 919.

Dansinger, M. L., Gleason, J. A., Griffith, J. L., Selker, H. P., & Schaefer, E. J. (2005). Comparison of the Atkins, Ornish, weight watchers, and zone diets for weight loss and heart disease risk reduction: A randomized trial. *JAMA*, *293*(1), 43–53.

Daval, M., Foufelle, F., & Ferré, P. (2006). Functions of AMP-activated protein kinase in adipose tissue. *The Journal of Physiology*, *574*(1), 55–62.

Di Pietro, N., Di Tomo, P., & Pandolfi, A. (2016). Carotenoids in cardiovascular disease prevention. *JSM Atherosclerosis*, *1*(1), 1–13.

Dufosse, L., Galaup, P., Yaron, A., Arad, S. M., Blanc, P., Murthy, K. N. C., et al. (2005). Microorganisms and microalgae as sources of pigments for food use: A scientific oddity or an industrial reality? *Trends in Food Science & Technology*, *16*(9), 389–406.

El-Sohemy, A., Baylin, A., Kabagambe, E., Ascherio, A., Spiegelman, D., & Campos, H. (2002). Individual carotenoid concentrations in adipose tissue and plasma as biomarkers of dietary intake. *The American Journal of Clinical Nutrition*, *76*(1), 172–179.

Erdman, J. W., Bierer, T. L., & Gugger, E. T. (1993). Absorption and transport of carotenoids. *Annals of the New York Academy of Sciences*, *691*(1), 76–85.

Eugster, C. H. (1995). History: 175 years of carotenoid chemistry. *Carotenoids*, *1*, 1–11.

Fajas, L. (2003). Adipogenesis: A cross-talk between cell proliferation and cell differentiation. *Annals of Medicine*, *35*(2), 79–85.

Faure, H., Fayol, V., Galabert, C., Grolier, P., Le Moel, G., Steghens, J. P., et al. (1999). Les caroténoïdes: 1. Métabolisme et physiologie. *Annales de Biologie Clinique*, *57*(2), 169–183.

Fedorenko, A., Lishko, P. V., & Kirichok, Y. (2012). Mechanism of fatty-acid-dependent UCP1 uncoupling in brown fat mitochondria. *Cell*, *151*(2), 400–413.

Fenni, S., Hammou, H., Astier, J., Bonnet, L., Karkeni, E., Couturier, C., et al. (2017). Lycopene and tomato powder supplementation similarly inhibit high-fat diet induced obesity, inflammatory response, and associated metabolic disorders. *Molecular Nutrition & Food Research*, *61*(9), 1–10.

Field, B. C., Chaudhri, O. B., & Bloom, S. R. (2009). Obesity treatment: Novel peripheral targets. *British Journal of Clinical Pharmacology*, *68*(6), 830–843.

Fonseca-Alaniz, M. H., Takada, J., Alonso-Vale, M. I. C., & Lima, F. B. (2007). Adipose tissue as an endocrine organ: From theory to practice. *Jornal de Pediatria, 83*(5), S192–S203.

Ganesan, P., Noda, K., Manabe, Y., Ohkubo, T., Tanaka, Y., Maoka, T., et al. (2011). Siphonaxanthin, a marine carotenoid from green algae, effectively induces apoptosis in human leukemia (HL-60) cells. *Biochimica et Biophysica Acta (BBA)—General Subjects, 1810*(5), 497–503.

Gerster, H. (1997). The potential role of lycopene for human health. *Journal of the American College of Nutrition, 16*(2), 109–126.

Gesta, S., Tseng, Y. H., & Kahn, C. R. (2007). Developmental origin of fat: Tracking obesity to its source. *Cell, 131*(2), 242–256.

Goossens, G. H. (2008). The role of adipose tissue dysfunction in the pathogenesis of obesity-related insulin resistance. *Physiology & Behavior, 94*(2), 206–218.

Goran, M. I. (2000). Energy metabolism and obesity. *Medical Clinics of North America, 84*(2), 347–362.

Gouranton, E., Thabuis, C., Riollet, C., Malezet-Desmoulins, C., El Yazidi, C., Amiot, M. J., et al. (2011). Lycopene inhibits proinflammatory cytokine and chemokine expression in adipose tissue. *Journal of Nutritional Biochemistry, 22*(7), 642–648.

Grundy, S. M. (2012). Pre-diabetes, metabolic syndrome, and cardiovascular risk. *Journal of the American College of Cardiology, 59*(7), 635–643.

Gul, T., Balkhi, H. M., & Haq, E. (2017). Inhibition of adipocyte differentiation by crocin in in vitro model of obesity. *Haya: The Saudi Journal of Life Sciences, 2*(8), 306–311.

Halford, J. C., Boyland, E. J., Blundell, J. E., Kirkham, T. C., & Harrold, J. A. (2010). Pharmacological management of appetite expression in obesity. *Nature Reviews Endocrinology, 6*(5), 255.

Harman-Boehm, I., Blüher, M., Redel, H., Sion-Vardy, N., Ovadia, S., Avinoach, E., et al. (2007). Macrophage infiltration into omental versus subcutaneous fat across different populations: Effect of regional adiposity and the comorbidities of obesity. *Journal of Clinical Endocrinology & Metabolism, 92*(6), 2240–2247.

Heal, D. J., Gosden, J., & Smith, S. L. (2009). Regulatory challenges for new drugs to treat obesity and comorbid metabolic disorders. *British Journal of Clinical Pharmacology, 68*(6), 861–874.

Hebebrand, J., & Hinney, A. (2009). Environmental and genetic risk factors in obesity. *Child and Adolescent Psychiatric Clinics of North America, 18*(1), 83–94.

Higuchi, N., Kato, M., Shundo, Y., Tajiri, H., Tanaka, M., Yamashita, N., et al. (2008). Liver X receptor in cooperation with SREBP-1c is a major lipid synthesis regulator in nonalcoholic fatty liver disease. *Hepatology Research, 38*(11), 1122–1129.

Holubková, A., Penesová, A., Šturdík, E., Mošovská, S., & Mikušová, L. (2012). Phytochemicals with potential effects in metabolic syndrome prevention and therapy. *Acta Chimica Slovaca, 5*(2), 186–199.

Ikeuchi, M., Koyama, T., Takahashi, J., & Yazawa, K. (2007). Effects of astaxanthin in obese mice fed a high-fat diet. *Bioscience, Biotechnology, and Biochemistry, 71*(4), 893–899.

Inoue, M., Tanabe, H., Matsumoto, A., Takagi, M., Umegaki, K., Amagaya, S., et al. (2012). Astaxanthin functions differently as a selective peroxisome proliferator-activated receptor γ modulator in adipocytes and macrophages. *Biochemical Pharmacology, 84*(5), 692–700.

Ip, B. C., Hu, K. Q., Liu, C., Smith, D. E., Obin, M. S., Ausman, L. M., et al. (2013). Lycopene metabolite, Apo-10′-lycopenoic acid, inhibits diethylnitrosamine-initiated, high fat diet-promoted hepatic inflammation and tumorigenesis in mice. *Cancer Prevention Research, 6*(12), 1–13.

Jackson, H., Braun, C. L., & Ernst, H. (2008). The chemistry of novel xanthophyll carotenoids. *American Journal of Cardiology, 101*, S50–S57.

Jewell, C., & O'Brien, N. M. (1999). Effect of dietary supplementation with carotenoids on xenobiotic metabolizing enzymes in the liver, lung, kidney and small intestine of the rat. *British Journal of Nutrition, 81*(3), 235–242.

Jo, S. J., Kim, J. W., Choi, H. O., Kim, J. H., Kim, H. J., Woo, S. H., et al. (2017). Capsanthin inhibits both adipogenesis in 3T3-L1 preadipocytes and weight gain in high-fat diet-induced obese mice. *Biomolecules & Therapeutics, 25*(3), 329.

Johnson, E. J. (2002). The role of carotenoids in human health. *Nutrition in Clinical Care, 5*(2), 56–65.

Jump, D. B., Clarke, S. D., Thelen, A., & Liimatta, M. (1994). Coordinate regulation of glycolytic and lipogenic gene expression by polyunsaturated fatty acids. *Journal of Lipid Research, 35*(6), 1076–1084.

Kameji, H., Mochizuki, K., Miyoshi, N., & Goda, T. (2010). β-Carotene accumulation in 3T3-L1 adipocytes inhibits the elevation of reactive oxygen species and the suppression of genes related to insulin sensitivity induced by tumor necrosis factor-α. *Nutrition, 26*(11–12), 1151–1156.

Kennett, G. A., & Clifton, P. G. (2010). New approaches to the pharmacological treatment of obesity: Can they break through the efficacy barrier? *Pharmacology Biochemistry and Behavior, 97*(1), 63–83.

Kianbakht, S., & Hashem Dabaghian, F. (2015). Anti-obesity and anorectic effects of saffron and its constituent crocin in obese Wistar rat. *Medicinal Plants, 1*(53), 25–33.

Kim, H., Hwang, H., Hong, J. W., Lee, Y. N., Ahn, I. P., Yoon, I. S., et al. (2011). A rice orthologue of the ABA receptor, OsPYL/RCAR5, is a positive regulator of the ABA signal transduction pathway in seed germination and early seedling growth. *Journal of Experimental Botany, 63*(2), 1013–1024.

Kiokias, S., Proestos, C., & Varzakas, T. (2016). A review of the structure, biosynthesis, absorption of carotenoids-analysis and properties of their common natural extracts. *Current Research in Nutrition and Food Science Journal, 4*, 25–37. Special Issue Carotenoids March 2016.

Kotake-Nara, E., Hase, M., Kobayashi, M., & Nagao, A. (2016). 3′-Hydroxy-ε, ε-caroten-3-one inhibits the differentiation of 3T3-L1 cells to adipocytes. *Bioscience, Biotechnology, and Biochemistry, 80*(3), 518–523.

Kovary, K., Louvain, T. S., Costa e Silva, M. C., Albano, F., Pires, B. B., Laranja, G. A., et al. (2001). Biochemical behaviour of norbixin during in vitro DNA damage induced by reactive oxygen species. *British Journal of Nutrition, 85*(4), 431–440.

Kozak, L. P., & Anunciado-Koza, R. (2009). UCP1: Its involvement and utility in obesity. *International Journal of Obesity, 32*(S7), S32.

Kral, J. G., & Näslund, E. (2007). Surgical treatment of obesity. *Nature Reviews Endocrinology, 3*(8), 574.

Krauss, S., Zhang, C. Y., & Lowell, B. B. (2005). The mitochondrial uncoupling-protein homologues. *Nature Reviews Molecular Cell Biology, 6*(3), 248.

Lago, F., Dieguez, C., Gómez-Reino, J., & Gualillo, O. (2007). Adipokines as emerging mediators of immune response and inflammation. *Nature Reviews Rheumatology, 3*(12), 716.

Lago, F., Gómez, R., Gómez-Reino, J. J., Dieguez, C., & Gualillo, O. (2009). Adipokines as novel modulators of lipid metabolism. *Trends in Biochemical Sciences, 34*(10), 500–510.

Lawlor, D. A., & Chaturvedi, N. (2006). Treatment and prevention of obesity-are there critical periods for intervention? *International Journal of Epidemiology, 35*(1), 3–9.

LeBlanc, E. S., O'connor, E., Whitlock, E. P., Patnode, C. D., & Kapka, T. (2011). Effectiveness of primary care-relevant treatments for obesity in adults: A systematic evidence review for the US Preventive Services Task Force. *Annals of Internal Medicine, 155*(7), 434–447.

Lee, M. J., Wu, Y., & Fried, S. K. (2010). Adipose tissue remodeling in pathophysiology of obesity. *Current Opinion in Clinical Nutrition and Metabolic Care, 13*(4), 371.

Lefterova, M. I., & Lazar, M. A. (2009). New developments in adipogenesis. *Trends in Endocrinology and Metabolism, 20*(3), 107–114.

Li, Z. S., Noda, K., Fujita, E., Manabe, Y., Hirata, T., & Sugawara, T. (2014). The green algal carotenoid siphonaxanthin inhibits adipogenesis in 3T3-L1 preadipocytes and the accumulation of lipids in white adipose tissue of KK-ay Mice1–3. *The Journal of Nutrition, 145*(3), 490–498.

Liu, H., Wang, J., Liu, M., Zhao, H., Yaqoob, S., Zheng, M., et al. (2018). Anti-obesity effects of ginsenoside Rg1 on 3T3-L1 preadipocytes and high fat diet-induced obese mice mediated by AMPK. *Nutrients, 10*(7), 830.

Lobo, G. P., Amengual, J., Li, H. N. M., Golczak, M., Bonet, M. L., Palczewski, K., et al. (2010). β, β-carotene decreases peroxisome proliferator receptor γ activity and reduces lipid storage capacity of adipocytes in a β, β-carotene-oxygenase 1-dependent manner. *Journal of Biological Chemistry, 285*(36), 27891–27899.

Luvizotto, R.D.A.M., Nascimento, A. F., Imaizumi, E., Pierine, D. T., Conde, S. J., Correa, C. R., et al. (2013). Lycopene supplementation modulates plasma concentrations and epididymal adipose tissue mRNA of leptin, resistin and IL-6 in diet-induced obese rats. *British Journal of Nutrition, 110*(10), 1803–1809.

Maeda, H., Hosokawa, M., Sashima, T., Takahashi, N., Kawada, T., & Miyashita, K. (2006). Fucoxanthin and its metabolite, fucoxanthinol, suppress adipocyte differentiation in 3T3-L1 cells. *International Journal of Molecular Medicine, 18*(1), 147–152.

Maeda, H., Kanno, S., Kodate, M., Hosokawa, M., & Miyashita, K. (2015). Fucoxanthinol, metabolite of fucoxanthin, improves obesity-induced inflammation in adipocyte cells. *Marine Drugs, 13*(8), 4799–4813.

Maeda, H., Saito, S., Nakamura, N., & Maoka, T. (2013). Paprika pigments attenuate obesity-induced inflammation in 3T3-L1 adipocytes. *ISRN Inflammation, 2013*, 1–9.

Mamun, A. A., Kinarivala, M., O'Callaghan, M. J., Williams, G. M., Najman, J. M., & Callaway, L. K. (2010). Associations of excess weight gain during pregnancy with long-term maternal overweight and obesity: Evidence from 21 y postpartum follow-up. *The American Journal of Clinical Nutrition, 91*(5), 1336–1341.

Marcotorchino, J., Romier, B., Gouranton, E., Riollet, C., Gleize, B., Malezet-Desmoulins, C., et al. (2012). Lycopene attenuates LPS-induced TNF-α secretion in macrophages and inflammatory markers in adipocytes exposed to macrophage-conditioned media. *Molecular Nutrition & Food Research, 56*(5), 725–732.

Mata-Gómez, L. C., Montañez, J. C., Méndez-Zavala, A., & Aguilar, C. N. (2014). Biotechnological production of carotenoids by yeasts: An overview. *Microbial Cell Factories, 13*(1), 12.

Mathieu, P., Lemieux, I., & Després, J. P. (2010). Obesity, inflammation, and cardiovascular risk. *Clinical Pharmacology & Therapeutics, 87*(4), 407–416.

Melnikova, I., & Wages, D. (2006). Anti-obesity therapies. *Nature Reviews Drug Discovery, 5*, 369–370.

Nicholls, D. G., & Rial, E. (1999). A history of the first uncoupling protein, UCP1. *Journal of Bioenergetics and Biomembranes, 31*(5), 399–406.

Ntambi, J. M., & Young-Cheul, K. (2000). Adipocyte differentiation and gene expression. *Journal of Nutrition, 130*(12), 3122S–3126S.

O'Brien, P. E., MacDonald, L., Anderson, M., Brennan, L., & Brown, W. A. (2013). Long-term outcomes after bariatric surgery: Fifteen-year follow-up of adjustable gastric banding and a systematic review of the bariatric surgical literature. *Annals of Surgery, 257*(1), 87–94.

Okada, T., Nakai, M., Maeda, H., Hosokawa, M., Sashima, T., & Miyashita, K. (2008). Suppressive effect of neoxanthin on the differentiation of 3T3-L1 adipose cells. *Journal of Oleo Science, 57*(6), 345–351.

Olmedilla, B., Granado, F., Blanco, I., & Rojas-Hidalgo, E. (1994). Seasonal and sex-related variations in six serum carotenoids, retinol, and α-tocopherol. *The American Journal of Clinical Nutrition, 60*(1), 106–110.

Paiva, S. A., & Russell, R. M. (1999). β-Carotene and other carotenoids as antioxidants. *Journal of the American College of Nutrition, 18*(5), 426–433.

Pantavos, A., Ruiter, R., Feskens, E. F., de Keyser, C. E., Hofman, A., Stricker, B. H., et al. (2015). Total dietary antioxidant capacity, individual antioxidant intake and breast cancer risk: The Rotterdam study. *International Journal of Cancer, 136*(9), 2178–2186.

Park, H. J., Lee, M. K., Park, Y. B., Shin, Y. C., & Choi, M. S. (2011). Beneficial effects of *Undaria pinnatifida* ethanol extract on diet-induced-insulin resistance in C57BL/6J mice. *Food and Chemical Toxicology, 49*(4), 727–733.

Payne, V. A., Au, W. S., Lowe, C. E., Rahman, S. M., Friedman, J. E., ORahilly, S., et al. (2010). C/EBP transcription factors regulate SREBP1c gene expression during adipogenesis. *Biochemical Journal, 425*(1), 215–224.

Pol, A., Gross, S. P., & Parton, R. G. (2014). Biogenesis of the multifunctional lipid droplet: Lipids, proteins, and sites. *Journal of Cell Biology, 204*(5), 635–646.

Pories, W. J. (2008). Bariatric surgery: Risks and rewards. *Journal of Clinical Endocrinology & Metabolism, 93*(11), 89–96.

Pryor, W. A., Stahl, W., & Rock, C. L. (2000). Beta carotene: From biochemistry to clinical trials. *Nutrition Reviews, 58*(2), 39–53.

Rao, A. V., & Rao, L. G. (2007). Carotenoids and human health. *Pharmacological Research, 55*(3), 207–216.

Riccioni, G., Gammone, M. A., & D'Orazio, N. (2015). Carotenoids and cardiovascular prevention: An update. *Journal of Nutrition & Food Sciences, 6*(1), 1–5.

Rodgers, R. J., Holch, P., & Tallett, A. J. (2010). Behavioural satiety sequence (BSS): Separating wheat from chaff in the behavioural pharmacology of appetite. *Pharmacology Biochemistry and Behavior, 97*(1), 3–14.

Rosen, E. D., & MacDougald, O. A. (2006). Adipocyte differentiation from the inside out. *Nature Reviews Molecular Cell Biology, 7*(12), 885.

Rosen, E. D., & Spiegelman, B. M. (2000). Molecular regulation of adipogenesis. *Annual Review of Cell and Developmental Biology, 16*(1), 145–171.

Saely, C. H., Geiger, K., & Drexel, H. (2012). Brown versus white adipose tissue: A mini-review. *Gerontology, 58*(1), 15–23.

Sam, S., & Mazzone, T. (2014). Adipose tissue changes in obesity and the impact on metabolic function. *Translational Research, 164*(4), 284–292.

Sargent, B. J., & Moore, N. A. (2009). New central targets for the treatment of obesity. *British Journal of Clinical Pharmacology, 68*(6), 852–860.

Sharma, H., & Chandola, H. M. (2011). Prameha in ayurveda: Correlation with obesity, metabolic syndrome, and diabetes mellitus. Part 1—Etiology, classification, and pathogenesis. *The Journal of Alternative and Complementary Medicine, 17*(6), 491–496.

Shi, S. Q., Ansari, T. S., McGuinness, O. P., Wasserman, D. H., & Johnson, C. H. (2013). Circadian disruption leads to insulin resistance and obesity. *Current Biology, 23*(5), 372–381.

Shirakura, Y., Takayanagi, K., Mukai, K., Tanabe, H., & Inoue, M. (2011). β-Cryptoxanthin suppresses the adipogenesis of 3T3-L1 cells via RAR activation. *Journal of Nutritional Science and Vitaminology*, *57*(6), 426–431.

Siersbæk, M. S., Loft, A., Aagaard, M. M., Nielsen, R., Schmidt, S. F., Petrovic, N., et al. (2012). Genome-wide profiling of peroxisome proliferator-activated receptor γ in primary epididymal, inguinal, and brown adipocytes reveals depot-selective binding correlated with gene expression. *Molecular and Cellular Biology*, *32*(17), 3452–3463.

Sjöström, L., Narbro, K., Sjöström, C. D., Karason, K., Larsson, B., Wedel, H., et al. (2007). Effects of bariatric surgery on mortality in Swedish obese subjects. *New England Journal of Medicine*, *357*(8), 741–752.

Stephens, J. M. (2012). The fat controller: Adipocyte development. *PLoS Biology*, *10*(11), 1–3.

Stöger, R. (2008). Epigenetics and obesity. *Pharmacogenomics*, *9*(12), 1851–1860.

Sugawara, T., Ganesan, P., Li, Z., Manabe, Y., & Hirata, T. (2014). Siphonaxanthin, a green algal carotenoid, as a novel functional compound. *Marine Drugs*, *12*(6), 3660–3668.

Sugiura, M., Nakamura, M., Ikoma, Y., Yano, M., Ogawa, K., Matsumoto, H., et al. (2006). The homeostasis model assessment-insulin resistance index is inversely associated with serum carotenoids in non-diabetic subjects. *Journal of Epidemiology*, *16*(2), 71–78.

Sun, K., Kusminski, C. M., & Scherer, P. E. (2011). Adipose tissue remodeling and obesity. *The Journal of Clinical Investigation*, *121*(6), 2094–2101.

Sun, K., & Scherer, P. E. (2010). *Adipose tissue dysfunction: A multistep process*. In *Novel insights into adipose cell functions*. Berlin, Heidelberg: Springer.(pp. 67–75).

Takaichi, S. (2011). Carotenoids in algae: Distributions, biosyntheses and functions. *Marine Drugs*, *9*(6), 1101–1118.

Tan, C. P., & Hou, Y. H. (2014). First evidence for the anti-inflammatory activity of fucoxanthin in high-fat-diet-induced obesity in mice and the antioxidant functions in PC12 cells. *Inflammation*, *37*(2), 443–450.

Tomas, E., Tsao, T. S., Saha, A. K., Murrey, H. E., Cheng Zhang, C., Itani, S. I., et al. (2002). Enhanced muscle fat oxidation and glucose transport by ACRP30 globular domain: Acetyl-CoA carboxylase inhibition and AMP-activated protein kinase activation. *Proceedings of the National Academy of Sciences*, *99*(25), 16309–16313.

Townsend, K. L., & Tseng, Y. H. (2014). Brown fat fuel utilization and thermogenesis. *Trends in Endocrinology and Metabolism*, *25*(4), 168–177.

Trayhurn, P., & Beattie, J. H. (2001). Physiological role of adipose tissue: White adipose tissue as an endocrine and secretory organ. *Proceedings of the Nutrition Society*, *60*(3), 329–339.

Tsukui, T., Konno, K., Hosokawa, M., Maeda, H., Sashima, T., & Miyashita, K. (2007). Fucoxanthin and fucoxanthinol enhance the amount of docosahexaenoic acid in the liver of KKAy obese/diabetic mice. *Journal of Agricultural and Food Chemistry*, *55*(13), 5025–5029.

Vickers, S. P., & Cheetham, S. C. (2007). *Preclinical developments in antiobesity drugs*. In vol. 13. *Appetite and body weight*. (pp. 323–336).

Wang, Y., Ausman, L. M., Greenberg, A. S., Russell, R. M., & Wang, X. D. (2010). Dietary lycopene and tomato extract supplementations inhibit nonalcoholic steatohepatitis-promoted hepatocarcinogenesis in rats. *International Journal of Cancer*, *126*(8), 1788–1796.

Wang, Y., Viscarra, J., Kim, S. J., & Sul, H. S. (2015). Transcriptional regulation of hepatic lipogenesis. *Nature Reviews Molecular Cell Biology*, *16*(11), 678.

Weisberg, S. P., McCann, D., Desai, M., Rosenbaum, M., Leibel, R. L., & Ferrante, A. W. (2003). Obesity is associated with macrophage accumulation in adipose tissue. *The Journal of Clinical Investigation*, *112*(12), 1796–1808.

White, U. A., & Stephens, J. M. (2010). Transcription factors that promote formation of white adipose tissue. *Molecular and Cellular Endocrinology*, *318*(1–2), 10–14.

Wilding, J. (2007). *Clinical investigations of anti-obesity drugs*. In: *Appetite and body weight*, vol.14, Academic Press.(pp. 337–355).

Williams, D. J., Edwards, D., Hamernig, I., Jian, L., James, A. P., Johnson, S. K., et al. (2013). Vegetables containing phytochemicals with potential anti-obesity properties: A review. *Food Research International*, *52*(1), 323–333.

Wing, R. R., Tate, D. F., Gorin, A. A., Raynor, H. A., & Fava, J. L. (2006). A self-regulation program for maintenance of weight loss. *New England Journal of Medicine*, *355*(15), 1563–1571.

Wirth, A., Wabitsch, M., & Hauner, H. (2014). The prevention and treatment of obesity. *Deutsches Ärzteblatt International*, *111*(42), 705.

Withrow, D., & Alter, D. A. (2011). The economic burden of obesity worldwide: A systematic review of the direct costs of obesity. *Obesity Reviews*, *12*(2), 131–141.

Woo, M. N., Jeon, S. M., Kim, H. J., Lee, M. K., Shin, S. K., Shin, Y. C., et al. (2010). Fucoxanthin supplementation improves plasma and hepatic lipid metabolism and blood glucose concentration in high-fat fed C57BL/6N mice. *Chemico-Biological Interactions*, *186*(3), 316–322.

Wozniak, S. E., Gee, L. L., Wachtel, M. S., & Frezza, E. E. (2009). Adipose tissue: The new endocrine organ? A review article. *Digestive Diseases and Sciences*, *54*(9), 1847–1856.

Wu, J., Cohen, P., & Spiegelman, B. M. (2013). Adaptive thermogenesis in adipocytes: Is beige the new brown? *Genes & Development*, *27*(3), 234–250.

Xi, L., Qian, Z., Xu, G., Zhou, C., & Sun, S. (2007). Crocetin attenuates palmitate-induced insulin insensitivity and disordered tumor necrosis factor-α and adiponectin expression in rat adipocytes. *British Journal of Pharmacology*, *151*(5), 610–617.

Xu, H., Barnes, G. T., Yang, Q., Tan, G., Yang, D., Chou, C. J., et al. (2003). Chronic inflammation in fat plays a crucial role in the development of obesity-related insulin resistance. *The Journal of Clinical Investigation*, *112*(12), 1821–1830.

Yim, M. J., Hosokawa, M., Mizushina, Y., Yoshida, H., Saito, Y., & Miyashita, K. (2011). Suppressive effects of amarouciaxanthin A on 3T3-L1 adipocyte differentiation through down-regulation of PPARγ and C/EBPα mRNA expression. *Journal of Agricultural and Food Chemistry*, *59*(5), 1646–1652.

Zeng, Z., He, W., Jia, Z., & Hao, S. (2017). Lycopene improves insulin sensitivity through inhibition of STAT3/Srebp-1c-mediated lipid accumulation and inflammation in mice fed a high-fat diet. *Experimental and Clinical Endocrinology & Diabetes*, *125*(09), 610–617.

Zhao, L., Gregoire, F., & Sul, H. S. (2000). Transient induction of ENC-1, a Kelch-related actin-binding protein, is required for adipocyte differentiation. *Journal of Biological Chemistry*, *275*(22), 16845–16850.

Zheng, J., Li, Z., Manabe, Y., Kim, M., Goto, T., Kawada, T., et al. (2018). Siphonaxanthin, a carotenoid from green algae, inhibits lipogenesis in hepatocytes via the suppression of liver X receptor α activity. *Lipids*, *53*(1), 41–52.

Further reading

Akoh, C. C. (2017). *Food lipids: Chemistry, nutrition, and biotechnology* (4th ed). CRC Press.1–1047.

Flier, J. S. (2004). Obesity wars: Molecular progress confronts an expanding epidemic. *Cell*, *116*(2), 337–350.

Hwang, C. S., Loftus, T. M., Mandrup, S., & Lane, M. D. (1997). Adipocyte differentiation and leptin expression. *Annual Review of Cell and Developmental Biology*, *13*(1), 231–259.

Maeda, H., Hosokawa, M., Sashima, T., Murakami-Funayama, K., & Miyashita, K. (2009). Anti-obesity and anti-diabetic effects of fucoxanthin on diet-induced obesity conditions in a murine model. *Molecular Medicine Reports*, *2*(6), 897–902.

McArdle, M. A., Finucane, O. M., Connaughton, R. M., McMorrow, A. M., & Roche, H. M. (2013). Mechanisms of obesity-induced inflammation and insulin resistance: Insights into the emerging role of nutritional strategies. *Frontiers in Endocrinology*, *4*, 52.

Pfander, H. (1992). *Carotenoids: An overview*. In Vol. 213. *Methods in enzymology* (pp. 3–13): Academic Press.

Silva, L. V., Nelson, D. L., Drummond, M. F. B., Dufossé, L., & Glória, M. B. A. (2005). Comparison of hydrodistillation methods for the deodorization of turmeric. *Food Research International*, *38*(8–9), 1087–1096.

Spiegelman, B. M., & Flier, J. S. (1996). Adipogenesis and obesity: Rounding out the big picture. *Cell*, *87*(3), 377–389.

Van den Berg, H., Faulks, R., Granado, H. F., Hirschberg, J., Olmedilla, B., Sandmann, G., et al. (2000). The potential for the improvement of carotenoid levels in foods and the likely systemic effects. *Journal of the Science of Food and Agriculture*, *80*(7), 880–912.

Underutilized sources of carotenoids

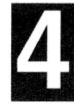

María del Mar Contreras-Gámez, *Ana María Gómez-Caravaca*[†]
*Department of Chemical, Environmental and Materials Engineering, University of Jaén, Jaén, Spain, [†]Department of Analytical Chemistry, Faculty of Sciences, University of Granada, Granada, Spain

Chapter outline

Introduction

Carotenoids are tetraterpenic pigments widely distributed in nature (Graça Dias et al., 2018). More than 1000 different carotenoids have been identified so far, in a wide range of different natural environments, including the plant kingdom, but this number can still be increased (Yabuzaki, 2017). There are two classes of carotenoids in plants: the carotenes, which are hydrocarbon compounds, and their oxygenated derivatives, xanthophylls (Pallett & Young, 2017). In the green tissues of plants, carotenoids are located in the chloroplasts. Moreover, carotenoids are also responsible for the yellow to red pigmentation of roots, flowers, fruits, etc., located in plastids as chromoplasts (Pallett & Young, 2017).

The distribution of carotenoids in plants food matrices and their levels have been recently reviewed (Graça Dias et al., 2018; Saini, Nile, & Park, 2015). Some of the most frequent carotenoids in plant foods are antheraxanthin, α-carotene, β-carotene, β-cryptoxanthin, lutein, lycopene, neoxanthin, phytoene, violaxanthin, and zeaxanthin

Table 1 Examples of carotenoids frequently found in food plants

Carotenoid	Molecular formula[a–d]	Molecular weight (g/mol)[a–d]	Some biological function[a,d]	Industrial application[d]	Chemical structure[a]
Antheraxanthin, antheraxanthin A	$C_{40}H_{56}O_3$	584.848	Photosynthetic pigment, photoprotective activity, membrane stabilizer in chloroplasts, energy source, antioxidant.	Surfactant, emulsifier	
α-Carotene	$C_{40}H_{56}$	536.888	Membrane stabilizer, energy source, provitamin A, anticarcinogenic activity, antioxidant.	Surfactant, emulsifier	
β-Carotene	$C_{40}H_{56}$	536.888	Photosynthetic pigment, photoprotective agent, provitamin A, antioxidant, anticarcinogenic activity, cell differentiation and proliferation promoter, immune response enhancement, brownish yellow color, membrane stabilizer.	Surfactant, emulsifier, pharmaceutical application	
β-Cryptoxanthin	$C_{40}H_{56}O$	552.848	Provitamin A activity, anticarcinogenic activity, antioxidant, anti-obesity effects, stimulates the repair of DNA oxidation damage, yellow food coloring.	Surfactant, emulsifier	

Lutein, lutein A	$C_{40}H_{56}O_2$	568.848	Photosynthetic pigment, photoprotective activity, anti-photosensitizing agent, anticarcinogenic activity, antioxidant, food coloring, yellowish green/brown color, nonprovitamin A.	Surfactant, emulsifier, drug	
Lycopene	$C_{40}H_{56}$	536.848	Membrane stabilizer, energy source, photoprotector, radioprotector against γ-radiation-induced cellular damages, antioxidant, anticarcinogenic activity, antiinflammatory activity, bright pink/brick red color, orange-red food coloring, nonprovitamin A.	Surfactant, emulsifier, pharmaceutical application	
Neoxanthin	$C_{40}H_{56}O_4$	600.848	Membrane stabilizer, energy source, photosynthetic pigment of higher plants, antimicrobial activity, anticarcinogenic activity, nonprovitamin A.	Surfactant, emulsifier	
Phytoene	$C_{40}H_{64}$	544.912	Membrane stabilizer, energy source, colorless carotenoid.	Surfactant, emulsifier	

Continued

Table 1 Continued

Carotenoid	Molecular formula[a–d]	Molecular weight (g/mol)[a–d]	Some biological function[a,d]	Industrial application[d]	Chemical structure[a]
Violaxanthin	$C_{40}H_{56}O_4$	600.848	Membrane stabilizer, energy source, photoprotective activity, photosynthetic pigment, anticarcinogenic activity, nonprovitamin A, yellow food coloring.	Surfactant, emulsifier	
Zeaxanthin	$C_{40}H_{56}O_2$	568.848	Membrane stabilizer, energy source, photosynthetic pigment, photoprotective activity, antiphotosensitizing agent, anticarcinogenic activity, antioxidant, eye protection from oxidative stress, yellow food coloring, nonprovitamin A.	Surfactant, emulsifier, pharmaceutical application	

[a] https://carotenoiddb.jp.
[b] https://pubchem.ncbi.nlm.nih.gov/.
[c] https://www.genome.jp/kegg/.
[d] http://www.hmdb.ca/.

(Graça Dias et al., 2018; Saini et al., 2015). Table 1 shows their molecular formula, molecular weight, chemical structure, biological functions, phytochemical classification, and industrial applications, which were retrieval from several databases. Some carotenoids are essential nutrients (e.g., α-carotene, β-carotene, and β-cryptoxanthin possess provitamin A activity). Just as a note, vitamin A deficiency affects over 250 million preschool children worldwide and from 250,000 to 500,000 vitamin A-deficient children become blind every year (World Health Organization, 2018). This highlights the importance of finding new sources rich in these carotenoids.

In addition, the relevance of carotenoids in agro-food and pharmaceutical industries has attracted the interest of many researchers because carotenoid rich diet is frequently associated with a lower risk of developing several diseases (Viuda-Martos et al., 2013). In fact, a recent review by Fiedor and Burda (2014) suggested that data from epidemiological studies and clinical trials (mainly from experiments with β-carotene, lycopene, lutein, and zeaxanthin) support that an adequate carotenoid supplementation may reduce and/or prevent the risk of several disorders mediated by reactive oxygen species (cancer, cardiovascular, photosensitivity disorders, etc.). Moreover, there are others carotenoids relevant due to their inherent ability as pigments, such as astaxanthin, which is added to fish feed to obtain a desirable pink flesh color (Berman et al., 2015). As an example of the current interest of carotenoids, in the EU a health claim for β-carotene was approved about the promotion of the maintenance of normal vision, skin, and mucosa, because of its relationship with vitamin A (EFSA Panel on Dietetic Products, 2010). In the case of this and other carotenoids, they can be used as food additives [Commission Regulation (EU) N° 231/, 2012] and cosmetics [Regulation (EC) N° 1223/, 2009].

Carotenoids can be obtained via industrial fermentation using microorganisms, plant extraction, and chemical synthesis. Currently, carotenoids produced by chemical synthesis dominate the global market, but their obtaining from natural sources is growing (Berman et al., 2015). In fact, the importance of natural food additives is increasing as an alternative to synthetic additives in foods, cosmetics, and pharmaceuticals according to EU directives (Viuda-Martos et al., 2013). Moreover, the potential of those carotenoids as health promoters has increased the possibilities of using them in functional foods and nutraceuticals.

In this context, by-products from plants can also be natural sources of carotenoids. Agro-food by-products can be derived from crop residues (primary biomass residues), which are nonedible plant parts from crops generated in the farm after harvesting, and from agro-industrial residues (secondary biomass residues), which are generated during postharvest process and food processing (Santana-Méridas, González-Coloma, & Sánchez-Vioque, 2012). The first type includes leaves, stalks, roots, branches, pruning, etc., whereas the second comprises discarded whole pieces, husks, hulls, peels, seeds, bagasse, pomace, pulp, etc. Therefore, depending on the vegetable and fruit source, some of these residues can be considered as a low-cost source to obtain carotenoids. Fig. 1 shows some critical stages of the vegetables and fruit processing in which wastes are generated. These promising sources are often ignored, underappreciated, and generally discarded without being further used. Furthermore, the exploitation of these microcomponents can be integrated into a biorefinery chain. This means that besides obtaining biofuels and bioenergy (heat and/or power) from biomass macrocomponents,

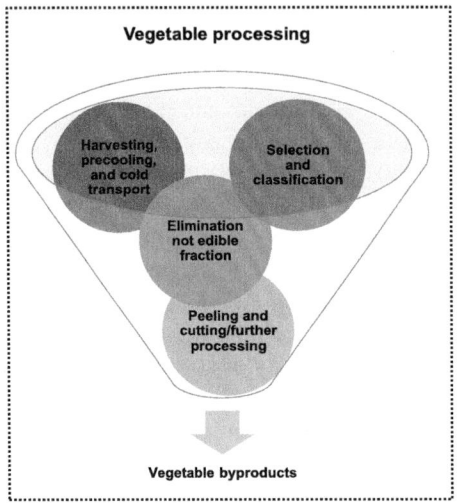
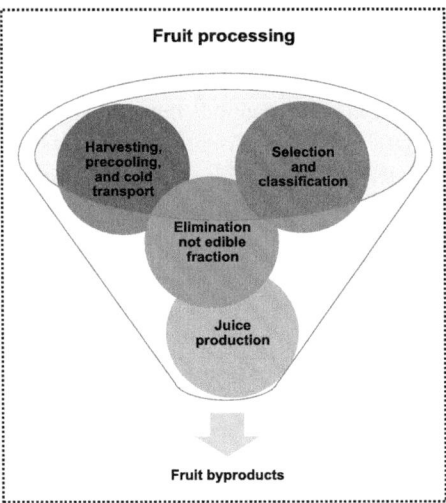

Fig. 1 Examples of processing stages of vegetables and fruits, in which residues are generated.

the exploitation of high-value microcomponents makes it possible to obtain additional economic benefits and to generate a more sustainable agroindustry. For these reasons, this chapter screens the occurrence of carotenoids in agro-food by-products.

Vegetable by-products as sources of carotenoids

Rejected and deteriorated vegetables

Interestingly, the percentage of the initial weight of vegetables and fruits that are lost or discarded is over 40% or even higher in many developing countries. Among them, the losses in agricultural production range between 15% and 20% for industrialized regions, such as Europe, North America, and industrialized Asia, mostly due to vegetable and fruit grading caused by quality standards set by retailers previous to distribution (De Ancos, Colina-Coca, González-Peña, & Sánchez-Moreno, 2015).

This means that if these vegetables and fruits are not intended for consumption, they can be valorized for their carotenoids content instead being discarded. Table 2 shows examples of raw vegetables rich in carotenoids to give an idea of their amounts and potential to be explored. Among vegetables, red pepper cultivars are interesting sources of carotenoids for their content in antheraxanthin (3318–4408 μg/100 g), β-carotene (798–9951 μg/100 g), β-cryptoxanthin (199–3559 μg/100 g), phytoene (1698 μg/100 g), violaxanthin (793–8417 μg/100 g), and zeaxanthin (1516–197,800 μg/100 g). Orange varieties also contain a great amount of these carotenoids, being generally richer than red ones (Kim, Geon, Park, Pyo, & Kim, 2016). Concerning other carotenoids, pumpkin, and carrot are rich in α-carotene (up to 7299 μg/100 g), kale, chicory, and Chinese cabbage in lutein (up to 10,470 μg/100 g), tomato in lycopene (up to 10,290

Table 2 Examples of vegetables rich in carotenoids

Carotenoid	Plant food source	Species	Concentration in edible parts (μg/100 g, fresh weight)	Reference
Antheraxanthin	Red pepper	*Capsicum annuum* L.	3318–4408	Graça Dias et al. (2018) and Minguez-Mosquera and Hornero-Mendez (1993)
α-Carotene	Pumpkin	*Cucurbita moschata* Duch/A	6706–7299	Graça Dias et al. (2018) and Jaeger de Carvalho et al. (2012)
	Carrot	*Daucus carota* L.	830–3860	Graça Dias et al. (2018), Guerra-Vargas, Jaramillo-Flores, Dorantes-Alvarez, and Hernández-Sánchez (2006), and Monge-Rojas, Campos, and Rica (2011)
β-Carotene	Kale	*Brassica oleracea* L.	2280–6000	De Azevedo and Rodriguez-Amaya (2005), Graça Dias et al. (2018), and Mercandante and Rodriguez-Amaya (1991)
	Red pepper	*Capsicum annuum* L.	798–9951	Graça Dias et al. (2018), Minguez-Mosquera and Hornero-Mendez (1993), and Reif, Arrigoni, Schärer, Nyström, and Hurrell (2013)
	Mentruz	*Lepidium pseudodidymum* Thell. ex Druce	11,400	Graça Dias et al. (2018) and Hornero-Méndez, Costa-García, and Mínguez-Mosquera (2002)
	Carrot	*Daucus carota* L.	3078–6820	Graça Dias et al. (2018), Guerra-Vargas et al. (2006), and Reif et al. (2013)
	Spinach	*Spinacia oleracea* L.	5340–7280	Reif et al. (2013)
β-Cryptoxanthin	Red pepper	*Capsicum annuum* L.	199–3559	Graça Dias et al. (2018), Granado, Olmedilla, Blanco, and Rojas-hidalgo (1992), and Minguez-Mosquera and Hornero-Mendez (1993)

Continued

Table 2 Continued

Carotenoid	Plant food source	Species	Concentration in edible parts (μg/100 g, fresh weight)	Reference
Lutein	Kale	*Brassica oleracea* L.	3290–5740	De Azevedo and Rodriguez-Amaya (2005) and Graça Dias et al. (2018)
	Chicory	*Cichorium intybus* L.	1760–8400	Reif et al. (2013)
	Chinese cabbage	*Brassica rapa* L.	1260–10,470	Reif et al. (2013)
Lycopene	Tomato	*Lycopersicon esculentum* Mill.	10,290[a]	Graça Dias et al. (2018) and Murillo and Meléndez-Martínez (2010)
	Tomato	*Lycopersicon esculentum* Mill.	1000–62,273[b]	Graça Dias et al. (2018), Granado et al. (1992), and Murillo and Meléndez-Martínez (2010)
Neoxanthin	Chicory	*Cichorium intybus* L.	1500–2050	Graça Dias et al. (2018), Kobori and Amaya (2008), and Niizu and Rodriguez-Amaya (2005)
	Lettuce	*Lactuca sativa* L.	250–9900	Graça Dias et al. (2018) and Kobori and Amaya (2008)
Phytoene	Carrot	*Daucus carota* L.	1399	Biehler et al. (2012)
	Red pepper	*Capsicum annuum* L.	1698	Biehler et al. (2012)
	Tomato	*Lycopersicon esculentum* Mill.	1388	Biehler et al. (2012)
Violaxanthin	Mentruz	*Lepidium pseudodidymum* Thell. ex Druce	6200	Graça Dias et al. (2018) and Hornero-Méndez et al. (2002)
	Red pepper	*Capsicum annuum* L.	793–8417	Graça Dias et al. (2018) and Minguez-Mosquera and Hornero-Mendez (1993)
Zeaxanthin	Red pepper	*Capsicum annuum* L.	1516–197,800	Biehler et al. (2012), Graça Dias et al. (2018), and Hornero-Méndez et al. (2002)

[a] *E*-isomers.
[b] *Z*-isomers.

and 62,273 µg/100 g of *E*- and *Z*-isomers), as well as chicory and lettuce in neoxanthin (up to 9900 µg/100 g). Nevertheless, it should bear in mind that generally the content of these carotenoids is highly variable depending on the cultivar/variety and the study (Graça Dias et al., 2018; Kantar et al., 2016). Moreover, peppers also contain other carotenoids such as capsanthin, capsanthin 5,6-epoxide, capsorubin, cucurbitaxanthin A, cucurbitaxanthin B, and latoxanthin (Fig. 2) up to 668,700 µg/g (fresh weight), depending on the cultivar and the carotenoid type (see review by Graça Dias et al., 2018). In the case of cucurbitaxanthin A (2700 µg/100 g of flesh) and cucurbitaxanthin B (800 µg/100 g of flesh), they were also isolated from the pumpkin *Cucurbita maxima* (Matsuno, Tani, Maoka, Matsuo, & Komori, 1986). Among them, the red pigment capsanthin, which is characteristic of *Capsicum* spp., could exert a potent inhibitory effect on colon carcinogenesis as suggested the review by Kim, Ha, and Hwang (2009).

Closer to reality, Allen and Rusnack (2009) have shown that reject tomatoes and sorting table tomatoes (or wet waste solids) can be valorized for their lycopene content compared to other by-products such as vines and wastewater (Table 3). Nevertheless, carotenoid content in deteriorated, split, and poor quality vegetables requires further study and more real cases. In any case, it should bear in mind that off-odor compounds responsible for quality loss of minimally processed vegetables, such as alkanes, could derive from carotenoid degradation (Díaz-Mula, Marín, Jordán, & Gil, 2017). This can be extrapolated to poor quality vegetables.

Underused vegetable parts obtained in the farm and after processing: Leaves, skins, peels, and seeds

In the case of vegetables, leaves, peels (or rinds), and seeds are generally the main studied by-products sources of carotenoids (Table 3). In some cases, leaves can be even richer in carotenoids than edible parts. As an example, the study of Liu et al. has shown that broccoli leaves, which represent above the 47% of the biomass weight, have higher concentration of carotenoids (total, 109,500 µg/100 dry weight) and other phytochemicals than the edible parts, the florets (total, 18,100 µg/100 dry weight) (Liu et al., 2018). This implies that broccoli leaves accounted for above 32% and 43% of the recommended daily allowance (RDA) of vitamin A for males and females (>14 years), respectively. Nevertheless, this fact depends on the vegetable type and the cultivar. In this way, another study evidenced that leaves of two cultivars of *Cucurbita pepo* L., with white and yellow-orange fruits, had higher carotenoid content than fruits. A contrary fact was observed for the green cultivar "MU-CU16," even though it had the highest level compared to the other cultivars (Fig. 3) (Obrero et al., 2013). In addition, leaves from sweet potato contain mainly lutein, β-carotene, and violaxanthin as well as *cis*-isomers and epoxy forms of these carotenoids in lower amounts (Chen & Chen, 1993). The content in leaves is higher than in other underused parts from this plant, such as stems (Ishiguro & Yoshimoto, 2006).

Rinds, peels, and skins from vegetables are also a source of carotenoids, as commented before. Obrero et al. (2013) suggested that the carotenoid content in the skin of zucchini depends on the cultivar, with even higher levels of carotenoids than leaves.

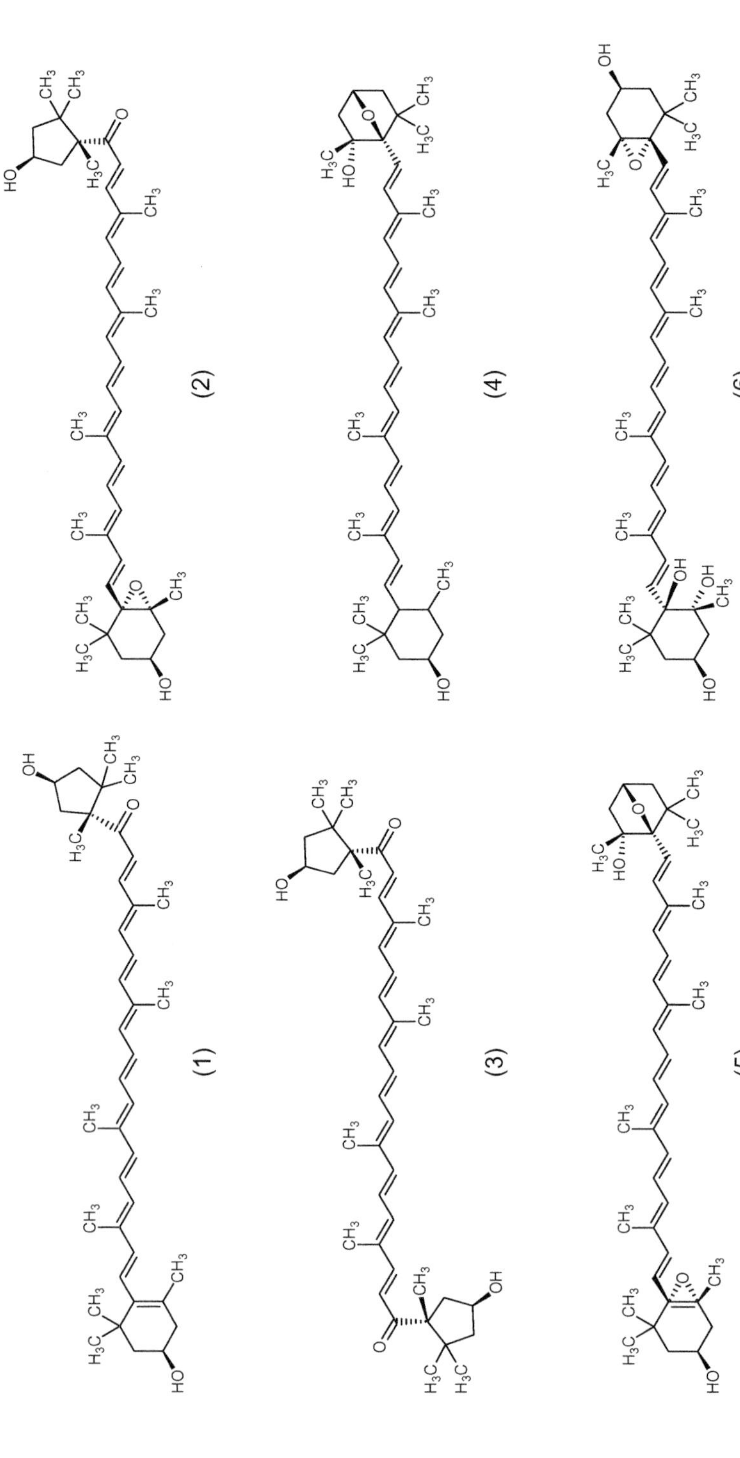

Fig. 2 Chemical structures of capsanthin (1), capsanthin 5,6-epoxide (2), capsorubin (3), cucurbitaxanthin A (4), cucurbitaxanthin B (5), and latoxanthin (6).

Table 3 Carotenoid composition of several agro-food by-products from vegetables: α-carotene (**α**-car), β-carotene (**β**-car), lutein (**lut**), β-cryptoxanthin (**β**-cryp), lycopene (**lyc**), neoxanthin (**neo**), violaxanthin (**vio**), zeaxanthin (**zea**) and total carotenoids (**car**)

Vegetable type	Scientific name[a]	By-product	Processing	Extraction method[a]	α-Car	β-Car	Lut	β-Cryp	Lyc	Neo	Vio	Zea	Total car[c]	Reference
Brassica vegetables														
Broccoli	B. oleracea var. italica	Stems	Freeze-drying	SLE, LLE/ UAE		0.0[b]	1080[b]			480[b]	0.0[b]			Liu, Zhang, Ser, Cumming, and Ku (2018)
Broccoli	B. oleracea var. italica	Leaves	Freeze-drying	SLE, LLE/ UAE		24,840[b]	48,410b			15,620[b]	20,630[b]			Liu et al. (2018)
Fruit vegetables														
Scallop	C. pepo L. ssp. ovifera cv. Scallop	Leaves	Freeze-drying	SLE		22,430								Obrero et al. (2013)
Zucchini	C. pepo L. ssp. pepo cv. MU_CU16	Leaves	Freeze-drying	SLE		30,860								Obrero et al. (2013)
	C. pepo L. ssp. pepo cv. MU_CU16	Skins	Freeze-drying	SLE			Up to ≈40,000							Obrero et al. (2013)
	C. pepo L. ssp. pepo cv. Parador	Leaves	Freeze-drying	SLE		23,790								Obrero et al. (2013)
Pumpkin	C. maxima L.	Seeds flour	Drying and milling	SLE		ND			ND				5400[b]	Silva, Simão, Marques, Leal, and Corrêa (2014)
Melon	C. melo L.	Rinds	Drying, milling	UAE		5643[b]	6324[b]	ND			Traces		12,461[b]	Benmeziane et al. (2018)
Pepper	C. annum L., var. piquillo	Seeds, skin leftovers and stems	Freeze-drying, crushing and sieving	SFE		260,923[d]								Romo-Huadle, Yetano-Cunchillos, González-Ferrero, Sáiz-Abajo, and González-Navarro (2012)

Continued

Table 3 Continued

Vegetable type	Scientific name[a]	By-product	Processing	Extraction method[a]	α-Car	β-Car	Lut	β-Cryp	Lyc	Neo	Vio	Zea	Total car[c]	Reference
Tomato	L. esculentum Mill.	Vines	Mincing	SLE					10,750[e]						Allen and Rusnack (2009)
	L. esculentum Mill.	Rejected tomatoes	Mincing	SLE					28,490e						Allen and Rusnack (2009)
	L. esculentum Mill.	Sorter table tomatoes	Mincing	SLE					26,950[e]						Allen and Rusnack (2009)
	L. esculentum Mill.	Seeds (with fruit rests)	Neutralization, drying and milling	SLE and LLE	40	1440	650		13,000			100			Knoblich, Anderson, and Latshaw (2005)
	L. esculentum Mill.	Peels (with fruit rests) removed with warmed and diluted NaOH, from canned tomatoes	Neutralization, drying and milling	SLE and LLE	0	2930	1450		73,400			370			Knoblich et al. (2005)
	L. esculentum Mill. cv. Stella, Topaz, Aquarius F1, Jacqueline, Marigold and Carobeta	Peels from hand-peeled tomatoes	Blanching, drying, grinding and sieving	UAE		32,520–293,360e	2270–21,220e		14,510–241,140e						Nikolova, Taneva, Prokopov, and Hadjikinova (2017)
	L. esculentum Mill.	Peels from industry	Drying, grinding and sieving	SLE and LLE										128,000[e]	Rizk, El-kady, and El-bialy (2014)
	L. esculentum Mill.	Peels from industry recovered with caustic lye	Neutralization and griding	MAE					13,592[b,f]						Ho, Ferruzzi, Liceaga, and San Martín-González (2015)

Species	Material	Pretreatment	Extraction method				Reference
L. esculentum Mill.	Peels	Blanching, drying, grinding	EAE		440,000		Lavecchia and Zuorro (2008)
L. esculentum Mill. var. Pachino	Peels	Pulsed electric field and steam blanching	SLE	37,900			Pataro et al. (2018)
L. esculentum Mill.	Skins with seeds (30%) and 3% moisture	Grinding	SLE/SFE		2390[e-g]		Kassama, Shi, and Mittal (2008)
L. esculentum Mill.	Wastewater by-product solids	Mincing	SLE		9350[e]		Allen and Rusnack (2009)
L. esculentum Mill.	Dry pumice (seeds, peels and vegetable parts)	Mincing	SLE		11,030[e]		Allen and Rusnack (2009)
L. esculentum Mill.	Pomace from tomato paste industry	Drying and milling	SLE/SFE		30,960[b,h]	29,600[b,h]	Baysal, Ersus, and Starmans (2000)
L. esculentum Mill.	Industrial pomace from cold break tomato paste industry	Freeze-drying	SLE		41,370[b]	14,980[b]	Kalogeropoulos, Chiou, Pyriochou, Peristeraki, and Karathanos (2012)
L. esculentum Mill. var. canario	Pomace (seeds, skins, part of the pulp) obtained using a laboratory peeler-pulper	Drying and grinding	UAE	14080[b,i]			Luengo, Condón-abanto, Condón, Álvarez, and Raso (2014)

Continued

Table 3 Continued

Vegetable type	Scientific name[a]	By-product	Processing	Extraction method[a]	α-Car	β-Car	Lut	β-Cryp	Lyc	Neo	Vio	Zea	Total car[c]	Reference
	L. esculentum Mill.	By-product of steam peeling (seeds and peels) from tomato sauce industry		SLE/SFE					1180/2450[b,j]					Rozzi, Singh, Vierling, and Watkins (2002)
	L. esculentum Mill.	Tomato processing waste (seeds and peels)	Drying, grinding and sieving	SLE									3750	Strati and Oreopoulou (2011)
	L. esculentum Mill. cv. Red Sea	Tomato processing waste (seeds and peels)	Drying, grinding and sieving	EAE and HP					8940b k				12700[b,k]	Strati, Gogou, and Oreopoulou (2015)
Starchy and nonstarchy root vegetables														
Sugar beet	B. vulgaris L.	Sugar beet pulp				21[b]								Habeeb et al. (2017)
Carrot	D. carota L., Nantes carrots	Peels	Freeze drying, milling and sieving	SLE and LLE/SFE	6760[e,l]	12,780[e,l]	190[e,l]		840[e,l]					Lima, Charalampopoulos, and Chatzifragkou (2018)
	D. carota L.	Peels	Grinding/powder, drying, blanching	SLE and LLE		8810–20,450[b]								Chantaro, Devahastin, and Chiewchan (2008)

	Species	Part	Pretreatment	Extraction method					Reference
	D. carota L. var. sativa	Peels	Blanching and grinding	MAE	>120,000[b,m]				Chummanpaisont, Niammuy, and Devahastin (2014)
	D. carota L. var. sativa	Peels	Blanching and grinding	MAE	Up to 132,700 and 136,000[b,n] 3920			Up to 289,200 and 274,110[b,n]	Hiranvarachat and Devahastin (2014)
	D. carota L.	Pulp waste from juice extraction	Drying and grinding	SLE					Shyamala and Jamuna (2010)
Sweet potato	I. batatas L.	Leaves	Raw	SLE	15,237e	20,966e	10,056e		Chen and Chen (1993)
	I. batatas L. cv. Suioh	Leaves	Freeze drying	SLE	3680	3680			Ishiguro and Yoshimoto (2006)
	I. batatas L. cv. Suioh	Stems	Freeze drying	SLE	180				Ishiguro and Yoshimoto (2006)
	I. batatas L. cv. Suioh	Petioles	Freeze drying	SLE	160				Ishiguro and Yoshimoto (2006)

[a] Abbreviations for scientific names: Beta vulgaris (B. vulgaris); Brassica oleracea (B. oleracea); Capsicum annum (C. annum); Cucumis melo (C. melo); Cucurbita maxima (C. maxima); Cucurbita pepo (C. pepo); Daucus carota (D. carota); Ipomoea batatas (I. batatas); Lycopersicon esculentum (L. esculentum). Abbreviations for the extraction methods: EAE, enzymatic-assisted extraction; HP, high-pressure-assisted extraction; LLE, liquid-liquid extraction; MAE, microwave-assisted extraction; MET, microemulsion technique; SFE, supercritical fluid extraction; SLE, solid-liquid extraction; UAE, ultrasounds assisted extraction. The extraction method was before saponification step (when it was required).

[b] μg/100 g dry weight.

[c] Determined spectrophotmetrically.

[d] Red pepper extract. Extraction yield was 68.1% at 4 MPa, 60°C, 120 min and 0.2–0.5 mm particle size.

[e] Not defined the weight basis.

[f] At 1:20 solid:liquid ratio, 400 W, 24 kJ equivalents for 60 s using ethyl acetate.

[g] This value corresponds to a recovery of 33.04% at 68.6°C, 41.8 Pa and 1.76% as modifier concentration (ethanol) using CO_2 as extractant and compared to a SLE control.

[h] At CO_2 flow rate of 4 kg/h, 55°C and 300 bar, with the addition of 5% ethanol a maximum of 53.93% of this content of lycopene was extracted. Half of the this amount of β-carotene was extracted in 2 h at 4 kg/h of CO_2, 65°C and 300 bar, also with the addition of 5% ethanol.

[i] At manosonication assisted extraction (50 kPa; 94 mm), 45°C, 50% hexane/50% ethanol.

[j] At 86°C and 34.47 MPa, 500 mL of CO_2 at a flow rate of 2.5 mL/min resulted in extracting 61.0% of this lycopene amount.

[k] With ethyl lactate.

[l] At 59.0°C, 349 bar and with the aid of 15.5% of ethanol, the maximum carotenoid recovery of the sum of these carotenoids was 86.1% at lab and 96.2% when scaling-up the conditions.

[m] Depending on the applied conditions and the time.

[n] 300 W/75 mL continuous and 300 W/150 mL intermittent conditions, depending on the time.

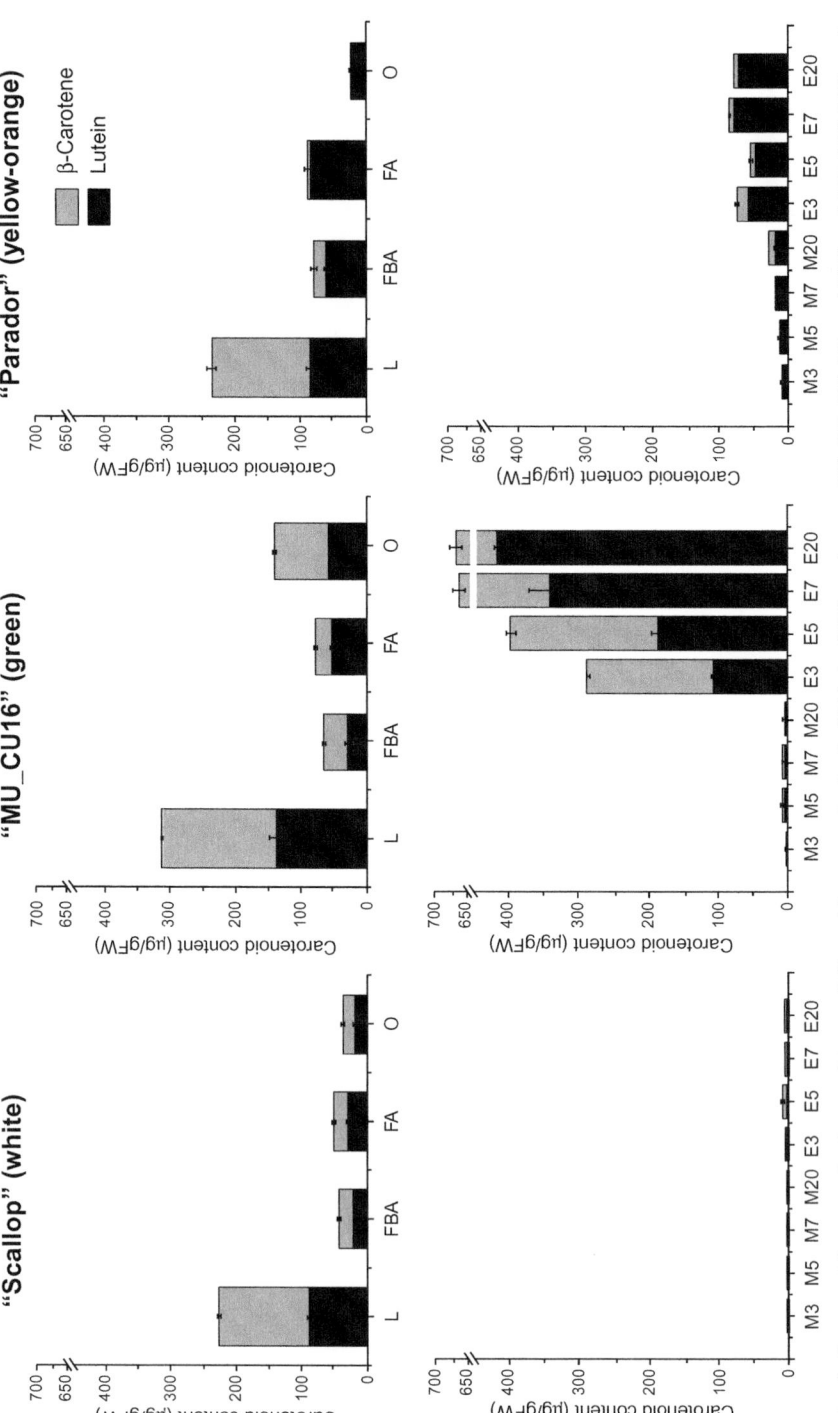

Fig. 3 Carotenoid content in three cultivars of *Cucurbita pepo*. Anthesis (FA), leaf (L), and ovary (O). E3, E5, E7, and E20 and M3, M5, M7, and M20 represent different stages of the fruits (3, 4, 5, and 20 days after pollination). Reprinted (adapted) with permission from Obrero, A., González-Verdejo, C. I., Die, J. V., et al. (2013). Carotenogenic gene expression and carotenoid accumulation in three varieties of *Cucurbita pepo* during fruit development. *Journal of Agricultural and Food Chemistry*. Copyright (2013) American Chemical Society.

For example, the content of lutein could be up to 40,000 µg/100 g of fresh weight, which is also higher than that in edible parts of lutein-rich vegetables (Tables 2 and 3).

Another important source of lutein together with β-carotene and lycopene is tomato peels (skin and outer pericarp tissue), which are generated during the tomato peeling operation applied in the processing industry. Tomato peels obtained from fresh red-ripe tomatoes can vary from 2.45% to 5.33% (Nikolova et al., 2017). Skins can also be separated from tomato pomace by a continuous floatation-cum-sedimentation system (Kaur, Wani, Oberoi, & Sogi, 2008). The contents of these carotenoids in peels and skins vary depending on the study and the type of raw material and tomato cultivar, with amounts up to 21,220 (lutein), 293,360 (β-carotene), 241,140 (lycopene) µg/100 g of dry weight. Lavecchia and Zuorro (2008) recovered 440,000 µg/100 g of lycopene from dry tomato peels (Table 3). Tomato peels may also present *cis*-lycopene, γ-carotene, phytofluene, and phytoene (Ho et al., 2015; Knoblich et al., 2005; Rizk et al., 2014). Moreover, in these studies, besides common solid-liquid extraction (SLE) methods (Kaur et al., 2008; Kehili et al., 2017), more "green" extraction methods have been developed to recover carotenoids: microwave-assisted extraction (MAE) for all-*trans* and *cis*-isomers of lycopene (Ho et al., 2015), supercritical fluid extraction (SFE) using CO_2 as extractant agent for lycopene and β-carotene (Kehili et al., 2017), and enzyme-assisted extraction (EAE) for lycopene (Lavecchia & Zuorro, 2008). Among them, MAE using ethyl acetate offered high yield results, even than SLE, but certain limitations could be regarding the consumer preference against solvent use and challenges with scaling up (Ho et al., 2015). EAE also required the use of solvents, but extracting considerable amounts of carotenoids (61,000–440,200 µg/100 g) (Munde et al., 2017). In the case of SFE, the recovery yields were medium, up to 61% for lycopene and 59% for β-carotene (Kehili et al., 2017), but it is possible to be scaled-up.

The utility of carotenoids from these sources can be exemplified with another study of the latter authors (Kehili, Choura, Zammel, Allouche, & Sayadi, 2018). In this study, lycopene from tomato peels was evaluated to stabilize refined olive and sunflower oils. For that a lycopene-rich oleoresin extracted with hexane was investigated for 5 months, under accelerated shelf-life, compared to the synthetic antioxidant, butylated hydroxytoluene. Their results suggested the highest efficiency of 250 and 2000 µg/g of this extract for the oxidative stabilization of the latter oils and correlated with the lycopene content, that is, 5 and 40 µg/g of lycopene, respectively.

Carrots peels, which represent above 11% of the total vegetable in the processing of carrots, have considerably high carotenoid contents: approximately, lutein, 190 µg/100 g; lycopene 840 µg/100 g; α-carotene, 6760 µg/100 g; β-carotene, 12,780 µg/100 g. It amounts to around 60% of that in the flesh (Lima et al., 2018). For that reason, several studies have focused on this matrix to study the recovering of carotenoids using green technologies as SFE with CO_2 and ethanol as cosolvent (Lima et al., 2018) and MAE with 50% (v/v) hexane, 25% (v/v) acetone, and 25% (v/v) ethanol (Chumnanpaisont et al., 2014; Hiranvarachat & Devahastin, 2014). It seems that SFE had better recovery results than the method of control based on SLE and LLE (liquid-liquid extraction), but higher amounts of β-carotene can be obtained with MAE (Table 3).

Moreover, seeds are other potential by-product underused. For example, the seed content of pumpkin fruits varies from 3.52% to 4.27%, being often used as animal feed, ground up for fertilizer or discarded (Devi, Prasad, & Sagarika, 2018). Its consumption after being salted and roasted and in bread, it is a guarantee of their safety for humans. The amount of carotenoids is above 5400 µg/100 g (dry weight). Seeds from tomato by-products also contain carotenoids, but in lower amounts than peels (Table 3).

Other by-products obtained from the processing industry of vegetables

There are other by-products derived from the processing industry of vegetables, which consisted of a mix of different vegetable parts, and so containing carotenoids. In this sense, a potential by-product could be derived from red peppers canned industry, comprising seeds, skin leftovers, and stems with above 15.9%, 34.7%, and 49.4% of the total weight, respectively (Romo-Hualde et al., 2012). The latter authors have employed SFE to extract vitamin C and β-carotene from this whole by-product, recovering 272,669 and 260,923 µg/100 g, respectively. Therefore, on the basis of their carotenoid content and production worldwide (>56 million tons, FAOSTAT, 2016), not only peppers may have a role to play in reducing nutrient deficiencies (Kantar et al., 2016), but also their by-products (see Tables 2 and 3 for comparison).

Tomato (*Lycopersicon esculentum* L.) is also a highly consumed vegetable worldwide, with >233 million tons produced in 2016 (FAOSTAT, 2016). It has been estimated that >80% of tomatoes grown are consumed in the form of processed products such as canned tomatoes, sauce, juice, soup, concentrate, puree, dry tomato, ketchup, or paste (Kaur et al., 2008). Besides peels and seeds, the processing of tomato generate a large amount of by-products such as tomato pomace, a mixture of peels and seeds, whose management is one of the most important sustainability-related issues faced by the industry due to their potential negative effects in the environment (Viuda-Martos et al., 2013). As an example, 10%–40% of the whole tomato processed in the paste plants is believed to be tomato pomace (Amiri-Rigi, Abbasi, & Scanlon, 2016). On a dry weight basis, this by-product contains significantly lower amounts of lycopene (413,700 µg/100 g) and increased amounts of β-carotene (14,980 µg/100 g) than whole tomatoes (101,320 and 8610 µg/100 g, respectively). On the fresh basis, both the content of carotenoids in both by-products is higher (Kalogeropoulos et al., 2012). Probably, for these reasons several studies have explored different extraction techniques to recover lycopene and other carotenoids from tomato pomace and other processing by-products (Table 3). Thus, as for peels, several extraction procedures have been applied as an alternative to the conventional SLE with solvents: SFE to extract β-carotene and lycopene from tomato pomace (Baysal et al., 2000) and from the by-product of steam peeling (seeds and peels) of a tomato sauce industry (Rozzi et al., 2002), SFE to extract lycopene from skins containing seeds (30%) and 3% moisture (Kassama et al., 2008), ultrasounds-assisted extraction (UAE) under pressure to recover carotenoids from tomato pomace (Luengo et al., 2014), EAE and high pressure-assisted extraction to recover carotenoids from tomato processing waste (Strati et al., 2015), as well as the combination of UAE, EAE, and microemulsion technique (MET) to obtain lycopene from tomato paste waste pomace (Amiri-Rigi et al., 2016). Since the carotenoids content has been determined by different methods, spectrophotometrically and using liquid chromatography, and the results have been expressed in several ways (% recovery, % yield vs control conditions, concentration values, etc.), it is difficult to conclude which extraction method gave the best results. In any case, the content of carotenoids is different depending on the by-product and processing type (Table 3).

Other studied sources have been investigated for their β-carotene content, such as sugar beet pulp (Habeeb et al., 2017) and carrot pulp waste from juice extraction (Shyamala & Jamuna, 2010), but they contained lower amounts than by-products from tomato processing (Table 3).

Factors affecting the content of carotenoids in vegetable by-products

Besides the heterogeneous starting material that can be found when extracting carotenoids, there are several aspects to keep in mind for underused vegetables and the aforementioned by-products. The crop year, harvest date, genotype, maturity stage, and the cultivation conditions (e.g., soil, soilless, conventional farm, organic farm, etc.) may affect the levels of carotenoids in vegetable tissues (De Azevedo & Rodriguez-Amaya, 2005; Graça Dias et al., 2018; Kim et al., 2016; Žnidarčič, Ban, & Šircelj, 2011). As an example, Nikolova et al. (2017) have highlighted that both the percentage of peels obtained from fresh red-ripe tomatoes and the lycopene content is affected by the genotype and the crop year, whereas the β-carotene and lutein contents were affected mainly by the tomato genotype. Alternatively, under very similar micro-climate conditions in the greenhouse, the crop year and the interaction of species/cultivars and year did not affect the concentration of carotenes and xanthophylls in several leafy vegetables as shown by Žnidarčič et al. (2011). Other aspects to be considered are the effects of the pretreatment of the vegetable, for example, before peeling. In this sense, a recent study have suggested that steam blanching and pulsed electric field (PEF), as pretreatments prior to peeling, increased the carotenoid content of the peels compared to untreated peels, up to 189% and 188%, respectively (Pataro et al., 2018). Nevertheless, depending on the conditions, thermal degradation during blanching should be controlled (Chantaro et al., 2008). In this sense, Pataro et al. (2018) concluded that an electroporation effect induced by PEF (E, 0.5 kV/cm; WT, 1 kJ/kg; T) prior to the thermal treatment enables intensifying the recovery of carotenoids at lower blanching temperature (up to 60°C) (Table 3). No evidences of isomerization or degradation of lycopene was found.

Moreover, the extraction method can affect not only the recovery of carotenoids but also their degradation (Ho et al., 2015; Seo, Burri, Quan, & Neidlinger, 2005). The method used for drying can also lead to the degradation of carotenoids in vegetable by-products (Albanese, Adiletta, Acunto, Cinquanta, & Di Matteo, 2014). As an example, the latter authors have suggested that hot air drying at 50°C and freeze drying are suitable methods to preserve carotenoids compounds and antioxidant activity in tomato peels. However, hot air drying (60–80°C) caused a decrease in the contents of β-carotene and other antioxidants (Chantaro et al., 2008). Furthermore, the storage may also affect the initial carotenoid content (Romo-Hualde et al., 2012), as well as the light and heat (Albanese et al., 2014). Microencapsulation by spray drying could be a strategy to increase the stability of carotenoids extracted from vegetables over storage time (Romo-Hualde et al., 2012), with relatively cost efficiency.

Fruits by-products as sources of carotenoids

Fruit by-products mainly come from raw material that is discarded during fruit processing in the food industry (fruit pulp, juice, nectar, puree, chutneys, fermented products, dehydrated fruit, etc.). Among them, the main fruit by-products can be found in peels, seeds, and bagasse. Only the juice industry produces wastes that range about 20%–60% of raw material (Amaya-Cruz et al., 2015). As an example, it can be said that around 53% of tropical fruit consumed in Brazil (principal world producer) is processed, producing consequently high amounts of wastes (Da Silva et al., 2014).

These fruit by-products are rich in micronutrients such as vitamins, fibers, minerals, and other secondary phytochemicals such as phenolic compounds, carotenoids, tocopherols, etc. Because of that, they could be recovered and reused to obtain added-value extracts for the production of nutraceuticals and functional foods; indeed, this fact would contribute positively to the environment, industry, and economy (Ayala-Zavala et al., 2011).

Despite that secondary metabolites such as carotenoids in fruit by-products have not been studied in depth; most bibliography makes reference to tropical and citric fruits. Table 4 summarizes the main fruit by-products and their carotenoids content.

Tropical fruits

Among tropical fruits, mango seems to be the most revalorized product. Mango peel stands out because it contains lutein as major carotenoid, followed by β-carotene and violaxanthin (Ajila et al., 2010; Ruales et al., 2018). Its content, among other environmental and agronomic factors, is highly influenced by ripening; in fact, Ajila et al. reported that carotenoids content of ripe Raspuri and Badami mango varieties were 43,600 and 19,400 µg/100 g dry weight, respectively, compared to 7350 and 8100 µg/100 g dry weight in raw Raspuri and Badami mango varieties (Ajila, Bhat, & Prasada Rao, 2007). Garcia-Mendoza et al. demonstrated that SFE with CO_2 reported a higher recovery of total carotenes than a conventional extraction with ethanol. The concentration using SFE was 560,000 µg β-carotene/100 g dry weight compared to 70,000 µg β-carotene/100 g dry weight obtained using conventional extraction (Garcia-Mendoza et al., 2015).

Mango by-products have also been used as ingredients in the formulation of different food. Mango peel powder was added to macaroni preparations at three different levels (2.5%, 5.0%, 7.5%) and studied its effect on the cooking properties, firmness, nutraceutical, and sensory characteristics of macaroni. Regarding carotenoids it was observed that they increased from 500 to 8400 µg/100 g in macaroni with 7.5% incorporation of mango peel powder; indeed, it was possible to enhance the nutritional

Table 4 Carotenoid composition of several agro-food by-products from tropical and other fruits: **α**-carotene (**α**-car), **β**-carotene (**β**-car), lutein (lut), **β**-cryptoxanthin (**β**-cryp), lycopene (lyc), neoxanthin (neo), violaxanthin (vio), zeaxanthin (zea) and total carotenoids (car)

Vegetable type	Scientific name[a]	By-product	Processing	Extraction method	α-Car	β-Car	Lut	β-Cryp	Lyc	Neo	Vio	Zea	Total car[c]	Reference
Tropical fruits														
Mango	*Mangifera indica* L.	Peel	Fresh										8100–19400a	Ajila, Jaganmohan Rao, and Prasada Rao (2010)
Mango	*Mangifera indica* L.	Peel	Freeze-drying			278	326				158		762a	Ruales et al. (2018)
Mango	*Mangifera indica* L.	Peel											7350–43,600a	Ajila, Naidu, Bhat, and Prasada Rao (2007)
Mango	*Mangifera indica* L.	Peel	Freeze-drying										36,500–394,500	Ajila, Bhat, and Prasada Rao (2007)
Mango	*Mangifera indica* L.	Peel	Freeze-drying	SFE									560,000a	Garcia-Mendoza, Paula, Paviani, Cabral, and Martinez-Correa (2015)
Mango	*Mangifera indica* L.	Mango seed kernel	Freeze-drying			50					18		107a	Ruales et al. (2018)
Avocado	*Persea americana*	Peel	Freeze-drying										2585–17,000	Vinha, Moreira, and Barreira (2013) and Wang, Bostic, and Gu (2010)

Continued

Table 4 Continued

Vegetable type	Scientific name[a]	By-product	Processing	Extraction method	α-Car	β-Car	Lut	β-Cryp	Lyc	Neo	Vio	Zea	Total car[c]	Reference
Avocado	*Persea americana*	Seed	Freeze-drying										700–6300	Vinha et al. (2013) and Wang et al. (2010)
Pink guava	*Psidium guajava*	Refiner, siever and decanter	Freeze-drying						2860–5510					Kong and Ismail (2011)
Pink guava	*Psidium guajava*	Decanter	Oven-drying						14,000[a]					Kong, Ismail, Tan, and Rajab (2010)
Guava	*Psidium guajava*	Peel flour	Oven-drying			37.76			26.72					Bertagnolli, Silveira, Fogaça, Umann, and Penna (2014)
Guava	*Psidium guajava*	Peel, pulp's leftovers, and seed	Freeze-drying			26.67			18.11					Da Silva et al. (2014)
Guava	*Psidium guajava*	By-products not specified	Oven-drying			791			477					Casarotti, Borgonovi, Batista, and Penna (2018)
Peach palm fruit	*Bactris gasipaes*	Peel	Oven-drying	Ultrasound assisted extraction									163,470[a]	Ordóñez-Santos, Pinzón-Zarate, and González-Salcedo (2015)
Peach palm fruit	*Bactris gasipaes*	Peel	Fresh			7300							33,690	Noronha Matos, Praia Lima, Pereira Barbosa, Zerlotti Mercadante, and Campos Chisté (2019)

Common name	Scientific name	Part	Drying method											Reference
Tucumã	Astrocaryum vulgare	Peel	Fresh			7800							18.060	Noronha Matos et al. (2019)
Pineapple	Ananas comosus L.	Rind and core	Not specified		Rind 89[a]	Rind 2537[a] Core 994[a]	Rind 288[a]							Freitas et al. (2015)
Pineapple	Ananas comosus L.	Peel and pulp's leftover	Freeze-drying			156.10[a]								Da Silva et al. (2014)
Cherimoya	Annona cherimola	Peel	Fresh		87.3–174		129–232							Albuquerque et al. (2016)
Pindo palm	Butia Capitata	Pomace	Not specified		82[a]	21.899[a]	362[a]	1268[a]				395[a]		
Pequi fruit	Caryocar Brasilense	Peel flours	Oven-drying										2116.52–3499.03[a]	Leão, França, Oliveira, Bastos, and Coimbra (2017)
Banana	Musa spp.	Peel	Freeze-drying		84[a]								186[a]	Yan et al. (2016)
Banana	Musa spp.	Peel	Freeze-drying				311.5–1188.1[a]						1906.4–8987.3[a]	Borges et al. (in press)
Banana	Musa spp.	Peel	Freeze	Ripe 124.57 Unripe 156.17	Ripe 183.56 Unripe 196.90	Ripe 1584.39 Unripe 1573.27							Ripe 1877.09 Unripe 1751.65	Aquino et al. (2018)
Banana	Musa spp.	Red and yellow peel	Freeze	10%–22% of total	15%–20% of total	58%–74% of total							Red 4415 Yellow 2964	Fu et al. (2018)
Buriti fruit	Mauritia flexuosa	Peel and endocarp	Freeze-drying										Peel 88300[a] Endocarp 19100[a]	Pereira-Freire et al. (2018)
Buriti fruit	Mauritia flexuosa	Peel and endocarp flours	Oven-drying										Peel 1186.7[a] Endocarp 291.2[a]	Resende, França, and Oliveira (2019)
Acerola	Malpighia emarginata	Seed	Freeze-drying		272.83[a,c]									Da Silva et al. (2014)

Continued

Table 4 Continued

Vegetable type	Scientific name[a]	By-product	Processing	Extraction method	α-Car	β-Car	Lut	β-Cryp	Lyc	Neo	Vio	Zea	Total car[c]	Reference
Cashew apple	*Anacardium occidentale* L.	Peel and pulp's leftovers	Freeze-drying		174.14[a]									Da Silva et al. (2014)
Cashew apple	*Anacardium occidentale* L.	Bagasse	Freeze										29.2 mg/L	Macedo, Robrigues, Pinto, and De Brito (2015)
Cashew apple	*Anacardium occidentale* L.	Concentrate from fibrous residue	Fresh		60	250	470	80				560	5420	De Abreu et al. (2013)
Papaya	*Carica papaya*	Peel, pulp's leftovers, and seed	Freeze-drying		490.29[a]				85.52[a]					Da Silva et al. (2014)
Passion fruit	*Passiflora edulis*	Peel, pulp's leftovers, and seed	Freeze-drying		57.93									Da Silva et al. (2014)
Passion fruit	*Passiflora edulis*	By-products not specified	Oven-drying		5607				2857					Casarotti et al. (2018)
Surinam cherry	*Eugenia uniflora* L.	Pulp's leftovers	Freeze-drying		1110.85				693.26					Da Silva et al. (2014)
Sapodilla	*Manikara zapota* L.	Peel, pulp's leftovers, and seed	Freeze-drying						36.48					Da Silva et al. (2014)
Other fruits														
Raspberry	*Rubus idaeus* L.	Seed oil											23,000 μg/100 g oil	Oomah, Ladet, Godfrey, Liang, and Girard (2000)
Blackberry Raspberry	*Rubus fruticosus* L. *Rubus idaeus* L.	Seed oil	Pomace air dried and pomace oven dried										Blackberry: 3230–3392 Raspberry: 3906–4144	Dimić, Vujasinović, Radočaj, and Pastor (2012)

Fruit	Species	Material	Method					Content	References
Raspberry Strawberry Chokeberry	*Rubus idaeus* L. *Fragaria x ananassa* *Aronia melanocarpa*	Seed oil (6 fractions)	Supercritical CO$_2$ extraction					12–109 mg/L 8–115 mg/L 6–99 mg/L	Milala et al. (2018)
Prickly pear	*Opuntia ficus-indica*	Peel	Freeze-drying					254000[a]	Ramadan and Mörsel (2003)
Prickly pear	*Opuntia ficus-indica*	Peel	- Conventional hot air drying - Instant controlled pressure drop (DIC)					Control: 169,320[a] DIC: 1,071,640	Namir, Elzahar, Ramadan, and Allaf (2017)
Apricot	*Prunus armeniaca*	Bagasse	Supercritical fluid extraction					4000–6000[a]	Döker, Salgin, Şanal, Mehmetoğlu, and Çalimli (2004)
Peach	*Prunus persica*	Mixture of fruit pieces, pulp and peels	Ethanol extraction	6755	220	8675	1208	16,859	de Vargas, Jablonski, Flôres, and Rios (2017)
Sour cherry	*Prunus cerasus*	Seed oil	Hexane and SC-CO$_2$ (both + ethanol)					Hexane: 8.47–10.03 mg/L SC-CO$_2$: 5.65–6.00 mg/L	Yilmaz and Gökmen (2013)
Sour cherry	*Prunus cerasus*	Seed oil	Freeze-dried seeds					510–1750 µg/100 g oil	Górnaś, Rudzińska, Raczyk, Mišina, and Segliņa (2016)
Sour cherry	*Prunus cerasus*	Seed						170–390[a]	Radenkovs and Feldmane (2017)
Sweet cherry	*Prunus avium*	Seed oil	Freeze-dried seeds					380–620 µg/100 g oil	Górnaś et al. (2016)

[a] µg/100 g dry weight.

quality of macaroni without affecting its textural and sensory properties (Jahurul et al., 2015).

Other authors studied muffins enriched in dried mango pulp fiber waste, one of the main by-products of mango juice industry. The addition of this mango by-product (3050 µg β-carotene/100 g dry weight) at 25% in bakery products as muffins allowed preserving shape, grain, texture, and overall quality and, moreover, muffins still contained carotenoids after baking (3550 µg β-carotene/100 g dry weight) improving their nutritional value (Sudha, Indumathi, Sumanth, Rajarathnam, & Shashirekha, 2015).

Mango seed kernel represents 45%–85% of the seed and approximately 20% of the whole fruit. Bibliography about carotenoids in mango seed kernel is scarce, maybe because its content is not enough relevant. β-carotene is the main carotene present in mango seed kernel, whereas the most important xanthophyll is violaxanthin and, according to Ruales et al. the total carotenoids content is 107 µg β-carotene/100 g dry weight (Ruales et al., 2018).

Avocado peel and seed have also been investigated in terms of carotenoids. Avocado peel mainly contains lutein (about 56%), followed by β-carotene (11%) (Gross, Gabai, Lifshitz, & Sklarz, 1973) and its total carotenoids content is much higher than avocado pulp. Peel obtained from ripe fruits of six cultivars of Florida avocados vary from 8900 to 17,000 µg/100 g dry weight (Wang et al., 2010), whereas avocado peel from Hass cultivar grown in Algarve (Portugal) showed 2585 µg/100 g dry weight (Vinha et al., 2013). However, avocado seed revealed lower carotenoids contents, similar to avocado pulp (700–6300 µg/100 g dry weight).

Lycopene has been described as the main carotenoid of pink guava, contributing around 80% of total carotenoids. The industry of pink guava puree generates about 25% wastes of the total loading fruit, these by-products are produced at three different stages and they can be classified as refiner, siever, and decanter. Total lycopene content on wet basis and determined by high-performance liquid chromatography (HPLC) has been reported to be 37,800, 28,600, 33,500, and 55,100 µg/100 g in fruits, refiner, siever, and decanter, respectively. Thus, these by-products could be used as a source of lycopene (Kong & Ismail, 2011). Besides, oven drying has been optimized as drying method for decanter obtained from pink guava puree and authors obtained the minimum lycopene degradation at 43.8°C for 6.4 h, being the lycopene content 14,000 µg/100 g (Kong et al., 2010).

Other studies that do not report the color of guava (probably white guava) presents a much lower content in carotenoids than pink guava, some authors have reported that fruit by-products contain 791 µg β-carotene/100 g dry weight and 477 µg lycopene/100 g dry weight (Casarotti et al., 2018), and other authors have described even lower carotenoids content (Bertagnolli et al., 2014; Da Silva et al., 2014).

By-products from other tropical fruits such as peach palm fruit, pineapple, cherimoya, pindo palm fruit, pequi fruit, banana, buriti fruit, tucumã, acerola, cashew apple, papaya, passion fruit, Surinam cherry, and sapodilla also contain carotenoids (Table 4). Nevertheless, carotenoids in by-products from tropical fruits is a field that could be studied more in depth in order to revalorize low-cost renewable resources, reduce industrial wastes, and provide positive economic and environmental impacts.

Citrus fruits

Citrus species are also known as fruits with the most complex carotenoid profiles. During the processing of citrus fruit for juice, peels are the main by-product. These peels become a waste and, if they are not reused, they give cause to an important source of environmental pollution.

Citrus species peels contain a high number of carotenoids, being the major ones (9Z)-violaxanthin (8%–33%), β-citraurin (11%–28%), and β-cryptoxanthin (3%–23%). The lutein content in the peel of all citrus species is 4%–8%. Some furanoids (neochrome, luteoxanthin, auroxanthin) and Z-isomers were also detected. The extract of green citrus peel such as lime contains high concentration of chloroplast pigments: lutein (46%), β-carotene (24.2%), α-carotene (8.5%), (9Z/9′Z)-lutein (3.4%), (13Z/13′Z)-lutein (1.8%), β-cryptoxanthin (3.4%), and (Z)-β-cryptoxanthin (0.9%) (Agócs et al., 2007).

Wang et al. studied the carotenoids content in peels of eight species of citrus fruits and they found that the contents ranged from 2100 to 204,000 µg/100 g d.w., being *Citrus reticulata* Blanco (mandarin orange) the species with the highest carotenoid content. The carotenoids identified by HPLC in these citrus species were lutein, zeaxanthin, β-cryptoxanthin, and β-carotene. β-Cryptoxanthin (3050 µg/100 g dry weight) and β-carotene (6920 µg/100 g dry weight) were the main carotenoids in *Citrus reticulata* Blanco peel (Wang, Chuang, & Hsu, 2008).

Fresh pomace (peels and segment walls) of naranjita fruit (*Citrus mitis* B.) showed a similar carotenoid content to *Citrus reticulata* Blanco peel described above (200,300 µg/100 g dry weight). An air-drying process was optimized for naranjita pomace but an important decrease in retention of total carotenoids was observed (about 40%) (Delgado-Nieblas et al., 2017).

Among citrus genus, orange is widely processed to obtain natural juices, pulps, candies, and extracts for manufacturing industries. This processing generates a huge amount of wastes that reach approximately 50% of the fruits (Hernández-Montoya, Montes-Morán, & Elizalde-González, 2009). Peel extracts from Valencia and Navel orange varieties demonstrated that Valencia orange peels was rich in apocarotenoids representing >60% of the total carotenoids. Besides, it contains β-cryptoxanthin and, in minor quantities, dihydroxycarotenoids (zeaxanthin and its epoxides). However, Navel peels showed β-cryptoxanthin as the main carotenoid, but ζ-carotene and some dihydroxy derivatives were also present. Apocarotenoids in this variety were in low concentrations. This study demonstrated how variety highly influences the carotenoid profile (Chedea, Kefalas, & Socaciu, 2010).

Orange seed oil from four different cultivars showed carotenoid contents that ranged between 1164 and 2669 µg β-carotene/100 g. Thus, these oils (that also contain high concentration of other bioactive compounds) could be used as specialty oil in diets (Jorge, Da Silva, & Aranha, 2016). Recently, Raman spectroscopy has revealed to be a good technique for rapid and nondestructive chemical mapping of carotenoids. This fact makes this technique a sustainable alternative for the revalorization of citrus wastes (Yang et al., 2017). *Citrus ichangensis* × *C. reticulate* peels and seeds flours have been extracted by supercritical CO_2 extraction for obtaining citrus peels and seeds oils. Peel oil presented 146,300 µg carotenoids/100 g oil and the concentration of the mixture of seed + peel oil was even higher (195,200 µg carotenoids/100 g oil). Therefore, this methodology represents a good revalorization strategy to obtain bioactive oils (Ndayishimiye & Chun, 2017). There are evidences about the use of orange by-products for obtaining bioactive enriched foods. Orange vesicles flour has been used for the production of snack foods containing corn flour and potato starch. The addition of orange by-products increases the content of carotenoids in the snacks (43.3 µg carotenoids/100 g sample using the predicted optimum conditions) (Tovar-Jiménez et al., 2015). Orange epicarp has also been used as a food additive to enrich fish burgers. The extract of the orange by-product was microencapsulated by spray-drying and 50 g/kg was added to fish burgers. The spray-drying microencapsulation process demonstrated to improve the bio-accessibility of bioactive compounds such as carotenoids because a higher release of carotenoids and other bioactives was observed in the enriched samples compared to control samples (Spinelli, Lecce, Likyova, Del Nobile, & Conte, 2018).

Other fruits

Some other fruit by-products contain considerable amounts of carotenoids. Among fruits, these can be found in berries, apricot, peach, prickly pear, or cherries. Table 4 shows the carotenoids content of the wastes generated by these fruits processing industry.

Cereals by-products as sources of carotenoids

Cereals constitute one of the main contributions to human nutrition, being an important source of proteins and energy, particularly in developing countries. Among cereals, rice and wheat are the main human food crops, and they represent more than half of the cereals produced in the world. Similarly to other plant crops, cereals and their by-products are rich in phytochemicals that have demonstrated antioxidative, antimutagenic, and anticarcinogenic activities (Smuda, Mohsen, Olsen, & Aly, 2018). It is important to take into account that most phytochemicals are concentrated in the outer layers compared to the internal layers of the cereals, but during the grain-refining process, the bran is removed causing the loss of high contents of bioactives such as dietary fiber, vitamins, minerals, tannins, carotenoids, and phenolic compounds (Verardo, Gómez-Caravaca, Messia, Marconi, & Caboni, 2011). Thus, cereals by-products are also considered a good source for the production of value added products such as food ingredients and nutraceuticals. Despite the fact that carotenoids are minor component in cereals, some of them contain higher concentrations of carotenoids compared to fruits and vegetables (Humphries & Khachik, 2003). The main carotenoids that have been found in cereals are α + β-carotene, β-cryptoxanthin, lutein, and zeaxanthin (Panfili, Fratianni, & Irano, 2004).

Wheat bran, one of the major by-products of the cereals industry, contains very low concentrations of carotenoids compared to other cereals. Stevenson et al. reported a value of 0.72 mg/100 g of total carotenoids in wheat bran (Stevenson, Phillips, O'sullivan, & Walton, 2012). Other authors also described similar carotenoids content in wheat bran, 0.42 mg/100 g (Smuda et al., 2018), or even lower (0.074 mg/100 g) (Ndolo & Beta, 2013). However, wheat germ, which only constitutes about 2%–3% of the whole wheat kernel, presents much higher carotenoids quantities that wheat bran (0.9–1.5 mg/100 g) (Ndolo & Beta, 2013; Smuda et al., 2018).

Carotenoids are strongly related to the different wheat genotypes; in fact significant differences in the content of carotenoids have been found in purple and black wheat genotypes. Lutein and zeaxanthin could be determined by HPLC and the sum of both of them resulted in 0.146 mg/100 g and 0.08 mg/100 g, in purple wheat bran and black wheat bran, respectively (Siebenhandl et al., 2007). Rice by-products can be divided in husk, bran, and germ. Rice husk is the by-product that presents the highest concentrations in carotenoids (around 0.2 mg/100 g), followed by rice bran and germ (around 0.1 and 0.05 mg/100 g, respectively) (Smuda et al., 2018). β-Carotene, lutein, and zeaxanthin are the major carotenoids described in rice and all of them diminish its concentration with the increase of milling time (increase of the outer rice layers removing) (Lamberts & Delcour, 2008). Maize is one of the cereals with the highest content in carotenoids. Among its by-products, bran, germ, and germ meal can be found. Maize germ meal shows the highest content of carotenoids (5.79 mg/100 g) followed by maize bran (3.2 mg/100 g) and maize germ (2.1 mg/100 g) (Smuda et al., 2018). However, according to Ndolo et al. yellow maize bran contains lower concentrations of carotenoids than yellow maize germ (0.05 and 0.38 mg/100 g, respectively), being lutein and zeaxanthin the determined carotenoids in these maize by-products (Ndolo & Beta, 2013).

Concerning barley, the sum of lutein and zeaxanthin of two different cultivars of black barley bran was reported to be around 0.12 mg/100 g (Siebenhandl et al., 2007). This data are in agreement with results obtained for nonpigmented barley bran (0.12 mg/100 g) and purple barley bran (0.32 mg/100 g), whereas barley germ showed a higher carotenoid content (1.47 and 1.27 mg/100 g for nonpigmented barley bran and purple barley bran, respectively) (Ndolo & Beta, 2013).

Opportunities: Inclusion of agro-food wastes in a biorefinery scheme

As an analogous concept to the petroleum refinery, biorefinery aims to integrate processes of renewable biomass conversion for obtaining biofuels and bioenergy (powers and/or heat) together with a wide range of bio-based products (Xiu, Zhang, & Shahbazi, 2011). In this way, biofuel and/or bioenergy are manufactured together with another range of bio-products in a set of interrelated processes, which make it possible to generate a more sustainable and competitive industry through obtaining economic benefits by various complementary ways. This has been the objective of innovative approaches for microalgal biorefinery, which can perform the production of several products, including carotenoids and biofuels (biodiesel, bioethanol, biogas, etc.) (Zhu, 2015).

In this context, there are different ways to take advantage of agro-food residues. As an example, Albarelli et al. (2018) proposed product diversification in the sugarcane biorefinery through the combination of algae growth and supercritical CO_2 extraction. Microalgae growth in the sugarcane biorefinery enabled CO_2 capture of 64.2 kg of CO_2/t sugarcane increasing investment on 1.8% compared with the biorefinery without microalgae growth, while SFE from microalgae could be used to extract lipids and carotenoids. In another study, the microalgae *Phormidium autumnale* was cultivated using agro-industrial wastes to produce and separate carotenoids, for example, all-*trans*-β-carotene (70.22 μg/g), all-*trans*-zeaxanthin (26.25 μg/g), all-*trans*-lutein (21.92 μg/g) were the major ones (Rodrigues et al., 2014). Another example could be the utilization of hydrothermally pretreated wheat straw for production of bioethanol and carotene-enriched biomass. For that, using the red yeast strain *Sporobolomyces roseus* on the pretreated wheat straw hydrolysates, 115,000–417,000 μg/100 g of ergosterol, a precursor of vitamin D2, and 123,000–156,000 μg g/g of β-carotene were obtained (Petrik, Kádár, & Márová, 2013).

Alternatively, a third way to valorize vegetables and fruits wastes is the extraction of carotenoids integrated into a biorefinery chain, as it has been proposed for microalgae sources. As an example, Kehili et al. (2016) valorized tomato by-products, peels and seeds, of a Tunisian industry for the recovery of value-added compounds using biorefinery cascade processing. The process integrated supercritical CO_2 extraction of carotenoids within the oil fractions of the aforementioned sources, protein extraction, and the pretreatment of the lignocellulosic residue for bioethanol production. Using supercritical CO_2, 5.79% oleoresin, 410.53 mg lycopene/kg, and 31.38 mg β-carotene/kg were extracted from tomato peels and 26.29% oil, 27.84 mg lycopene/kg, and 5.25 mg β-carotene/kg from tomato seeds, on dry weights. Protein extraction yields using alkaline extraction were close to 30% of the initial protein contents (13.28% in tomato peels and 39.26% in tomato seeds). Finally, liquid hot water treatment of the lignocellulosic residue at 160°C, 50 bar for 30 min was the most adequate for cellulose and hemicellulose hydrolysis, while keeping the degradation products low (Kehili et al., 2016).

Similarly, a potential approach to a grain biorefinery is based on supercritical CO_2. This approach involves the utilization of all components of a grain to produce value-added products and/or ingredients. In this process, lipid is first extracted from the grain using supercritical CO_2, and the extracted lipid mixture is sent directly to a fractionation column to separate high-value minor lipids such as carotenoids, tocopherols, and phytosterol. The residue after lipid extraction with increased amounts of carbohydrates and protein could be subsequently utilized (Temelli & Ciftci, 2015). In another study, corn distiller's dried grains with soluble, a by-product of the bioethanol industry, were also extracted using supercritical CO_2 at 50–70°C, 34.5–49.6 MPa, and constant CO_2 flow rate of 1 L/min. The highest yield of total lipids (9.2%, w/w) was obtained at 49.6 MPa and 70°C. The extract contained 10,700 μg/100 g carotenoids, 153,800 μg/100 g tocochromanols, and 1,590,400 μg/100 g phytosterols. Thus, supercritical CO_2 extraction can be used as a "green" process to recover lipids and valuable minor lipid components from inexpensive sources, as commented before (Ciftci, Calderon, & Temelli, 2012).

Palm-pressed mesocarp fiber constitutes about 15.7% of the solid biomass of fresh fruit bunch (Lau, Choo, Ma, & Chuah, 2008). Bear in mind that palm oil is the most consumed oil worldwide (59.97 million metric tons in 2016/2017; Statistica, 2018) and so a huge amount of residue is generated. This cellulosic material traps about 5%–7% of residue oil after screw-press extraction of crude palm oil. Traditionally, it is used as solid fuel to generate electricity for the mill, but before it could be subjected to extraction of palm minor components. For that, Lau and coworkers used continuous supercritical CO_2 the extraction at 40°C in three stages; firstly to extract vitamin E and squalene enhanced fraction at 10 MPa, secondly to remove bulk triglycerides at 20 MPa, and thirdly to produce carotene enriched fraction at 30 MPa, with recoveries higher than 90% (Lau et al., 2008).

Other sources

The biorefinery concept can be extended to medicinal plants with the view of developing a more sustainable business model for biomass producers and extractors. In a recent study, Lapkin et al. (2014) evaluated *Artemisia annua* L. cultivated or harvested in the wild for extraction of artemisinin, an antimalarial compound, and drug precursor, comprising on average 1% dry weight of the plant biomass. Moreover, depending on the geographic region of the plants, several co-metabolites, including β-carotene (492–14,989 μg/100 g) and xanthophylls (129–575 μg/100 g), could be extracted along with artemisinin. This could be the basis of a multistep extraction-fractionation sequence to be transferred to a large scale and focused on leaving no residues that could adversely affect downstream lignocellulose fermentation, but more studies are required on the latter topic. Remarkably, an approach based on this idea could face the unstable business environment followed by farmers to abandon cultivation of *Artemisia annua* L., which creates further uncertainty over the future availability of the drug precursor and over its prices.

In another context, Temelli and Ciftci (2015) have reviewed commercial examples of lipid-based oils obtained from different plant materials, where the use of supercritical CO_2 as the extraction solvent is promoted by several companies worldwide. These products are specialty oils, with high added-value due to their high content of polyunsaturated fatty acids and bioactive phytochemicals, including like carotenoids, phytosterols, tocopherols, and tocotrienols. Some of these oils are based on seeds of berries, for example, blackcurrant, lingonberry, sea buckthorn berries, saw palmetto, primrose, etc., and some of them are underused.

Conclusions

Agro-food by-products are a low-cost source and, thus, obtaining carotenoids extracts from these by-products can be the basis of the formulation of new natural pharmacological active ingredients to be used in pharmaceutical and cosmeceutical products, foods, and animal production, as an alternative to synthetic carotenoids. As an example, the nutritional quality of macaroni was enhanced using mango peel powder without affecting its textural and sensory properties (Jahurul et al., 2015). Moreover, besides the use of vegetables and fruits by-products as source of provitamin A in the food industry, antioxidant enrichment for protection of fresh-cut fruits, fruit beverages, salads, etc. using their own by-products could be another application. Alternatively, the use of carotenoids as natural colorants and antioxidants of other products is also feasible as demonstrated Rizk et al. (2014) when supplemented ice-cream with tomato peels carotenoids.

Therefore, agro-food by-products are a valuable stock material to be used for recovering carotenoids. In fact, there are some vegetable by-products with high levels of one or various carotenoids, for example, leaves of broccoli (β-carotene, lutein, neoxanthin, and violaxanthin), skin of zucchini (lutein), carrots peels (α- and β-carotene), as well as red peppers (β-carotene), and tomato processing by-products (β-carotene and lycopene). In the case of by-products of vegetables, there could be other minor carotenoids, such as antheraxanthin, *cis*- isomers, etc., which go unnoticed in most of studies because they are minor compounds or simply not studied. Concerning fruit by-products, it is interesting to highlight the great concentration in carotenoids of mango peel (lutein, β-carotene, and violaxanthin) and, among cereals, maize by-products have shown the highest carotenoids content (lutein and zeaxanthin). Moreover, deteriorated vegetables and fruits could be considered for the extraction of carotenoids, but further studies are required to demonstrate their potential and safety. Nevertheless, the requirement of standardization should be considered when extracting carotenoids from these underused sources due to the heterogeneous starting material that can be found.

The suitability of the pretreatment, drying, and extraction methods to improve the recovery of carotenoids and reduce their degradation is also another aspect to be studied for each by-product as a cost efficiency factor and environmental adequacy as well as taking into account the application purpose (human nutrition, animal nutrition, cosmetics, etc.).

Finally, the integration of carotenoids extraction into a biorefinery processing cascade for also obtaining biofuel/bioenergy and other coproducts seems promising since it could lead to a more sustainable and competitive industry. However, there are still few examples in the literature and further demonstration projects could be initiated on this promising topic.

Funding

M.d.M. Contreras thanks the postdoctoral grant funded by the "Acción 6 del Plan de Apoyo a la Investigación de la Universidad de Jaén, 2017–19."

References

Agócs, A., Nagy, V., Szabó, Z., Márk, L., Ohmacht, R., & Deli, J. (2007). Comparative study on the carotenoid composition of the peel and the pulp of different citrus species. *Innovative Food Science and Emerging Technologies, 8*, 390–394.

Ajila, C. M., Bhat, S. G., & Prasada Rao, U. J. S. (2007). Valuable components of raw and ripe peels from two Indian mango varieties. *Food Chemistry, 102*, 1006–1011.

Ajila, C. M., Jaganmohan Rao, L., & Prasada Rao, U. J. S. (2010). Characterization of bioactive compounds from raw and ripe *Mangifera indica* L. peel extracts. *Food and Chemical Toxicology, 48*, 3406–3411.

Ajila, C. M., Naidu, K. A., Bhat, S. G., & Prasada Rao, U. J. S. (2007). Bioactive compounds and antioxidant potential of mango peel extract. *Food Chemistry, 105*, 982–988.

Albanese, D., Adiletta, G., Acunto, M. D., Cinquanta, L., & Di Matteo, M. (2014). Tomato peel drying and carotenoids stability of the extracts. *International Journal of Food Science and Technology*, 2458–2463.

Albarelli, J. Q., Santos, D. T., Ensinas, A. V., Marechal, F., Cocero, M. J., & Meireles, M. A. A. (2018). Product diversification in the sugarcane biorefinery through algae growth and supercritical CO_2 extraction: thermal and economic analysis. *Renewable Energy, 129*(Part B), 776–785.

Albuquerque, T. G., Santos, F., Sanches-Silva, A., Oliveira, M. B., Bento, A. C., & Costa, H. S. (2016). Nutritional and phytochemical composition of *Annona cherimola* Mill. fruits and by-products: Potential health benefits. *Food Chemistry, 193*, 187–195.

Allen, S.D., Rusnack, M.R., 2009. Composition resulting from process for extracting carotenoids from fruit and vegetable processing waste. Patent No US 7,527,820 B2.

Amaya-Cruz, D. M., Rodríguez-González, S., Pérez-Ramírez, I. F., Loarca-Piña, G., Amaya-Llano, S., Gallegos-Corona, M. A., et al. (2015). Juice by-products as a source of dietary fibre and antioxidants and their effect on hepatic steatosis. *Journal of Functional Foods, 17*, 93–102.

Amiri-Rigi, A., Abbasi, S., & Scanlon, M. G. (2016). Enhanced lycopene extraction from tomato industrial waste using microemulsion technique: Optimization of enzymatic and ultrasound pre-treatments. *Innovative Food Science and Emerging Technologies, 35*, 160–167.

Aquino, C. F., Salomao, L. C. C., Pinheiro-Sant'Ana, H. M., Ribeiro, S. M. R., De Siqueira, D. L., & Cecon, P. R. (2018). Carotenoids in the pulp and peel of bananas from 15 cultivars in two ripening stages. *Revista Ceres, 65*, 217–226.

Ayala-Zavala, J. F., Vega-Vega, V., Rosas-Domínguez, C., Palafox-Carlos, H., Villa-Rodriguez, J. A., Siddiqui, M. W., et al. (2011). Agro-industrial potential of exotic fruit by-products as a source of food additives. *Food Research International, 44*, 1866–1874.

Baysal, T., Ersus, S., & Starmans, D. A. J. (2000). Supercritical CO_2 extraction of β-carotene and lycopene from tomato paste waste. *Journal of Agricultural and Food Chemistry, 48*, 5507–5511.

Benmeziane, A., Boulekbache-Makhlouf, L., Mapelli-Brahm, P., Khaled Khodja, N., Remini, H., Madani, K., et al. (2018). Extraction of carotenoids from cantaloupe waste and determination of its mineral composition. *Food Research International, 111*, 391–398.

Berman, J., Zorrilla-López, U., Farre, G., Zhu, C., Sandmann, G., Twyman, R. M., et al. (2015). Nutritionally important carotenoids as consumer products. *Phytochemistry Reviews, 14*, 727–743.

Bertagnolli, S. M. M., Silveira, M. L. R., Fogaça, A.d.O., Umann, L., & Penna, N. G. (2014). Bioactive compounds and acceptance of cookies made with Guava peel flour. *Food Science and Technology, 34*, 303–308.

Biehler, E., Alkaweri, A., Hoffmann, L., Krause, E., Guillaume, M., Lair, M.-L., et al. (2012). Contribution of violaxanthin, neoxanthin, phytoene and phytofluene to total carotenoid intake: Assessment in Luxembourg. *Journal of Food Composition and Analysis, 25*, 56–65.

Borges C.V., Minatel I.O., Amorim E.P., Belin M.A.F., Gomez-Gomez H.A., Correa C.R., et al., Ripening and cooking processes influence the carotenoid content in bananas and plantains (*Musa spp.*), *Food Research International* in press, https://doi.org/10.1016/j.foodres.2018.08.022.

Casarotti, S. N., Borgonovi, T. F., Batista, C.L.F.M., & Penna, A. L. B. (2018). Guava, orange and passion fruit by-products: Characterization and its impacts on kinetics of acidifi cation and properties of probiotic fermented products. *LWT—Food Science and Technology, 98*, 69–76.

Chantaro, P., Devahastin, S., & Chiewchan, N. (2008). Production of antioxidant high dietary fiber powder from carrot peels. *LWT—Food Science and Technology, 41*, 187–1994.

Chedea, V. S., Kefalas, P., & Socaciu, C. (2010). Patterns of carotenoid pigments extracted from two orange peel wastes (Valencia and Navel var.). *Journal of Food Biochemistry, 34*, 101–110.

Chen, B. H., & Chen, Y. Y. (1993). Stability of chlorophylls and carotenoids in sweet potato leaves during microwave cooking. *Journal of Agricultural and Food Chemistry, 41*, 1315–1320.

Chumnanpaisont, N., Niamnuy, C., & Devahastin, S. (2014). Mathematical model for continuous and intermittent microwave-assisted extraction of bioactive compound from plant material: Extraction of β-carotene from carrot peels. *Chemical Engineering Science, 116*, 442–451.

Ciftci, O. N., Calderon, J., & Temelli, F. (2012). Supercritical carbon dioxide extraction of corn distiller's dried grains with solubles: Experiments and mathematical modeling. *Journal of Agricultural and Food Chemistry, 60*, 12482–12490.

Commission Regulation (EU). (2012). No 231/2012 of 9 March 2012 laying down specifications for food additives listed in annexes II and III to regulation (EC) no 1333/2008 of the European Parliament and of the council. *Official Journal of the European Union, L83*, 1–290.

Da Silva, L. M. R., De Figueiredo, E. A. T., Ricardo, N.M.P.S., Vieira, I. G. P., De Figueiredo, R. W., Brasil, I. M., et al. (2014). Quantification of bioactive compounds in pulps and by-products of tropical fruits from Brazil. *Food Chemistry, 143*, 398–404.

De Abreu, F. P., Dornier, M., Dionisio, A. P., Carail, M., Caris-Veyrat, C., & Dhuique-Mayer, C. (2013). Cashew apple (*Anacardium occidentale* L.) extract from by-product of juice processing: A focus on carotenoids. *Food Chemistry, 138*, 25–31.

De Ancos, B., Colina-Coca, C., González-Peña, D., & Sánchez-Moreno, C. (2015). Bioactive compounds from vegetable and fruit by-products. In V. Kumar Gupta, et al. (Eds.), *Biotechnology of bioactive compounds: Sources and applications* (pp. 3–36). Wiley-Blackwell.

De Azevedo, C. H., & Rodriguez-Amaya, D. B. (2005). Carotenoid composition of kale as influenced by maturity, season and minimal processing. *Journal of the Science of Food and Agriculture, 85*, 591–597.

de Vargas, E. F., Jablonski, A., Flôres, S. H., & Rios, A.d.O. (2017). Waste from peach (*Prunus persica*) processing used for optimisation of carotenoids ethanolic extraction. *International Journal of Food Science and Technology, 52*, 757–762.

Delgado-Nieblas, C. I., Zazueta-Morales, J. J., Ahumada-Aguilar, J. A., Aguilar-Palazuelos, E., Carrillo-López, A., Jacobo-Valenzuela, N., et al. (2017). Optimization of an air-drying process to obtain a dehydrated naranjita (*Citrus mitis* B.) pomace product with high bioactive compounds and antioxidant capacity. *Journal of Food Process Engineering, 40*, e12338.

Devi, N. M., Prasad, R. V., & Sagarika, N. (2018). A review on health benefits and nutritional composition of pumpkin seeds. *International Journal of Chemical Studies, 6*, 1154–1157.

Díaz-Mula, H. M., Marín, A., Jordán, M. J., & Gil, M. I. (2017). Off-odor compounds responsible for quality loss of minimally processed baby spinach stored under MA of low

O_2 and high CO_2 using GC–MS and olfactometry techniques. *Postharvest Biology and Technology*, *129*, 129–135.

Dimić, E. B., Vujasinović, V. B., Radočaj, O. F., & Pastor, O. P. (2012). Characteristics of blackberry and raspberry seeds and oils. *Acta Periodica Technologica*, (43), 1–9.

Döker, O., Salgin, U., Şanal, I., Mehmetoğlu, Ü., & Çalimli, A. (2004). Modeling of extraction of β-carotene from apricot bagasse using supercritical CO_2 in packed bed extractor. *Journal of Supercritical Fluids*, *28*, 11–19.

EFSA Panel on Dietetic Products, N. and A. (NDA). (2010). Scientific opinion on the substantiation of health claims related to vitamin A (including β-carotene) and maintenance of normal vision (ID 4239, 4701), maintenance of normal skin and mucous membranes (ID 4660, 4702), and maintenance of normal hair (ID 46). *EFSA Journal*, *8*(10), 1754. 1–13.

FAOSTAT. (2016). http://www.fao.org/faostat/en/#data (Accessed August 2018).

Fiedor, J., & Burda, K. (2014). Potential role of carotenoids as antioxidants in human health and disease. *Nutrients*, *6*, 466–488.

Freitas, A., Moldão-Martins, M., Costa, H. S., Albuquerque, T. G., Valente, A., & Sanches-Silva, A. (2015). Effect of UV-C radiation on bioactive compounds of pineapple (*Ananas comosus* L. Merr.) by-products. *Journal of the Science of Food and Agriculture*, *95*, 44–52.

Fu, X., Cheng, S., Liao, Y., Huang, B., Du, B., Zeng, W., et al. (2018). Comparative analysis of pigments in red and yellow banana fruit. *Food Chemistry*, *239*, 1009–1018.

Garcia-Mendoza, M. P., Paula, J. T., Paviani, L. C., Cabral, F. A., & Martinez-Correa, H. A. (2015). Extracts from mango peel by-product obtained by supercritical CO_2 and pressurized solvent processes. *LWT—Food Science and Technology*, *62*, 131–137.

Górnaś, P., Rudzińska, M., Raczyk, M., Mišina, I., & Segliņa, D. (2016). Impact of cultivar on profile and concentration of lipophilic bioactive compounds in kernel oils recovered from sweet cherry (*Prunus avium* L.) by-products. *Plant Foods for Human Nutrition*, *71*, 158–164.

Górnaś, P., Rudzińska, M., Raczyk, M., Mišina, I., Soliven, A., & Segliņa, D. (2016). Composition of bioactive compounds in kernel oils recovered from sour cherry (*Prunus cerasus* L.) by-products: Impact of the cultivar on potential applications. *Industrial Crops and Products*, *82*, 44–50.

Graça Dias, M., Olmedilla-Alonso, B., Hornero-Méndez, D., Mercandante, A. Z., Osorio, C., Vargas-Murga, L., et al. (2018). Comprehensive database of carotenoid contents in ibero-american foods. A valuable tool in the context of functional foods and the establishment of recommended intakes of bioactives. *Journal of Agricultural and Food Chemistry*, *66*, 5055–5107.

Granado, F., Olmedilla, B., Blanco, I., & Rojas-hidalgo, E. (1992). Carotenoid composition in raw and cooked Spanish vegetables. *Journal of Agricultural and Food Chemistry*, *40*, 2135–2140.

Gross, J., Gabai, M., Lifshitz, A., & Sklarz, B. (1973). Carotenoids in pulp, peel and leaves of *Persea americana*. *Phytochemistry*, *12*, 2259–2263.

Guerra-Vargas, M., Jaramillo-Flores, M. E., Dorantes-Alvarez, L., & Hernández-Sánchez, H. (2006). Carotenoid retention in canned pickled jalapeño peppers and carrots as affected by sodium chloride, acetic acid, and pasteurization. *Journal of Food Science*, *66*, 620–626.

Habeeb, A. A. M., Gad, A. E., Mustafa, M. M., Atta, M. A. A., Division, R. A., & Authority, A. E. (2017). *Using of sugar beet pulp by-product in farm animals feeding*. 3 (pp. 107–120. IJSRST.

Hernández-Montoya, V., Montes-Morán, M. A., & Elizalde-González, M. P. (2009). Study of the thermal degradation of citrus seeds. *Biomass and Bioenergy*, *33*, 1295–1299.

Hiranvarachat, B., & Devahastin, S. (2014). Enhancement of microwave-assisted extraction via intermittent radiation: Extraction of carotenoids from carrot peels. *Journal of Food Engineering, 126*, 17–26.

Ho, K.K.H.Y., Ferruzzi, M. G., Liceaga, A. M., & San Martín-González, M. F. (2015). Microwave-assisted extraction of lycopene in tomato peels: Effect of extraction conditions on all-trans and cis-isomer yields. *LWT—Food Science and Technology, 62*, 160–168.

Hornero-Méndez, D., Costa-García, J., & Mínguez-Mosquera, M. I. (2002). Characterization of carotenoid high-producing *Capsicum annuum* cultivars selected for paprika production. *Journal of Agricultural and Food Chemistry, 50*, 5711–5716.

Humphries, J. M., & Khachik, F. (2003). Distribution of lutein, zeaxanthin, and related geometrical isomers in fruit, vegetables, wheat, and pasta products. *Journal of Agricultural and Food Chemistry, 51*, 1322–1327.

Ishiguro, K., & Yoshimoto, M. (2006). Content of an eye-protective nutrient lutein in sweet potato leaves. *Acta Horticulturae*, (703), 253–256.

Jaeger de Carvalho, L. M., Barros Gomes, P., De Oliveira Godoy, R. L., Pacheco, S., Fernandes do Monte, P. H., Viana De Carvalho, J. L., et al. (2012). Total carotenoid content, α-carotene and β-carotene, of landrace pumpkins (*Cucurbita moschata* Duch): A preliminary study. *Food Research International, 47*, 337–340.

Jahurul, M. H. A., Zaidul, I. S. M., Ghafoor, K., Al-Juhaimi, F. Y., Nyam, K. L., Norulaini, N. A. N., et al. (2015). Mango (*Mangifera indica* L.) by-products and their valuable components: A review. *Food Chemistry, 183*, 173–180.

Jorge, N., Da Silva, A. C., & Aranha, C. P. M. (2016). Antioxidant activity of oils extracted from orange (*Citrus sinensis*) seeds. *Anais da Academia Brasileira de Ciências, 88*, 951–958.

Kalogeropoulos, N., Chiou, A., Pyriochou, V., Peristeraki, A., & Karathanos, V. T. (2012). Bioactive phytochemicals in industrial tomatoes and their processing by-products. *LWT—Food Science and Technology, 49*, 213–216.

Kantar, M. B., Anderson, J. E., Lucht, S. A., Mercer, K., Bernau, V., Case, K. A., et al. (2016). Vitamin variation in *Capsicum* spp. provides opportunities to improve nutritional value of human diets. *PLoS ONE, 11*, 1–12.

Kassama, L. S., Shi, J., & Mittal, G. S. (2008). Optimization of supercritical fluid extraction of lycopene from tomato skin with central composite rotatable design model. *Separation and Purification Technology, 60*, 278–284.

Kaur, D., Wani, A. A., Oberoi, D. P. S., & Sogi, D. S. (2008). Effect of extraction conditions on lycopene extractions from tomato processing waste skin using response surface methodology. *Food Chemistry, 108*, 711–718.

Kehili, M., Choura, S., Zammel, A., Allouche, N., & Sayadi, S. (2018). Oxidative stability of refined olive and sunflower oils supplemented with lycopene-rich oleoresin from tomato peels industrial by-product, during accelerated shelf-life storage. *Food Chemistry, 246*, 295–304.

Kehili, M., Kammlott, M., Choura, S., Zammel, A., Zetzl, C., Smirnova, I., et al. (2017). Supercritical CO_2 extraction and antioxidant activity of lycopene and β-carotene-enriched oleoresin from tomato (*Lycopersicum esculentum* L.) peels by-product of a Tunisian industry. *Food and Bioproducts Processing, 102*, 340–349.

Kehili, M., Schmidt, L. M., Reynolds, W., Zammel, A., Zetzl, C., Smirnova, I., et al. (2016). Biorefinery cascade processing for creating added value on tomato industrial by-products from Tunisia. *Biotechnology for Biofuels, 9*, 261. 1–12.

Kim, J., Geon, C., Park, J., Pyo, Y., & Kim, S. (2016). Carotenoid profiling from 27 types of paprika (*Capsicum annuum* L.) with different colors, shapes, and cultivation methods. *Food Chemistry, 201*, 64–71.

Kim, S., Ha, T. Y., & Hwang, I. K. (2009). Analysis, bioavailability, and potential healthy effects of capsanthin, natural red pigment from *Capsicum* spp. *Food Review International, 25,* 198–213.

Knoblich, M., Anderson, B., & Latshaw, D. (2005). Analyses of tomato peel and seed by-products and their use as a source of carotenoids. *Journal of the Science of Food and Agriculture, 85,* 1166–1170.

Kobori, C. N., & Amaya, D. B. R. (2008). Uncultivated Brazilian green leaves are richer sources of carotenoids than are commercially produced leafy vegetables. *Food and Nutrition Bulletin, 29,* 320–328.

Kong, K. W., & Ismail, A. (2011). Lycopene content and lipophilic antioxidant capacity of by-products from *Psidium guajava* fruits produced during puree production industry. *Food and Bioproducts Processing, 89,* 53–61.

Kong, K. W., Ismail, A., Tan, C. P., & Rajab, N. F. (2010). Optimization of oven drying conditions for lycopene content and lipophilic antioxidant capacity in a by-product of the pink guava puree industry using response surface methodology. *LWT—Food Science and Technology, 43,* 729–735.

Lamberts, L., & Delcour, J. A. (2008). Carotenoids in raw and parboiled brown and milled rice. *Journal of Agricultural and Food Chemistry, 56,* 11914–11919.

Lapkin, A., Adou, E., Mlambo, B. N., Chemat, S., Suberu, J., Collis, A. E. C., et al. (2014). Integrating medicinal plants extraction into a high-value biorefinery: An example of *Artemisia annua* L. *Comptes Rendus Chimie, 17,* 232–241.

Lau, H. L. N., Choo, Y. M., Ma, A. N., & Chuah, C. H. (2008). Selective extraction of palm carotene and vitamin E from fresh palm-pressed mesocarp fiber (*Elaeis guineensis*) using supercritical CO_2. *Journal of Food Engineering, 84,* 289–296.

Lavecchia, R., & Zuorro, A. (2008). Improved lycopene extraction from tomato peels using cell-wall degrading enzymes. *European Food Research and Technology, 228,* 153–158.

Leão, D. P., Franca, A. S., Oliveira, L. S., Bastos, R., & Coimbra, M. A. (2017). Physicochemical characterization, antioxidant capacity, total phenolic and proanthocyanidin content of flours prepared from Pequi (*Caryocar brasilense* Camb.) fruit by-products. *Food Chemistry, 225,* 146–153.

Lima, M. D. A., Charalampopoulos, D., & Chatzifragkou, A. (2018). Optimisation and modelling of supercritical CO_2 extraction process of carotenoids from carrot peels. *Journal of Supercritical Fluids, 133,* 94–102.

Liu, M., Zhang, L., Ser, S. L., Cumming, J. R., & Ku, K.-M. (2018). Comparative phytonutrient analysis of broccoli by-products: The potentials for broccoli by-product utilization. *Molecules, 23*(4), 900.

Luengo, E., Condón-abanto, S., Condón, S., Álvarez, I., & Raso, J. (2014). Improving the extraction of carotenoids from tomato waste by application of ultrasound under pressure. *Separation and Purification Technology, 136,* 130–136.

Macedo, M., Robrigues, R. D. P., Pinto, G. A. S., & De Brito, E. S. (2015). Influence of pectinolyttic and cellulotyc enzyme complexes on cashew bagasse maceration in order to obtain carotenoids. *Journal of Food Science and Technology, 52,* 3689–3693.

Matsuno, T., Tani, Y., Maoka, T., Matsuo, K., & Komori, T. (1986). Isolation and structural elucidation of cucurbitaxanthin A and B from pumpkin *Cucurbita maxima. Phytochemistry, 25,* 2837–2840.

Mercandante, A. Z., & Rodriguez-Amaya, D. B. (1991). Carotenoid composition of a leafy vegetable in relation to some agricultural variables. *Journal of Agricultural and Food Chemistry, 39,* 1094–1097.

Milala, J., Grzelak-Błaszczyk, K., Sójka, M., Kosmala, M., Dobrzyńska-Inger, A., & Rój, E. (2018). Changes of bioactive components in berry seed oils during supercritical CO_2 extraction. *Journal of Food Processing & Preservation, 42,* 1–7.

Minguez-Mosquera, M. I., & Hornero-Mendez, D. (1993). Separation and quantification of the carotenoid pigments in red peppers (*Capsicum annuum* L.), paprika, and oleoresin by reversed-phase HPLC. *Journal of Agricultural and Food Chemistry, 41*, 1616–1620.

Monge-Rojas, R., Campos, H., & Rica, C. (2011). Tocopherol and carotenoid content of foods commonly consumed in Costa Rica. *Journal of Food Composition and Analysis, 24*, 202–216.

Munde, P. J., Muley, A. B., Ladole, M. R., Pawar, A. V., Talib, M. I., & Parate, V. R. (2017). Optimization of pectinase-assisted and tri-solvent-mediated extraction and recovery of lycopene from waste tomato peels. *3 Biotech, 7*, 1–10.

Murillo, E., & Meléndez-Martínez, A. J. (2010). Screening of vegetables and fruits from Panama for rich sources of lutein and zeaxanthin. *Food Chemistry, 122*, 167–172.

Namir, M., Elzahar, K., Ramadan, M. F., & Allaf, K. (2017). Cactus pear peel snacks prepared by instant pressure drop texturing: Effect of process variables on bioactive compounds and functional properties. *Journal of Food Measurement and Characterization, 11*, 388–400.

Ndayishimiye, J., & Chun, B. S. (2017). Optimization of carotenoids and antioxidant activity of oils obtained from a co-extraction of citrus (*Yuzu ichandrin*) by-products using supercritical carbon dioxide. *Biomass and Bioenergy, 106*, 1–7.

Ndolo, V. U., & Beta, T. (2013). Distribution of carotenoids in endosperm, germ, and aleurone fractions of cereal grain kernels. *Food Chemistry, 139*, 663–671.

Niizu, P. Y., & Rodriguez-Amaya, D. B. (2005). New data on the carotenoid composition of raw salad vegetables. *Journal of Food Composition and Analysis, 18*, 739–749.

Nikolova, M., Taneva, D., Prokopov, T., & Hadjikinova, M. (2017). Influence of genotype and crop year on carotenoids content of peels from Bulgarian tomato cultivars. *Ukrainian Journal of Food Science, 6*, 470–479.

Noronha Matos, K. A., Praia Lima, D., Pereira Barbosa, A. P., Zerlotti Mercadante, A., & Campos Chisté, R. (2019). Peels of tucumã (*Astrocaryum vulgare*) and peach palm (*Bactris gasipaes*) are by-products classified as very high carotenoid sources. *Food Chemistry, 272*, 216–221.

Obrero, A., González-Verdejo, C. I., Die, J. V., Gómez, P., Del Río-Celestino, M., & Román, B. (2013). Carotenogenic gene expression and carotenoid accumulation in three varieties of cucurbita pepo during fruit development. *Journal of Agricultural and Food Chemistry, 61*, 6393–6403.

Oomah, B. D., Ladet, S., Godfrey, D. V., Liang, J., & Girard, B. (2000). Characteristics of raspberry (*Rubus idaeus* L.) seed oil. *Food Chemistry, 69*, 187–193.

Ordóñez-Santos, L. E., Pinzón-Zarate, L. X., & González-Salcedo, L. O. (2015). Optimization of ultrasonic-assisted extraction of total carotenoids from peach palm fruit (*Bactris gasipaes*) by-products with sunflower oil using response surface methodology. *Ultrasonics Sonochemistry, 27*, 560–566.

Pallett, K. E., & Young, A. J. (2017). Carotenoids. In R. G. Alscher & J. L. Hess (Eds.), *Antioxidants in higher plants* (p. 31). London: Taylor & Francis.

Panfili, G., Fratianni, A., & Irano, M. (2004). Improved normal-phase high-performance liquid chromatography procedure for the determination of carotenoids in cereals. *Journal of Agricultural and Food Chemistry, 52*, 6373–6377.

Pataro, G., Carullo, D., Siddique, A. B., Falcone, M., Donsì, F., & Ferrari, G. (2018). Improved extractability of carotenoids from tomato peels as side benefits of PEF treatment of tomato fruit for more energy-efficient steam-assisted peeling. *Journal of Food Engineering, 233*, 65–73.

Pereira-Freire, J. A., Oliveira, G.L.D.S., Lima, L. K. F., Ramos, C. L. S., Arcanjo-Medeiros, S. R., De Lima, A. C. S., et al. (2018). In vitro and ex vivo chemopreventive action of

Mauritia flexuosa products. *Evidence-based Complementary and Alternative Medicine, 2018*, 1–12. Article ID 2051279.

Petrik, S., Kádár, Z., & Márová, I. (2013). Utilization of hydrothermally pretreated wheat straw for production of bioethanol and carotene-enriched biomass. *Bioresource Technology, 133*, 370–377.

Radenkovs, V., & Feldmane, D. (2017). Profile of lipophilic antioxidants in the by-products recovered from six cultivars of sour cherry (*Prunus cerasus* L.). *Natural Product Research, 31*, 2549–2553.

Ramadan, M. F., & Mörsel, J. T. (2003). Recovered lipids from prickly pear [*Opuntia ficus-indica* (L.) Mill.] peel: A good source of polyunsaturated fatty acids, natural antioxidant vitamins and sterols. *Food Chemistry, 83*, 447–456.

Regulation (EC). (2009). No 1223/2009 of the European parliament and of the council of 30 November 2009 on cosmetic products. *Official Journal of the European Union, L342*, 59–209.

Reif, C., Arrigoni, E., Schärer, H., Nyström, L., & Hurrell, R. F. (2013). Carotenoid database of commonly eaten Swiss vegetables and their estimated contribution to carotenoid intake. *Journal of Food Biochemistry, 29*, 64–72.

Resende, L. M., Franca, A. S., & Oliveira, L. S. (2019). Buriti (*Mauritia flexuosa* L. f.) fruit by-products flours: Evaluation as source of dietary fibers and natural antioxidants. *Food Chemistry, 270*, 53–60.

Rizk, E. M., El-kady, A. T., & El-bialy, A. R. (2014). Characterization of carotenoids (lyco-red) extracted from tomato peels and its uses as natural colorants and antioxidants of ice cream. *Annals of Agricultural Science, 59*, 53–61.

Rodrigues, D. B., Flores, E. M. M., Barin, J. S., Mercadante, A. Z., Jacob-Lopes, E., & Zepka, L. Q. (2014). Production of carotenoids from microalgae cultivated using agroindustrial wastes. *Food Research International, 65*(Part B), 144–148.

Romo-Hualde, A., Yetano-Cunchillos, A. I., González-Ferrero, C., Sáiz-Abajo, M. J., & González-Navarro, C. J. (2012). Supercritical fluid extraction and microencapsulation of bioactive compounds from red pepper (*Capsicum annum* L.) by-products. *Food Chemistry, 133*, 1045–1049.

Rozzi, N. L., Singh, R. K., Vierling, R. A., & Watkins, B. A. (2002). Supercritical fluid extraction of lycopene from tomato processing by-products. *Journal of Agricultural and Food Chemistry, 50*, 2638–2643.

Ruales, J., Baenas, N., Moreno, D. A., Stinco, C. M., Meléndez-Martínez, A. J., & García-Ruiz, A. (2018). Biological active ecuadorian mango 'Tommy Atkins' ingredients—An opportunity to reduce agrowaste. *Nutrientes, 10*, 1–14.

Saini, R. K., Nile, S. H., & Park, S. W. (2015). Carotenoids from fruits and vegetables: Chemistry, analysis, occurrence, bioavailability and biological activities. *Food Research International, 76*, 735–750.

Santana-Méridas, O., González-Coloma, A., & Sánchez-Vioque, R. (2012). Agricultural residues as a source of bioactive natural products. *Phytochemistry Reviews, 11*, 447–466.

Seo, J. S., Burri, B. J., Quan, Z., & Neidlinger, T. R. (2005). Extraction and chromatography of carotenoids from pumpkin. *Journal of Chromatography A, 1073*, 371–375.

Shyamala, B. N., & Jamuna, P. (2010). Nutritional content and antioxidant properties of pulp waste from *Daucus carota* and *Beta vulgaris*. *Malaysian Journal of Nutrition, 16*, 397–408.

Siebenhandl, S., Grausgruber, H., Pellegrini, N., Del Rio, D., Fogliano, V., Pernice, R., et al. (2007). Phytochemical profile of main antioxidants in different fractions of purple and blue wheat, and black barley. *Journal of Agricultural and Food Chemistry, 55*, 8541–8547.

Silva, J. S., Simão, A. A., Marques, T. R., Leal, R. S., & Corrêa, A. D. (2014). Chemical constituents of the pumpkin seeds flour. *Journal of Biotechnology and Biodiversity*, *5*, 148–156.

Smuda, S. S., Mohsen, S. M., Olsen, K., & Aly, M. H. (2018). Bioactive compounds and antioxidant activities of some cereal milling by-products. *Journal of Food Science and Technology*, *55*, 1134–1142.

Spinelli, S., Lecce, L., Likyova, D., Del Nobile, M. A., & Conte, A. (2018). Bioactive compounds from orange epicarp to enrich fish burgers. *Journal of the Science of Food and Agriculture*, *98*, 2582–2586.

Statistica. (2018). https://www.statista.com/statistics/263937/vegetable-oils-global-consumption/ [accessed November 2018].

Stevenson, L., Phillips, F., O'sullivan, K., & Walton, J. (2012). Wheat bran: Its composition and benefits to health, a European perspective. *International Journal of Food Sciences and Nutrition*, *63*, 1001–1013.

Strati, I. F., Gogou, E., & Oreopoulou, V. (2015). Enzyme high pressure assisted extraction of carotenoids from tomato waste. *Food and Bioproducts Processing*, *94*, 668–674.

Strati, I. F., & Oreopoulou, V. (2011). Process optimisation for recovery of carotenoids from tomato waste. *Food Chemistry*, *129*, 747–752.

Sudha, M. L., Indumathi, K., Sumanth, M. S., Rajarathnam, S., & Shashirekha, M. N. (2015). Mango pulp fibre waste: Characterization and utilization as a bakery product ingredient. *Journal of Food Measurement and Characterization*, *9*, 382–388.

Temelli, F., & Ciftci, N. (2015). Developing an integrated supercritical fluid biorefinery for theprocessing of grains. *Journal of Supercritical Fluids*, *96*, 77–85.

Tovar-Jiménez, X., Caro-Corrales, J., Gómez-Aldapa, C. A., Zazueta-Morales, J., Limón-Valenzuela, V., Castro-Rosas, J., et al. (2015). Third generation snacks manufactured from orange by-products: Physicochemical and nutritional characterization. *Journal of Food Science and Technology*, *52*, 6607–6614.

Verardo, V., Gómez-Caravaca, A. M., Messia, M. C., Marconi, E., & Caboni, M. F. (2011). Development of functional spaghetti enriched in bioactive compounds using barley coarse fraction obtained by air classification. *Journal of Agricultural and Food Chemistry*, *59*, 9127–9134.

Vinha, A. F., Moreira, J., & Barreira, S. V. P. (2013). Physicochemical parameters, phytochemical composition and antioxidant activity of the algarvian avocado (*Persea americana* Mill.). *Journal of Agricultural Science*, *5*, 100–109.

Viuda-Martos, M., Sanchez-Zapata, E., Sayas-Barberá, E., Sendra, E., Pérez-Álvarez, J. A., & Fernández-López, J. (2013). Tomato and tomato by-products. Human health benefits of lycopene and its application to meat products: A review. *Critical Reviews in Food Science and Nutrition*, *54*(8), 1032–1049.

Wang, W., Bostic, T. R., & Gu, L. (2010). Antioxidant capacities, procyanidins and pigments in avocados of different strains and cultivars. *Food Chemistry*, *122*, 1193–1198.

Wang, Y. C., Chuang, Y. C., & Hsu, H. W. (2008). The flavonoid, carotenoid and pectin content in peels of citrus cultivated in Taiwan. *Food Chemistry*, *106*, 277–284.

World Health Organization (WHO). (2018). *Micronutrient deficiencies. Vitamin A deficiency*-http://www.who.int/nutrition/topics/vad/en/ [accessed September 2018].

Xiu, S., Zhang, B., & Shahbazi, A. (2011). Biorefinery processes for biomass conversion to liquid fuel. In M. A. Dos Santos Bernardes (Ed.), *Biofuel's engineering process technology* (pp. 167–190). London: InTech.

Yabuzaki, J. (2017). Carotenoids database: Structures, chemical fingerprints and distribution among organisms. *Database*, *2017*, 1–11.

Yan, L., Fernando, W.M.A.D.B., Brennan, M., Brennan, C. S., Jayasena, V., & Coorey, R. (2016). Effect of extraction method and ripening stage on banana peel pigments. *International Journal of Food Science and Technology*, *51*, 1449–1456.

Yang, Y., Wang, X., Zhao, C., Tian, G., Zhang, H., Xiao, H., et al. (2017). Chemical mapping of essential oils, flavonoids and carotenoids in citrus peels by Raman microscopy. *Journal of Food Science*, *82*, 2840–2846.

Yilmaz, C., & Gökmen, V. (2013). Compositional characteristics of sour cherry kernel and its oil as influenced by different extraction and roasting conditions. *Industrial Crops and Products*, *49*, 130–135.

Zhu, L. (2015). Biorefinery as a promising approach to promote microalgae industry: An innovative framework. *Renewable and Sustainable Energy Reviews*, *41*, 1376–1384.

Žnidarčič, D., Ban, D., & Šircelj, H. (2011). Carotenoid and chlorophyll composition of commonly consumed leafy vegetables in Mediterranean countries. *Food Chemistry*, *129*, 1164–1168.

Carotenoids from microalgae

5

T. Lafarga*, I. Clemente†, M. Garcia-Vaquero‡
*IRTA, XaRTA-Postharvest, Parc Científic i Tecnològic Agroalimentari de Lleida, Lleida, Spain, †School of Agriculture and Food Science, University College Dublin, Dublin 4, Ireland, ‡School of Veterinary Medicine, University College Dublin, Dublin 4, Ireland

Chapter Outline

Introduction

The oceans are the Earth's most valuable natural resource and because of their phenomenal biodiversity, marine resources are gaining an increased importance in the context of the European bioeconomy. At the beginning of the 21st century, the hypothesis that microalgae could be a suitable candidate for the production of biofuels as an alternative to the costly fossil fuels motivated a significant monetary investment in this field by large energy companies (Garrido-Cardenas, Manzano-Agugliaro, Acien-Fernandez, & Molina-Grima, 2018). The production yield of biofuels from the microalgal industries is still far from the initially predicted outcomes. However, the large investment made over those years has led to an exponential increase in the technological aspects as well as in the production capacity of the microalgal industry. This permitted, for example, to reduce the cost of production of microalgal biomass to 5 € per kg (Garrido-Cardenas et al., 2018) or even to <1 € per kg when the culture of these cells was combined with wastewater treatment, using CO_2 capture from industrial flue gases (Acién, Fernández, Magán, & Molina, 2012). Microalgae biotechnology is a relatively new area which has grown exponentially over the last two decades, especially since 2005 (Garrido-Cardenas et al., 2018). Nowadays, commercially cultivated microalgae for food use is a mature industry that focuses primarily on the cultivation of several microalgae from *Chlorella, Spirulina, Dunaliella, Nannochloris, Nitzschia, Crypthecodinium, Schizochytrium, Tetraselmins*, and *Skeletonema* species (Ejike et al., 2017). Most of the companies currently commercializing dried microalgae or compounds derived thereof, are based in Australia, Israel, Germany, Spain, the Netherlands, and the United States (Cuellar-Bermudez et al., 2015).

Microalgae live in complex habitats and are exposed to extreme conditions, thus producing a wide variety of specific and valuable compounds (Hamed, Özogul, Özogul, & Regenstein, 2015). In fact, the large amount of valuable molecules that can be obtained from microalgae, with potential for being used in a wide variety of applications including food, nutraceutical, and pharmaceutical industries, is what makes microalgae particularly attractive. High-value compounds from microalgae include proteins, carbohydrates, oils, and pigments. Major groups of natural pigments include chlorophylls, carotenoids, anthocyanins, and betanins which are responsible for the green, yellow/orange/red, red/blue, and red color of microalgae, plants, fruits, or vegetables (Rodriguez-Amaya, 2016). Despite the enormous efforts being made to find novel natural sources and to increase yields of the production of pigments and colorants, only few natural food color additives have reached the market. The main reasons for the limited exploitation of natural colorants include the lower stability and limited range of colors (hues) of natural compounds compared to chemically synthesized food-grade colorants (Rodriguez-Amaya, 2016). However, natural food colorants such as carotenoids have important biological functions including provitamin A, antioxidant, gene transcription regulation, enhancement of gap junction communication, and enhancement of the immune function (Cooperstone & Schwartz, 2016). Moreover, they currently offer certain advantages such as lower cost of production and toxicity risk together with higher customer preference of these products when used as medicine or supplements over the chemically synthesized carotenoids (Gong & Bassi, 2016; Praveenkumar, Lee, Lee, & Oh, 2015).

Carotenoids are lipophilic colored compounds which are the most widely spread and diverse pigments found in nature (Sasso, Pohnert, Lohr, Mittag, & Hertweck, 2012). Most carotenoids share a common C40 backbone structure of isoprene units and are divided into two main groups namely carotenes and xanthophylls. Depending on the function of the compounds on the microalgal cells, these compounds can be divided as primary carotenoids (i.e., lutein), which absorb light and are strongly linked to the photosynthetic processes or secondary carotenoids (such as astaxanthin and canthaxanthin) that play a major role in cell protective mechanisms (Gong & Bassi, 2016). Astaxanthin and β-carotene are the two most recognized carotenoids and make up almost half of the global carotenoid market (Gong & Bassi, 2016), which was estimated to be 1.2 billion USD in 2016 and is expected to increase to over 1.5 billion USD by 2021 (Sathasivam & Ki, 2018). Other reports suggested that the global carotenoid market would reach 1.8 billion USD by 2019 (Gong & Bassi, 2016). The market prices of carotenoids can vary from 300 to 3000 USD per kg of β-carotene and from 2500 to 10,000 USD per kg of astaxanthin (Taucher et al., 2016). The most relevant natural source and process to obtain β-carotene is the culture of *Dunaliella salina*, which can accumulate up to 12% of β-carotene on a dry weight basis depending on the cultivation conditions (Del Campo, García-González, & Guerrero, 2007). Industrial production of β-carotene from microalgae started in the 1980s in Israel, Australia, and the United States and expanded later to other countries including India and China (Borowitzka, 2013). In addition, *Haematococcus pluvialis* accumulates astaxanthin inside their extra-plastidial lipid bodies at a concentration of approximately 4% on a wet weight basis (Wayama et al., 2013) and approximately 300 tons of *Haematococcus* biomass have been produced annually as a natural source of astaxanthin (Brennan & Owende, 2010).

Microalgae cells are covered by dynamic, complex, carbohydrate-rich cell walls which difficult the extraction of carotenoids and other valuable compounds derived from microalgae (Kim et al., 2016). Cell disruption is a necessary step to increase the yields of recovery of carotenoids. Different nonconventional cell disruption methods including pulsed electric fields (PEFs), high-pressure homogenization (HPH), or ultrasounds (USs) have been evaluated as novel strategies to improve the extraction yields and purity of microalgal carotenoids. Chemical and biological methods for weakening and/or breaking the cell wall of microalgae have also been carried out, either alone or in combination with nonconventional techniques (Kim et al., 2016). Other key steps in the downstream processing of microalgal carotenoids include the cultivation, harvesting, extraction, and purification of the compounds (Gong & Bassi, 2016).

This chapter describes in detail the recent advances of carotenoid production at multiple downstream processing stages such as cultivation and harvesting (i.e., cultivation systems, conditions, and stresses), pretreatments (drying and cell disruption methods), extraction techniques (conventional and innovative technologies), and purification and storage conditions necessary to produce microalgal carotenoids. The challenges of the microalgal carotenoid industry such as the recent advances in the chemical synthesis and the cost of production of microalgae were also described in detail together with the developments in certain molecular approaches (metabolic and transcriptional engineering) to increase the synthesis of microalgal carotenoids.

Cultivation and harvesting of microalgae

The process of production of carotenoids from microalgae is represented in Fig. 1. The production of high-value compounds from microalgae includes the processes of cultivation of the microalgal biomass (i.e., choice of cultivation systems and application of stresses to improve the yields of the molecules and/or biomass), harvest, or concentration of the algal cells followed by further downstream processing strategies (cell disruption techniques, extraction, purification, and storage of the compounds of interest) that will influence greatly the cost of production of microalgal carotenoids (Khanra et al., 2018; Li, Zhu, Niu, Shen, & Wang, 2011; Molina Grima, Belarbi, Acién

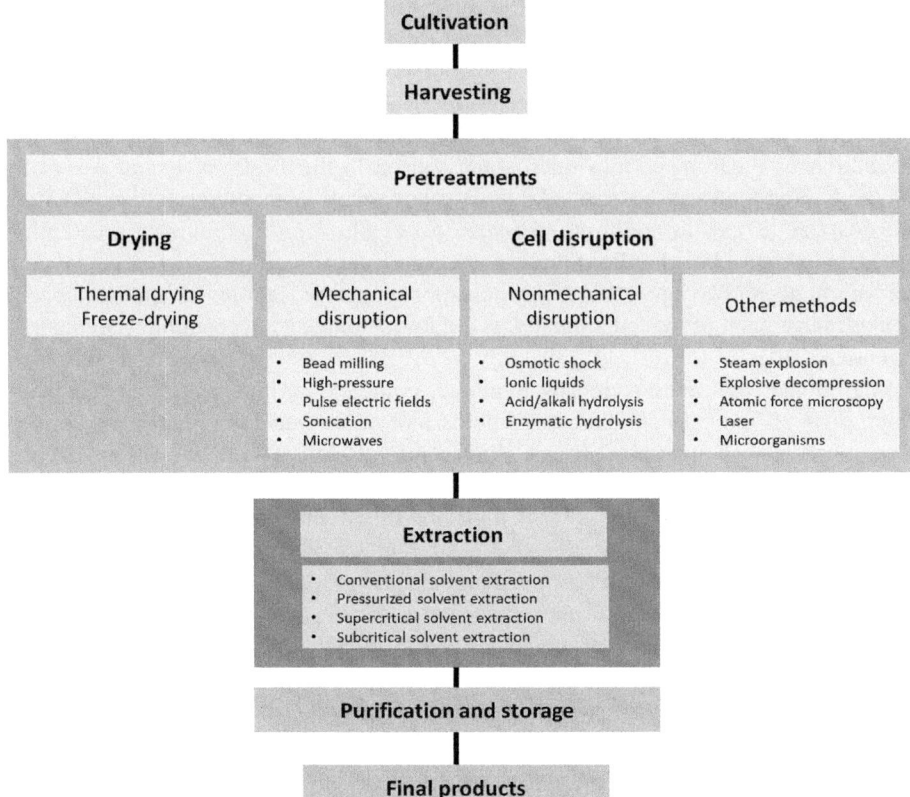

Fig. 1 Schematic representation of the downstream processing stages to obtain microalgal carotenoids.

Fernández, Robles Medina, & Chisti, 2003).

Large-scale production of microalgae can be obtained using multiple cultivation systems classified as open and closed systems depending on the contact of the microalgal biomass with the environment (Acién et al., 2018). Open cultivation strategies include the use of artificial ponds, tanks, raceways, and thin-layer (i.e., inclined-surfaces) systems. These methods were successfully used in the cultivation of several economically relevant microalgae species such as *Chlorella*, *Scenedesmus*, *Nannochloropsis*, *Arthrospira*, and *Dunaliella* (Acién et al., 2018). Open systems offer certain advantages for the production of microalgal biomass such as a low cost of production, easy cleaning, self-cooling, and low oxygen accumulation (Acién et al., 2018). However, the production of biomass is extremely dependent on the climatological conditions and more importantly there is an increased risk of microbial contamination of the algal biomass. Alternatively, closed photobioreactors were developed allowing the manipulation of the cultivation conditions while decreasing the risk of contamination of microalgae. The most commonly used closed cultivation systems include bubble columns, tubular loops, airlift, and flat panels (Khanra et al., 2018) that are currently used successfully to cultivate sensible strains such as *Haematococcus pluvialis, Isochrysis galbana*, and *Porphyridium cruentum* (Acién et al., 2018). The design and operation of different cultivation systems, the optimization of the cultivation conditions in each system, and the adaptation of the cultivation to different biological needs of multiple microalgal species and strains have been discussed extensively in the literature (Acién et al., 2018; Pruvost, Le Gouic, Lepine, Legrand, & Le Borgne, 2016).

Manipulation of the cultivation conditions

Microalgae display great adaptability to different abiotic stresses due to the production of secondary metabolites. Environmental factors (i.e., modifications of temperature, light, salinity, and nutrient deprivation) and the use of additives in the media (i.e., iron and copper) have been explored to increase the production of carotenoids and other high-value compounds (Liang, Zhu, & Jiang, 2018; Paliwal et al., 2017). The recent scientific advances in the field of genomics, transcriptomics, and proteomics have provided increased evidence on key genes and metabolic pathways in microalgal physiology to develop novel metabolic and transcriptional engineering strategies to enhance the accumulation of carotenoids and other metabolites from microalgae (Bajhaiya, Moreira, & Pittman, 2017; Liang et al., 2018). In fact, Chen et al. (2017) emphasized the use of abiotic stresses, omics technologies, and genetic engineering to enhance the efficiency of the biorefinery process to obtain biofuels, energy, and high-value products (see Fig. 2).

The manipulation of several cultivation conditions including nitrogen (N), light intensity, carbon source, salinity, and other environmental stresses together with their effect on the production of carotenoids in several microalgae species is summarized in Table 1.

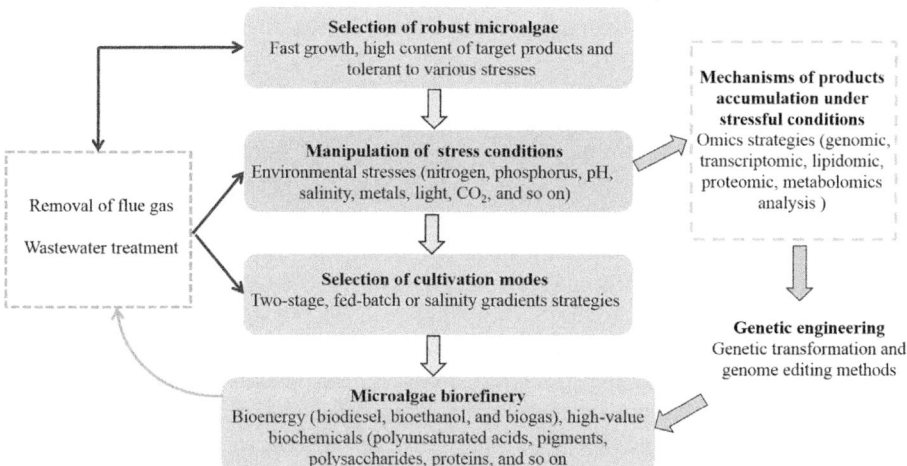

Fig. 2 Diagram from Chen et al. (2017) showing the use of stress manipulation strategies during the cultivation of microalgae to improve the biorefinery concept.

The limitation of N has been considered as one of the main factors influencing the production of lipids and carotenoids in several microalgae species. Zhang et al. (2017) studied the effect of different levels of N (ranging from 0 to $2.48 \times 10^5 \mu g/L$) on the accumulation of carotenoids in *Chlorella vulgaris* measured using Raman spectroscopy. These authors reported that moderate N stress facilitated the synthesis of carotenoids, while an excessive stress resulted in low photosynthetic activity. Similarly, *Haematococcus pluvialis* cultures with limited N or phosphate resulted in an increased astaxanthin content of the biomass (up to 2.6 g astaxanthin per L) after 8 days of N depletion or 14 days in the case of phosphate (Boussiba, Bing, Yuan, Zarka, & Chen, 1999). Moreover, Abe et al. (2007) discovered the ability of microalgae *Coelastrella striolata* var. *multistriata* to change from green to reddish orange color in response to limited N in the media, due to an increase in the production of β-carotene, canthaxanthin, and astaxanthin. The reddish orange cells accumulated levels of up to 47.5 mg of canthaxanthin per g of dried biomass.

Light parameters including the photoperiod and intensity of light radiation influenced the growth of the biomass and the production of carotenoids and other metabolites in microalgae (Minhas, Hodgson, Barrow, & Adholeya, 2016). Under favorable culture conditions, *Haematococcus pluvialis* cells remain in a macrozooid life cycle stage and an increase in the light intensity from 20 to 400 μmol photon/m²/s during 2 days transformed the cells into their hematocysts stage, an increased accumulation of total carotenoids from 1.5 to 6.22 μg per mL together with a significant reduction of total chlorophyll contents of the cells (Gwak et al., 2014). *Dunaliella salina* increases the production of β-carotene in response to high light intensities, reaching a maximum level of β-carotene (17 g per L cell volume) after 2 days of light stress (Lamers et al., 2010). Moreover the combination of high light intensities with other stressors resulted in increased production of carotenoids. The application of light stress combined with N deficiency and salt, resulted in an overproduction of esterified carotenoids in *Coelastrella* sp. (Saeki et al., 2017) and high light intensity together with N and phosphorous depletion increased the synthesis of astaxanthin in *Haematococcus pluvialis* (Chekanov et al., 2014).

The levels of CO_2 in the atmosphere are normally a limiting factor for the growth of microalgae and the cells usually need enrichment with CO_2 to boost their growth and photosynthetic activity (Chekanov et al., 2017). The tolerance of microalgae to CO_2 depends on the species and the growth conditions of the cultured cells within the same species. Microalgae can be classified based on the tolerance to CO_2 as: sensitive or intolerant microalgae if the cell growth is inhibited at levels of <2%–5% of CO_2; tolerant microalgae if the cells can resist levels of up to 20% CO_2; and extremely CO_2-tolerant species if the cells tolerate levels higher than 20% of CO_2 (Solovchenko & Khozin-Goldberg, 2013). The tolerance of microalgae to CO_2 has recently acquired scientific relevance due to the possibility to use microalgae as a biomitigation tool against the continuous rise in anthropogenic CO_2 emission (Solovchenko & Khozin-Goldberg, 2013). The biological sequestration of CO_2 by microalgae is thought to be the most environmentally safe and sustainable way to mitigate the rise in atmospheric CO_2 levels (Borowitzka & Moheimani, 2013; Kumar, Dasgupta, Nayak, Lindblad, &

Table 1 Summary of the effects of cultivation stresses (nitrogen (N), light intensity, carbon source, salinity and multiple stresses combined) on the production of carotenoids in several microalgae species

Stress condition	Species	Effects on microalgal pigments	References
Nitrogen limitation (N)	*Chlorella vulgaris*	Low and excessive N stress increased and inhibited the synthesis of carotenoids, respectively	Zhang et al. (2017)
	Coelastrella striolata	N limitation increased the carotenoid contents (β-carotene, canthaxanthin, and astaxanthin) changing the color of the cells from green to red	Abe, Hattori, and Hirano (2007)
Light	*Haematococcus pluvialis*	An increase in light irradiance from 20 to 400 μmol photon/m^2/s increased 3.15- fold the amount of total carotenoids in microalgae	Gwak et al. (2014)
	Dunaliella salina	An increase in light irradiance induced an increased production of intracellular β-carotene after 2 days of stress	Lamers et al. (2010)
Source carbon (CO_2)	*Haematococcus pluvialis* mutant	High light and 15% CO_2 produced an increase of 2.7-fold in astaxanthin production in microalgae with respect to the control group receiving high light and air as control	Cheng et al. (2017)
	Haematococcus pluvialis BM 1	Moderate CO_2 levels increased astaxanthin accumulation in the biomass in comparison with high levels (≥10%) that caused impaired photosynthesis and a reduction in astaxanthin accumulation	Chekanov, Schastnaya, Solovchenko, and Lobakova (2017)
Salt	*Chlorella protothecoides*	The addition of 20 g NaCl/L increased the production of carotenoids	Campenni' et al. (2013)
	Dunaliella sp.	An increase in salinity from the optimum NaCl concentration (2 M) increased the production of carotenoids in *Dunaliella salina*. *Dunaliella viridis* cultured under the same conditions produced low levels of carotenoids	Hadi, Shariati, and Afsharzadeh (2008)

Continued

Table 1 Continued

Stress condition	Species	Effects on microalgal pigments	References
Multiple-stresses	*Coelastrella* sp. KGU-Y002	Using N deficient and high light intensity culture conditions, the supplementation with KCl enhanced the synthesis of esterified astaxanthin, adonixanthin, and zeaxanthin	Saeki, Aburai, Aratani, Miyashita, and Abe (2017)
	Haematococcus pluvialis BM 1	High light together with N and phosphorus deprivation increased the synthesis of astaxanthin	Chekanov et al. (2014)

Das, 2011; Solovchenko & Khozin-Goldberg, 2013; Yoo, Jun, Lee, Ahn, & Oh, 2010). Microalgae have been successfully cultivated using CO_2 from a power plant (Koberg, Cohen, Ben-Amotz, & Gedanken, 2011) or wastewater effluents from dairy farms (Hena, Fatimah, & Tabassum, 2015). Considerable efforts and advances have been made in the area of CO_2 biomitigation, renewing the interest in the discovery of novel species or strains extremely tolerant to CO_2 (40%–100% CO_2) or in establishing the tolerance of different microalgae species and strains to CO_2, to determine the amount of carbon that can be used or fixed by the biomass for potential industrial bioremediation applications (Cabello, Morales, & Revah, 2017; Solovchenko & Khozin-Goldberg, 2013). Moreover, the use of high levels of CO_2 requires important modifications in the cells' metabolism and synthesis of multiple compounds. Different gas mixtures have been examined to increase the production of neutral lipids such as triacylglycerol to use the biomass as precursors of biofuels (Gouveia et al., 2017; Madadi, Tabatabaei, Aghbashlo, Zahed, & Pourbabaee, 2018). In the case of carotenoids, levels of 15% CO_2 were used to increase the synthesis of astaxanthin in *Haematococcus pluvialis* (Cheng et al., 2017). Moderately high levels of CO_2 (up to 5%) increased the growth and synthesis of astaxanthin in *Haematococcus pluvialis* BM 1, while an increase in CO_2 to 10% or 20% reduced the growth, photosynthesis, and carbon assimilation by the biomass (Chekanov et al., 2017).

Furthermore, several microalgae species are able to adapt to the salinity of the media by producing an excess of β-carotene and glycerol to maintain the osmotic balance of the cells (Hadi et al., 2008). The microalgae *Chlorella protothecoides* cultured in N-depleted media showed high synthesis of carotenoids using 20 g of NaCl per L, with total carotenoids levels of 0.8% on wet weight basis (Campenni' et al., 2013). Canthaxanthin was the main carotenoid accumulated by *Chlorella* under those cultivation conditions, representing 23.3% of the total carotenoids accumulated by the microalgae; although other carotenoids were also present at different concentrations, for example, echinenone (14.7%), free astaxanthin (7.1%), and lutein-zeaxanthin (4.1%) (Campenni' et al., 2013). *Dunaliella salina* and *Dunaliella viridis* biomasses showed optimum growth at 2 and 1 M NaCl, respectively (Hadi et al., 2008). *Dunaliella salina* biomass increased the synthesis of glycerol and carotenoids at high salinity levels changing the color of the biomass to the characteristic orange-red, while the levels of both compounds remain unaltered in *Dunaliella viridis* under the same culture conditions (Hadi et al., 2008).

In addition to all these optimization of stresses, the application of certain chemicals to the media has shown promising results to enhance the accumulation of carotenoids (see Table 2).

These chemicals could be classified as precursors of certain molecules that intervene in the biosynthetic pathway of carotenoids (i.e., pyruvate, citrate, and malic acid), phytohormones, and chemical analogs that increase the production of carotenoids (i.e., indole-3-butyric acid, methyl jasmonate, and gibberellins), inhibitors that regulate the biosynthetic pathway (trimethylamine, nicotine, imidazole and 2-methylimidazole, diphenylamine, squalene epoxidase, and terbinafine), and other chemicals that induce oxidative stress responses in the cells (hydrogen peroxide, iron, and ethanol) (Liang et al., 2018).

These cultivation strategies to increase the production of multiple high-value compounds were recently reviewed in detail by many authors in the scientific literature (Chen et al., 2017; Liang et al., 2018; Minhas et al., 2016; Sun, Guan, Kong, Geng, & Wang, 2016). More efforts are needed to uncover the impact of multiple cultivation stresses on the synthesis of high-value products and understanding the genetic mechanisms underlying the adaptation of the microalgal cells to those stresses for an efficient industrial use of the biomass (Chen et al., 2017).

Recovery of the microalgal biomass

The harvesting or recovery processes of the microalgal biomass face several difficulties due to the small size of the cells (3–30 μm diameter), the density of the cultures that is similar to that of water, and the high dilution of the cells that are normally grown at low dry cell concentrations (0.05–18 g per L); thus, depending on the cultivation system of choice, the recovery of the microalgal biomass will require the treatment of large volumes (Molina Grima et al., 2003). The selection of the appropriate harvesting method will depend on the microalgae species and the market value of the final product of interest, as the microalgal harvest could contribute significantly to the total cost of production (Gerde, Yao, Lio, Wen, & Wang, 2014; Khanra et al., 2018; Molina Grima et al., 2003).

The biomass can be recovered by centrifugation, flotation, and filtration preceded or not by a flocculation step to concentrate the biomass previous to the harvest (Dickinson et al., 2017; Lam et al., 2017; Molina Grima et al., 2003). The advantages and disadvantages of the different harvesting strategies are summarized in Table 3.

The use of sedimentation tanks or settling ponds to perform gravity sedimentation is a strategy commonly used to obtain low-value products and biomass from sewage-based cultivation ponds. The final products achieved using this method are more diluted than in the case of centrifugal recovery (Molina Grima et al., 2003).

The preconcentration of the microalgae cultures using flocculation is used to reduce the cost of centrifugation harvesting of diluted microalgal cultures (i.e., open ponds) in

Table 2   Summary of the main additives or chemical stresses used to enhance the accumulation of several carotenoids in microalgae

Carotenoid product enhanced	*Microalgae* sp.	Chemicals	References
Astaxanthin	*Haematococcus pluvialis*	Ethanol	Wen et al. (2015)
	Haematococcus pluvialis	Epibrassinolide	Gao et al. (2013)
	Haematococcus pluvialis	Jasmonic acid and salicylic acid	Gao, Z., Meng, C., Zhang, X., Xu, D., Zhao, et al. (2012b) and Gao, Z., Meng, C., Zhang, X., Xu, D., Miao, et al. (2012a)
	Haematococcus pluvialis	Methyl jasmonate, gibberellic acid	Lu et al. (2010)
	Chlorella zofingiensis	Pyruvate, citrate and malic acid	Chen, Wei, Chen, Wang, and Chen (2009)
	Haematococcus pluvialis	Salicylic acid and methyl jasmonate	Vidhyavathi, Venkatachalam, Sarada, and Ravishankar (2008)
	Chlorococcum sp.	Hydrogen peroxide, methyl viologen and iron	Yin-Nin Ma and Chen (2001)
	Chlorella zofingiensis	Hydrogen peroxide and sodium hypochlorite	Ip and Chen (2005)
Carotenoids	*Spirulina platensis*	Hydrogen peroxide	Abd El-Baky, El Baz, and EL-Baroty (2009)
	Nannochloropsis oceanica	Terbinafine	Lu et al. (2014)
	Haematococcus pluvialis	Sodium acetate, sodium chloride, iron and methyl viologen	Steinbrenner and Linden (2001)
β-Carotene	*Dunaliella salina*	Iron, acetate and malonate	Mojaat, Pruvost, Foucault, and Legrand (2008)
Lutein	*Dunaliella salina*	2-Methylimidazole	Yildirim, Akgun, and Dalay (2017)
Lycopene	*Dunaliella bardawil*	Triethylamine	Liang, Hao, Li, Liang, and Jiang (2016)
	Chlorella regularis Y-21	Nicotine	Ishikawa and Abe (2004)
	Dunaliella salina CCAP 19/18	Nicotine	Fazeli et al. (2009)

Table 3 Summary of the advantages and disadvantages of the use of different harvesting methods during the downstream processing of microalgae

Harvesting method	Description	Advantages	Disadvantages
Centrifugation	Use of centrifugal force to sediment microalgae	Very high concentration efficiency, no contamination	High energy, cost
Flotation	Use of microbubbles to carry microalgae to the surface	Can use very low energy, moderate concentration efficiency	Can be costly if flocculant is needed, depends on the characteristics of microalgae
Filtration	Biomass filtered through pores	High concentration efficiency, moderate energy usage, no contamination	Fouling of the filter needs constant maintenance
Flocculation	Substance is added to the culture to sediment the cells	Low energy, moderate concentration efficiency, low expense	Can contaminate microalgae, need to remove flocculant

Reproduced from Dickinson, S., Mientus, M., Frey, D., Amini-Hajibashi, A., Ozturk, S., Shaikh, F., Sengupta, D. & El-Halwagi, M. M. 2017. A review of biodiesel production from microalgae. *Clean Technologies and Environmental Policy, 19*, 637–668.

which the centrifugation can represent up to 20%–25% of the total cost of cultivation of microalgae (Lam, Vermuë, Eppink, Wijffels, & Van Den Berg, 2018; Molina Grima et al., 2003). Flocculation is the result of the collision and charge interaction forces between the flocculation agents and the cell surface of microalgae present in a liquid medium (Gerde et al., 2014). Microalgae suspended in water could carry a positive or negative charge due to the presence of carboxylic (−COOH) or amine (−NH$_2$) groups on the cell surface. These charged groups will attract ions with an opposite charge at their surface forming an electrical double layer of dense counter ions. These different layers of counter ions could be divided as those in close contact to the cells and non-accessible to other ions, an outer layer namely Stern layer and a cloud of counter ions further away from the microalgal surface (Vandamme, Foubert, & Muylaert, 2013) as represented in Fig. 3.

The dispersed counter ions surrounding the charged particles result in an electrical repulsion between the particles present in the same suspension. The zeta potential is the difference in charge between the fluid and the layer of counter ions associated with the charged microalgae when the cells are moving in a solution (see Fig. 3). At high zeta potential (>25 mV, positive or negative), the electrical repulsion between the microalgae is strong and when the zeta potential decreases and it is close to zero, the cells will approach and aggregate and the process of flocculation occurs (Vandamme et al., 2013). Different flocculation techniques have been successfully applied in freshwater and marine cultures of microalgae such as the use of chemicals (inorganic-organic flocculants and cationic polymers), approaches based on the biology of microalgae

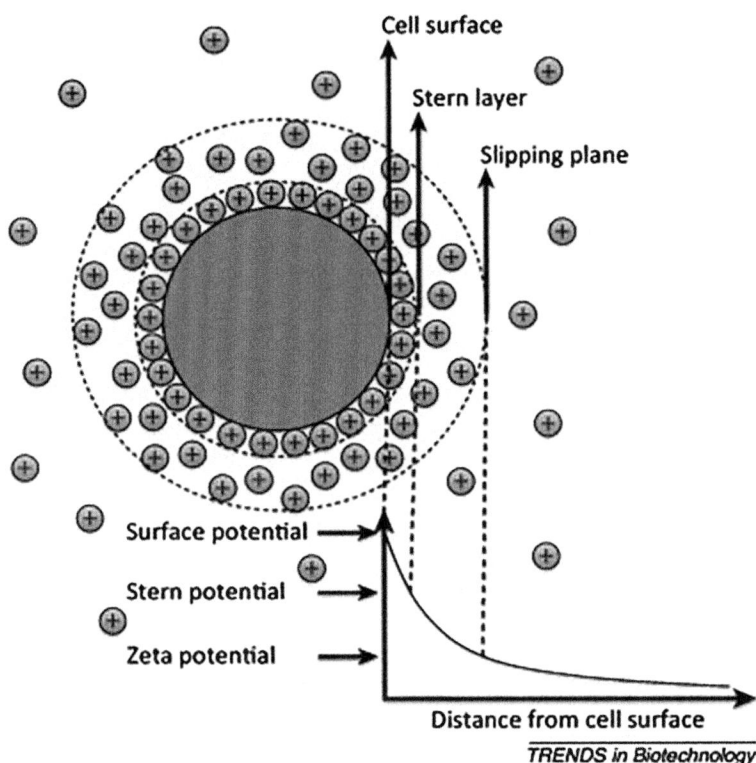

Fig. 3 Schematic representation provided by Vandamme et al. (2013) of an electrical double layer of charged ions in solution surrounding a negatively charged microalgal cell and the zeta potential that will influence the application of flocculation harvesting strategies.

(bioflocculation), and emerging technologies such as magnetically charged nanoparticles (Lam et al., 2018; Vandamme et al., 2013). One of the major issues when using flocculants is the residual traces of these chemicals in the final biomass that could interfere with the final applications of the biomass (i.e., food or feed) or the next processing steps needed to extract the compounds of interest (Vandamme et al., 2013). The advantages and disadvantages of the use of inorganic flocculants (i.e., aluminum and iron salts), organic flocculants (i.e., polyacrylamides and other polymers such as chitosan and vegetable starches), bioflocculants (such as bacteria or fungi), and magnetite (Fe_2O_3) nanoparticles are described in detail by several scientific publications (Gerde et al., 2014; Lam et al., 2018; Srivastava, Seo, Ko, Ahn, & Oh, 2018; Ummalyma et al., 2017; Vandamme et al., 2013).

Centrifugation requires large energy and high operation cost; however, this technique is commonly used due to the possibility to recover microalgae without contaminating the biomass (Dickinson et al., 2017). This technique can be used to harvest microalgae without using preconcentration steps when harvesting biomass from more concentrated cell suspensions such as closed photobioreactors (Lam et al., 2018). Ruiz et al. (2016) estimated the centrifugation costs in 0.2–0.3 € per kg DW when using a close photobioreactor system, representing approximately between 5% and 7% of the total cultivation costs.

Flotation uses air microbubbles (10–30 µm), generated by dissolved air flotation, electrolytic flotation, or dispersed air flotation, to transport the microalgal cells to the surface of the media for collection (Dickinson et al., 2017). The effectivity of the flotation process will depend on the size and surface characteristics of the microalgae and on the size of the bubbles to carry the cells effectively. Flotation is less energy intensive and expensive than centrifugation although further advances in microbubble production are needed to expand the applications of this harvesting strategy at industrial level (Dickinson et al., 2017).

Several membrane filtration methods were also used to harvest microalgae including ultrafiltration (pore size ranging from 0.02 to 0.2 µm) and microfiltration (0.1–10 µm) (Milledge & Heaven, 2013). Gerardo, Zanain, and Lovitt (2015) optimized the process of cross-flow microfiltration to harvest Chlorella minutissima taking into consideration the scale-up effects and modeling the scenario at industrial level. Under optimized conditions, this microfiltration technique consumed 1.27 kWh per kg of microalgae and reduced the cost of harvest in approximately 57% without using chemicals that could complicate the next downstream processing stages.

Hydrophobic membranes such as polyvinyl fluoride phase inverted membranes have been commonly used to harvest microalgae. Due to the hydrophobic nature of these polymers, polyvinyl membranes normally experience fouling processes due to the sorption, deposition, and irreversible attachment of hydrophobic macromolecules to the polymer (Marbelia, Bilad, Maes, Arafat, & Vankelecom, 2018). Several strategies are recently being investigated to reduce the fouling of membranes including hydrophilic coating, surface grafting, in situ polymerization of monomers, and in situ dope blending with amphiphilic copolymers (Bilad et al., 2018). Recently, researchers are exploring the potential of nanofiber membranes to harvest microalgae. These membranes possess an appropriate surface chemistry to reduce the fouling process of membranes (Bilad et al., 2018). Azizo, Wirzal, Bilad, and Yusoff (2017) used novel nylon 6, 6 nanofiber hydrophilic membranes to harvest C. vulgaris and the nanofilter had higher surface pore size and population when compared to the phase inverted polyvinylidene fluoride membranes, increasing the permeability of clean water and the productivity of the harvesting process.

Biomass processing to recover high valuable compounds

As previously described in Fig. 1, after the cultivation and harvesting of the biomass, the most commonly used pretreatments include the biomass drying and the use of cell disruption techniques to increase the efficiency of extraction of carotenoids (Khanra et al., 2018). Drying techniques including thermal and freeze-drying and cell disruption techniques such as mechanical methods (e.g., bead milling, high pressure, PEFs, soni-cation, and microwaves), nonmechanical techniques (i.e., osmotic shock, ionic liquids, chemical, and enzymatic hydrolysis), and other methods are discussed below.

Biomass drying

The use of dehydration or drying of the biomass at this stage could benefit the extraction of high-value molecules. For instance, the extraction of oils from wet and undisrupted cells is difficult compared to freeze-dried biomass (Molina Grima et al., 2003). Due to the high water content of microalgae, sun-drying is not con-sidered as an effective drying methodology (Rizwan, Mujtaba, Memon, Lee, & Rashid, 2018) being necessary to use other strategies depending on the desired final product and the nature of the compounds of interest as these techniques could influ-ence significantly the shelf life of the compounds. Spray-, freeze-, and drum-drying have been successfully used to dry *Dunaliella* sp. rich in β-carotenes to produce a uniform powder and increase the stability of the final product (Molina Grima et al., 2003). *Isochrysis galbana* and *Nannochloropsis oculata* spray-dried at different temperatures (ranging from 150°C to 200°C) were used to dry the biomass for its later incorporation in chewing gums and enrich these products in chlorophylls and carotenoids (Palabiyik et al., 2018). Spray-drying is the preferred method for dry-ing high-value compounds, however, it can cause damage to algal pigments, thus freeze-drying have been widely used to obtain pigments at laboratory scale (Molina Grima et al., 2003).

Cell wall disruption methods

The composition and chemical nature of the microalgal cell walls are important fac-tors to consider in order to select the appropriate disruption method to recover valu-able intracellular products such as carotenoids (Cheng, Labavitch, & Vandergheynst, 2015). For example, Yoo, Park, Kim, Choi, and Yang (2012) reported significantly higher lipid recoveries on cell wall-less mutant stains and senescent cell phases. The response of the cell wall to changes in the growth environment is also an important aspect to consider during species selection (Praveenkumar et al., 2015). Major bot-tlenecks limiting the expansion of microalgae biotechnology are the high production costs and the small scale of the currently successful production strategies (Garrido-Cardenas et al., 2018). Less than 20,000 tons of biomass are produced worldwide at a cost close to 5 €/kg (Borowitzka, 2013). Although cell disruption pretreatments introduce additional processing costs, these are key steps which allow increasing the recovery yield of carotenoids by several folds (Gong & Bassi, 2016). There have been several attempts to obtain effective cell wall disruption methods to extract carotenoids and other valuable compounds from microalgae. Cell wall disruption methods can be divided into two main groups based on the working mechanisms of cellular disintegra-tion namely mechanical and nonmechanical methods. Cell wall disruption strategies as well as the main advantages and disadvantages of these methods that are briefly summarized in Table 4.

Table 4 Table provided by Günerken et al. (2015) comparing the key aspects of the main cell disruption methods in microalgae

Disruption method	Mildness	Selective product recovery	Optimum dry cell weight concentration	Energy consumption	Practical scalability	Repeatability
Bead milling	Yes/no	No	Concentrated	High/medium	Yes	High
High pressure homogenization	Yes/no	No	Diluted/concentrated	High/medium	Yes	High
High speed homogenizer	No	No	Diluted	High/medium	Yes	High/medium
Ultrasound	Yes/no	No	Diluted	Medium/low	Yes/no	Medium
Microwave	Yes/no	No	Diluted	High/medium	Yes/no	Medium
Enzymatic lysis	Yes	Yes	Diluted	Low	Yes	High
Chemical treatment	Yes/no	Yes	Diluted/concentrated	Medium/low	Yes	High
Pulsed electric field	Yes/no	No	Very diluted/diluted	High/medium/low	Yes/no	Medium

Mechanical disruption methods

Bead milling is the most commonly used cell wall disruption method due to its high efficiency in short-time single-pass operations, high-through output, high biomass loading, ease to scale-up, low labor intensity, and the high availability of commercial equipment. Cell walls are disrupted in the bead collision zones by compaction of shear forces with energy transfer from the beads to the cells (Günerken et al., 2015). As highlighted previously, the energy requirements of cell wall disruptive pretreatments are of key importance. Postma et al. (2015) reported that energy consumption of bead milling could be kept under 5 kWh per kg. The authors also reported a linear increase in the specific energy consumption in time and a threefold increase in energy consumption when increasing the speed from 6 to 12 m/s. The energy consumption of bead milling operation of *Chlorella* sp. was 0.85 kWh/kg of dry weight after single pass (Doucha & Lívanský, 2008) and 81 kWh/kg of dry weight after a batch operation (Postma et al., 2015). In practice, the energy consumption of this method will depend on several factors including the concentration of the biomass, microalgae species, and growth conditions (Günerken et al., 2015). Several studies also evaluated bead milling as a cell disruption method rather than from an economical point of view. For example, Taucher et al. (2016) evaluated the effects of several mechanical and nonmechanical disruption methods on *Haemotococcus pluvialis*, *Chromochloris zofingiensis*, and *Chlorella sorokiniana* and the highest disruption yields on *Chromochloris zofingiensis* and *Chlorella sorokiniana* were obtained by bead milling. Safi et al. (2014) observed a complete disruption of the cell wall after bead milling for 1 h as shown in the microscope images shown in Fig. 4.

In that study, the disruption of the cell walls was conducted using 0.3–0.5 mm Y_2O_3-stabilized ZrO_2 grinding beads for 1 h with a 1:13 solid-to-water ratio (*w/v*) operating in batch mode with temperature control to not to exceed 33°C. Overall, several parameters affected the cell disruption efficiency including the suspension feed rate (for continuous operations) or process time (for batch operations), agitator speed, agitator disk design, biomass concentration, growth phase (depending on the cultivation conditions), time, bead diameter, bead density, and bead filling (Günerken et al., 2015). Therefore, optimum conditions need to be assessed for each homogenizer and process independently. Doucha and Lívanský (2008) reported that the optimum bead diameter ranged between 0.3 and 0.5 mm or 0.5 and 0.7 mm when using a Dyno-Mill or a LabStar LS1 homogenizer, respectively. In addition, high-density beads have shown to be more effective in high-viscosity samples, while low-density beads resulted in higher cell disruption in low-viscosity media (Günerken et al., 2015). Higher speed also resulted in higher disintegration rates caused by the increase of the forces and frequency of the impacts (Postma et al., 2015).

HPH is a purely mechanical process during which a liquid dispersion is forced by high pressure, generally between 50 and 300 MPa, to pass through a micrometric disruption chamber (Carullo et al., 2018). As the suspension exits the chamber, the pressure drastically decreases and the velocity increases, leading the occurrence of intense fluid-mechanical stresses that physically disrupt the cell walls and membranes (Yap, Dumsday, Scales, & Martin, 2015). Process parameters for this technology include

I. **II.**

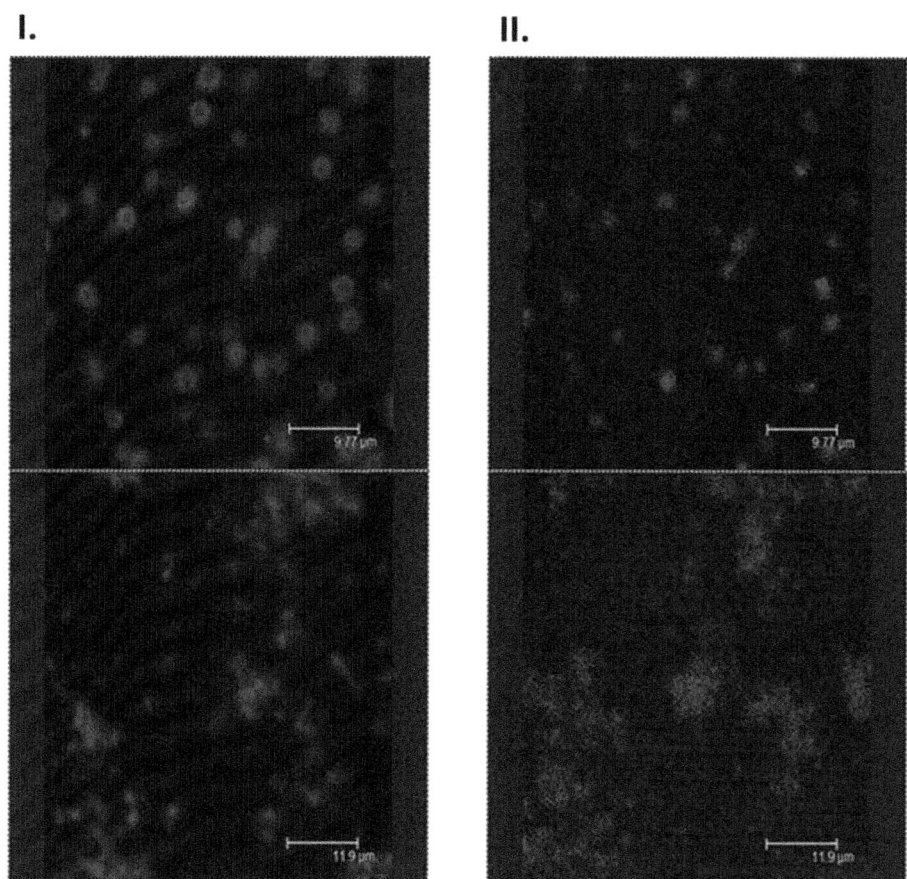

Fig. 4 Confocal microscopic images provided by Safi et al. (2014) of microalgae before (upper pictures, scale 9.77 μm) and after (lower pictures, scale 11.9 μm) a bead milling treatment. (I) The pictures on the left were obtained at 488 nm excitation wavelength showing the cell walls in a *light blue color* (gray in print versions). (II) The pictures on the right were taken at 633 nm and show the internal parts of the cells in *red* (gray in print versions).

cycle number, flow rate, homogenizers' design, and pressure (Günerken et al., 2015). This strategy showed high cell wall disruption efficiency in several studies. Thereby, Carullo et al. (2018) reported an instantaneous and complete release of all the intracellular material of *Chlorella vulgaris* after HPH of the concentrated biomass (12 g per L). The pressure drop across the orifice of the homogenizer and the volumetric flow rate were 150 MPa and 155 mL/min, respectively. Xie et al. (2016) obtained highest carotenoid extraction yields after both, bead-beating and HPH of the thermotolerant microalga *Desmodesmus* sp. F51. In that study, both the homogenization pressure (10–40 psi) and cycle number (1–4) affected the degree of cell disruption.

PEFs consist of a short time (from nanoseconds to milliseconds) electrical treatment with PEF strength from 100 to 300 V/cm to 20–80 kV/cm (Barba et al., 2015). This technology is based on the fact that cell membranes, when exposed to intense electric fields during short duration, undergo an electrical breakdown making them permeable. Depending on the treatment conditions, membranes can either become transiently or permanently permeable (Luengo, Martínez, Bordetas, Álvarez, & Raso, 2015). The process parameters to control in this technology include the conductivity (electrolyte concentration), biomass concentration, growth phase, microalgae type, oscillation, and time (Günerken et al., 2015). Luengo et al. (2015) obtained 3.5–4.2 times higher lutein extraction yields after PEFs processing at 25 kV/cm and 100 μs at 25–30°C compared to the untreated control. Parniakov et al. (2015) studied a two-stage extraction procedure which included PEFs processing at 20 kV/cm in water as pretreatment and a second step which included using binary mixtures of dimethyl sulfoxide and ethanol. In that study, using PEFs as a pretreatment allowed reaching higher levels of extracted nondegraded proteins and pigments including carotenoids. This strategy also allowed effective extraction using less concentrated mixtures of organic solvents. Luengo, Condón-Abanto, Álvarez, and Raso (2014) reported that the application of PEFs at 20 kV/cm for 75 μs increased the extraction yield of carotenoids and chlorophylls a and b. The authors of that study did not observe further increments in the yields of extraction with increased field strength and treatment time. Although this technology is promising, some authors suggested that it is not competitive with other conventional mechanical processes for some compounds and results reported so far are controversial. For example, Lam et al. (2017) observed that PEFs processing of *Chlorella vulgaris* and *Neochloris oleoabundans* permitted a 13% release of proteins from the microalgae cells compared to the 45%–50% obtained after bead milling. Parniakov, Barba, et al. (2015) reported lower pigment extraction yields after PEFs processing compared to sonication and an overall extraction yield for various compounds comparable with that for aqueous extraction in a basic medium. In addition, Grimi et al. (2014) suggested that although PEFs processing at 20 kV/cm and 1–4 ms allowed selective extraction of water-soluble ionic components, water-soluble proteins and microelements, this technology was ineffective for increased recovery of chlorophylls and carotenoids.

Sonication works by generating sonic waves at frequencies beyond 18 kHz at specific intensities and amplitudes (Bevilacqua et al., 2018). Cell disruption caused by sonication is due to a phenomenon known as cavitation which is caused by the rapid compression and decompression cycles of sonic waves. Cell disruption occurs when cavitations undergo unsteady oscillations and explodes, creating extremely localized shock waves and high temperatures in a process known as transient cavitation (Lee, Lewis, & Ashman, 2012). Although sonicators were design for batch operations, these can be adapted for continuous operations by the addition of flow cells (Lee et al., 2012). Process parameters of sonication include cycle number and time, power of US, growth phase, and microalgae species (Günerken et al., 2015). This technology has been repeatedly used to increase the extraction of valuable compounds from a wide variety of natural sources including seaweed (Garcia-Vaquero, Rajauria, O'doherty, & Sweeney, 2017; Garcia-Vaquero, Rajauria, Tiwari, Sweeney, & O'Doherty, 2018), fruits (Moorthy et al., 2017), and pulses (Lafarga, Álvarez, Bobo, & Aguiló-Aguayo, 2018). Sonication has also been used to increase the recovery of high-value compounds from microalgae. McMillan, Watson, Ali, and Jaafar (2013) observed 67% cell wall disruption efficiency after US processing. However, in that study, the disruption efficiency did not compare well with that obtained after laser treatment (96%), microwave processing (94%), thermolysis (87%), and mechanical solid shear (92%). Parniakov et al. (2015) obtained a fivefold and ninefold higher recovery of phenolic compounds or chlorophylls after sonication of *Nannochloropsis* spp. at 24 kHz and 400 W for 15 or 7.5 min, respectively. Similar results were reported by Dey and Rathod (2013), who obtained a 47.1% recovery of β-carotene from *Spirulina platensis* after sonicating 1.5 g of biomass (presoaked in methanol for 2 min) in 50 mL heptane at 30°C, 167 W/cm^2, and 61.5% duty cycle for 8 min. The authors observed a 12-fold increase in the extraction yield by presoaking the microalgae in methanol for 2 min. Zou, Jia, Li, Wang, and Wu (2013) used a response surface methodology for increased extraction of astaxanthin from *Haematococcus pluvialis* and identified the optimal extraction conditions as 48% ethanol in ethyl acetate, liquid-to-solid ratio of 20:1 (*v/w*) and extraction conditions maintained for 16 min at 41.1°C and 200 W of ultrasonic power. At these optimized conditions, the yields of astaxanthin were 27.58 ± 0.40 mg/g. Moreover, Jaeschke, Rech, Marczak, and Mercali (2017) evaluated the effect of sonication at 20 kHz in combination with ethanol for increased lipid and carotenoid extraction from *Heterochlorella luteoviridis*. In that study, the authors reported that regarding carotenoid extraction there is an optimal extraction region at 40%–80% of US intensity and 60%–75% of ethanol concentration. Deenu, Naruenartwongsakul, and Kim (2013) optimized the process of enzymatic hydrolysis alone or in combination with sonication to obtain lutein from *Chlorella vulgaris*. In that study, the authors reported the optimal US conditions as 35 kHz, 56.58 W/cm^2, 37.7°C, and a solvent-to-solid ratio of 31 mL/g at 37.7°C. With those conditions, the authors recovered 3.16 mg/g of lutein from the microalgal biomass. Moreover, the application of US processing technologies led to an increased recovery of other compounds including lipids (Araujo et al., 2013; Martinez-Guerra, Gude, Mondala, Holmes, & Hernandez, 2014) and chlorophylls (Kong et al., 2014).

Microwaves can be also used as a pretreatment to enhance the extraction of carotenoids. The heating phenomenon is obtained when a matrix containing polar molecules (generally water) is place under the influence of oscillating electric fields (at frequencies of MHz-GHz), generating vibrations of these polar molecules. This leads to inter- and intramolecular friction, which together with the collision of charged ions results in rapid heating, pressurization, and electroporation of cell membranes (Balasubramanian, Allen, Kanitkar, & Boldor, 2011). Process parameters of microwave treatments include temperature, solid-liquid ratio, dielectric properties of the sample, and processing time (Balasubramanian et al., 2011). The main advantages of microwave processing include short processing times, high disruption efficiency, and relatively low-energy consumption (Cheng et al., 2013). Indeed, Pasquet et al. (2011) suggested that microwave-assisted extraction was the best extraction process for *Cylondrotheca closterium* pigments as it combined rapidity, reproducibility, homogeneous heating, and high extraction yields. In that study, microwave-assisted extraction at 50W for 3–5 min allowed total extraction of fucoxanthin with a maximal extraction yield of 4.29 mg/g. Microwave-assisted extraction at 75°C for 5 min resulted in an astaxanthin recovery from *Haematococcus pluvialis* of 74% previously (Ruen-Ngam, Shotipruk, & Pavasant, 2010). McMillan et al. (2013) reported 94% disruption efficiency after microwave processing of *Nannochloropsis oculata*. In addition, microwaves can operate in continuous mode. Balasubramanian et al. (2011) utilized a 1.2 kW, 2450 MHz resonant continuous microwave processing systems for oil extraction from *Scenedesmus obliquus*. In that study, maximum oil yield was achieved at 95°C for 30 min and was calculated as 76%–77% of total recoverable oil (43%–47% recoveries were obtained for water bath control). Both conditions, extraction time and temperature, had a significant influence on the yield of extraction. Even higher recoveries were obtained by Pan et al. (2016). The authors of that study reported that microwave irradiation could promote the extraction rate over 15 times from *Chlorella sorokiniana*, 10 times from *Galdieria sulphuraria,* and several hundred percent from *Nannochloropsis salina.*

Nonmechanical disruption methods

The presence of moisture significantly affects the extraction process as the contact between the organic solvents and the biomass dispersed in water is limited. Osmotic shock-based cell disruption has been studied as an alternative to conventional mechanical disruption methods, due to the possibility to avoid the cost-intensive process of drying the microalgal cells (Lee, Cho, Chang, & Oh, 2017). Although some studies utilized this strategy to obtain increased recoveries of lipids and other valuable compounds, to the best of our knowledge, it has not yet been studied to recover carotenoids. For example, Yoo et al. (2012) assessed the effects of varied strengths of osmotic shock on the direct lipid extraction from *Chlamydomonas reinhardtii*. Different osmotic strengths were obtained by dissolving sodium chloride, ranging from 0 to 1 g per 5 mL of algal culture. The authors of that study reported a twofold increase in the recovery of lipids compared to other conventional solvent extraction methods. However, it must be highlighted that different microalgae species have different mechanisms of adaptation to osmotic stress (Lee et al., 2017). Other chemical disruption strategies such as ionic liquids have shown to be effective cell destabilizers. Different ionic liquids have been extensively studied but their high price, energy requirements, and toxicity have prevented their industrial application (Gong & Bassi, 2016).

The acid hydrolysis of the sugar polymers in microalgal cell walls has been effectively applied as a pretreatment before applying further cell disruption techniques. The most commonly utilized acid is sulfuric acid due to its efficacy and low cost (Lee & Han, 2015). Other hydrolytic strategies such as enzymatic hydrolyses have shown promising potential as the enzymes decrease the activation energy needed for further chemical reactions, the high selectivity of the enzymes and the mild conditions of operation that decrease the generation of coproducts and degradation of compounds during the reactions (Gong & Bassi, 2016). The high price of the enzymes together with the need to maintain stable conditions during long processing times, currently limits the potential application of this strategy at large scale. However, enzymatic hydrolysis was effectively used to increase the extraction yields of carotenoids in several microalgae species. Deenu et al. (2013) optimized enzymatic hydrolysis alone (using Viscozyme) or in combination with sonication for the extraction of lutein from *Chlorella vulgaris*. In that study, the authors reported the optimal enzymatic pretreatment conditions as 2 h of processing time, pH 4.5, 50°C, and enzyme concentration 1.23% (*w/v*). When combined with USs, the extraction yield of lutein was 3.36 mg/g, higher than using both treatments alone. Zheng et al. (2011) evaluated the potential of 10 different disruption methods in microalgae including enzymatic hydrolysis using multiple enzymes (snailase, cellulase, and lysozyme). Of all the methods evaluated by these authors to recover lipids, the highest recoveries were obtained by grinding the biomass in liquid nitrogen, while the second highest method consisted in enzymatic treatments with lysozyme and cellulose. The hydrolysis using snailase resulted in low extraction yields of lipids compared to other methods such as microwaves or USs (Zheng et al., 2011).

Other novel strategies

Steam explosion is another form of cell disruption, which works by exposing the biomass at temperatures (ranging from 160°C to 260°C) and vapor pressures (1.03–3.45 MPa) generating a cell wall lysis by depressurization when bringing the cells to ambient temperature (Khanra et al., 2018). Lorente, Farriol, and Salvadó (2015) compared the effect of steam explosion, autoclaving, sonication, and MW processing and reported highest lipid recoveries after steam explosion followed by n-hexane extraction. Similar results were also obtained by Nurra et al. (2014) at a 53-m^3 microalgae pilot plant with semi-closed photobioreactors operating in batch mode. In that study, when the extraction was carried out using hexane, an increase from 0.3 to 3.6 and 8.8% was observed when operating at 120°C or 180°C, respectively. This strategy has been reported to be species specific and suitable for large-scale operation due to its efficiency together with its low operational costs and environmental impacts (Khanra et al., 2018). However, this method is relatively new and it is currently under investigation at laboratory scale for biogas production and more studies will be needed to its efficiency to attain high-value compounds (Khanra et al., 2018).

Novel strategies including explosive decompression, atomic force microscopy, and laser treatments have been effectively used for microalgal cell disruption. For example, Dierkes, Steinhagen, Bork, Lütge, and Knez (2012) obtained 72%–92% and 80%–100% astaxanthin and lipid recoveries using explosive decompression with carbon dioxide, propane, or butane. McMillan et al. (2013) obtained 96.5% disruption when using 16 MJ/L of laser power. Disruption using this technique is induced by the high temperatures and shear forces generated during the treatment. However, this technology is not scalable and laser treatments are not suitable disruption methods for microalgae biorefineries (Günerken et al., 2015).

Finally, the cultivation of microalgae together with algicidal microorganisms (i.e., bacteria or viruses) has been suggested as a potential alternative to conventional cell wall disruption strategies. For example, Chen, Bai, and Chang (2013) suggested cultivating *Chlorella vulgaris* ESP-31 in conjunction with the indigenous bacterium

Flammeovirga yaeyamensis, which secretes specific digestive enzymes that degrade the cell wall of microalgae to increase the recovery of lipids. The authors of that study obtained approximately a 100% increase in lipid extraction efficiency and observed the damage in the microalgae cell walls caused by the bacterial treatment using scanning electron microscopy. Overall, mechanical processes, despite their high energetic costs, generally provide high product recovery yields as well as good process controllability and scalability (Lee et al., 2017). These methods are generally less dependent on the microalgae species and are also less likely to lead to contamination of the product (Lee et al., 2012).

Carotenoid extraction methods

Harvesting and extraction processes are the two most expensive steps during the production of microalgal carotenoids (Gong & Bassi, 2016; Kim et al., 2013). The extraction of carotenoids using conventional solvent extraction together with super- and subcritical extraction processes is discussed below.

Conventional and pressurized solvent extraction

Solvents with a similar polarity to those of carotenoids are vital for an efficient recovery of these molecules from complex mixtures. The most commonly studied solvents include methanol, hexane, ethanol, and acetone. Binary extraction systems using dichloromethanol/methanol, chloroform/methanol, and acetone/petroleum ether attained better results compared to the use of those solvents alone for the extraction of carotenoids from *Desmodesmus* sp. (Soares, Marques Júnior, Lopes, Derner, & Antoniosi Filho, 2016). Some studies suggested that acetone is able to extract the majority of photosynthetic pigments of various polarities and its use is also recommended at a concentration of 90% for the analyses of pigments from phytoplankton (Pasquet et al., 2011). Acetone combined with USs or microwaves also gave the best astaxanthin extraction yields from *Haematococcus pluvialis* when compared to the use of individual solvents including methanol, ethanol, and acetonitrile (Ruen-Ngam et al., 2010). However, other researchers obtained the highest yields of carotenoids by using dichloromethane at 60°C (Taucher et al., 2016). Overall, several factors affect the extraction efficiency of solvents such as the temperature, nature of the organic solvent, extraction time, agitation, and number of cycles. The Bligh and Dyer method and Soxhlet are the most commonly adopted for small-scale operations using solvents (Gong & Bassi, 2016).

Pressurized liquid extraction is a relatively novel extraction technique which needs less solvent and uses less time to extract high yields of high-value compounds. This technology involves retaining the sample in an oxygen- and light-free environment and it is based on the use of conventional solvents at controlled temperatures and pressures. Pressure does not significantly affect the extraction efficiency and this parameter generally ranges between 1500 and 2000 psi (Denery, Dragull, Tang, & Li, 2004). Pressurized liquid extraction has been proposed as an efficient technique for carotenoid extraction from microalgae. Denery et al. (2004) used pressurized liquid extraction as new method to extract carotenoids from *Haematococcus pluvialis* and *Dunaliella salina* and observed higher extraction yields when compared to traditional solvent extractions, maintaining the integrity of chemical components. The authors of that study suggested that this strategy could be interesting for labile and light-sensitive compounds. Jaime et al. (2010) used this extraction method after a mechanical cell wall disruption at freezing temperatures for extracting carotenoids from *Haematococcus pluvialis*. In that study, the authors used hexane and ethanol as extracting solvents and the extraction temperatures ranged from 50°C to 200°C. The highest yield was measured as 37.1% and was obtained operating at 200°C and using ethanol as the extraction solvent.

Super- and subcritical solvent extraction

Conventional solvent extraction is cheap and easy to scale-up; however, solvent extraction is nonenvironmental-friendly, time consuming, and requires long procedures with multiple steps of evaporation and concentration. Therefore, efforts are being made to look for novel environmental-friendly extraction techniques, which do not include harmful solvents such as super- and subcritical solvent extraction.

At critical conditions, substances have the density of the liquid state and the viscosity of gaseous state (Khanra et al., 2018). CO_2 is generally utilized as a fluid because of its low price and availability and also because it is inert and nonflammable (Hosikian, Lim, Halim, & Danquah, 2010). The advantages and potential of supercritical solvent extractions have been reviewed by Yen, Yang, Chen, Jesisca, and Chang (2015). Main factors affecting these extraction methods include the pressure, temperature, fluid flow rate, and use of cosolvents (Chen et al., 2012). Several studies have been performed for extracting carotenoids from microalgae using supercritical CO_2 extraction. For example, Macías-Sánchez et al. (2009) obtained higher selectivity and comparable carotenoid yields when using supercritical CO_2 extraction compared to the application of sonication procedures using methanol as solvent. CO_2 has a low polarity which makes it not suitable for extraction of polar compounds; however, this strategy can be combined with other conventional solvents for increasing yields and allowing extraction of polar compounds. Thereby, Macías-Sánchez et al. (2008) utilized supercritical CO_2 extraction in combination with ethanol to obtain valuable compounds from *Nannochloropsis gaditana, Synechococcus* sp., and *Dunaliella salina*. In order to obtain high yields of compounds, the authors operate at temperatures and pressures ranging between 50°C and 60°C and 300–500 bar, respectively. Higher carotenoid/chlorophyll ratios were achieved using supercritical fluid extraction combined with a cosolvent instead of the conventional solvent extraction. Moreover, Goto, Kanda, and Machmudah (2015) also obtained high yields of carotenoid from macroalgae using supercritical CO_2. The authors of that study also evaluated the potential of subcritical dimethyl ether (DME) as solvent at around 0.59 MPa. DME has been approved as a safe solvent for use in the extraction of food-grade components by the European Food Safety Authority (EFSA), the United States Food and Drug Administration (FDA), and Food Standards Australia New Zealand (Hosikian et al., 2010). In the study previously mentioned by Goto et al. (2015), subcritical extraction of carotenoids using 286 g DME resulted in a fucoxanthin yield of 390 mg/g of *Undaria pinnatifida*. Subcritical CO_2 extraction has also been studied for the extraction of lutein, β-carotene, and astaxanthin (Gong & Bassi, 2016). Other extraction processes such as switchable solvent extraction, which refers to the use of solvents that can switch their polarity under different atmospheres or electromagnetic separation have been proposed as potential methods for recovering valuable compounds from microalgae. However, these methodologies are not capable to efficiently extract carotenoids from microalgae to date (Gong & Bassi, 2016).

Purification and storage of carotenoids

After the process of extraction of carotenoids, further strategies are needed in order to purify the compounds of interest, eliminate the remaining cell debris, and to preserve the molecules so the final carotenoids keep their properties intact when reaching the consumer (see Fig. 1).

The purification of carotenoids from microalgae does not differ from those obtained from other natural sources. The classical method to purify carotenoids is based on the Willstatter method (Gong & Bassi, 2016). This purification strategy uses salts (NaOH or KOH) as saponification agents at low temperatures (below 60°C to avoid the degradation of the products), followed by organic solvents (i.e., hexane or mixtures of ethanol, water, and dichloromethane) that will be later removed to obtain the final carotenoid products (Gong & Bassi, 2016). This purification strategy is time consuming and it is being currently replaced by multiple chromatographic protocols summarized and explained in detail in multiple publications (Mercadante, Rodrigues, Petry, & Mariutti, 2017; Rodriguez-Amaya, 2001; Saini, Nile, & Park, 2015).

Once the carotenoids are extracted and purified, the degradation of the final products obtained could be induced by oxygen, light, or heat (Gong & Bassi, 2016). Dias, Camões, and Oliveira (2014) studied the effect of the temperature on the stability of carotenoids (α- and β-carotene, β-cryptoxanthin, lutein, lycopene, and zeaxanthin) in fruits and different standard solution concentrations once the carotenoids were extracted. This study concluded that the carotenoid standard solutions (0.05–5 μg/mL) did not show degradation and could be stored 6 months at −70°C with the exception of lycopene. Chen et al. (2016) microencapsulated whole cells of *Haematococcus pluvialis* using HPH and spray drying to improve the stability of asthaxanthin. The changes in different carotenoids during storage and the different strategies currently used to prevent the degradation of these high-value compounds in a wide variety of food products, including microalgae, were summarized and detailed further by multiple authors (Behsnilian & Mayer-Miebach, 2017; Camacho-Rodríguez, Macías-Sánchez, Cerón-García, Alarcón, & Molina-Grima, 2018; Gong & Bassi, 2016; Ortiz, Ponrajan, Bonnet, Rocheford, & Ferruzzi, 2018; Safafar, Langvad, Møller, & Jacobsen, 2017).

Recent advances in the synthesis of carotenoids

Microalgae are excellent sources of carotenoids and continuous efforts are being made to improve multiple downstream processing stages to achieve high-value compounds. Currently, chemically synthesized carotenoids dominate the global market, although several issues concerning their use have favored the exploitation of carotenoids extracted from natural sources. Moreover, recent advances in genomics, transcriptomics, and proteomics of microalgae have led to the characterization of key genes and regulators of the metabolic pathways of microalgal carotenoid production with promising industrial applications.

Chemical synthesis carotenoids

The total chemical synthesis of β-carotene was developed independently for three major research teams in 1950 (Gong & Bassi, 2016) concluding successfully with the development of two total synthesis approaches namely Roche and BASF synthesis represented in Fig. 5.

The first scaled up method was the Roche synthesis developed by F. Hoffman-La Roche & Co. Ltd. in 1954. This synthesis was performed by assembling the C40 backbone of β-carotene by a reaction of C19 + C2 + C19 using Grignard coupling, elimination, and partial hydrogenation. In 1960, Badische Anilin and Soda-Fabrik developed a new method to obtain higher yields of compounds namely BASF synthesis. This synthetic pathway is based on a Wittig condensation reaction assembling the carbons in a symmetrical manner (C20 + C20). In this reaction, an aldehyde-ketone reacts with triphenyl phosphonium ylide nucleophile and the reaction produces an alkene and triphenylphosphine oxide (Álvarez, Vaz, Gronemeyer, & De Lera, 2014; Berman et al., 2015; Gong & Bassi, 2016). After the development and optimization of the Roche and BASF syntheses, many other synthetic pathways have been developed successfully. The commercial production of β-carotene for the food industry is currently dominated by two major companies (BASF and DSM) that produce approximately 200 Tm of carotene per year, accounting for approximately 85% of the world supplies (Álvarez et al., 2014). The synthesis of other carotenoids such as astaxanthin can also achieved by a Wittig reaction between 2 C15-phosphonium and a C10-dialdehyde or by a dienol ether condensation reaction in a symmetrical manner (C10 + C20 + C10). Approximately 97% of commercial production of astaxanthin is done through chemical synthesis due to the high price of obtaining this product from natural resources (Berman et al., 2015).

Four other carotenoids—8′-apo-β-carotenal (C30), ethyl 8′-apo-β-carotenoate (C30), citranaxanthin (C33), and canthaxanthin (C40)—are also produced synthetically and commercially produced and sold as cosmetics, nutraceuticals, vitamin supplements, and feed additives for poultry, aquaculture, and other livestock. The chemical synthesis of other carotenoids with commercial value such as lycopene, zeaxanthin, and capsorubin has also been developed. However, several of these carotenoids are still extracted and commercialized from their natural resources, that is, capsorubin

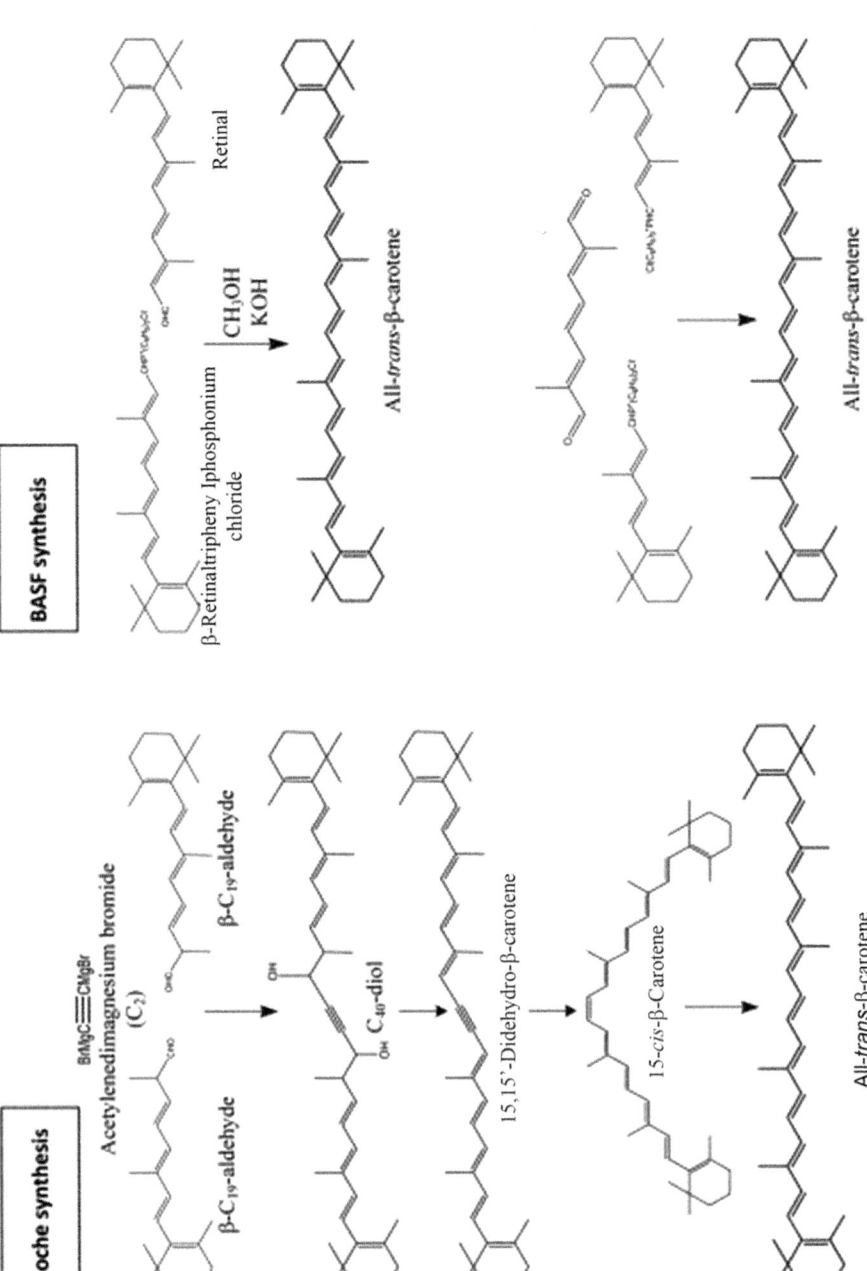

Fig. 5 Pathways for the chemical synthesis of carotenoids developed by Roche and BASF. Image provided by Gong, M. & Bassi, A. 2016. Carotenoids from microalgae: A review of recent developments. *Biotechnology Advances, 34*, 1396–1412.

from paprika extracts and lutein from marigold flowers (Álvarez et al., 2014). The chemical synthesis of over 200 carotenoids has been reported and the methodologies and advances in the field extensively described in detail in several monographs and reviews (Álvarez et al., 2014; Britton, Pfander, & Liaaen-Jensen, 1996; Ito, Yamano, Tode, & Wada, 2009).

Although the chemical synthesis of carotenoids is a well-established market, the natural products are considered safer for human consumption. The carotenoids extracted from their natural sources are normally constituted by complex mixtures of isomers together with other bioactive compounds, unlike the chemically synthesized carotenoids that are normally *trans*-isomers. Several studies emphasized the potential health risk of certain chemically synthesized carotenoids and other antioxidants (Gong & Bassi, 2016; Patrick, 2000; Sen & Chakraborty, 2015). Thus, natural compounds currently offer certain advantages such as lower cost of production and toxicity risks, together with higher customer preference of these products when used as medicine or supplements over the chemically synthesized carotenoids (Gong & Bassi, 2016; Praveenkumar et al., 2015). However, the market of β-carotene is currently dominated by the chemically synthesized compounds, while natural compounds represent only 2% of the total global market (Gong & Bassi, 2016). The current scientific advances in the knowledge of the biosynthetic pathways and molecular strategies to untap the potential industrial exploitation of natural carotenoids from microalgae are detailed below.

Biosynthesis of microalgal carotenoids

The consumer preferences for natural additives and the potentially lower cost of production of natural carotenoids have recently increased the scientific interest in obtaining these compounds using microorganisms including yeast, bacteria, mold, and microalgae (Das et al., 2007). Moreover, the recent knowledge of the natural pathways and genes involved in carotenoid production from carotenogenic microbes has opened the possibility to produce these compounds in other noncarotenogenic microbes (Das et al., 2007). The synthesis of carotenoids in microalgae can be obtained via two different metabolic pathways namely the 2-*C*-methyl-D-eryhritol 4-phophate (MEP) pathway and the mevalonate (MVA) pathway represented in detail in Fig. 6.

Microalgae, using the energy of light can trap CO_2 in the chloroplasts and via the Calvin cycle generate glyceraldehyde 3-phosphate (GAP) to synthesize pyruvate that will be used as the precursor of multiple cellular compounds including glucose, starch, fatty acids, and terpenoids (Liang et al., 2018). Microalgal cells can generate C5 isoprenoid precursors such as isopentenyl diphosphate (IPP) and its isomer dimethylallyl diphosphate (DMAPP) from the acetyl-CoA present in the cytosol via the MVA pathway or from the previously described pyruvate present in the chloroplast following the MEP pathway (Liang et al., 2018; Moise et al., 2014). These precursors will follow a cascade of reactions that will conclude with the production of different hemiterpenes (C5), monoterpenes (C10), sesquiterpenes (C15), diterpenes (C20), triterpenes (C30), and tetraterpenes (C40). The main reactions of both metabolic pathways in microalgae for the production of multiple carotenoids have been recently reviewed in detail by Liang et al. (2018).

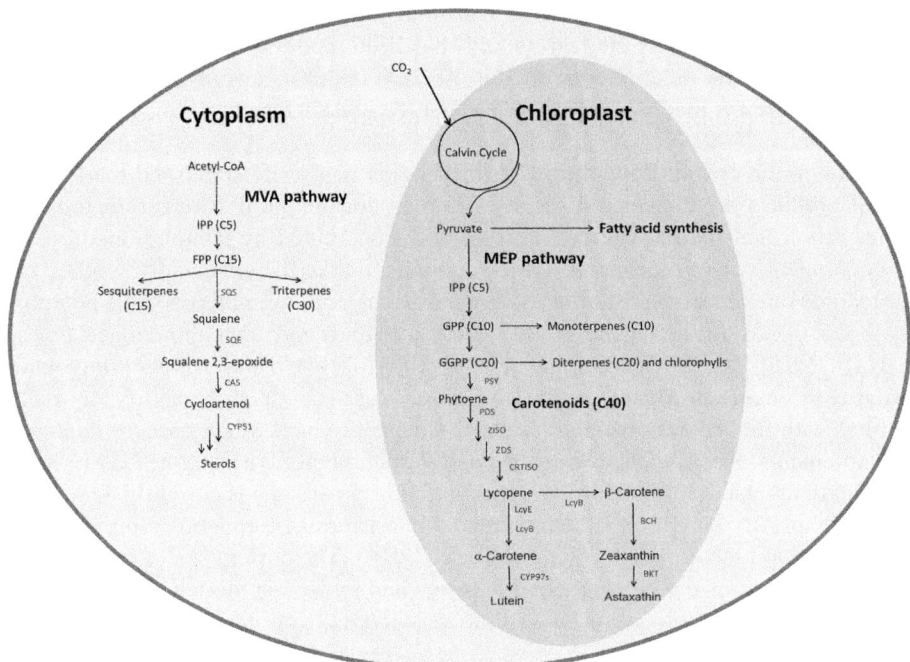

Fig. 6 Schematic representation of the biosynthesis of carotenoids in microalgal cells adapted from Liang et al. (2018) and Moise, Al-Babili, and Wurtzel (2014). The full name of the enzymes abbreviated in the figure are: *BCH*, β-carotene hydroxylase; *BKT*, β-carotene ketolase; *CAS*, cycloartenol synthase; *CRTISO*, carotenoid isomerase; *CYP97s*, cytochrome P450-type carotenoid hydroxylases; *CYPS1*, cytochrome P450-type carotenoid hydroxylases; *LcyB*, lycopene β-cyclase; *LcyE*, lycopene ε-cyclase; *PDS*, phytoene desaturase; *PSY*, phytoene synthase; *SQE*, squalene epoxidase; *SQS*, squalene synthase; *ZDS*, ζ-carotene desaturase; *ZISO*, 15-*cis*-ζ-carotene isomerase.

The recent scientific developments in genomics, transcriptomics, and proteomics of microalgae have led to the characterization of key genes and regulators of the metabolic pathways for carotenoid production, making a major breakthrough in the field due to the possibilities to increase the biosynthesis of carotenoids and other high-value products through metabolic or transcriptional engineering (Liang et al., 2018). Examples of metabolic engineering are the recent studies on the genes PSY and PDS. The overexpression of the PSY gen from *Dunaliella salina* in *Chlamydomonas reinhardtii* resulted in an increase of total carotenoids with respect to nontransformed cells (Couso, Vila, Rodriguez, Vargas, & Leon, 2011), while the overexpression of PSY from *Chlorella zofingiensis* in *Chlamydomonas reinhardtii* increased the production of violaxanthin and lutein (Cordero, Couso, León, Rodríguez, & Vargas, 2011). Moreover, a modification of the PDS gen in *Haematococcus pluvialis* increased significantly the production of astaxanthin compared to nonmodified cells (Steinbrenner & Sandmann, 2006). Regulatory proteins such as transcriptional factors and regulators may play important roles regulating gene transcription of carotenoids in response to abiotic stress in plants and microalgae. The transcription factor AtRAP2.2 binds to PSY and PDS genes in the plant Arabidopsis thaliana and modified the synthesis of carotenoids (Welsch, Maass, Voegel, Dellapenna, & Beyer, 2007). In microalgae *Dunaliella bardawil* the transcription factor WRKY can act as a regulator of carotenoid synthesis under salt stresses and may act as an activator to regulate the expression of carotenogenic genes under salt stress (Liang & Jiang, 2017).

Future of microalgal carotenoid industry

Hundreds of microalgae strains have been reported in the literature as rich sources of carotenoids. However, most of these trains have not yet achieved commercial-scale production mainly because of a lack of strain robustness or low productivity under outdoor conditions. Low production capacity and high production costs limit microalgae biomass applications. Garrido-Cardenas et al. (2018) recently suggested that to solve these problems, the current production capacities must be increased by several orders of magnitude, developing more robust-efficient systems and reducing the cost of production by increasing the production capacity. For example, the costs of microalgal production could be reduced to <1 €/kg when the production of the biomass is coupled with wastewater treatment using CO_2 capture from flue gases (Acién et al., 2012).

Microalgal carotenoids namely astaxanthin and β-carotene are being currently commercialized (Leu & Boussiba, 2014). Natural astaxanthin is currently approved by the FDA for direct human consumption. Li et al. (2011) predicted the cost of producing natural astaxanthin from *Haematococcus pluvialis* in 718 USD per kg. These results are encouraging to the microalgal industry as the estimated cost of production of synthetic astaxanthin is about 1000 USD per kg with a market price above 2000 USD/kg. Moreover, the potential application at large scale of stress manipulation, omics-based technologies, and molecular approaches that are feasible at the laboratory scale, offer an interesting scenario to lower the future cost of microalgae production and downstream processing to obtain carotenoids (Liang et al., 2018). Thereby, molecular approaches including metabolic and transcriptional engineering of microalgae have shown promising results to increase the production of carotenoids. The negative impacts of genetically modified organisms for the human health and ecological systems are considered the main limitations that hinder the exploitation of these techniques (Liang et al., 2018).

In addition, synthetic carotenoids are dominantly all-trans compounds and have occupied the majority of the market mainly as for animal feed production, as colorants, or preservatives. In turn, natural carotenoids are usually complex mixtures of various isomers and are also generally found mixed with other bioactive compounds (Gong & Bassi, 2016). The intake of certain synthetic carotenoid isomers such as β-carotene is considered not as safe as the intake of the naturally obtained one (Patrick, 2000).

Lastly, more interdisciplinary studies are needed to evaluate the different aspects regarding the production of high-value products such as carotenoids, including an economic and environmental evaluations and life cycle analyses in an attempt to achieve more environmental-friendly production while reducing the cost of production and downstream processing of carotenoids (Chew et al., 2017).

Conclusions

Microalgae are a rich source of multiple high-value compounds such as carotenoids. This chapter summarizes the recent advances developed at different downstream processing stages including cultivation (cultivation systems, conditions, and stresses), harvesting of microalgae, pretreatments of the biomass (drying and cell disruption), extraction techniques (conventional and innovative technologies), and purification and storage conditions to achieve the final microalgal carotenoids. The challenges of the microalgal carotenoid industry such as the recent advances in the chemical synthesis of multiple molecules, with over 200 carotenoids chemically synthesized to date, were also described in detail together with the recent knowledge on the biosynthetic pathways of microalgal carotenoids. Promising developments in the field of genomics, transcriptomics, and proteomics that led to a greater knowledge of the metabolic pathways for carotenoid production are also discussed together with the novel molecular approaches to increase the synthesis of microalgal carotenoids. Despite the recent advances in the production of high-value products from microalgae, more efforts are needed in order to reduce the cost of at all the stages of microalgae production and downstream processing to obtain carotenoids, while using more environmental-friendly techniques and processes.

Acknowledgments

Marco Garcia-Vaquero works within the project "Macroalgal Fibre Initiative" funded by Science Foundation Ireland (SFI) [grant number: 14/IA/2548]. Tomás Lafarga is in receipt of *Juan de la Cierva* contract awarded by the Spanish Ministry of Economy, Industry, and Competitiveness (FJCI-2016-29541).

References

Abd El-Baky, H. H., El Baz, F. K., & EL-Baroty, G. S. (2009). Enhancement of antioxidant production in *Spirulina platensis* under oxidative stress. *Acta Physiologiae Plantarum*, *31*, 623.

Abe, K., Hattori, H., & Hirano, M. (2007). Accumulation and antioxidant activity of secondary carotenoids in the aerial microalga *Coelastrella striolata var. multistriata. Food Chemistry*, *100*, 656–661.

Acién, F., Fernández, J., Magán, J., & Molina, E. (2012). Production cost of a real microalgae production plant and strategies to reduce it. *Biotechnology Advances*, *30*, 1344–1353.

Acién, F., Molina, E., Reis, A., Torzillo, G., Zittelli, G., Sepúlveda, C., et al. (2018). Photobioreactors for the production of microalgae. In *Microalgae-based biofuels and bioproducts*: Elsevier.

Álvarez, R., Vaz, B., Gronemeyer, H., & De Lera, Á.R. (2014). Functions, therapeutic applications, and synthesis of retinoids and carotenoids. *Chemical Reviews*, *114*, 1–125.

Araujo, G. S., Matos, L. J., Fernandes, J. O., Cartaxo, S. J., GonÇalves, L. R., Fernandes, F. A., et al. (2013). Extraction of lipids from microalgae by ultrasound application: Prospection of the optimal extraction method. *Ultrasonics Sonochemistry*, *20*, 95–98.

Azizo, A. S., Wirzal, M. D. H., Bilad, M. R., & Yusoff, A. R. M. (2017). Assessment of nylon 6, 6 nanofibre membrane for microalgae harvesting. *AIP Conference Proceedings*, 020032.

Bajhaiya, A. K., Moreira, J. Z., & Pittman, J. K. (2017). Transcriptional engineering of microalgae: Prospects for high-value chemicals. *Trends in Biotechnology*, *35*, 95–99.

Balasubramanian, S., Allen, J. D., Kanitkar, A., & Boldor, D. (2011). Oil extraction from *Scenedesmus obliquus* using a continuous microwave system-design, optimization, and quality characterization. *Bioresource Technology*, *102*, 3396–3403.

Barba, F. J., Parniakov, O., Pereira, S. A., Wiktor, A., Grimi, N., Boussetta, N., et al. (2015). Current applications and new opportunities for the use of pulsed electric fields in food science and industry. *Food Research International*, *77*, 773–798.

Behsnilian, D., & Mayer-Miebach, E. (2017). Impact of blanching, freezing and frozen storage on the carotenoid profile of carrot slices (*Daucus carota* L. cv. *Nutri Red*). *Food Control*, *73*, 761–767.

Berman, J., Zorrilla-López, U., Farré, G., Zhu, C., Sandmann, G., Twyman, R. M., et al. (2015). Nutritionally important carotenoids as consumer products. *Phytochemistry Reviews*, *14*, 727–743.

Bevilacqua, A., Petruzzi, L., Perricone, M., Speranza, B., Campaniello, D., Sinigaglia, M., et al. (2018). Nonthermal technologies for fruit and vegetable juices and beverages: Overview and advances. *Comprehensive Reviews in Food Science and Food Safety*, *17*, 2–62.

Bilad, M. R., Azizo, A. S., Wirzal, M. D. H., Jia Jia, L., Putra, Z. A., Nordin, N.A.H.M., et al. (2018). Tackling membrane fouling in microalgae filtration using nylon 6,6 nanofiber membrane. *Journal of Environmental Management*, *223*, 23–28.

Borowitzka, M. A. (2013). High-value products from microalgae—Their development and commercialisation. *Journal of Applied Phycology*, *25*, 743–756.

Borowitzka, M. A., & Moheimani, N. R. (2013). Sustainable biofuels from algae. *Mitigation and Adaptation Strategies for Global Change*, *18*, 13–25.

Boussiba, S., Bing, W., Yuan, J.-P., Zarka, A., & Chen, F. (1999). Changes in pigments profile in the green alga *Haeamtococcus pluvialis* exposed to environmental stresses. *Biotechnology Letters*, *21*, 601–604.

Brennan, L., & Owende, P. (2010). Biofuels from microalgae—A review of technologies for production, processing, and extractions of biofuels and co-products. *Renewable and Sustainable Energy Reviews*, *14*, 557–577.

Britton, G., Pfander, H., & Liaaen-Jensen, S. (1996). Carotenoids. *Synthesis*: Vol. 2. Springer Science & Business Media.

Cabello, J., Morales, M., & Revah, S. (2017). Carbon dioxide consumption of the microalga *Scenedesmus obtusiusculus* under transient inlet CO_2 concentration variations. *Science of the Total Environment*, *584-585*, 1310–1316.

Camacho-Rodríguez, J., Macías-Sánchez, M., Cerón-García, M., Alarcón, F., & Molina-Grima, E. (2018). Microalgae as a potential ingredient for partial fish meal replacement in aquafeeds: Nutrient stability under different storage conditions. *Journal of Applied Phycology*, *30*, 1049–1059.

Campenni', L., Nobre, B. P., Santos, C. A., Oliveira, A. C., Aires-Barros, M. R., Palavra, A. M. F., et al. (2013). Carotenoid and lipid production by the autotrophic microalga *Chlorella protothecoides* under nutritional, salinity, and luminosity stress conditions. *Applied Microbiology and Biotechnology*, *97*, 1383–1393.

Carullo, D., Abera, B. D., Casazza, A. A., Donsì, F., Perego, P., Ferrari, G., et al. (2018). Effect of pulsed electric fields and high pressure homogenization on the aqueous extraction of intracellular compounds from the microalgae *Chlorella vulgaris*. *Algal Research, 31,* 60–69.

Chekanov, K., Lobakova, E., Selyakh, I., Semenova, L., Sidorov, R., & Solovchenko, A. (2014). Accumulation of astaxanthin by a new *Haematococcus pluvialis* strain BM1 from the white sea coastal rocks (Russia). *Marine Drugs, 12,* 4504.

Chekanov, K., Schastnaya, E., Solovchenko, A., & Lobakova, E. (2017). Effects of CO2 enrichment on primary photochemistry, growth and astaxanthin accumulation in the chlorophyte *Haematococcus pluvialis*. *Journal of Photochemistry and Photobiology B: Biology, 171,* 58–66.

Chen, C.-Y., Bai, M.-D., & Chang, J.-S. (2013). Improving microalgal oil collecting efficiency by pretreating the microalgal cell wall with destructive bacteria. *Biochemical Engineering Journal, 81,* 170–176.

Chen, M., Liu, T., Chen, X., Chen, L., Zhang, W., Wang, J., et al. (2012). Subcritical co-solvents extraction of lipid from wet microalgae pastes of *Nannochloropsis* sp. *European Journal of Lipid Science and Technology, 114,* 205–212.

Chen, L., Liu, X., Li, D., Chen, W., Zhang, K., & Chen, S. (2016). Preparation of stable microcapsules from disrupted cell of *Haematococcus pluvialis* by spray drying. *International Journal of Food Science & Technology, 51,* 1834–1843.

Chen, B., Wan, C., Mehmood, M. A., Chang, J.-S., Bai, F., & Zhao, X. (2017). Manipulating environmental stresses and stress tolerance of microalgae for enhanced production of lipids and value-added products–a review. *Bioresource Technology, 244,* 1198–1206.

Chen, T., Wei, D., Chen, G., Wang, Y., & Chen, F. (2009). Employment of organic acids to enhance astaxanthin formation in heterotrophic *Chlorella zofingiensis*. *Journal of Food Processing and Preservation, 33,* 271–284.

Cheng, Y. S., Labavitch, J., & Vandergheynst, J. (2015). Elevated CO_2 concentration impacts cell wall polysaccharide composition of green microalgae of the genus *Chlorella*. *Letters in Applied Microbiology, 60,* 1–7.

Cheng, J., Li, K., Zhu, Y., Yang, W., Zhou, J., & Cen, K. (2017). Transcriptome sequencing and metabolic pathways of astaxanthin accumulated in *Haematococcus pluvialis* mutant under 15% CO_2. *Bioresource Technology, 228,* 99–105.

Cheng, J., Sun, J., Huang, Y., Feng, J., Zhou, J., & Cen, K. (2013). Dynamic microstructures and fractal characterization of cell wall disruption for microwave irradiation-assisted lipid extraction from wet microalgae. *Bioresource Technology, 150,* 67–72.

Chew, K. W., Yap, J. Y., Show, P. L., Suan, N. H., Juan, J. C., Ling, T. C., et al. (2017). Microalgae biorefinery: High value products perspectives. *Bioresource Technology, 229,* 53–62.

Cooperstone, J., & Schwartz, S. (2016). Recent insights into health benefits of carotenoids. In *Handbook on natural pigments in food and beverages*: Elsevier.

Cordero, B. F., Couso, I., León, R., Rodríguez, H., & Vargas, M.Á. (2011). Enhancement of carotenoids biosynthesis in *Chlamydomonas reinhardtii* by nuclear transformation using a phytoene synthase gene isolated from *Chlorella zofingiensis*. *Applied Microbiology and Biotechnology, 91,* 341–351.

Couso, I., Vila, M., Rodriguez, H., Vargas, M., & Leon, R. (2011). Overexpression of an exogenous phytoene synthase gene in the unicellular alga *Chlamydomonas reinhardtii* leads to an increase in the content of carotenoids. *Biotechnology Progress, 27,* 54–60.

Cuellar-Bermudez, S. P., Aguilar-Hernandez, I., Cardenas-Chavez, D. L., Ornelas-Soto, N., Romero-Ogawa, M. A., & Parra-Saldivar, R. (2015). Extraction and purification of high-value metabolites from microalgae: Essential lipids, astaxanthin and phycobiliproteins. *Microbial Biotechnology, 8,* 190–209.

Das, A., Yoon, S.-H., Lee, S.-H., Kim, J.-Y., Oh, D.-K., & Kim, S.-W. (2007). An update on microbial carotenoid production: Application of recent metabolic engineering tools. *Applied Microbiology and Biotechnology*, *77*, 505.

Deenu, A., Naruenartwongsakul, S., & Kim, S. M. (2013). Optimization and economic evaluation of ultrasound extraction of lutein from *Chlorella vulgaris*. *Biotechnology and Bioprocess Engineering*, *18*, 1151–1162.

Del Campo, J. A., García-González, M., & Guerrero, M. G. (2007). Outdoor cultivation of microalgae for carotenoid production: Current state and perspectives. *Applied Microbiology and Biotechnology*, *74*, 1163–1174.

Denery, J. R., Dragull, K., Tang, C., & Li, Q. X. (2004). Pressurized fluid extraction of carotenoids from *Haematococcus pluvialis* and *Dunaliella salina* and kavalactones from *Piper methysticum*. *Analytica Chimica Acta*, *501*, 175–181.

Dey, S., & Rathod, V. K. (2013). Ultrasound assisted extraction of β-carotene from *Spirulina platensis*. *Ultrasonics Sonochemistry*, *20*, 271–276.

Dias, M. G., Camões, M.F.G.F.C., & Oliveira, L. (2014). Carotenoid stability in fruits, vegetables and working standards—Effect of storage temperature and time. *Food Chemistry*, *156*, 37–41.

Dickinson, S., Mientus, M., Frey, D., Amini-Hajibashi, A., Ozturk, S., Shaikh, F., et al. (2017). A review of biodiesel production from microalgae. *Clean Technologies and Environmental Policy*, *19*, 637–668.

Dierkes, H., Steinhagen, V., Bork, M., Lütge, C. & Knez, Z. 2012. Cell lysis of plant or animal starting materials by a combination of a spray method and decompression for the selective extraction and separation of valuable intracellular materials. Patent no. Ep 2315825 A1.

Doucha, J., & Lívanský, K. (2008). Influence of processing parameters on disintegration of *Chlorella* cells in various types of homogenizers. *Applied Microbiology and Biotechnology*, *81*, 431.

Ejike, C. E., Collins, S. A., Balasuriya, N., Swanson, A. K., Mason, B., & Udenigwe, C. C. (2017). Prospects of microalgae proteins in producing peptide-based functional foods for promoting cardiovascular health. *Trends in Food Science & Technology*, *59*, 30–36.

Fazeli, M. R., Tofighi, H., Madadkar-Sobhani, A., Shahverdi, A. R., Nejad-Sattari, T., Mirzaie, S., et al. (2009). Nicotine inhibition of lycopene cyclase enhances accumulation of carotenoid intermediates by *Dunaliella salina* Ccap 19/18. *European Journal of Phycology*, *44*, 215–220.

Gao, Z., Meng, C., Gao, H., Zhang, X., Xu, D., Su, Y., et al. (2013). Analysis of mRNA expression profiles of carotenogenesis and astaxanthin production of *Haematococcus pluvialis* under exogenous 2, 4-epibrassinolide (EBR). *Biological Research*, *46*, 201–206.

Gao, Z., Meng, C., Zhang, X., Xu, D., Miao, X., Wang, Y., et al. (2012a). Induction of salicylic acid (SA) on transcriptional expression of eight carotenoid genes and astaxanthin accumulation in Haematococcus pluvialis. *Enzyme and Microbial Technology*, *51*, 225–230.

Gao, Z., Meng, C., Zhang, X., Xu, D., Zhao, Y., Wang, Y., et al. (2012b). Differential expression of carotenogenic genes, associated changes on astaxanthin production and photosynthesis features induced by JA in *H. pluvialis*. *PLoS ONE*, *7*, e42243.

Garcia-Vaquero, M., Rajauria, G., O'doherty, J. V., & Sweeney, T. (2017). Polysaccharides from macroalgae: Recent advances, innovative technologies and challenges in extraction and purification. *Food Research International*, *99*, 1011–1020.

Garcia-Vaquero, M., Rajauria, G., Tiwari, B., Sweeney, T., & O'Doherty, J. (2018). Extraction and yield optimisation of fucose, glucans and associated antioxidant activities from *Laminaria digitata* by applying response surface methodology to high intensity ultrasound-assisted extraction. *Marine Drugs*, *16*, 257.

Garrido-Cardenas, J. A., Manzano-Agugliaro, F., Acien-Fernandez, F. G., & Molina-Grima, E. (2018). Microalgae research worldwide. *Algal Research*, *35*, 50–60.

Gerardo, M. L., Zanain, M. A., & Lovitt, R. W. (2015). Pilot-scale cross-flow microfiltration of *Chlorella minutissima*: A theoretical assessment of the operational parameters on energy consumption. *Chemical Engineering Journal*, *280*, 505–513.

Gerde, J. A., Yao, L., Lio, J., Wen, Z., & Wang, T. (2014). Microalgae flocculation: Impact of flocculant type, algae species and cell concentration. *Algal Research*, *3*, 30–35.

Gong, M., & Bassi, A. (2016). Carotenoids from microalgae: A review of recent developments. *Biotechnology Advances*, *34*, 1396–1412.

Goto, M., Kanda, H., & Machmudah, S. (2015). Extraction of carotenoids and lipids from algae by supercritical CO_2 and subcritical dimethyl ether. *The Journal of Supercritical Fluids*, *96*, 245–251.

Gouveia, L., Oliveira, A. C., Congestri, R., Bruno, L., Soares, A. T., Menezes, R. S., et al. (2017). 10—Biodiesel from microalgae. In C. Gonzalez-Fernandez & R. MuÑoz (Eds.), *Microalgae-based biofuels and bioproducts*: Woodhead Publishing.

Grimi, N., Dubois, A., Marchal, L., Jubeau, S., Lebovka, N., & Vorobiev, E. (2014). Selective extraction from microalgae *Nannochloropsis* sp. using different methods of cell disruption. *Bioresource Technology*, *153*, 254–259.

Günerken, E., D'Hondt, E., Eppink, M., Garcia-Gonzalez, L., Elst, K., & Wijffels, R. (2015). Cell disruption for microalgae biorefineries. *Biotechnology Advances*, *33*, 243–260.

Gwak, Y., Hwang, Y.-S., Wang, B., Kim, M., Jeong, J., Lee, C.-G., et al. (2014). Comparative analyses of lipidomes and transcriptomes reveal a concerted action of multiple defensive systems against photooxidative stress in *Haematococcus pluvialis*. *Journal of Experimental Botany*, *65*, 4317–4334.

Hadi, M. R., Shariati, M., & Afsharzadeh, S. (2008). Microalgal biotechnology: Carotenoid and glycerol production by the green algae *Dunaliella* isolated from the Gave-Khooni salt marsh, Iran. *Biotechnology and Bioprocess Engineering*, *13*, 540.

Hamed, I., Özogul, F., Özogul, Y., & Regenstein, J. M. (2015). Marine bioactive compounds and their health benefits: A review. *Comprehensive Reviews in Food Science and Food Safety*, *14*, 446–465.

Hena, S., Fatimah, S., & Tabassum, S. (2015). Cultivation of algae consortium in a dairy farm wastewater for biodiesel production. *Water Resources and Industry*, *10*, 1–14.

Hosikian, A., Lim, S., Halim, R., & Danquah, M. K. (2010). Chlorophyll extraction from microalgae: A review on the process engineering aspects. *International Journal of Chemical Engineering*, *2010*.

Ip, P.-F., & Chen, F. (2005). Employment of reactive oxygen species to enhance astaxanthin formation in *Chlorella zofingiensis* in heterotrophic culture. *Process Biochemistry*, *40*, 3491–3496.

Ishikawa, E., & Abe, H. (2004). Lycopene accumulation and cyclic carotenoid deficiency in heterotrophic *Chlorella* treated with nicotine. *Journal of Industrial Microbiology and Biotechnology*, *31*, 585–589.

Ito, M., Yamano, Y., Tode, C., & Wada, A. (2009). Carotenoid synthesis: Retrospect and recent progress. *Archives of Biochemistry and Biophysics*, *483*, 224–228.

Jaeschke, D. P., Rech, R., Marczak, L. D. F., & Mercali, G. D. (2017). Ultrasound as an alternative technology to extract carotenoids and lipids from *Heterochlorella luteoviridis*. *Bioresource Technology*, *224*, 753–757.

Jaime, L., Rodríguez-Meizoso, I., Cifuentes, A., Santoyo, S., Suarez, S., Ibáñez, E., et al. (2010). Pressurized liquids as an alternative process to antioxidant carotenoids' extraction from *Haematococcus pluvialis* microalgae. *LWT—Food Science and Technology*, *43*, 105–112.

Khanra, S., Mondal, M., Halder, G., Tiwari, O. N., Gayen, K., & Bhowmick, T. K. (2018). Downstream processing of microalgae for pigments, protein and carbohydrate in industrial application: A review. *Food and Bioproducts Processing, 110*, 60–84.

Kim, D.-Y., Vijayan, D., Praveenkumar, R., Han, J.-I., Lee, K., Park, J.-Y., et al. (2016). Cell-wall disruption and lipid/astaxanthin extraction from microalgae: *Chlorella* and *Haematococcus*. *Bioresource Technology, 199*, 300–310.

Kim, J., Yoo, G., Lee, H., Lim, J., Kim, K., Kim, C. W., et al. (2013). Methods of downstream processing for the production of biodiesel from microalgae. *Biotechnology Advances, 31*, 862–876.

Koberg, M., Cohen, M., Ben-Amotz, A., & Gedanken, A. (2011). Bio-diesel production directly from the microalgae biomass of *Nannochloropsis* by microwave and ultrasound radiation. *Bioresource Technology, 102*, 4265–4269.

Kong, W., Liu, N., Zhang, J., Yang, Q., Hua, S., Song, H., et al. (2014). Optimization of ultrasound-assisted extraction parameters of chlorophyll from *Chlorella vulgaris* residue after lipid separation using response surface methodology. *Journal of Food Science and Technology, 51*, 2006–2013.

Kumar, K., Dasgupta, C. N., Nayak, B., Lindblad, P., & Das, D. (2011). Development of suitable photobioreactors for CO_2 sequestration addressing global warming using green algae and cyanobacteria. *Bioresource Technology, 102*, 4945–4953.

Lafarga, T., Álvarez, C., Bobo, G., & Aguiló-Aguayo, I. (2018). Characterization of functional properties of proteins from Ganxet beans (*Phaseolus vulgaris* L. var. *Ganxet*) isolated using an ultrasound-assisted methodology. *LWT—Food Science and Technology, 98*, 106–112.

Lam, G. P. T., Postma, P. R., Fernandes, D. A., Timmermans, R. A. H., Vermuë, M. H., Barbosa, M. J., et al. (2017). Pulsed electric field for protein release of the microalgae *Chlorella vulgaris* and *Neochloris oleoabundans*. *Algal Research, 24*, 181–187.

Lam, G. P., Vermuë, M. H., Eppink, M. H. M., Wijffels, R. H., & Van Den Berg, C. (2018). Multi-product microalgae biorefineries: From concept towards reality. *Trends in Biotechnology, 36*, 216–227.

Lamers, P. P., Van De Laak, C. C. W., Kaasenbrood, P. S., Lorier, J., Janssen, M., De Vos, R. C. H., et al. (2010). Carotenoid and fatty acid metabolism in light-stressed *Dunaliella salina*. *Biotechnology and Bioengineering, 106*, 638–648.

Lee, S. Y., Cho, J. M., Chang, Y. K., & Oh, Y.-K. (2017). Cell disruption and lipid extraction for microalgal biorefineries: A review. *Bioresource Technology, 244*, 1317–1328.

Lee, I., & Han, J.-I. (2015). Simultaneous treatment (cell disruption and lipid extraction) of wet microalgae using hydrodynamic cavitation for enhancing the lipid yield. *Bioresource Technology, 186*, 246–251.

Lee, A. K., Lewis, D. M., & Ashman, P. J. (2012). Disruption of microalgal cells for the extraction of lipids for biofuels: Processes and specific energy requirements. *Biomass and Bioenergy, 46*, 89–101.

Leu, S., & Boussiba, S. (2014). *Advances in the production of high-value products by microalgae.*

Li, J., Zhu, D., Niu, J., Shen, S., & Wang, G. (2011). An economic assessment of astaxanthin production by large scale cultivation of *Haematococcus pluvialis*. *Biotechnology Advances, 29*, 568–574.

Liang, M.-H., Hao, Y.-F., Li, Y.-M., Liang, Y.-J., & Jiang, J.-G. (2016). Inhibiting lycopene cyclases to accumulate lycopene in high β-carotene-accumulating *Dunaliella bardawil*. *Food and Bioprocess Technology, 9*, 1002–1009.

Liang, M.-H., & Jiang, J.-G. (2017). Analysis of carotenogenic genes promoters and WRKY transcription factors in response to salt stress in *Dunaliella bardawil*. *Scientific Reports, 7*, 37025.

Liang, M.-H., Zhu, J., & Jiang, J.-G. (2018). High-value bioproducts from microalgae: Strategies and progress. *Critical Reviews in Food Science and Nutrition*, 01–53.

Lorente, E., Farriol, X., & Salvadó, J. (2015). Steam explosion as a fractionation step in biofuel production from microalgae. *Fuel Processing Technology*, *131*, 93–98.

Lu, Y., Jiang, P., Liu, S., Gan, Q., Cui, H., & Qin, S. (2010). Methyl jasmonate- or gibberel-lins A3-induced astaxanthin accumulation is associated with up-regulation of transcription of β-carotene ketolase genes (bkts) in microalga *Haematococcus pluvialis*. *Bioresource Technology*, *101*, 6468–6474.

Lu, Y., Zhou, W., Wei, L., Li, J., Jia, J., Li, F., et al. (2014). Regulation of the cholesterol biosyn-thetic pathway and its integration with fatty acid biosynthesis in the oleaginous microalga *Nannochloropsis oceanica*. *Biotechnology for Biofuels*, *7*, 81.

Luengo, E., Condón-Abanto, S., Álvarez, I., & Raso, J. (2014). Effect of pulsed electric field treatments on permeabilization and extraction of pigments from *Chlorella vulgaris*. *Journal of Membrane Biology*, *247*, 1269–1277.

Luengo, E., Martínez, J. M., Bordetas, A., Álvarez, I., & Raso, J. (2015). Influence of the treatment medium temperature on lutein extraction assisted by pulsed electric fields from *Chlorella vulgaris*. *Innovative Food Science & Emerging Technologies*, *29*, 15–22.

Macías-Sánchez, M. D., Mantell, C., Rodríguez, M., Martínez De La Ossa, E., Lubián, L. M., & Montero, O. (2009). Comparison of supercritical fluid and ultrasound-assisted extraction of carotenoids and chlorophyll a from *Dunaliella salina*. *Talanta*, *77*, 948–952.

Macías-Sánchez, M. D., Mantell Serrano, C., Rodríguez Rodríguez, M., Martínez De La Ossa, E., Lubián, L. M., & Montero, O. (2008). Extraction of carotenoids and chlorophyll from microalgae with supercritical carbon dioxide and ethanol as cosolvent. *Journal of Separation Science*, *31*, 1352–1362.

Madadi, R., Tabatabaei, M., Aghbashlo, M., Zahed, M. A., & Pourbabaee, A. A. (2018). Biodiesel from microalgae. In *Waste to Wealth*. Springer.

Marbelia, L., Bilad, M. R., Maes, S., Arafat, H. A., & Vankelecom, I. F. J. (2018). Poly(vinylidene fluoride)-based membranes for microalgae filtration. *Chemical Engineering & Technology*, *41*, 1305–1312.

Martinez-Guerra, E., Gude, V. G., Mondala, A., Holmes, W., & Hernandez, R. (2014). Microwave and ultrasound enhanced extractive-transesterification of algal lipids. *Applied Energy*, *129*, 354–363.

McMillan, J. R., Watson, I. A., Ali, M., & Jaafar, W. (2013). Evaluation and comparison of algal cell disruption methods: Microwave, waterbath, blender, ultrasonic and laser treatment. *Applied Energy*, *103*, 128–134.

Mercadante, A. Z., Rodrigues, D. B., Petry, F. C., & Mariutti, L. R. B. (2017). Carotenoid esters in foods—A review and practical directions on analysis and occurrence. *Food Research International*, *99*, 830–850.

Milledge, J. J., & Heaven, S. (2013). A review of the harvesting of micro-algae for biofuel pro-duction. *Reviews in Environmental Science and Bio/Technology*, *12*, 165–178.

Minhas, A. K., Hodgson, P., Barrow, C. J., & Adholeya, A. (2016). A review on the assess-ment of stress conditions for simultaneous production of microalgal lipids and carotenoids. *Frontiers in Microbiology*, *7*, 546.

Moise, A. R., Al-Babili, S., & Wurtzel, E. T. (2014). Mechanistic aspects of carotenoid biosyn-thesis. *Chemical Reviews*, *114*, 164–193.

Mojaat, M., Pruvost, J., Foucault, A., & Legrand, J. (2008). Effect of organic carbon sources and Fe^{2+} ions on growth and β-carotene accumulation by *Dunaliella salina*. *Biochemical Engineering Journal*, *39*, 177–184.

Molina Grima, E., Belarbi, E. H., Acién Fernández, F. G., Robles Medina, A., & Chisti, Y. (2003). Recovery of microalgal biomass and metabolites: Process options and economics. *Biotechnology Advances, 20*, 491–515.

Moorthy, I. G., Maran, J. P., Ilakya, S., Anitha, S. L., Sabarima, S. P., & Priya, B. (2017). Ultrasound assisted extraction of pectin from waste *Artocarpus heterophyllus* fruit peel. *Ultrasonics Sonochemistry, 34*, 525–530.

Nurra, C., Torras, C., Clavero, E., Ríos, S., Rey, M., Lorente, E., et al. (2014). Biorefinery concept in a microalgae pilot plant. Culturing, dynamic filtration and steam explosion fractionation. *Bioresource Technology, 163*, 136–142.

Ortiz, D., Ponrajan, A., Bonnet, J. P., Rocheford, T., & Ferruzzi, M. G. (2018). Carotenoid stability during dry milling, storage, and extrusion processing of biofortified maize genotypes. *Journal of Agricultural and Food Chemistry, 66*, 4683–4691.

Palabiyik, I., Durmaz, Y., Öner, B., Toker, O. S., Coksari, G., Konar, N., et al. (2018). Using spray-dried microalgae as a natural coloring agent in chewing gum: Effects on color, sensory, and textural properties. *Journal of Applied Phycology, 30*, 1031–1039.

Paliwal, C., Mitra, M., Bhayani, K., Bharadwaj, S. V. V., Ghosh, T., Dubey, S., et al. (2017). Abiotic stresses as tools for metabolites in microalgae. *Bioresource Technology, 244*, 1216–1226.

Pan, J., Muppaneni, T., Sun, Y., Reddy, H. K., Fu, J., Lu, X., et al. (2016). Microwave-assisted extraction of lipids from microalgae using an ionic liquid solvent [BMIM][HSO$_4$]. *Fuel, 178*, 49–55.

Parniakov, O., Apicella, E., Koubaa, M., Barba, F. J., Grimi, N., Lebovka, N., et al. (2015). Ultrasound-assisted green solvent extraction of high-added value compounds from microalgae *Nannochloropsis* spp. *Bioresource Technology, 198*, 262–267.

Parniakov, O., Barba, F. J., Grimi, N., Marchal, L., Jubeau, S., Lebovka, N., et al. (2015). Pulsed electric field assisted extraction of nutritionally valuable compounds from microalgae *Nannochloropsis* spp. using the binary mixture of organic solvents and water. *Innovative Food Science & Emerging Technologies, 27*, 79–85.

Pasquet, V., Chérouvrier, J.-R., Farhat, F., Thiéry, V., Piot, J.-M., Bérard, J.-B., et al. (2011). Study on the microalgal pigments extraction process: Performance of microwave assisted extraction. *Process Biochemistry, 46*, 59–67.

Patrick, L. (2000). Beta-carotene: The controversy continues. *Alternative Medicine Review, 5*, 530–545.

Postma, P. R., Miron, T. L., Olivieri, G., Barbosa, M. J., Wijffels, R. H., & Eppink, M. H. M. (2015). Mild disintegration of the green microalgae *Chlorella vulgaris* using bead milling. *Bioresource Technology, 184*, 297–304.

Praveenkumar, R., Lee, K., Lee, J., & Oh, Y.-K. (2015). Breaking dormancy: An energy-efficient means of recovering astaxanthin from microalgae. *Green Chemistry, 17*, 1226–1234.

Pruvost, J., Le Gouic, B., Lepine, O., Legrand, J., & Le Borgne, F. (2016). Microalgae culture in building-integrated photobioreactors: Biomass production modelling and energetic analysis. *Chemical Engineering Journal, 284*, 850–861.

Rizwan, M., Mujtaba, G., Memon, S. A., Lee, K., & Rashid, N. (2018). Exploring the potential of microalgae for new biotechnology applications and beyond: A review. *Renewable and Sustainable Energy Reviews, 92*, 394–404.

Rodriguez-Amaya, D. B. (2001). *A guide to carotenoid analysis in foods*. Washington: ILSI Press.

Rodriguez-Amaya, D. B. (2016). Natural food pigments and colorants. *Current Opinion in Food Science, 7*, 20–26.

Ruen-Ngam, D., Shotipruk, A., & Pavasant, P. (2010). Comparison of extraction methods for recovery of astaxanthin from *Haematococcus pluvialis*. *Separation Science and Technology*, *46*, 64–70.

Ruiz, J., Olivieri, G., De Vree, J., Bosma, R., Willems, P., Reith, J. H., et al. (2016). Towards industrial products from microalgae. *Energy & Environmental Science*, *9*, 3036–3043.

Saeki, K., Aburai, N., Aratani, S., Miyashita, H., & Abe, K. (2017). Salt-stress and plant hormone-like responses for selective reactions of esterified xanthophylls in the aerial microalga *Coelastrella* sp. KGU-Y002. *Journal of Applied Phycology*, *29*, 115–122.

Safafar, H., Langvad, S., Møller, P., & Jacobsen, C. (2017). Storage conditions affect oxidative stability and nutritional composition of freeze-dried *Nannochloropsis salina*. *European Journal of Lipid Science and Technology*, *119*, 1600477.

Safi, C., Camy, S., Frances, C., Varela, M. M., Badia, E. C., Pontalier, P.-Y., et al. (2014). Extraction of lipids and pigments of *Chlorella vulgaris* by supercritical carbon dioxide: Influence of bead milling on extraction performance. *Journal of Applied Phycology*, *26*, 1711–1718.

Saini, R. K., Nile, S. H., & Park, S. W. (2015). Carotenoids from fruits and vegetables: Chemistry, analysis, occurrence, bioavailability and biological activities. *Food Research International*, *76*, 735–750.

Sasso, S., Pohnert, G., Lohr, M., Mittag, M., & Hertweck, C. (2012). Microalgae in the postgenomic era: A blooming reservoir for new natural products. *FEMS Microbiology Reviews*, *36*, 761–785.

Sathasivam, R., & Ki, J. S. (2018). A review of the biological activities of microalgal carotenoids and their potential use in healthcare and cosmetic industries. *Marine Drugs*, *16*.

Sen, S., & Chakraborty, R. (2015). Antioxidant supplements: Friend or foe? In *Free radicals in human health and disease*. Springer.

Soares, A. T., Marques Júnior, J. G., Lopes, R. G., Derner, R. B., & Antoniosi Filho, N. R. (2016). Improvement of the extraction process for high commercial value pigments from *Desmodesmus* sp. microalgae. *Journal of the Brazilian Chemical Society*, *27*, 1083–1093.

Solovchenko, A., & Khozin-Goldberg, I. (2013). High-CO_2 tolerance in microalgae: Possible mechanisms and implications for biotechnology and bioremediation. *Biotechnology Letters*, *35*, 1745–1752.

Srivastava, A., Seo, S.-H., Ko, S.-R., Ahn, C.-Y., & Oh, H.-M. (2018). Bioflocculation in natural and engineered systems: Current perspectives. *Critical Reviews in Biotechnology*, *38*, 1176–1194.

Steinbrenner, J., & Linden, H. (2001). Regulation of two carotenoid biosynthesis genes coding for phytoene synthase and carotenoid hydroxylase during stress-induced astaxanthin formation in the green alga *Haematococcus pluvialis*. *Plant Physiology*, *125*, 810–817.

Steinbrenner, J., & Sandmann, G. (2006). Transformation of the green alga *Haematococcus pluvialis* with a phytoene desaturase for accelerated astaxanthin biosynthesis. *Applied and Environmental Microbiology*, *72*, 7477–7484.

Sun, H., Guan, B., Kong, Q., Geng, Z., & Wang, N. (2016). Repeated cultivation: Non-cell disruption extraction of astaxanthin for *Haematococcus pluvialis*. *Scientific Reports*, *6*, 20578.

Taucher, J., Baer, S., Schwerna, P., Hofmann, D., Hümmer, M., Buchholz, R., et al. (2016). Cell disruption and pressurized liquid extraction of carotenoids from microalgae. *Journal of Thermodynamics & Catalysis*, *7*, 158.

Ummalyma, S. B., Gnansounou, E., Sukumaran, R. K., Sindhu, R., Pandey, A., & Sahoo, D. (2017). Bioflocculation: An alternative strategy for harvesting of microalgae—An overview. *Bioresource Technology*, *242*, 227–235.

Vandamme, D., Foubert, I., & Muylaert, K. (2013). Flocculation as a low-cost method for harvesting microalgae for bulk biomass production. *Trends in Biotechnology, 31*, 233–239.

Vidhyavathi, R., Venkatachalam, L., Sarada, R., & Ravishankar, G. A. (2008). Regulation of carotenoid biosynthetic genes expression and carotenoid accumulation in the green alga *Haematococcus pluvialis* under nutrient stress conditions. *Journal of Experimental Botany, 59*, 1409–1418.

Wayama, M., Ota, S., Matsuura, H., Nango, N., Hirata, A., & Kawano, S. (2013). Three-dimensional ultrastructural study of oil and astaxanthin accumulation during encystment in the green alga *Haematococcus pluvialis*. *PLoS ONE, 8*, e53618.

Welsch, R., Maass, D., Voegel, T., Dellapenna, D., & Beyer, P. (2007). Transcription factor RAP2. 2 and its interacting partner SINAT2: Stable elements in the carotenogenesis of *Arabidopsis* leaves. *Plant Physiology, 145*, 1073–1085.

Wen, Z., Liu, Z., Hou, Y., Liu, C., Gao, F., Zheng, Y., et al. (2015). Ethanol induced astaxanthin accumulation and transcriptional expression of carotenogenic genes in *Haematococcus pluvialis*. *Enzyme and Microbial Technology, 78*, 10–17.

Xie, Y., Ho, S.-H., Chen, C.-N.N., Chen, C.-Y., Jing, K., Ng, I. S., et al. (2016). Disruption of thermo-tolerant *Desmodesmus* sp. F51 in high pressure homogenization as a prelude to carotenoids extraction. *Biochemical Engineering Journal, 109*, 243–251.

Yap, B. H. J., Dumsday, G. J., Scales, P. J., & Martin, G. J. O. (2015). Energy evaluation of algal cell disruption by high pressure homogenisation. *Bioresource Technology, 184*, 280–285.

Yen, H.-W., Yang, S.-C., Chen, C.-H., Jesisca, & Chang, J.-S. (2015). Supercritical fluid extraction of valuable compounds from microalgal biomass. *Bioresource Technology, 184*, 291–296.

Yildirim, A., Akgun, I., & Dalay, M. (2017). Converted carotenoid production in *Dunaliella salina* by using cyclization inhibitors 2-methylimidazole and 3-amino-1, 2, 4-triazole. *Turkish Journal of Biology, 41*, 213–219.

Yin-Nin Ma, R., & Chen, F. (2001). Induction of astaxanthin formation by reactive oxygen species in mixotrophic culture of *Chlorococcum* sp. *Biotechnology Letters, 23*, 519–523.

Yoo, C., Jun, S.-Y., Lee, J.-Y., Ahn, C.-Y., & Oh, H.-M. (2010). Selection of microalgae for lipid production under high levels carbon dioxide. *Bioresource Technology, 101*, S71–S74.

Yoo, G., Park, W.-K., Kim, C. W., Choi, Y.-E., & Yang, J.-W. (2012). Direct lipid extraction from wet *Chlamydomonas reinhardtii* biomass using osmotic shock. *Bioresource Technology, 123*, 717–722.

Zhang, P., Li, Z., Lu, L., Xiao, Y., Liu, J., Guo, J., et al. (2017). Effects of stepwise nitrogen depletion on carotenoid content, fluorescence parameters and the cellular stoichiometry of *Chlorella vulgaris*. *Spectrochimica Acta Part A: Molecular and Biomolecular Spectroscopy, 181*, 30–38.

Zheng, H., Yin, J., Gao, Z., Huang, H., Ji, X., & Dou, C. (2011). Disruption of *Chlorella vulgaris* cells for the release of biodiesel-producing lipids: A comparison of grinding, ultrasonication, bead milling, enzymatic lysis, and microwaves. *Applied Biochemistry and Biotechnology, 164*, 1215–1224.

Zou, T. B., Jia, Q., Li, H. W., Wang, C. X., & Wu, H. F. (2013). Response surface methodology for ultrasound-assisted extraction of astaxanthin from *Haematococcus pluvialis*. *Marine Drugs, 11*, 1644–1655.

Analysis and metabolomics of carotenoids

Patricia Regal, Alexandre Lamas, Cristina A. Fente, Carlos M. Franco, A. Cepeda
Department of Analytical Chemistry, Nutrition and Bromatology, Faculty of Veterinary Science, University of Santiago de Compostela, Lugo, Spain

Chapter outline

Keys to carotenoid analysis

Carotenoids are a group of >700 fat-soluble pigments ubiquitous in nature and responsible for orange-yellow and/or red pigmentation in animals, plants, and microorganisms (Ngamwonglumlert & Devahastin, 2019). These compounds can be synthesized by plants, algae, yeast, fungi, and photosynthetic bacteria. Conversely, animals and humans cannot produce carotenoids themselves, so they have to obtain them from the diet. The prime universal classification of carotenoids recognizes two classes: carotenes and xanthophylls. Accordingly, these terpenoids take the form of C14 polyene hydrocarbon chains that may (xanthophylls) or may not (carotenes) have oxygen atoms attached. In this sense, xanthophylls represent all the hydroxy-, epoxy-, oxy-, and furanoxy-derivatives of the carotenes. Lutein and zeaxanthin are classical examples of xanthophylls, as β-carotene and lycopene are so for carotenes (Amorim-Carrilho, Cepeda, Fente, & Regal, 2014). Carotenoids may also be classified as acyclic, monocyclic, and bicyclic compounds, depending on the number of rings present in the molecule. Their color is strictly related to their structure, and more precisely, to their conjugated backbone. Other important carotenoid properties, such as antioxidant and provitamin A activities are also related to their molecular architecture.

Almost all carotenoids, in a greater or lesser degree, show scavenging properties against extensive numbers of diverse reactive oxygen species (ROS) that may be produced over the course of the cellular life cycle in animals. This antioxidant capacity has been the most investigated and it has been suggested as the main mechanism of action of carotenoids in the prevention of human diseases (Khalid, Saeed-ur-Rahman,

Carotenoids: Properties, Processing and Applications. https://doi.org/10.1016/B978-0-12-817067-0.00006-3

Iqbal, & Huang, 2019). In addition to the previous, individual carotenoids may also act through other mechanisms, for example, provitamin A activity. The three most important provitamin A components of most carotenoid-containing foods are α-carotene, β-cryptoxanthin, and β-carotene (Eggersdorfer & Wyss, 2018). Vitamin A deficiency remains a health problem in developing countries, and it can result in visual malfunction and impaired immune function. Another example of carotenoid roles in human health is the presence of lutein, zeaxanthin, and the isomer *meso*-zeaxanthin in the human retina. Concentrated in the macula, these compounds are known as macular pigment (Lima, Rosen, & Farah, 2016). In this context, carotenoids are considered effective health-promoting compounds present in human diet and have been proposed to reduce the incidence of chronic diseases, such as cardiovascular diseases, cancer, and eye/eyesight problems such as cataracts and macular degeneration (Eggersdorfer & Wyss, 2018; Khalid et al., 2019).

Carotenoids are present in many common human foods but deeply pigmented fruits and vegetables constitute their major dietary sources. Yellow-orange vegetables and fruits provide most of the β-carotene and α-carotene of the human diet, orange fruits provide mostly α-cryptoxanthin, dark green vegetables and egg yolk provide lutein and zeaxanthin, and tomatoes supply lycopene (Amorim-Carrilho et al., 2014). Carotenoids can also be found in animals, for instance in birds plumage, fish, crustaceans, and insects. The exposure of carotenoid-containing food to heat, light, and oxygen are detrimental to their stability and these factors can lead to structural changes and degradation of carotenoids, resulting in the losses of their antioxidant and provitamin A activities (Ngamwonglumlert & Devahastin, 2019). On the other hand, carotenoid composition varies qualitatively and quantitatively among different fruits and vegetables and even in a given food, it can be affected not only by ripening, cultivar, climate, part of the plant, and production techniques but also by postharvest handling, processing, and storage (Rodriguez-Amaya, 2003; Saini, Nile, & Park, 2015). Apart from the above, the literature strongly supports that when ingested by animals, the bioaccessibility and bioavailability of carotenoids are dependent on several factors (Rodriguez-Amaya, 2010; Saini et al., 2015). As a matter of fact, factors influencing their bioavailability and bioconversion have been summarized in the mnemonic "SLAMENGHI": species of carotenoids, linkages at molecular levels, amount of carotenoid, matrix, effectors, nutrients status, genetics, host-related factors, and interactions among these variables (West & Castenmiller, 1998). Bioaccessibility and bioavailability of bioactive compounds contained in food can be determined using in vivo and in vitro procedures, taking into account the strengths and limitations of each experimental technique (Carbonell-Capella, Buniowska, Barba, Esteve, & Frígola, 2014).

Due to the strong evidence of their biological importance in human nutrition and health, the food content of provitamin A carotenoids (α-carotene, β-carotene, and β-cryptoxanthin), and nonprovitamin A carotenoids (lycopene, lutein, and zeaxanthin) have been extensively studied (Amorim-Carrilho et al., 2014). In this sense, a lot of effort has been directed toward ensuring accurate and reliable carotenoid analysis and current knowledge on the carotenoid composition (qualitatively and quantitatively) of foods is truly broad and comprehensive (Amorim-Carrilho et al., 2014; Rodriguez-Amaya, 2010). Apocarotenoids (APOs), carotenoid-derived molecules, add variety and complexity to the analysis of carotenoids. Even if they do not strictly belong to the group of their precursors, these isoprenoids have also important functions in plants and in mammals, closely related to carotenoid roles (Beltran & Stange, 2016; Harrison & Quadro, 2018). Out of the more than seven hundred carotenoids known to date, lycopene, β-carotene, and zeaxanthin are the precursors of the main APOs described to date, which include bixin, crocin, picrocrocin, abscisic acid, strigolactone, and mycorradicin (Beltran & Stange, 2016). These derivatives are generated on enzymatic and nonenzymatic cleavage of carotenes and xanthophylls in plants or animals (Harrison & Quadro, 2018). Both retinoids and nonretinoid APOs have attracted much attention in plant and biomedical research, implying an emerging need for comprehensive and modern analytical methods to accurately quantify these compounds and their precursors in different matrices (Mi, Jia, Wang, & Al-Babili, 2018; Zoccali, Giuffrida, Salafia, Giofrè, & Mondello, 2018).

Analytical methods for carotenoids

A variety of guides, manuals, and/or reviews on the analysis of carotenoids in food and other biological matrices is available in the literature (Amorim-Carrilho et al., 2014; Arvayo-Enríquez, Mondaca-Fernández, Gortárez-Moroyoqui, López-Cervantes, & Rodríguez-Ramírez, 2013; Giuffrida, Donato, Dugo, & Mondello, 2018; Islam & Schweigert, 2015; Kopec, Cooperstone, Cichon, & Schwartz, 2012; Mercadante, Rodrigues, Petry, & Mariutti, 2017; Rivera & Canela-Garayoa, 2012; Rodriguez-Amaya, 2003; Rodriguez-Amaya, 2016). The wide array of structures and poor stability of carotenes and xanthophylls greatly contribute to the inherent difficulty of carotenoid analysis and, therefore, there is not a reference method to analyze them all. In addition, the lack of commercially available standards, the low concentrations of some carotenoids, and the presence of interfering compounds in biological samples add difficulty to the development of reliable analytical methods to identify and quantify carotenoids in real samples (Amorim-Carrilho et al., 2014; Oliver & Palou, 2000). On the other hand, APOs have emerged as very important cleavage products of carotenoids with different bioactive properties in plants (Hou, Rivers, León, McQuinn, & Pogson, 2016) and animals (Harrison & Quadro, 2018). Relatively few methods are available in the literature for the analysis of APOs and their esters in a fast and efficient way (Giuffrida, Zoccali, Giofrè, Dugo, & Mondello, 2017). Hence, analytical methods for determining not only carotenoids but also APOs profiles in plant material are required to better understand their biological functions (Kyriakoudi & Tsimidou, 2018; Mi, Jia, Balakrishna, Wang, & Al-Babili, 2019).

Considerable effort and research have been invested so far in developing methods for reliable analysis of carotenoids present in food and in other biological matrices (plasma, serum, red blood cells, breast milk, human/animal tissues, etc.), and significant progress has been achieved (Amorim-Carrilho et al., 2014; Giuffrida, Donato, et al., 2018; Rodriguez-Amaya, 2010). A standard analytical method for carotenoid analysis in biological matrices comprises the following steps, with some variations: sample homogenization, carotenoid extraction and/or saponification, and instrumental measurement (usually, separation + detection). As Rodriguez-Amaya already stated several years ago (Rodriguez-Amaya, 2003), the carotenoid analysis is inherently difficult and error-prone, so the analyst must take advantage of all analytical advances and cutting-edge technologies available to avoid errors and obtain reliable quantitative data (Fig. 1).

Extraction methods

When it comes to carotenoid analysis, in the vast majority of cases, these bioactive compounds must be extracted from the matrix before their instrumental analysis and this step has proved far from easy so far. Unlike other analytes, carotenoid extraction in laboratories is not generally standardized (Riggi, 2010; Saini & Keum, 2018). Most types of samples require the first step of homogenization or grinding, in order to facilitate the access of extraction solvents and/or release the analytes from the matrix, usually composed of rigid plant/algae cell walls. After that, extractions with organic solvents (or combinations) or, to a lesser extent, with solid-phase sorbents are applied to collect carotenoids for further analysis (Saini & Keum, 2018).

The most common procedure is the one-step application of an organic solvent. Many different organic solvents and synergistic solvent combinations have been used

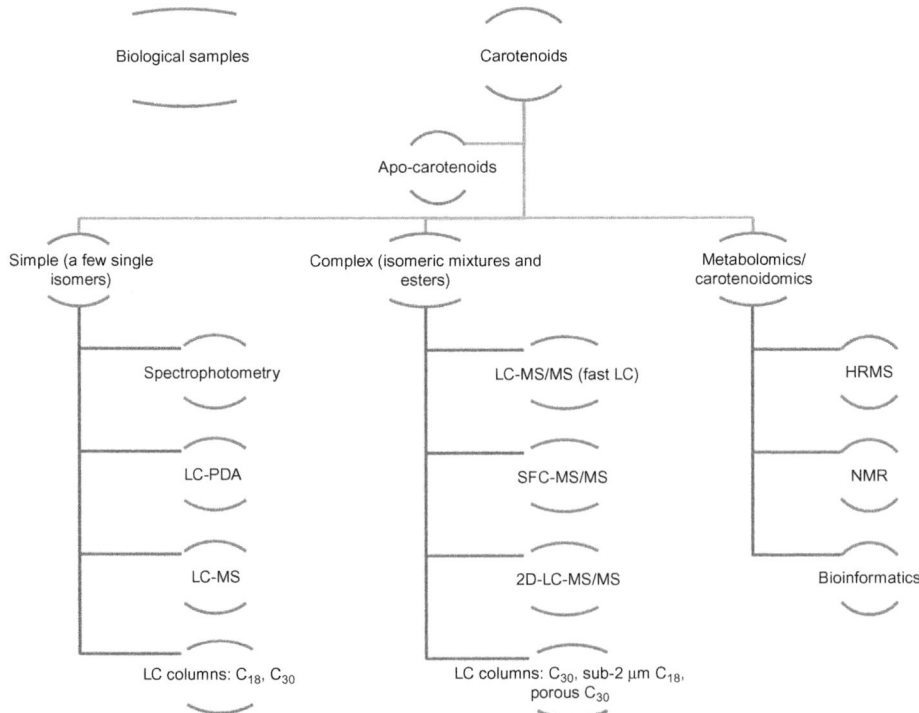

Fig. 1 Schematic overview of the most popular alternatives in carotenoid analysis and carotenoid-related metabolomics.

in the analysis of carotenoids and the selection of the appropriate option is one of the most critical factors for an efficient extraction (Amorim-Carrilho et al., 2014; Strati & Oreopoulou, 2011). The most popular nonpolar carotenoids, lacking polar functional groups in their hydrocarbon structure, are β-carotene, α-carotene, and lycopene (carotenes). The attachment of one or two polar oxygen-containing groups to the hydrocarbon chain (xanthophylls), such as epoxy (violaxanthin and neoxanthin) or hydroxyl (lutein and zeaxanthin) groups, increases the polarity of these carotenoids (Saini & Keum, 2018). In this context, nonpolar, and medium-polar solvents as hexane and ethyl acetate, respectively, are frequently selected for nonpolar (carotenes) or esterified carotenoids, while polar solvents as ethanol or acetone are more suitable for polar carotenoids (xanthophylls) (Amorim-Carrilho et al., 2014; Saini & Keum, 2018). All other matrix components, particularly water, play also an important role in solvent selection. Tri-mixtures of acetone, ethanol or methanol, and hexane are frequently found in the literature for the simultaneous extraction of polar and nonpolar carotenoids from plant matrices (Amorim-Carrilho et al., 2014; Saini & Keum, 2018). Hexane, ethanol, ethanol/hexane, and combinations of them with acetone, are, by far, the most commonly used solvents for carotenoid analysis in diverse biological matrices (Amorim-Carrilho et al., 2014; Arvayo-Enríquez et al., 2013; Saini & Keum, 2018). Ethanol and acetone are particularly efficient when high amount of water is present.

Solid-phase extraction (SPE) is a very simple and cost-effective alternative in the preparation of biological samples, as well as highly versatile thanks to the existence of multiple sorbents and formats. Unlike liquid extractions, SPE has been rarely reported in carotenoid studies (Amorim-Carrilho et al., 2014; Shen et al., 2009). The typical sorbents include C30 and C18, while diol and silica cartridges have only shown good retention for polar carotenoids as lutein (Shen et al., 2009). In this context, molecularly imprinted solid-phase extraction (MISPE) offers alternative sorbents with enhanced selection abilities in complicated matrices, including food (Regal, Díaz-Bao, Barreiro, Cepeda, & Fente, 2012). However, literature reporting MISPE for carotenoid analysis is scarce (Mohajeri, Hosseinzadeh, Keyhanfar, & Aghamohammadian, 2010; Zhu & Row, 2013), suggesting that there might be a need for further research in this field.

Besides the above-mentioned alternatives, many other different extraction techniques have been applied to food and human samples for carotenoid extraction, including atmospheric liquid extraction with maceration, Soxhlet extraction, supercritical fluid extraction (SFE), pressurized liquid extraction (PLE), accelerated solvent extraction (ASE), ultrasound-assisted extraction (UAE), microwave-assisted extraction (MAE), pressurized hot-water extraction (PHWF), pulsed electric field (PEF) and moderate electric field (MEF)-assisted extraction, enzyme-assisted extraction (EAE), and green solvents, among others (Saini & Keum, 2018). Soxhlet delivers the highest yield of carotenoids, while SFE has demonstrated to be the superior green alternative (Riggi, 2010; Saini & Keum, 2018). Recently, a very simple and sensitive dilute-and-shoot method has been developed for quantification of five common carotenoids in plasma by HPLC-MS/MS (Bukowski, Voeller, & Jahns, 2018). This work represents a clear improvement over previous techniques since no extraction or cleanup is required.

The susceptibility of carotenoids to oxidation and isomerization has also to be considered so that extraction and analysis must be performed as quickly as possible and under special conditions of light, temperature, oxygen, and pH. In this context, short extraction times under appropriate temperature conditions are preferred, in order to prevent degradation and enzymatic oxidation. Protection from direct exposure to UV light prevents photoisomerization and destruction of carotenoids. Additionally, samples must be protected from oxygen, in order to provide an inert environment. The addition of antioxidants during extraction can be considered routine in the carotenoid analysis. BHT is by far the most commonly used antioxidant added to extraction solvents to protect carotenoids, along with oxygen elimination (Amorim-Carrilho et al., 2014). Pyrogallol, butylhydroxyanisol (BHA), α-tocopherol (TOC), ascorbic acid, and tert-butylhydroquinone (TBHQ) are also used (Arvayo-Enríquez et al., 2013; Saini & Keum, 2018). Nevertheless, it has been suggested that the addition of antioxidants to the extraction solvents can be omitted provided that carotenoids are analyzed within 48 h of storage at −80°C (Rivera & Canela, 2012). Finally, calcium or magnesium carbonate or sodium bicarbonate can be added during the extraction to neutralize acids found in plant material and thus prevent structural changes (Arvayo-Enríquez et al., 2013; Saini & Keum, 2018).

Saponification

Xanthophylls can be found in their free form or in a more stable fatty acid esterified form, with a concurrent increase in the complexity of this group of carotenoids (Granado, Olmedilla, Gil-Martinez, & Blanco, 2001; Mariutti & Mercadante, 2018). Accordingly, sample saponification is commonly applied to carotenoid extracts from vegetables and fruits, in order to release esterified xanthophylls but also to eliminate interfering compounds as, for instance, chlorophylls and saponifiable lipids. This step not only simplifies the chromatographic separation but also adds valuable information about the nature and distribution of carotenoids in that particular matrix. The recommended procedures involve the addition of methanolic KOH to sample extracts, at room temperature, in the dark, under an atmosphere of nitrogen and/or with the addition of antioxidants, and with saponification performed overnight (Amorim-Carrilho et al., 2014; Kimura, Rodriguez-Amaya, & Godoy, 1990). This is a rather time-consuming step in the carotenoid analysis, involving the use of considerable volumes of solvents, potential occurrence of isomerization of carotenes and significant losses in total carotenoid content (Kimura et al., 1990). This step is not necessary for all samples but and despite all the existing drawbacks, saponification is still justified for certain matrices to improve analytical resolution and to reduce analytical time in chromatographic separations (Amorim-Carrilho et al., 2014; Inbaraj et al., 2008; Kimura et al., 1990). In this sense, simpler and gentle protocols of saponification have been proposed, such as reduced or "short-cut" protocols without loss of accuracy and precision (Granado et al., 2001). Another good example of these alternative solutions is the use of strongly basic resins instead of KOH, achieving complete removal of chlorophylls with hardly any losses of carotenoids (Larsen & Christensen, 2005). Alternatively, some chromatographic methods can separate the free carotenoids and their esters, hence they may be applied to analyze unsaponified extracts (Inbaraj et al., 2008; Mariutti & Mercadante, 2018).

Chromatographic separation and/or determination of carotenoids

Spectrophotometric methods and liquid chromatography (HPLC) separation, with the latter coupled to photodiode array detectors (PDA) or MSs, are commonly employed for identification and quantification of carotenoids in food and in other matrices (Amorim-Carrilho et al., 2014). The simplest option is the spectroscopic determination of total carotenoids as equivalents of β-carotene (AOAC methods). On the other hand, using HPLC instruments carotenoids can not only be quantified but individual carotenoids can be separated. These two options are considered reference methods to measure total carotenoids (Islam & Schweigert, 2015) even though other alternatives exist. For example, the so-called iCheck method (BioAnalyt GmbH, Germany), a rapid lab-independent spectrophotometric method that claims to be less time consuming and easy to operate than spectroscopy and HPLC. As a matter of fact, HPLC is the gold standard in terms of analytical resolution for carotenoid determination in biological and food samples (Amorim-Carrilho et al., 2014; Giuffrida, Donato, et al., 2018; Rivera & Canela-Garayoa, 2012; Rodríguez-Bernaldo de Quirós & Costa, 2006; Saini & Keum, 2018). On the basis of the inherent instability and low volatility of these compounds, gas chromatography is considered unsuitable for their analysis. Due to the chemical and physical properties of carotenoids, HPLC coupled to various absorbance detectors (UV, Vis, PDA) has been so far the most common analytical method for determining carotenoid profiles, both qualitatively and quantitatively, in food and other matrices (Rodríguez-Bernaldo de Quirós & Costa, 2006). However, the close structural similarities existing between the diverse members of the carotenoid family may result in the coelution of many of them during chromatography. As a consequence, their determination by absorbance is not possible anymore because their spectra are very similar, if not the same. In this context, many researchers have complemented their identification using mass spectrometry (MS).

Other analytical alternatives have been reported for the analysis of carotenoids, including infrared (IR), mid- and near-infrared spectroscopy (MIR and NIR), Raman, and nuclear magnetic resonance (NMR), among others. These technologies do not require a previous chromatographic separation of compounds, not even a previous extraction step, which means a great simplification of the analysis. In light of the above, these approaches are referred to as "nondestructive" and "rapid" carotenoid determinations. For instance, NIR-FT-Raman spectroscopy has been used to analyze carotenoids in situ in intact plant material, providing reliable information with regard to the structure and the individual carotenoid distribution in various plant tissues (Hara, Ishigaki, Kitahama, Ozaki, & Genkawa, 2018; Schulz, Baranska, & Baranski, 2005). Likewise, the visible and near-infrared (Vis-NIR) spectroscopy has been applied to obtain a fast and simultaneous measurement of six main types of lipid-soluble pigments in green tea (including chlorophylls, lutein, β-carotene, and pheophytin derivatives), demonstrating that spectroscopy combined with chemometrics is a powerful and nondestructive tool for rapid determination of these compounds (Li, Jin, Sun, Ye, & Liu, 2019). Authors obtained a clear clustering of different types of tea and spectroscopic data was correlated to results obtained by HPLC-UV/Vis. Similarly, NIR has been applied for rapid quantification of lycopene, β-carotene, and total soluble solids on single intact watermelon, predicting the quality of each fruit (Tamburini, Costa, Rugiero, Pedrini, & Marchetti, 2017). In the particular case of NMR, this technique provides a nondestructive, reliable alternative for characterization of structural and stereochemical variations of carotenoids, obtaining excellent carotenoid profiles in real samples with minimal purification procedures, with or without previous LC separations (Aman et al., 2005; Tiziani, Schwartz, & Vodovotz, 2006). Despite all their interesting applications, the use of the aforementioned technologies is unfrequent in carotenoid analysis, particularly in comparison to liquid chromatography coupled with UV/Vis, PDA or MS detectors.

Alternatives in chromatography

Conventional HPLC

High-performance liquid chromatography (HPLC) has certainly won the right to be considered the most commonly used methodology and hence the gold standard in carotenoid separations so far (Giuffrida, Donato, et al., 2018). HPLC is broadly used in carotenoid analysis (Bergantin et al., 2018; Bordiga et al., 2018; Inbaraj et al., 2008; Schimpf, Thompson, & Pan, 2018; Strati & Oreopoulou, 2011; Zeb, 2017; Zheng, Zhang, Quan, Zheng, & Xi, 2016; Zhong et al., 2016), mainly coupled with PDA and triple quadrupole MSs. It is well known that the separation of carotenoids is strongly influenced by the properties of the stationary phase. In this context, many types of stationary phases have been used for their analysis, including normal and reversed phase (RP) fillings; however, normal-phase offers poor separation of nonpolar carotenoids. The free forms of these natural pigments are usually separated on reversed-phase columns, and the same is true for acylated carotenoids (Mariutti & Mercadante, 2018; Mercadante et al., 2017).

Octadecyl (C_{18}) and triacontyl (C_{30}) ligands columns have been the preferred and more resolving phases for carotenoid analysis in sample extracts isolated from biological matrices (Amorim-Carrilho et al., 2014; Giuffrida, Donato, et al., 2018). The majority of articles published on carotenoid analysis have employed C_{18} LC columns but this phase does not resolve geometrical isomers and inefficiently resolves positional isomers, particularly lutein and zeaxanthin (Amorim-Carrilho et al., 2014). Although polymeric C_{18} columns offer improved separation of nonpolar carotenoids compared to monomeric counterparts, even better separations have been demonstrated with polymeric C_{30} columns (Fig. 2) (Sander, Sharpless, & Pursch, 2000). The effectiveness of this "carotenoid phase" to resolve both *cis/trans* and positional isomers has been widely demonstrated since its first application for carotenoid separation by its creators, in 1994 (Sander et al., 1994). On the other hand, chromatographic separation is a key step in the analysis of nonsaponified carotenoid extracts. In this respect, C_{30} stationary phases have been also the most widely used for xanthophyll ester separation (Mercadante et al., 2017), always applying gradient elutions with mobile phases mainly based on mixtures of methanol, methyl tert-butyl ether (MTBE), and water.

In 2016, Turcsi et al. presented a comprehensive database of the separation characteristics of 100 carotenoids and isomers (regio-, stereo-, and geometrical isomers) on C_{18} and C_{30} stationary phases (Turcsi, Nagy, & Deli, 2016). The information

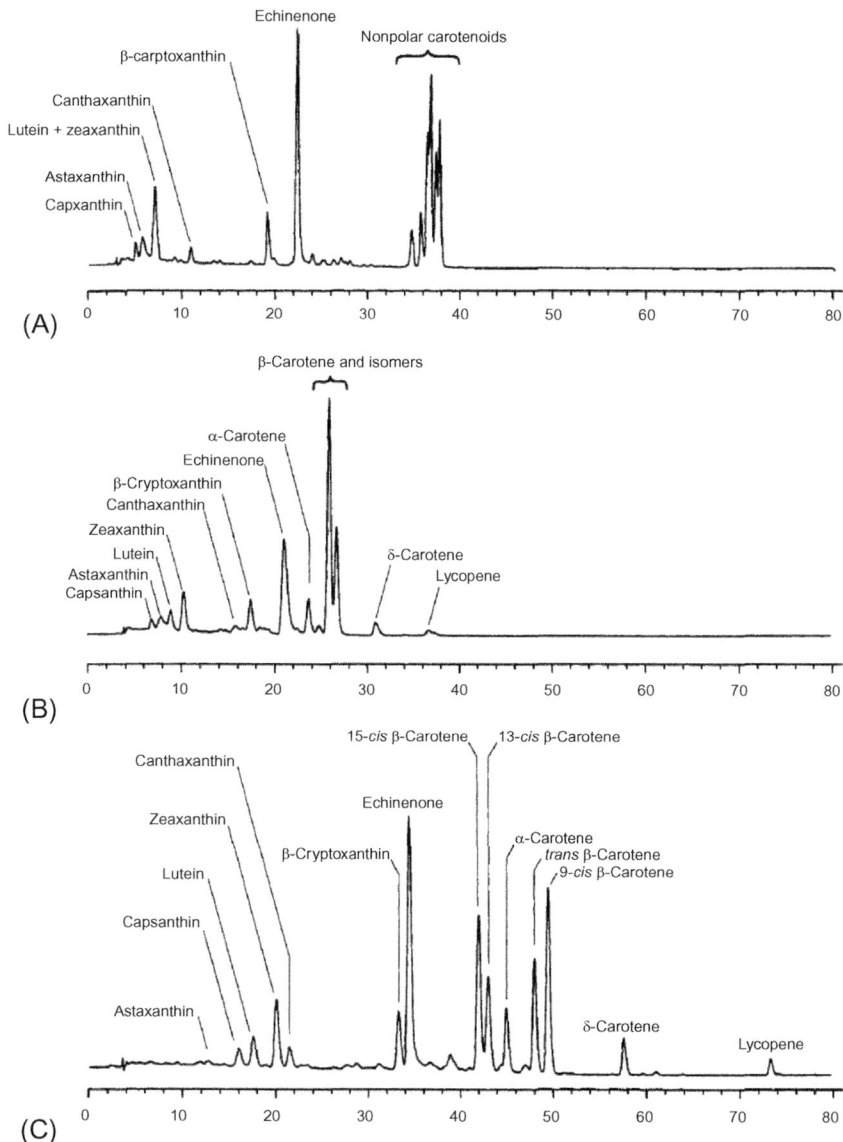

Fig. 2 LC-PDA chromatograms showing separation of carotenoid standards achieved using (A) monomeric and (B) polymeric C_{18} columns and (C) C_{30} column, set at 20°C. Reprinted with permission from Sander et al. (1994). Copyright 1994 American Chemical Society.

contained in the database can be used as a reference in the development of analytical methods, but also in the elucidation of unknown carotenoids. Interestingly enough, in reversed-phase chromatography, the sequence of elution reflects a decreasing polarity of eluted carotenoids, while on a C_{30} separation the retention behavior changes

(Sander et al., 2000; Turcsi et al., 2016). Nevertheless, the efficiency of C_{30} columns to resolve geometrical isomers usually requires longer run times resulting in low-throughput and being this its principal analytical limitation (Amorim-Carrilho et al., 2014). On the other hand, the use of column temperature to enhance carotenoid separation by LC has been widely recognized in the literature (see Table 1). Temperatures ranging from 20°C to 40°C are usually applied, and this is a noteworthy parameter in method development and optimization. When working with YMC C_{30} column and binary gradient, 23°C is the optimal temperature for most carotenoids, while some isomers show better resolution at higher temperatures (Böhm, 2001). As for the particle size, the more common columns applied to carotenoid analysis include 5, 3, and 3.5 μm fillings.

Most of the liquid mobile phases used for LC in carotenoid analysis are modifications of the primarily used acetonitrile and/or methanol (Amorim-Carrilho et al., 2014). A small percentage of a less polar solvent can be added as a modifier to obtain the desired retention, increase the solubility of carotenoids in the eluent and improve chromatographic resolution, for example, dichloromethane, tetrahydrofuran, methyl tert-butyl ether, ethyl acetate, hexane, acetone, other chlorinated solvents, and water. The addition of ammonium acetate buffer or triethylamine to acetonitrile-based phases improves carotenoid recovery, and tetrahydrofuran is the most beneficial modifier for methanol phases (Giuffrida, Donato, et al., 2018; Oliver & Palou, 2000).

Fast chromatography

In liquid chromatography, as the particle size of the stationary phase inside the column decreases to <2.5 μm, there is a significant gain in resolution efficiency. Thus, by using LC columns with smaller particles for carotenoid analysis, the speed and peak capacity of our method can be extended. In this context, new liquid chromatography was born, giving rise to what should be categorized as fast liquid chromatography. The terms rapid resolution liquid chromatography (RRLC), ultrafast liquid chromatography (UFLC), ultra performance liquid chromatography (UPLC), and ultrahigh-performance liquid chromatography (UHPLC) can be found in the literature, referring all of them to fast chromatography but from different manufacturers and working at various back pressures. These alternatives have greatly improved traditional HPLC methods.

UHPLC and/or UPLC use narrow-bore columns packed with sub-2-μm particles, and mobile-phase delivery systems operating at high backpressures, much higher than HPLC. Thus, this alternative offers several advantages over conventional HPLC systems, such as higher peak resolving capacities, narrower peaks (higher signal-to-noise ratio), faster analyses, and a gain sensitivity. The shorter analysis times also considerably save mobile phase solvents (Giuffrida, Donato, et al., 2018). UHPLC coupled with PDA, UV/Vis detector (Bertolín et al., 2018; Eriksen et al., 2017; Stout et al., 2018), and MSs (Abate-Pella et al., 2017; Lachowicz et al., 2018; Mi et al., 2018) has been successfully applied to the analysis of carotenoids in food and other biological matrices. However, the popular carotenoid (C_{30} stationary phase) columns are not commercially available for UHPLC, and for this reason, mostly C_{18} have been used instead. It is, therefore, important to be aware that UHPLC offers shorter run times in comparison to HPLC with C_{30} but also the poorer resolution of carotenoid *isomers*.

Table 1 Examples of current analytical methods reported in the literature for carotenoid analysis in various matrices (2017–19)

Matrices	Carotenoids	Analytical method	Aim(s)	Reference
Oils and fats from Amazonian oleaginous plants	Total carotene	HPLC-PDA, normal-phase Lichrospher column, at 20°C	Determination of carotene content (β-carotene as external calibrator)	Serra et al. (2019)
Human feces	α-Carotene, β-carotene, capsanthin, lycopene, lutein, phytoene, phytofluene, violaxanthin, zeaxanthin, and isomers (total: 25 compounds)	RRLC-UV/Vis/PDA, C30 YMC column, at 28°C	Isoprenoids bioaccessibility evaluation in human studies	Stinco, Benítez-González, Meléndez-Martínez, Hernanz, and Vicario (2019)
Human blood samples	Carotenoids and APOs (>10 compounds)	SFE-SFC-APCI-QqQ/MS, Ascentis Express C30 column, at 35°C	Quantification of dietary carotenoids and APOs; identification novel compounds	Zoccali et al. (2018)
Pumpkin (*Cucurbita máxima* "Delica" and *Cucurbita moschata* "Violina")	Violaxanthin, astaxanthin, antheraxanthin, zeaxanthin, lutein, lycopene, α-carotene, β-carotene	HPLC-UV/Vis-APCI-MS/MS, C30 Develosil RP-Aqueous column, at 23°C	Food traceability markers: quantification of carotenoids, before and after cooking	Bergantin et al. (2018)
Human plasma	α-Carotene, β-carotene, β-cryptoxanthin, lycopene, lutein/zeaxanthin	HPLC-ESI-MS/MS, YMC C30 column ("dilute-and-shoot")	Determination of carotenoids as biomarkers of vegetable and fruit intake	Bukowski et al. (2018)
Cantaloupe (*Cucumis melo* L.) waste	Lutein, β-carotene, violaxanthin, β-cryptoxanthin	TCC: UV-Vis spectrophotometer at 450nm (expressed as μg of β-carotene equivalent per g of dry weight) Individual carotenoids: RRLC-PDA, C18 Poroshell 120 column, at 28°C	Quantification of carotenoids in waste as health-promoting compounds	Benmeziane et al. (2018)

Continued

Table 1 Continued

Matrices	Carotenoids	Analytical method	Aim(s)	Reference
Ovine milk and tissues (meat, liver, and fat)	Lutein, β-carotene	UHPLC-PDA, silica-based bonded phase column (Acquity UPLC HSS), at 35°C	Quantification of carotenoids in different animal matrices	Bertolín, Joy, Rufino-Moya, Lobón, and Blanco (2018)
Different anatomical parts of wild garlic (*Allium ursinum*)	Neoxanthin, violaxanthin, all-*trans*-lutein, 13-*cis*-lutein, α-cryptoxanthin, β-cryptoxanthin, α-carotene, all-*trans* β-carotene, 9-*cis*-β-carotene, 13-*cis*-β-carotene, 15-*cis*-β-carotene (11 carotenoids)	UHPLC-PDA-ESI-Q/TOF-MS, RP C18 column (Acquity UPLC BEH), at 32°C	Influence of harvesting and anatomical parts in carotenoid content	Lachowicz, Oszmiański, and Wiśniewski (2018)
Cow milk	Lutein, β-carotene, zeaxanthin	UHPLC-PDA, C18 RP column (Acquity UPLC BEH), at 32°C	Determination of carotenoids	Stout, Benoist, and Drake (2018)
Infant, pediatric, and adult nutritionals	*cis* and *trans* isomers of lutein, β-carotene, lycopene	HPLC-UV-Vis, C30 column	Determination of carotenoids	Schimpf et al. (2018)
Red Habanero peppers (*Capsicum chinense* Jacq.)	Twenty-one carotenoids (free, monoesters, diesters)	SFE-SFC-APCI-QqQ/MS, Ascentis Express C30 column, at 35°C	Determination of carotenoids	Zoccali, Giuffrida, Dugo, and Mondello (2017)
Watermelon pulp	Lycopene	HPLC-PDA, YMC C30 column	Optimization of lycopene extraction from watermelon	Oberoi and Sogi (2017)
Leafy vegetables (*B. compestris*, *B. rapa*, *B. juncea*, *M. neglecta*, and two spinach varieties)	Twelve free carotenoids and one fatty acid ester (β-cryptoxanthin ester)	HPLC-PDA, Zorbax Eclipse C18, at 25°C	Determination of carotenoids	Zeb (2017)

Sample	Carotenoids	Method	Purpose	Reference
Fish and poultry feed	Astaxanthin, astaxanthin dimethyldisuccinate, adonirubin, canthaxanthin, β-carotene, capsanthin, ethyl ester of beta-apo-8′-carotenoic acid, citranaxanthin, lutein, zeaxanthin	HPLC-PDA, Suplex pKb-100 RP column, at 20°C	Control of carotenoids as feed additives	Vincent, Serano, and von Holst (2017)
Human plasma	β-Cryptoxanthin, lutein, zeaxanthin	UHPSFC-ESI-MS/MS, Viridis HSS C18 SB column, at 40°C	Determination of carotenoids circulating levels in humans (profiling of fat-soluble vitamers)	Petruzziello, Grand-Guillaume Perrenoud, Thorimbert, Fogwill, and Rezzi (2017)
Cooking oils (canola, sunflower, mixed, vegetable and coconut oil)	Lutein, lycopene, β-carotene	UHPSFC-PDA, HSS C18 SB column, at 40°C	Fast determination of carotenoids	Rathi, Liew, Fairulnizal, Isameyah, and Barknowitz (2017)
Algae (*Haematococcus pluvialis*)	13 Carotenoids	UHPLC-PDA, BEH C18 column, at 35°C	Carotenoid profiling in algae under environmental stresses	Jin, Lao, Zhou, Zhang, and Cai (2017)
Rainbow trout tissue (muscle and liver)	All-*trans*-lutein, all-*trans*-astaxanthin, all-*trans*-zeaxanthin, all-*trans*-β-cryptoxanthin, all-*trans*-canthaxanthin, all-*trans*-ζ-carotene, all-*trans*-β-carotene, all-*trans*-ϒ-carotene	HPLC-PDA-MS/MS, ProntoSIL C30 column, at 19°C	Quantification of carotenoids and tentative identification of unknowns	Pérez Fernández, Ventura, Tomai, Curini, and Gentili (2017)

Continued

Table 1 Continued

Matrices	Carotenoids	Analytical method	Aim(s)	Reference
Goldenberry (*Physalis peruviana* L.) peel, pulp, and calyx of ripe fruits	53 free carotenoids and esters (42 tentatively identified)	HPLC-UV/Vis-APCI-MS^n, C30 column, at 25°C	Characterization of carotenoid profiles at various ripening stages and in different tissues	Etzbach, Pfeiffer, Weber, and Schieber (2018)
Starchy staples (maize, plantain and tuber crops)	Lutein, zeaxanthin, β-cryptoxanthin, α-carotene, β-carotene	HPLC-PDA, RP C30 column	Microapproach to quantify carotenoids in starchy staples	Wald, Nohr, and Biesalski (2018)
Acrocomia aculeata fruits	25 carotenoids	HPLC-PDA-APCI/ESI-MS^n, YMC C30 RP column, at 23°C	Quantitation of carotenoids in different progressing maturity stages	Schex et al. (2018)
Tamarillo (*Solanum betaceum* Cav.)	Carotenoids and APOs (>30 compounds)	SFE-SFC-APCI-QqQ/MS, Ascentis Express C30 column, at 35°C	Characterization of carotenoids and APOs composition; identification of novel APOs	Giuffrida et al. (2018)
Plant tissues, rice, and spinach	Volatile and nonvolatile APOs	UHPLC-ESI-HRMS, Acquity UPLC BEH C18 column at 35°C	Profiling and quantification; structural elucidation of APOs based on HRMS and MS/MS data	Mi et al. (2018)
Snow algae	Lutein, β-carotene, astaxanthin	Micro-Raman spectroscopy	In situ measurements	Osterrothová et al. (2019)
Transgenic sweetpotato plants	Violaxanthin, lutein, zeaxanthin, β-cryptoxanthin, 13Z-β-carotene, β-carotene, 9Z-β-carotene, total carotenoid content	HPLC-PDA	Study of transgenic plants tolerance to abiotic stress	Ke et al. (2019)

Sample	Carotenoids	Method	Objective	Reference
Goldenberry (*Physalis peruviana* L.) puree	Total carotenoid content	UFLC-PDA, Accucore C30 column, at 25°C	Effects of thermal pasteurization and ultrasound treatment on carotenoid composition	Etzbach, Pfeiffer, Schieber, and Weber (2019)
Peels of tucumã (*Astrocaryum vulgare*) and peach palm (*Bactris gasipaes*)	TCC, all-*E*-β-carotene, all-*E*-δ-carotene, *Z*-γ-carotene, all-*E*-γ-carotene	HPLC-PDA-APCI-MS/MS, C30 YMC column, at 29°C	Study of new potential sources of carotenoids	Noronha Matos, Praia Lima, Pereira Barbosa, Zerlotti Mercadante, and Campos (2019)
Golden scallops (*Chlamys nobilis*)	TCC	UV-Vis spectrophotometer	Determination of carotenoids in aquatic animals	Cheng et al. (2019)
Colored-grain wheat flours	Antheraxanthin, lutein (and isomers), zeaxanthin, β-carotene, α-carotene, lutein esters	HPLC-PDA, YMC C30 column, at 25°C	Stability of carotenoids: dough, baking, and short-term storage of baked buns	Paznocht, Kotíková, Orsák, Lachman, and Martinek (2019)
Goji berries (*Lycium barbarum* L.)	Carotenoid fraction, zeaxanthin dipalmitate	CIELAB colorimetric assay; HPLC-PDA, RP18 column	Evaluating the differences among: varieties, harvesting periods, seasons, and extraction procedures	Patsilinakos, Ragno, Carradori, Petralito, and Cesa (2018)
Citrus juice sacs of: Satsuma mandarin (*Citrus unshiu* Marc), Valencia orange (*C. sinensis* Osbeck), Lisbon lemon (*C. limon* Burm.f.)	β-Carotene, β-cryptoxanthin, all-trans-violaxanthin, 9-*cis*-violaxanthin, lutein	HPLC-PDA, YMC Carotenoid S-5 column	Temperature influence on plant carotenoid metabolism (in vitro study)	Yungyuen et al. (2018)

Continued

Table 1 Continued

Matrices	Carotenoids	Analytical method	Aim(s)	Reference
Biomass (microalgae)	18 carotenoids	HPLC-PDA, RP Ultrasphere C-18 column, at 25°C	Carotenoid profiling in algae (potential sources of carotenoids)	Di Lena, Casini, Lucarini, and Lombardi-Boccia (2018)
Citrus fruits: "Beibei" 447 Jincheng orange (*Citrus sinensis* Osbeck), navel orange (*C. sinensis* Osbeck) and Ponkan mandarin (*C. reticulata* Blanco)	β-Carotene, lutein, β-cryptoxanthin, β-citraurin, zeaxanthin, α-carotene, violaxanthin	HPLC-PDA, YMC C30 column, at 30°C	Study of carotenoid metabolism transcriptome	Xie, Yao, Ming, Deng, and Zeng (2019)
Anolis sagrei lizard eggs	TCC	Spectrophotometry	Study of maternal allocation of carotenoids to eggs	Reinke, Erritouni, and Calsbeek (2018)
Carrot (*Daucus carota* L.) juice	TCC	Spectrophotometry	Processing influence on bioaccessibility	Liu et al. (2019)
Peel and pulp of persimmon (*Diospyros kaki* L.) "Kaki Tipo" cv	24 carotenoids and esters	HPLC-PDA-APCI/MS, YMC C30 column, at 35°C	Characterization of carotenoid profiles at various ripening stages	Bordiga et al. (2018)
Green tea	Lutein, β-carotene	Vis-NIR HPLC-UV/Vis, Diamonsil C18 column, at 35°C	Role of lipid-soluble pigments (including chlorophylls and pheophytins) in color formation of tea	Li et al. (2019)

Sample	Analytes	Method	Application	Reference
Commercial vegetable juice	Lycopene	NIR-Raman (portable spectrometer)	Discrimination of lycopene-rich vegetable juice	Hara et al. (2018)
Strawberry (*Fragaria vesca*) leaves, Avizant Red and Yellow chicken feed, *Chloroflexus aurantiacus* bacteria	α-Carotene, β-carotene, lutein, lycopene, α-cryptoxanthin, β-cryptoxanthin, asthaxanthin. Crocin, canthaxanthin, echinenone, capsanthin	UHPLC-APCI-QqQ/MS, cyano-propyl column, at 25°C	Determination of carotenoids	Abate-Pella, Freund, Slovin, Hegeman, and Cohen (2017)
Pharmaceutical formulations	Lycopene, β-carotene	HPLC-UV/Vis, core-shell C18 column, at 35°C (double injection, single run)	Determination of carotenoids, water- and fat-soluble vitamins	Melfi, Nardiello, Cicco, Candido, and Centonze (2018)
Human samples (serum, chylomicrons, feces), frozen spinach	Zeaxanthin, lutein, β-criptoxanthin, echinenone, lycopene, α-carotene, all-*E*-β-carotene	UHPLC-PDA, HSS C18 column, at 35°C	Determination of carotenoids	Eriksen, Madsen, Dragsted, and Arrigoni (2017)
Red chili pepper (*Capsicum annuum* L.)	50 carotenoids (including esters and isomers)	SFC×RP-UHPLC-PDA-Q-ToF MS-IMS, Ascentis ES Cyano, at 40°C×Acquity UPLC BEH C18, at 60°C	Carotenoid fingerprinting	Donato et al. (2018)

Continued

Table 1 Continued

Matrices	Carotenoids	Analytical method	Aim(s)	Reference
Animal and vegetable fats (extra-virgin olive oil, salted Azorean butter, vegetable margarine, food supplements, crude palm oil, sunflower oil, cannabis oil, fish oil-based supplements)	β-Carotene, lutein	HPLC-UV/Vis, NP silica column, at 22°C	Fingerprinting for authenticity purposes (without sample pretreatment)	Cruz and Casal (2018)
Chicory (*Cichorium intybus* L.) leaves	All-*E*-lutein, all-*E*-β-carotene, all-*E*-neoxanthin, all-*E*-violaxanthin, 9-*Z*-lutein, 9′-*Z*-lutein	HPLC-PDA, C18 RP column, at 25°C	Determination of cooking effect on carotenoids	Zeb, Haq, and Murkovic (2019)
Bacteria (701 strains)	Astaxanthin, canthaxanthin, zeaxanthin, lutein	HPLC-PDA-MS, C18 RP column, at 35°C	High throughput screening and profiling of carotenoids	Asker (2018)

APCI, atmospheric pressure chemical ionization; *APOs*, apocarotenoids; *HPLC*, high-performance liquid chromatography; *HRMS*, high-resolution mass spectrometry; *MS*, mass spectrometry; *NIR*, near infrared; *NP*, normal phase; *PDA*, photodiode array detector; *QqQMS*, triple quadrupole mass spectrometry; *RP*, reversed-phase; *RRLC*, rapid resolution liquid chromatography; *SFC*, supercritical fluid chromatography; *SFE*, supercritical fluid extraction; *TCC*, total carotenoid contents; *UFLC*, ultrafast liquid chromatography; *UHPSFC*, ultrahigh-performance supercritical fluid chromatography; *UV/Vis*, ultraviolet-visible spectroscopy.

With regard to RRLC, its performance is based on the use of small particle sizes (~2 μm) along with optimized LC instrumentation (Benmeziane et al., 2018; Stinco et al., 2019). RRLC also offers higher resolution and sensitivity, and shorter retention times than HPLC, with the advantage of achieving a good resolution of isomeric forms due to the usage of C_{30} column (Stinco et al., 2019). Compared with common HPLC and some UHPLC approaches, RRLC has even superior performance and offers reduced solvent consumption. In 2018, a comparative chromatographic study was performed by Giuffrida et al. (Giuffrida, Zoccali, et al., 2018) employing a novel partially porous C_{30} column of 2.7 μm particle size and a conventional C_{30} column packed with 3 μm particles. This novel approach using this "nearly-sub-2 μm" porous C_{30} showed a better compound resolution and shorter analysis time than conventional HPLC, and it could be considered an important tool for fast liquid chromatography of carotenoid and carotenoid esters. Alternatively, UFLC instruments have successfully achieved speed and separation performance levels that do not depend on high pressure. These equipment has already been used to fast determine carotenoids in goldenberry puree using a C_{30} column of 2.6 μm particle size (Etzbach et al., 2019).

Notwithstanding the above, C_{30} columns used for HPLC separations are the most popular choice for qualification and quantification of carotenoids and isomers. Additionally, shorter analytical runs seem to compromise resolution, particularly for isomers, leaving the analyst in a dilemma between resolving and fast-processing (Eriksen et al., 2017).

Supercritical fluid chromatography (SFC)

Supercritical fluid chromatography (SFC) is known since the early 1960s, but it has gained popularity since the beginning of the millennium, thanks to the significant improvements in instrumentation and analytical performance and robustness of equipment (Nováková et al., 2014; Pilařová, Plachká, Khalikova, Svec, & Nováková, 2019). It may be considered a hybrid of gas and liquid chromatographies, incorporating many features of both techniques. This technique is particularly attractive to resolve samples when faced with chemical complexity, offering an orthogonal selectivity compared to reversed-phase liquid chromatography, as long as the compounds are soluble in a CO_2-rich mobile phase. Additionally, the use of CO^2 as mobile phase offers enhanced safety and environmental advantages as compared to other predecessor techniques, such as HPCL or UHPLC (Sánchez-Camargo, Parada-Alonso, Ibáñez, & Cifuentes, 2019). On the other hand, ultrahigh-performance SFC (UHPSFC) is based on the use of columns packed with fully porous sub-2 μm particles with kinetic performance significantly better than that of the UHPLC (Grand-Guillaume Perrenoud et al., 2016; Petruzziello et al., 2017). In the literature, UHPSFC is sometimes referred to as "Ultra-Performance Convergence Chromatography" (UPC^2 by Waters) (Grand-Guillaume Perrenoud et al., 2013; Grand-Guillaume Perrenoud et al., 2016; Rathi et al., 2017). In this context, SFC and UHPSFC are considered powerful analytical techniques for the extensive characterization of complex mixtures of lipidic nature including, but not limited to, carotenoids and their isomers (Giuffrida, Donato, et al., 2018; Song, Liu, & Bai, 2017; Yamada & Bamba, 2017).

Both alternatives, SFC and UHPSFC, can be coupled with a wide array of detectors (UV, MS, HRMS, etc.). An interesting tutorial on the topic was published by Nováková et al. (2014), with guidelines and tips on stationary phase selection, mobile phase conditions, and best detection alternatives (Nováková et al., 2014). So far, very few reports are available in the literature on carotenoids separation using these technologies. For instance, a novel C_{30} fused-core particle column, with a particle size of 2.7 μm and consisting of a silica nucleus encircled by a thin porous shell of C_{30} stationary phase, has been used for supercritical separation of carotenoids, providing very high column efficiency (Zoccali et al., 2017; Zoccali et al., 2018). In this analytical design, the sample-containing CO^2 is directed to the SFC flow line after the first step of extraction in the SFE unit, for being analyzed in a triple quadrupole MS with APCI interface. Similarly, carotenoids and APOs can be determined simultaneously using this approach (Giuffrida et al., 2017; Giuffrida, Zoccali, et al., 2018).

Multidimensional chromatography

When one-dimensional or monodimensional chromatography is not sufficient for optimal separation of carotenoids in complex food samples or shows limitations, multidimensional alternatives provide extra resolution capabilities and help to reduce the usually extensive sample preparation protocols (Cacciola, Dugo, & Mondello, 2017). Despite the number of dimensions/separations being in theory unlimited, the vast majority of multidimensional methods reported to date for carotenoid analysis include two dimensions, for instance, 2D liquid chromatography (LC×LC) and comprehensive SFC coupled with liquid chromatography (SFC×LC) (Giuffrida, Donato, et al., 2018).

The combination of normal phase (NP)×RP columns could be considered the most orthogonal setup in LC×LC since it uses sorbents with different separation mechanisms. Recently, this NP-LC×RP-LC approach has been successfully applied to the analysis of both free and esterified carotenoids in fruit (Cacciola et al., 2012; Dugo et al., 2008), increasing the overall separation power and peak capacity of the chromatography. Alternatively, SFC×LC minimizes solvent immiscibility problems, thanks to the use of supercritical fluid CO_2, showing even more orthogonality than NP-LC×RP-LC (Giuffrida, Donato, et al., 2018). Because of its low polarity, supercritical CO_2 is considered particularly suitable for carotenoid separations, including free carotenoids, carotenoids monoesters, carotenoids diesters and ñs in a very fast "green" and efficient way (Giuffrida, Donato, et al., 2018; Mariutti & Mercadante, 2018). Despite its unquestionable potential, this multidimensional approach is still in its infancy, probably due to the inherent difficulty of handling two dimensions (instruments, software, and generated data). An excellent example of SFC×LC capabilities is the work developed by Bonaccorsi et al., reporting a method to identify 115 different compounds in peppers, belonging to chlorophylls, free xanthophylls, free carotenes, xanthophyll monoesters, and xanthophyll diesters (Bonaccorsi et al., 2016). Similarly, Donato et al. used SFC×LC for carotenoid fingerprinting in red chili pepper (Donato et al., 2018).

LC-PDA and LC-UV/Vis

Liquid chromatography coupled with PDA or UV/Vis detectors has been frequently applied for the analysis of carotenoids in vegetables, plants, microalgae, bacteria, and human and animal samples, among others (Asker, 2018; Benmeziane et al., 2018; Bertolín et al., 2018; Cruz & Casal, 2018; Jin et al., 2017; Patsilinakos et al., 2018; Schimpf et al., 2018; Serra et al., 2019; Stinco et al., 2019; Stout et al., 2018; Zeb, 2017; Zheng et al., 2016). Given the structural similarities existing between the diverse members of the carotenoid family, and consequently their close elution in chromatographic separations, the spectra provided by absorbance detectors may become insufficient for their identification. MS has provided the identification capability required in these situations, allowing significant advances in carotenoid analysis (Rivera, Christou, & Canela-Garayoa, 2014).

Yet, LC-PDA and LC-UV/Vis are the most popular and straightforward alternatives in carotenoid analytical chemistry. In this context, carotenoids are frequently determined simultaneously with fat-soluble vitamins and/or polyphenols (Bordiga et al., 2018; Cruz & Casal, 2018; Hrvolová et al., 2016; Melfi et al., 2018; Pérez Fernández et al., 2017; Schex et al., 2018; Serra et al., 2019), and/or chlorophylls and other natural pigments (Cruz & Casal, 2018; Di Lena et al., 2018; Schweiggert et al., 2016; Wald et al., 2018; Xie et al., 2019; Zeb et al., 2019), in most cases coupled with MS detectors to facilitate multi-class determinations.

LC-MS and LC-MS/MS

Since carotenoid LC-chromatograms in real samples are usually very complex, the identity of some compounds may not be possible solely on the basis of absorbance readings, requiring further confirmation by MS. With MS, the obtained mass spectra are compared with published data, mass spectral libraries, or mass spectra obtained from commercial standards analyzed in parallel (Amorim-Carrilho et al., 2014; Bergantin et al., 2018). The introduction of MS into the world of carotenoid analysis represented a huge step forward, leading to significant advances in the field, thanks to the ability of MSs to distinguish between coeluting compounds and to determine molecular weights (Rivera et al., 2014). This technology adds elucidation capabilities to carotenoid analysis and enables the discovery of new compounds belonging to the family. In the case of unknown carotenoids, esters or their metabolites, the combination of PDA or UV/Vis detectors with MS and MS/MS instruments, after chromatographic separation, has proven a very useful tool for accurate identification (Aman et al., 2005; Bergantin et al., 2018; Bordiga et al., 2018; García-de Blas, Mateo, Viñuela, & Alonso-Álvarez, 2011; Gentili et al., 2015; Inbaraj et al., 2008; Kopec, Carail, & Caris-Veyrat, 2018; Lachowicz et al., 2018; Mariutti & Mercadante, 2018; Pérez Fernández et al., 2017; Zhong et al., 2016). Actually, the analysis of carotenoid esters in food and human biological samples has been recently reviewed by Mariutti and Mercadante (2018) and Mercadante et al. (2017). In their reviews, the challenges usually faced in each analytical step are presented. It is important to highlight that identification of carotenoid esters requires elution order, UV/Vis and MSn data (Mariutti & Mercadante, 2018).

On the basis of the above-mentioned characteristics of MS, liquid chromatography-absorbance-MS setup has become very common nowadays in laboratories devoted to carotenoid research (Table 1). An excellent example of its capabilities was presented by Gentili et al. (2015), using a triple quadrupole–linear ion trap hybrid MS (QqQ-LIT) and a diode array detector for large-scale screening of carotenoids in tomato fruits [99]. This high-throughput analytical strategy fully exploited the potentialities of LC-PDA-MS combinations, since the relative abundance between the MRM transitions (ion ratio) was used for the first time as an extra tool for the distinction of structural isomers and related families of geometrical isomers. Additionally, only six authentic standards of carotenoids were analyzed, and their chromatographic behavior was used to optimize the separative LC conditions and to predict the chromatographic behavior of untargeted carotenoids (Gentili et al., 2015).

It becomes clear then that LC-MS/MS offers added selectivity and specificity to the more simple LC-MS configurations, allowing distinguishing between coeluting carotenoids (Rivera & Canela-Garayoa, 2012). Tandem MS also enables the development of improved preparative solutions with minimal sample handling, as in the case of the LC-MS/MS dilute-and-shoot alternative recently proposed by Bukowski et al. (Bukowski et al., 2018). Nevertheless, LC-MS systems have also contributed greatly to carotenoid analysis and as such, they are still used for characterization studies (Asker, 2018; Bordiga et al., 2018; Zhong et al., 2016). On the other hand, carotenoids are ideal candidates for SFC, and for this particular reason, SFC-MS methods have also appeared in the literature (Giuffrida et al., 2017; Giuffrida, Donato, et al., 2018; Pilařová et al., 2019; Zoccali et al., 2018).

High-resolution mass spectrometry (LC-HRMS)
Unlike conventional MS, high-resolution mass spectrometry (HRMS) provides accurate masses of detected ions (exact mass vs nominal mass provided by low-resolution MS), even though the accuracies vary significantly among the existing instruments. The three existing alternatives, that is, time-of-flight MS (TOF), Orbitrap MS, and Fourier Transform Ion Cyclotron Resonance (FT-ICR) MS are capable of resolving closely spaced spectral peaks. HRMS is a fast and sensitive approach to provide information on putative identities of a multitude of molecules (carotenoids) in one single experiment (Grand-Guillaume Perrenoud et al., 2016). Additionally, hybrid analyzers produce also MS/MS fragmentation patterns that add extra identification capabilities to HRMS. Liquid chromatography coupled with high-resolution instruments, in particular, TOF and Orbitrap, have been frequently used in the last decade for carotenoid analysis, greatly contributing to the discovery of new compounds and isomers, including APOs (Abate-Pella et al., 2017; Mi et al., 2018; Rivera & Canela-Garayoa, 2012).

LC-MS interfacing
Several interfacing strategies are available to enable the coupling of liquid chromatography with MSs. In this context, the existing literature on carotenoid analysis by LC-MS systems reports different interfaces, such as electron impact (EI), fast atom bombardment (FAB), matrix-assisted laser desorption/ionization (MALDI), electrospray (ESI), atmospheric pressure chemical ionization (APCI), and atmospheric pressure

photoionization (APPI) and atmospheric pressure solids analysis probe (ASAP) (Amorim-Carrilho et al., 2014). Among all these options, atmospheric pressure ionization interfaces are the most frequently used, particularly, ESI and APCI (Table 1). In general, APCI shows a greater ability to ionize nonpolar carotenoids, and ESI is preferred for more polar analytes.

Several authors have commented on how APCI offers distinct advantages over ESI and other interfaces, in both positive and negative mode (Rezanka, Olsovska, Sobotka, & Sigler, 2009; Rivera, Vilaró, & Canela, 2011; Van Breemen, Dong, & Pajkovic, 2012). Alternatively, several dopants can be used to enhance carotenoid signals under ESI or APPI (Amorim-Carrilho et al., 2014; Rivera et al., 2011). Nevertheless, LC-APCI-MS methods still are the most popular choice for a wide range of carotenoids and in different matrices (Abate-Pella et al., 2017; Bergantin et al., 2018; Bordiga et al., 2018; Etzbach et al., 2018; Giuffrida, Zoccali, et al., 2018; Noronha Matos et al., 2019; Schex et al., 2018; Zoccali et al., 2017). With regard to carotenoid metabolites, liquid chromatography in combination with PDA and MS/MS, with APCI interface, has been also applied to characterize a series of apo-luteinoids and apo-zeaxanthinoids chemically generated in the laboratory, providing a robust method to study these APOs in plants, foods, and animals (Kopec et al., 2018).

The successful SFC-MS hyphenation requires also an interface, taking into account the specific physicochemical properties and compressibility of the SFC mobile phase. Directing the SFC effluent into the ionization source of the MS is more challenging than in LC (Guillarme, Desfontaine, Heinisch, & Veuthey, 2018). For ESI, a splitter and makeup pump are requisites, while in APCI the splitter is not desired in the interface since it provides severe loss of sensitivity. Recently, a new APCI source has been reported by Ciclet et al. to hyphenate SFC to MS instruments (Ciclet et al., 2018). The so-called UniSpray source does not seem to be the most adequate option for carotenoid ionization.

Metabolomics in carotenoid analysis

Over the past two decades, foodomics has emerged as an innovative and promising discipline that includes different *omics* possibilities (epigenomics and genomics, transcriptomics, proteomics, metabolomics) applied to food research (Cifuentes, 2013). These high-throughput approaches join together different cutting-edge analytical platforms, big data output, and bioinformatics. In this context, and particularly in the case of metabolomics, MS and NMR-based systems have become essential tools for metabolome profiling (Courant, Antignac, Dervilly-Pinel, & Le Bizec, 2014; Larive, Barding, & Dinges, 2015). Metabolomics/metabonomics can be considered as chemical *profiling* of a biological matrix (cell, tissue, fluid, etc.) as it aims at systematically profiling the widest range of small metabolites, ideally the complete collection (metabolome), present in that matrix, all this following an untargeted, comprehensive, and quantitative approach. The ultimate goal of metabolomics studies is characterizing the metabolites found in a sample collected at a specific point in time and/or under a predefined biological situation. In many cases, these experiments also compare two or more different groups of samples seeking for metabolic differences and/or biomarkers of that difference. In order to accomplish this, HRMS has probably been the most widely used technology to provide the information required in metabolomics, providing also putative identities of multitude of metabolites, thanks to its high-resolution capabilities (Werner et al., 2008; Werner, Heilier, Ducruix, Ezan, & Junot, 2008). Strictly, the term metabolomics implies that the measurements are untargeted and the identity of the obtained metabolites/analytes is unknown, at least in the first instance. However, the previous application of a type of extraction or sample pretreatment can define somehow the chemical nature of those metabolites, contributing to their future structural elucidation (Drouin, Rudaz, & Schappler, 2018). For instance, choosing an appropriate extraction solvent is crucial for separating lipophilic and hydrophilic fractions.

Metabolomics untargeted approaches are also referred to as metabolic fingerprinting or profiling, aimed at comparing patterns of metabolites or analyzing a group of selected metabolites, respectively. These means that an initial untargeted experiment can be used to highlight a set of potential metabolites of interest (biomarkers) and further submit them to a quasi-targeted metabolomics approach to demonstrate their value, considering these experiments as discovery and validation studies, respectively (Khamis, Adamko, Purves, & El-Aneed, 2019). A third approach would be the targeted analysis of a wide range of known compounds (or a group of compounds), such as carotenoids, measuring them in different groups of samples, in a high-throughput manner. In this context, and considering that metabolomics is untargeted by nature, the proper way to proceed is to coin a new omics discipline, that is, *carotenoidomics*. Additional examples of a large-scale study of known small molecules are fatty acidomics, lipidomics, or glycomics, among others (Griffiths & Wang, 2009; Losito, Facchini, Valentini, Cataldi, & Palmisano, 2018; Smith, Cummings, & Song, 2019), but of course, these disciplines clearly cover fewer metabolites than the almighty and untargeted metabolimics. Regardless of the omics discipline in practice, chemometrics has been integrated into science throughout them (Trygg, Holmes, & Lundstedt, 2007). Chemometrics provides the mathematical and statistical tools required for evaluation of a large amount of collected data associated with omics and improves the biological understanding of this chemical information.

Metabolomics can be used to discover new carotenoid implications in diverse biological processes. For example, the application of this data-rich holistic approach in food science and nutrition can help to support relationships between diet and health concluded from clinical studies (Bayram et al., 2018; Woodside, Draper, Lloyd, & McKinley, 2017). Carotenoid metabolites can be characterized in vivo using metabolomics, although it requires substantial refining of analytical protocols. Till date, there are no detailed analytical techniques available to fingerprint carotenoid metabolites, mainly due to interference with complex biological matrices (Arathi, Sowmya, Vijay, Baskaran, & Lakshminarayana, 2015). Apart from the above, multidimensional (nontargeted and targeted) approaches combined with multivariate chemometric techniques have brought countless and invaluable benefits in authentication and hazard detection in condiments, that is, spices and herbs (Reinholds, Bartkevics, Silvis, van Ruth, & Esslinger, 2015). Ordoudi et al. used spectroscopic data obtained by FT-MIR for quality control in saffron (fraud, mislabeling, and storage effects) (Ordoudi, de los Mozos Pascual, & Tsimidou, 2014). The obtained data were submitted to principal component analysis (PCA), and APOs were highlighted as potential makers of saffron alterations, thanks to multivariate regression analysis. Plants produced by organic and conventional systems can also be differentiated using UHPLC-ESI-qTOF-MS metabolomics, as illustrated by Llano et al. (Llano, Muñoz-Jiménez, Jiménez-Cartagena, Londoño-Londoño, & Medina, 2018). Also, chemical changes and heat stability of extra-virgin olive oil have been assessed by UHPLC-qTOF-MS using this discipline, allowing identifying significant markers of frying process, including carotenoids, fatty acids, and phenolic compounds (Blasi et al., 2018). Alternatively, metabolomics can be used to investigate seasonal and/or genotype variations in the composition of certain foods and its potential relation to their bioactivity profile, leading to assisted breeding of crops and strategies that improve carotenoid production of various plants, algae, yeast, fungi, and bacteria (Alseekh, Bermudez, de Haro, Fernie, & Carrari, 2018; Bu, Sun, Shang, & Yan, 2017; Farré et al., 2016; Heavisides et al., 2018; Moresco et al., 2017). The previous are just a few examples of how metabolomics can contribute to food research, and in particular to increase knowledge about carotenoids and improve crop yield and quality.

When carotenoids are measured in a high-throughput manner, the approach could be called *carotenoidomics*. However, the number of compounds that should be measured simultaneously to use the term *omics* is large, usually hundreds to thousands of analytes, for this reason, the term *carotenoidomics* must be used carefully. "Large" is a rather subjective concept, but carotenoid analyst should include at least a few tens of compounds in a *carotenoidomics* study. In case of doubt, the term "carotenoid profiling" should be used instead. Notwithstanding the above, the dynamic measurement of multiple carotenoids simultaneously has also been used in favor of agriculture and food production and innovation. For example, carotenoid profiles in goldenberry (*Physalis peruviana* L.) fruits acquired by HPLC-DAD-APCI-MS[n] at various ripening stages and in different fruits fractions (peel, pulp, and calyx) demonstrated that the ripening stage and the part of the fruit should be considered in the production of carotenoid-rich products (Etzbach et al., 2018). In a similar approach, α-tocopherol and 25 carotenoids were determined by HPLC-PDA-APCI/ESI-MS[n] and PCA was used for pattern recognition among the Macauba fruit samples at three maturity stages (Schex et al., 2018). The study of carotenoids is also important in transcriptome evaluation of plants, and how they react under different conditions or gene modifications (Xie et al., 2019; Yungyuen et al., 2018).

Conclusion

LC coupled with absorbance detectors (UV, Vis, PDA) and/or MSs are currently the most common instrumental methods for carotenoid and APO analysis. SFC and comprehensive 2D LC (LC×LC) are interesting alternatives to conventional LC separations, as they show the extra capability to resolve complex mixtures of lipidic nature, including carotenoid isomers. However, these technologies require more specialized and expensive instruments and longer analytical times, nearly double than LC. On top of this, in the past decade, carotenoid analysis has moved from classical approaches to more modern and innovative solutions, as the high-throughput metabolomics. In this context, HRMS outstands out for its high-resolution and high mass accuracy.

References

Abate-Pella, D., Freund, D. M., Slovin, J. P., Hegeman, A. D., & Cohen, J. D. (2017). An improved method for fast and selective separation of carotenoids by LC–MS. *Journal of Chromatography B*, *1067*, 34–37.

Alseekh, S., Bermudez, L., de Haro, L. A., Fernie, A. R., & Carrari, F. (2018). Crop metabolomics: From diagnostics to assisted breeding. *Metabolomics*, *14*(11), 148.

Aman, R., Biehl, J., Carle, R., Conrad, J., Beifuss, U., & Schieber, A. (2005). Application of HPLC coupled with DAD, APcI-MS and NMR to the analysis of lutein and zeaxanthin stereoisomers in thermally processed vegetables. *Food Chemistry*, *92*, 753–763.

Amorim-Carrilho, K. T., Cepeda, A., Fente, C., & Regal, P. (2014). Review of methods for analysis of carotenoids. *Trac-Trends in Analytical Chemistry*, *56*, 49–73. APR.

Arathi, B. P., Sowmya, P. R., Vijay, K., Baskaran, V., & Lakshminarayana, R. (2015). Metabolomics of carotenoids: the challenges and prospects—A review. *Trends in Food Science and Technology*, *45*(1), 105–117.

Arvayo-Enríquez, H., Mondaca-Fernández, I., Gortárez-Moroyoqui, P., López-Cervantes, J., & Rodríguez-Ramírez, R. (2013). Carotenoids extraction and quantification: A review. *Analytical Methods*, *5*(12), 2916–2924.

Asker, D. (2018). High throughput screening and profiling of high-value carotenoids from a wide diversity of bacteria in surface seawater. *Food Chemistry*, *261*, 103–111.

Bayram, B., González-Sarrías, A., Istas, G., Garcia-Aloy, M., Morand, C., Tuohy, K., et al. (2018). Breakthroughs in the health effects of plant food bioactives: A perspective on microbiomics, nutri(epi)genomics, and metabolomics. *Journal of Agricultural and Food Chemistry*, *66*(41), 10686–10692.

Beltran, J. C. M., & Stange, C. (2016). Apocarotenoids: A new carotenoid-derived pathway. In *Carotenoids in nature*. In: Springer.

Benmeziane, A., Boulekbache-Makhlouf, L., Mapelli-Brahm, P., Khaled Khodja, N., Remini, H., Madani, K., et al. (2018). Extraction of carotenoids from cantaloupe waste and determination of its mineral composition. *Food Research International*, *111*, 391–398.

Bergantin, C., Maietti, A., Tedeschi, P., Font, G., Manyes, L., & Marchetti, N. (2018). HPLC-UV/Vis-APCI-MS/MS determination of major carotenoids and their bioaccessibility from "Delica"(*Cucurbita maxima*) and "Violina" (*Cucurbita moschata*) pumpkins as food traceability markers. *Molecules*, *23*(11), 2791.

Bertolín, J. R., Joy, M., Rufino-Moya, P. J., Lobón, S., & Blanco, M. (2018). Simultaneous determination of carotenoids, tocopherols, retinol and cholesterol in ovine lyophilised samples of milk, meat, and liver and in unprocessed/raw samples of fat. *Food Chemistry*, *257*, 182–188.

Blasi, F., Rocchetti, G., Montesano, D., Lucini, L., Chiodelli, G., Ghisoni, S., et al. (2018). Changes in extra-virgin olive oil added with *Lycium barbarum* L. carotenoids during frying: Chemical analyses and metabolomic approach. *Food Research International*, *105*, 507–516.

Böhm, V. (2001). Use of column temperature to optimize carotenoid isomer separation by C30 high performance liquid chromatography. *Journal of Separation Science*, *24*(12), 955–959.

Bonaccorsi, I., Cacciola, F., Utczas, M., Inferrera, V., Giuffrida, D., Donato, P., et al. (2016). Characterization of the pigment fraction in sweet bell peppers (*Capsicum annuum* L.) harvested at green and overripe yellow and red stages by offline multidimensional convergence chromatography/liquid chromatography–mass spectrometry. *Journal of Separation Science, 39*(17), 3281–3291.

Bordiga, M., Travaglia, F., Giuffrida, D., Mangraviti, D., Rigano, F., Mondello, L., et al. (2018). Characterization of peel and pulp proanthocyanidins and carotenoids during ripening in persimmon "Kaki tipo" cv, cultivated in italy. *Food Research International,* 800–809.

Bu, X., Sun, L., Shang, F., & Yan, G. (2017). Comparative metabolomics profiling of engineered *Saccharomyces cerevisiae* lead to a strategy that improving β-carotene production by acetate supplementation. *PLoS ONE, 12*(11), e0188385.

Bukowski, M. R., Voeller, K., & Jahns, L. (2018). Simple and sensitive dilute-and-shoot analysis of carotenoids in human plasma. *Journal of Chromatography B, 1095,* 32–38.

Cacciola, F., Donato, P., Giuffrida, D., Torre, G., Dugo, P., & Mondello, L. (2012). Ultra high pressure in the second dimension of a comprehensive two-dimensional liquid chromatographic system for carotenoid separation in red chili peppers. *Journal of Chromatography. A, 1255,* 244–251.

Cacciola, F., Dugo, P., & Mondello, L. (2017). Multidimensional liquid chromatography in food analysis. *Trends in Analytical Chemistry, 96,* 116–123.

Carbonell-Capella, J., Buniowska, M., Barba, F. J., Esteve, M. J., & Frígola, A. (2014). Analytical methods for determining bioavailability and bioaccessibility of bioactive compounds from fruits and vegetables: A review. *Comprehensive Reviews in Food Science and Food Safety, 13*(2), 155–171.

Cheng, D., Zhang, Y., Liu, H., Zhang, H., Tan, K., Ma, H., et al. (2019). An improving method for extracting total carotenoids in an aquatic animal chlamys nobilis. *Food Chemistry, 280,* 45–50.

Ciclet, O., Barron, D., Bajic, S., Veuthey, J., Guillarme, D., & Grand-Guillaume, P. A. (2018). Natural compounds analysis using liquid and supercritical fluid chromatography hyphenated to mass spectrometry: Evaluation of a new design of atmospheric pressure ionization source. *Journal of Chromatography B, 1083,* 1–11.

Cifuentes, A. (2013). Foodomics: Principles and applications. In A. Cifuentes (Ed.), *Foodomics: Advanced mass spectrometry in modern food science and nutrition* (p. 10). Madrid: John Wiley & Sons Inc.

Courant, F., Antignac, J., Dervilly-Pinel, G., & Le Bizec, B. (2014). Basics of mass spectrometry based metabolomics. *Proteomics, 14*(21–22), 2369–2388.

Cruz, R., & Casal, S. (2018). Direct analysis of vitamin A, vitamin E, carotenoids, chlorophylls and free sterols in animal and vegetable fats in a single normal-phase liquid chromatographic run. *Journal of Chromatography. A, 1565,* 81–88.

Di Lena, G., Casini, I., Lucarini, M., & Lombardi-Boccia, G. (2019). Carotenoid profiling of five microalgae species from large-scale production. *Food Research International, 120,* 810–818.

Donato, P., Giuffrida, D., Oteri, M., Inferrera, V., Dugo, P., & Mondello, L. (2018). Supercritical fluid chromatography × ultra-high pressure liquid chromatography for red chilli pepper fingerprinting by photodiode array, quadrupole-time-of-flight and ion mobility mass spectrometry (SFC × RP-UHPLC-PDA-Q-ToF MS-IMS). *Food Analytical Methods, 11*(12), 3331–3341.

Drouin, N., Rudaz, S., & Schappler, J. (2018). Sample preparation for polar metabolites in bioanalysis. *Analyst, 143*(1), 16–20.

Dugo, P., Herrero, M., Kumm, T., Giuffrida, D., Dugo, G., & Mondello, L. (2008). Comprehensive normal-phase×reversed-phase liquid chromatography coupled to photodiode array and mass spectrometry detection for the analysis of free carotenoids and carotenoid esters from mandarin. *Journal of Chromatography. A, 1189*(1), 196–206.

Eggersdorfer, M., & Wyss, A. (2018). Carotenoids in human nutrition and health. *Archives of Biochemistry and Biophysics, 652,* 18–26.

Eriksen, J. N., Madsen, P. L., Dragsted, L. O., & Arrigoni, E. (2017). Optimized, fast-throughput UHPLC-DAD based method for carotenoid quantification in spinach, serum, chylomicrons, and feces. *Journal of Agricultural and Food Chemistry, 65*(4), 973–980.

Etzbach, L., Pfeiffer, A., Schieber, A., & Weber, F. (2019). Effects of thermal pasteurization and ultrasound treatment on the peroxidase activity, carotenoid composition, and physicochemical properties of goldenberry (*Physalis peruviana* L.) puree. *LWT, 100,* 69–74.

Etzbach, L., Pfeiffer, A., Weber, F., & Schieber, A. (2018). Characterization of carotenoid profiles in goldenberry (*Physalis peruviana* L.) fruits at various ripening stages and in different plant tissues by HPLC-DAD-APCI-MSn. *Food Chemistry, 245,* 508–517.

Farré, G., Perez-Fons, L., Decourcelle, M., Breitenbach, J., Hem, S., Zhu, C., et al. (2016). Metabolic engineering of astaxanthin biosynthesis in maize endosperm and characterization of a prototype high oil hybrid. *Transgenic Research, 25*(4), 477–489.

García-de Blas, E., Mateo, R., Viñuela, J., & Alonso-Álvarez, C. (2011). Identification of carotenoid pigments and their fatty acid esters in an avian integument combining HPLC–DAD and LC–MS analyses. *Journal of Chromatography B, 879,* 341–348.

Gentili, A., Caretti, F., Ventura, S., Pérez-Fernández, V., Venditti, A., & Curini, R. (2015). Screening of carotenoids in tomato fruits by using liquid chromatography with diode array-linear ion trap mass spectrometry detection. *Journal of Agricultural and Food Chemistry, 63*(33), 7428–7439.

Giuffrida, D., Donato, P., Dugo, P., & Mondello, L. (2018). Recent analytical techniques advances in the carotenoids and their derivatives determination in various matrixes. *Journal of Agricultural and Food Chemistry, 66*(13), 3302–3307.

Giuffrida, D., Zoccali, M., Arigò, A., Cacciola, F., Roa, C. O., Dugo, P., et al. (2018). Comparison of different analytical techniques for the analysis of carotenoids in tamarillo (*Solanum betaceum* cav.). *Archives of Biochemistry and Biophysics, 646,* 161–167.

Giuffrida, D., Zoccali, M., Giofrè, S. V., Dugo, P., & Mondello, L. (2017). Apocarotenoids determination in *Capsicum chinense* jacq. cv. habanero, by supercritical fluid chromatography-triple-quadrupole/mass spectrometry. *Food Chemistry, 231,* 316–323.

Granado, F., Olmedilla, B., Gil-Martinez, E., & Blanco, I. (2001). A fast, reliable and low-cost saponification protocol for analysis of carotenoids in vegetables. *Journal of Food Composition and Analysis, 14,* 479–489.

Grand-Guillaume Perrenoud, A., Guillarme, D., Boccard, J., Veuthey, J., Barron, D., & Moco, S. (2016). Ultra-high performance supercritical fluid chromatography coupled with quadrupole-time-of-flight mass spectrometry as a performing tool for bioactive analysis. *Journal of Chromatography A, 1450,* 101–111.

Grand-Guillaume Perrenoud, A., Hamman, C., Goel, M., Veuthey, J., Guillarme, D., & Fekete, S. (2013). Maximizing kinetic performance in supercritical fluid chromatography using state-of-the-art instruments. *Journal of Chromatography A, 1314,* 288–297.

Griffiths, W. J., & Wang, Y. Q. (2009). Mass spectrometry: From proteomics to metabolomics and lipidomics. *Chemical Society Reviews, 38*(7), 1882–1896.

Guillarme, D., Desfontaine, V., Heinisch, S., & Veuthey, J. (2018). What are the current solutions for interfacing supercritical fluid chromatography and mass spectrometry? *Journal of Chromatography B, 1083,* 160–170.

Hara, R., Ishigaki, M., Kitahama, Y., Ozaki, Y., & Genkawa, T. (2018). Use of the product of mean intensity ratio (PMIR) technique for discriminant analysis of lycopene-rich vegetable juice using a portable NIR-excited raman spectrometer. *Food Chemistry*, *241*, 353–357.

Harrison, E. H., & Quadro, L. (2018). Apocarotenoids: Emerging roles in mammals. *Annual Review of Nutrition*, *38*, 153–172.

Heavisides, E., Rouger, C., Reichel, A. F., Ulrich, C., Wenzel-Storjohann, A., Sebens, S., et al. (2018). Seasonal variations in the metabolome and bioactivity profile of *Fucus vesiculosus* extracted by an optimised, pressurised liquid extraction protocol. *Marine Drugs*, *16*(12).

Hou, X., Rivers, J., León, P., McQuinn, R. P., & Pogson, B. J. (2016). Synthesis and function of apocarotenoid signals in plants. *Trends in Plant Science*, *21*(9), 792–803.

Hrvolová, B., Martínez-Huélamo, M., Colmán-Martínez, M., Hurtado-Barroso, S., Lamuela-Raventós, R. M., & Kalina, J. (2016). Development of an advanced HPLC–MS/MS method for the determination of carotenoids and fat-soluble vitamins in human plasma. *International Journal of Molecular Sciences*, *17*(10), 1719.

Inbaraj, B. S., Lu, H., Hung, C. F., Wu, W. B., Lin, C. L., & Chen, B. H. (2008). Determination of carotenoids and their esters in fruits of *Lycium barbarum* linnaeus by HPLC–DAD–APCI–MS. *Journal of Pharmaceutical and Biomedical Analysis*, *47*, 812–818.

Islam, K. M. S., & Schweigert, F. J. (2015). Comparison of three spectrophotometric methods for analysis of egg yolk carotenoids. *Food Chemistry*, *172*, 233–237.

Jin, H., Lao, Y. M., Zhou, J., Zhang, H. J., & Cai, Z. H. (2017). Simultaneous determination of 13 carotenoids by a simple C18 column-based ultra-high-pressure liquid chromatography method for carotenoid profiling in the astaxanthin-accumulating *Haematococcus pluvialis*. *Journal of Chromatography A*, *1488*, 93–103.

Ke, Q., Kang, L., Kim, H. S., Xie, T., Liu, C., Ji, C. Y., et al. Down-regulation of lycopene ε-cyclase expression in transgenic sweetpotato plants increases the carotenoid content and tolerance to abiotic stress. *Plant Science*, *281*, (2019). 52–60.

Khalid, M., Saeed-ur-Rahman, B. M., Iqbal, H. M. N., & Huang, D. (2019). Biosynthesis and biomedical perspectives of carotenoids with special reference to human health-related applications. *Biocatalysis and Agricultural Biotechnology*, *17*, 399–407.

Khamis, M. M., Adamko, D. J., Purves, R. W., & El-Aneed, A. (2019). Quantitative determination of potential urine Biomedical biomarkers of respiratory illnesses using new targeted metabolomic approach. *Analytica Chimica Acta*, *1047*, 81–92.

Kimura, M., Rodriguez-Amaya, D. B., & Godoy, H. T. (1990). Assessment of the saponification step in the quantitative determination of carotenoids and provitamins A. *Food Chemistry*, *35*, 187–195.

Kopec, R. E., Carail, M., & Caris-Veyrat, C. (2018). Production, separation, and characterization of apo-luteinoids by LC-MS/MS. *Journal of Chromatography B*, *1102–1103*, 45–51.

Kopec, R. E., Cooperstone, J. L., Cichon, M. J., & Schwartz, S. J. (2012). *Analysis methods of carotenoids*. In *Analysis of antioxidant-rich phytochemicals* (pp. 105–149). Hoboken: Chichester: Wiley-Blackwell.

Kyriakoudi, A. Z., & Tsimidou, M. (2018). Latest advances in the extraction and determination of saffron apocarotenoids. *Electrophoresis*, *39*(15), 1846–1859.

Lachowicz, S., Oszmiański, J., & Wiśniewski, R. (2018). Determination of triterpenoids, carotenoids, chlorophylls, and antioxidant capacity in *Allium ursinum* L. at different times of harvesting and anatomical parts. *European Food Research and Technology*, *244*(7), 1269–1280.

Larive, C. K., Barding, G. A., & Dinges, M. M. (2015). NMR spectroscopy for metabolomics and metabolic profiling. *Analytical Chemistry*, *87*(1), 133–146.

Larsen, E., & Christensen, L. P. (2005). Simple saponification method for the quantitative determination of carotenoids in green vegetables. *Journal of Agricultural and Food Chemistry, 53*(17), 6598–6602.

Li, X., Jin, J., Sun, C., Ye, D., & Liu, Y. (2019). Simultaneous determination of six main types of lipid-soluble pigments in green tea by visible and near-infrared spectroscopy. *Food Chemistry, 270*, 236–242.

Lima, V. C., Rosen, R. B., & Farah, M. (2016). Macular pigment in retinal health and disease. *International Journal of Retina and Vitreous, 2*(1), 19.

Liu, X., Liu, J., Bi, J., Yi, J., Peng, J., Ning, C., et al. (2019). Effects of high pressure homogenization on pectin structural characteristics and carotenoid bioaccessibility of carrot juice. *Carbohydrate Polymers, 203*, 176–184.

Llano, S. M., Muñoz-Jiménez, A. M., Jiménez-Cartagena, C., Londoño-Londoño, J., & Medina, S. (2018). Untargeted metabolomics reveals specific withanolides and fatty acyl glycoside as tentative metabolites to differentiate organic and conventional *Physalis peruviana* fruits. *Food Chemistry, 244*, 120–127.

Losito, I., Facchini, L., Valentini, A., Cataldi, T. R. I., & Palmisano, F. (2018). Fatty acidomics: Evaluation of the effects of thermal treatments on commercial mussels through an extended characterization of their free fatty acids by liquid chromatography—Fourier transform mass spectrometry. *Food Chemistry, 255*, 309–322.

Mariutti, L. R. B., & Mercadante, A. Z. (2018). Carotenoid esters analysis and occurrence: What do we know so far? *Archives of Biochemistry and Biophysics, 648*, 36–43.

Melfi, M. T., Nardiello, D., Cicco, N., Candido, V., & Centonze, D. (2018). Simultaneous determination of water- and fat-soluble vitamins, lycopene and beta-carotene in tomato samples and pharmaceutical formulations: Double injection single run by reverse-phase liquid chromatography with UV detection. *Journal of Food Composition and Analysis, 70*, 9–17.

Mercadante, A. Z., Rodrigues, D. B., Petry, F. C., & Mariutti, L. R. B. (2017). Carotenoid esters in foods—A review and practical directions on analysis and occurrence. *Food Research International, 99*, 830–850.

Mi, J., Jia, K., Balakrishna, A., Wang, J. Y., & Al-Babili, S. (2019).An LC-MS profiling method reveals a route for apocarotene glycosylation and shows its induction by high light stress in arabidopsis. *Analyst, 144*(4), 1197–1204.

Mi, J., Jia, K., Wang, J. Y., & Al-Babili, S. (2018). A rapid LC-MS method for qualitative and quantitative profiling of plant apocarotenoids. *Analytica Chimica Acta, 1035*, 87–95.

Mohajeri, S. A., Hosseinzadeh, H., Keyhanfar, F., & Aghamohammadian, J. (2010). Extraction of crocin from saffron (*Crocus sativus*) using molecularly imprinted polymer solid-phase extraction. *Journal of Separation Science, 33*(15), 2302–2309.

Moresco, R., Afonso, T., Uarrota, V. G., Navarro, B. B., Nunes, E. C., Rocha, M., et al. (2017). Classification tools for carotenoid content estimation in *Manihot esculenta* via metabolomics and machine learning. *Adv. Intell. Syst. Comput., 616*, 280–288.

Ngamwonglumlert, L., & Devahastin, S. (2019). *Carotenoids* (pp. 40–52) In L. Melton, F. Shahidi, & P. Varelis (Eds.), *Encyclopedia of food chemistry*. USA: Academic Press.

Noronha Matos, K. A., Praia Lima, D., Pereira Barbosa, A. P., Zerlotti Mercadante, A., & Campos, C. R. (2019). Peels of tucumã (*Astrocaryum vulgare*) and peach palm (*Bactris gasipaes*) are by-products classified as very high carotenoid sources. *Food Chemistry, 272*, 216–221.

Nováková, L., Grand-Guillaume Perrenoud, A., Francois, I., West, C., Lesellier, E., & Guillarme, D. (2014). Modern analytical supercritical fluid chromatography using columns packed with sub-2µm particles: A tutorial. *Analytica Chimica Acta, 824*, 18–35.

Oberoi, D. P. S., & Sogi, D. S. (2017). Utilization of watermelon pulp for lycopene extraction by response surface methodology. *Food Chemistry, 232*, 316–321.

Oliver, J., & Palou, A. (2000). Chromatographic determination of carotenoids in foods. *Journal of Chromatography A, 881*(1), 543–555.

Ordoudi, S. A., de los Mozos Pascual, M., & Tsimidou, M. Z. (2014). On the quality control of traded saffron by means of transmission fourier-transform mid-infrared (FT-MIR) spectroscopy and chemometrics. *Food Chemistry, 150*, 414–421.

Osterrothová, K., Culka, A., Němečková, K., Kaftan, D., Nedbalová, L., Procházková, L., et al. (2019). Analyzing carotenoids of snow algae by raman microspectroscopy and high-performance liquid chromatography. *Spectrochimica Acta. Part A, Molecular and Biomolecular Spectroscopy, 212*, 262–271.

Patsilinakos, A., Ragno, R., Carradori, S., Petralito, S., & Cesa, S. (2018). Carotenoid content of goji berries: CIELAB, HPLC-DAD analyses and quantitative correlation. *Food Chemistry, 268*, 49–56.

Paznocht, L., Kotíková, Z., Orsák, M., Lachman, J., & Martinek, P. (2019). Carotenoid changes of colored-grain wheat flours during bun-making. *Food Chemistry, 277*, 725–734.

Pérez Fernández, V., Ventura, S., Tomai, P., Curini, R., & Gentili, A. (2017). Determination of target fat-soluble micronutrients in rainbow trout's muscle and liver tissues by liquid chromatography with diode array-tandem mass spectrometry detection. *Electrophoresis, 38*(6), 886–896.

Petruzziello, F., Grand-Guillaume Perrenoud, A., Thorimbert, A., Fogwill, M., & Rezzi, S. (2017). Quantitative profiling of endogenous fat-soluble vitamins and carotenoids in human plasma using an improved UHPSFC-ESI-MS interface. *Analytical Chemistry, 89*(14), 7615–7622.

Pilařová, V., Plachká, K., Khalikova, M. A., Svec, F., & Nováková, L. (2019). Recent developments in supercritical fluid chromatography–Mass spectrometry: Is it a viable option for analysis of complex samples? *Trends in Analytical Chemistry, 112*, 212–225.

Rathi, D., Liew, C. Y., Fairulnizal, M. M., Isameyah, D., & Barknowitz, G. (2017). Fat-soluble vitamin and carotenoid analysis in cooking oils by ultra-performance convergence chromatography. *Food Analytical Methods, 10*(4), 1087–1096.

Regal, P., Díaz-Bao, M., Barreiro, R., Cepeda, A., & Fente, C. (2012). Application of molecularly imprinted polymers in food analysis: Clean-up and chromatographic improvements. *Central European Journal of Chemistry, 10*(3), 766–784.

Reinholds, I., Bartkevics, V., Silvis, I. C. J., van Ruth, S. M., & Esslinger, S. (2015). Analytical techniques combined with chemometrics for authentication and determination of contaminants in condiments: A review. *Journal of Food Composition and Analysis, 44*, 56–72.

Reinke, B. A., Erritouni, Y., & Calsbeek, R. (2018). Maternal allocation of carotenoids to eggs in an anolis lizard. *Comparative Biochemistry and Physiology. Part A, Molecular & Integrative Physiology, 218*, 56–62.

Rezanka, T., Olsovska, J., Sobotka, M., & Sigler, K. (2009). The use of APCI-MS with HPLC and other separation techniques for identification of carotenoids and related compounds. *Current Analytical Chemistry, 5*(1), 1–25.

Riggi, E. (2010). Recent patents on the extraction of carotenoids. *Recent Patents on Food, Nutrition & Agriculture, 2*(1), 75–82.

Rivera, S., & Canela, R. (2012). Influence of sample processing on the analysis of carotenoids in maize. *Molecules, 17*(9), 11255–11268.

Rivera, S. M., & Canela-Garayoa, R. (2012). Analytical tools for the analysis of carotenoids in diverse materials. *Journal of Chromatography A, 1224*, 1–10.

Rivera, S. M., Christou, P., & Canela-Garayoa, R. (2014). Identification of carotenoids using mass spectrometry. *Mass Spectrometry Reviews*, *33*(5), 353–372.

Rivera, S., Vilaró, F., & Canela, R. (2011). Determination of carotenoids by liquid chromatography/mass spectrometry: Effect of several dopants. *Analytical and Bioanalytical Chemistry*, *400*(5), 1339–1346.

Rodriguez-Amaya, D. B. (2003). Food carotenoids: Analysis, composition and alterations during storage and processing of foods. *Forum of Nutrition*, *56*, 35–37.

Rodriguez-Amaya, D. B. (2010). Quantitative analysis, in vitro assessment of bioavailability and antioxidant activity of food carotenoids—A review. *Journal of Food Composition and Analysis*, *23*, 726–740.

Rodriguez-Amaya, D. (2016). Structures and analysis of carotenoid molecules. In C. Stange (Ed.), *Carotenoids in nature: Biosynthesis, regulation and function*. Cham: Springer International Publishing. ID: Rodriguez-Amaya2016.

Rodríguez-Bernaldo de Quirós, A., & Costa, H. S. (2006). Analysis of carotenoids in vegetable and plasma samples: A review. *Journal of Food Composition and Analysis*, *19*, 97–111.

Saini, R. K., & Keum, Y. (2018). Carotenoid extraction methods: A review of recent developments. *Food Chemistry*, *240*, 90–103.

Saini, R. K., Nile, S. H., & Park, S. W. (2015). Carotenoids from fruits and vegetables: Chemistry, analysis, occurrence, bioavailability and biological activities. *Food Research International*, *76*, 735–750.

Sánchez-Camargo, A. P., Parada-Alonso, F., Ibáñez, E., & Cifuentes, A. (2019). Recent applications of on-line supercritical fluid extraction coupled to advanced analytical techniques for compounds extraction and identification. *Journal of Separation Science*, *42*(1), 243–247.

Sander, L. C., Sharpless, K. E., Craft, N. E., & Wise, S. A. (1994). Development of engineered stationary phases for the separation of carotenoid isomers. *Analytical Chemistry*, *66*(10), 1667–1674.

Sander, L. C., Sharpless, K. E., & Pursch, M. (2000). C30 stationary phases for the analysis of food by liquid chromatography. *Journal of Chromatography. A*, *880*(1), 189–202.

Schex, R., Lieb, V. M., Jiménez, V. M., Esquivel, P., Schweiggert, R. M., Carle, R., et al. (2018). HPLC-DAD-APCI/ESI-MSn analysis of carotenoids and α-tocopherol in costa rican *Acrocomia aculeata* fruits of varying maturity stages. *Food Research International*, *105*, 645–653.

Schimpf, K. J., Thompson, L. D., & Pan, S. (2018). Determination of carotenoids in infant, pediatric, and adult nutritionals by HPLC with UV-visible detection: Single-laboratory validation, first action 2017.04. *Journal of AOAC International*, *101*(1), 264–276.

Schulz, H., Baranska, M., & Baranski, R. (2005). Potential of NIR-FT-Raman spectroscopy in natural carotenoid analysis. *Biopolymers: Original Research on Biomolecules*, *77*(4), 212–221.

Schweiggert, R. M., Vargas, E., Conrad, J., Hempel, J., Gras, C. C., Ziegler, J. U., et al. (2016). Carotenoids, carotenoid esters, and anthocyanins of yellow-, orange-, and red-peeled cashew apples (*Anacardium occidentale* L.). *Food Chemistry*, *200*, 274–282.

Serra, J. L., AMdC, R., de Freitas, R. A., AJA, M., Darnet, S. H., & LHMd, S. (2019). Alternative sources of oils and fats from amazonian plants: Fatty acids, methyl tocols, total carotenoids and chemical composition. *Food Research International*, *116*, 12–19.

Shen, Y., Hu, Y., Huang, K., Yin, S., Chen, B., & Yao, S. (2009). Solid-phase extraction of carotenoids. *Journal of Chromatography. A*, *1216*(30), 5763–5768.

Smith, D. F., Cummings, R. D., & Song, X. (2019). History and future of shotgun glycomics. In *Biochemical Society Transactions*: Portland Press Ltd. BST20170487.

Song, S., Liu, H., & Bai, Y. (2017). Supercritical fluid chromatography and its application in lipid isomer separation. *Journal of Analysis and Testing*, *1*(4), 330–334.

Stinco, C. M., Benítez-González, A. M., Meléndez-Martínez, A. J., Hernanz, D., & Vicario, I. M. (2019). Simultaneous determination of dietary isoprenoids (carotenoids, chlorophylls and tocopherols) in human faeces by rapid resolution liquid chromatography. *Journal of Chromatography A*, *1583*, 63–72.

Stout, M. A., Benoist, D. M., & Drake, M. A. (2018). Technical note: Simultaneous carotenoid and vitamin analysis of milk from total mixed ration-fed cows optimized for xanthophyll detection. *Journal of Dairy Science*, *101*(6), 4906–4913. June 2018.

Strati, I. F., & Oreopoulou, V. (2011). Effect of extraction parameters on the carotenoid recovery from tomato waste. *International Journal of Food Science and Technology*, *46*(1), 23–29.

Tamburini, E., Costa, S., Rugiero, I., Pedrini, P., & Marchetti, M. G. (2017). Quantification of lycopene, β-carotene, and total soluble solids in intact red-flesh watermelon (*Citrullus lanatus*) using on-line near-infrared spectroscopy. *Sensors*, *17*(4), 746.

Tiziani, S., Schwartz, S. J., & Vodovotz, Y. (2006). Profiling of carotenoids in tomato juice by one-and two-dimensional NMR. *Journal of Agricultural and Food Chemistry*, *54*(16), 6094–6100.

Trygg, J., Holmes, E., & Lundstedt, T. (2007). Chemometrics in metabonomics. *Journal of Proteome Research*, *6*(2), 469–479.

Turcsi, E., Nagy, V., & Deli, J. (2016). Study on the elution order of carotenoids on endcapped C18 and C30 reverse silica stationary phases. A review of the database. *Journal of Food Composition and Analysis*, *47*, 101–112.

Van Breemen, R. B., Dong, L., & Pajkovic, N. D. (2012). Atmospheric pressure chemical ionization tandem mass spectrometry of carotenoids. *International Journal of Mass Spectrometry*, *312*, 163–172.

Vincent, U., Serano, F., & von Holst, C. (2017). Development and validation of a multi-analyte method for the regulatory control of carotenoids used as feed additives in fish and poultry feed. *Food Additives & Contaminants, Part A: Chemistry, Analysis, Control, Exposure & Risk Assessment*, *34*(8), 1285–1297.

Wald, J. P., Nohr, D., & Biesalski, H. K. (2018). Rapid and easy carotenoid quantification in ghanaian starchy staples using RP-HPLC-PDA. *Journal of Food Composition and Analysis*, *67*, 119–127.

Werner, E., Croixmarie, V., Umbdenstock, T., Ezan, E., Chaminade, P., Tabet, J. C., et al. (2008). Mass spectrometry-based metabolomics: Accelerating the characterization of discriminating signals by combining statistical correlations and ultrahigh resolution. *Analytical Chemistry*, *80*(13), 4918–4932.

Werner, E., Heilier, J., Ducruix, C., Ezan, E., & Junot, C. (2008). Mass spectrometry for the identification of the discriminanting signals from metabolomics: Current status and future trends. *Journal of Chromatography, B: Analytical Technologies in the Biomedical and Life Sciences*, *871*(2), 143–163.

West, C. E., & Castenmiller, J. J. (1998). Quantification of the "SLAMENGHI" factors for carotenoid bioavailability and bioconversion. *International Journal for Vitamin and Nutrition Research*, *68*(6), 371–377.

Woodside, J. V., Draper, J., Lloyd, A., & McKinley, M. C. (2017). Use of biomarkers to assess fruit and vegetable intake. *Proceedings of the Nutrition Society*, *76*(3), 308–315.

Xie, J., Yao, S., Ming, J., Deng, L., & Zeng, K. (2019). Variations in chlorophyll and carotenoid contents and expression of genes involved in pigment metabolism response to oleocellosis in citrus fruits. *Food Chemistry*, *272*, 49–57.

Yamada, T., & Bamba, T. (2017). Lipid profiling by supercritical fluid chromatography/ mass spectrometry. In P. Wood (Ed.), *Lipidomics*. New York, NY: Springer New York. ID: Yamada2017.

Yungyuen, W., Ma, G., Zhang, L., Futamura, M., Tabuchi, M., Yamawaki, K., et al. (2018). Regulation of carotenoid metabolism in response to different temperatures in citrus juice sacs in vitro. *Scientia Horticulturae*, *238*, 384–390.

Zeb, A. (2017). A simple, sensitive HPLC-DAD method for simultaneous determination of carotenoids, chlorophylls and α-tocopherol in leafy vegetables. *Journal of Food Measurement & Characterization*, *11*(3), 979–986.

Zeb, A., Haq, A., & Murkovic, M. (2019). Effects of microwave cooking on carotenoids, phenolic compounds and antioxidant activity of *Cichorium intybus* L. (chicory) leaves. *European Food Research and Technology*, *245*(2), 365–374.

Zheng, H., Zhang, Q., Quan, J., Zheng, Q., & Xi, W. (2016). Determination of sugars, organic acids, aroma components, and carotenoids in grapefruit pulps. *Food Chemistry*, *205*, 112–121.

Zhong, L., Gustavsson, K., Oredsson, S., Głąb, B., Yilmaz, J. L., & Olsson, M. E. (2016). Determination of free and esterified carotenoid composition in rose hip fruit by HPLC-DAD-APCI+-MS. *Food Chemistry*, *210*, 541–550.

Zhu, T., & Row, K. (2013). Optimization and application of liquid chromatography determination of dispersive liquid-liquid microextraction purified astaxanthin in shrimp waste. *Chemical Research in Chinese Universities*, *29*(3), 429–433.

Zoccali, M., Giuffrida, D., Dugo, P., & Mondello, L. (2017). Direct online extraction and determination by supercritical fluid extraction with chromatography and mass spectrometry of targeted carotenoids from red habanero peppers (*Capsicum chinense* jacq.). *Journal of Separation Science*, *40*(19), 3905–3913.

Zoccali, M., Giuffrida, D., Salafia, F., Giofrè, S. V., & Mondello, L. (2018). Carotenoids and apocarotenoids determination in intact human blood samples by online supercritical fluid extraction-supercritical fluid chromatography-tandem mass spectrometry. *Analytica Chimica Acta*, *1032*, 40–47.

Carotenoids degradation and precautions during processing

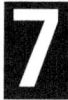

Wei Lu*,†,‡, Valentyn A. Maidannyk*,†, Aaron S.L. Lim*,†
*Food Chemistry & Technology Department, Teagasc Food Research Centre, Cork, Ireland, †School of Food and Nutritional Sciences, University College Cork, Cork, Ireland, ‡School of Agriculture and Biology, Shanghai Jiao Tong University, Shanghai, China

Chapter outline

Introduction

Carotenoids are well known for their health benefits as provitamin A, and as antioxidants to prevent many chronic diseases, for example, cancer, cardiovascular disease, and macular degeneration (Rodriguez-Amaya, 2015). However, carotenoids, for example, β-carotene or lycopene, are usually lipophilic due to the presence of long unsaturated aliphatic chains as in some fatty acids (Fig. 1), which makes them insoluble

Carotenoids: Properties, Processing and Applications. https://doi.org/10.1016/B978-0-12-817067-0.00007-5

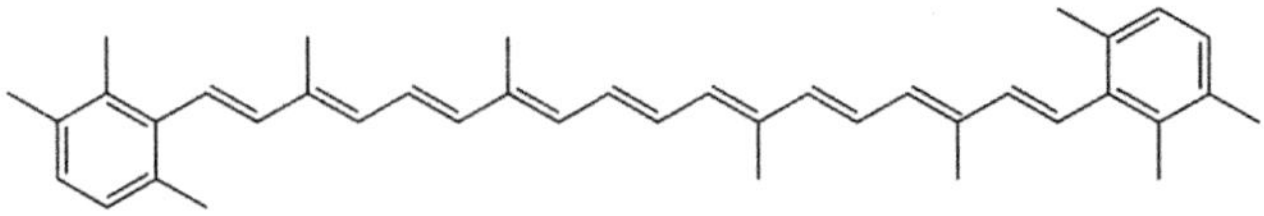

Fig. 1 General structure of a carotenoid: polyene with double bonds.

in water and liable to degradation (e.g., heat or light) (Subagio & Morita, 2001). In addition, naturally occurring carotenoids usually form complexes with biopolymers, such as proteins and polysaccharides, which restrain their adsorption by human body (Goodwin, 1984). The extreme pH environment in stomach can also result in the chemical instability of carotenoids. All these factors greatly affect the stability and the oral bioavailability of carotenoids, and protective delivery mechanisms of these compounds are, therefore, required. Utilization of microencapsulation and delivery technologies can achieve this, and numerous studies have been carried out to encapsulate carotenoids into different delivery systems, for example, liposome (Tan et al., 2014; Tan, Feng, Zhang, Xia, & Xia, 2016), emulsions (Lu, Kelly, & Miao, 2017a, 2017b; Mao, Wang, Liu, & Gao, 2018), nanoparticles (Yi, Lam, Yokoyama, Cheng, & Zhong, 2014a, 2014b, 2015), or powders (Desobry, Netto, & Labuza, 1997), with attempts of significantly maintaining their chemical stability and improving their oral bioavailability.

Microencapsulation utilizes wall materials to entrap and protect encapsulated materials such as carotenoids from environmental stresses for extended shelf life as well as enables controlled release of the encapsulated materials (Shahidi & Han, 1993). Both spray-drying and freeze-drying are dehydration methods commonly utilized for microencapsulation (Desobry et al., 1997; Harnkarnsujarit, Charoenrein, & Roos, 2012; Ré, 1998). There has been increasing interest in the use of layer-by-layer (LBL) interfacial structuring to further improve stability of O/W emulsion formed through electrostatic attraction between a charged primary layer with an oppositely charged secondary layer present (Guzey & McClements, 2006; Moreau, Kim, Decker, & McClements, 2003). The thicker and denser interfacial layer on the oil particles, lower van der Waals attraction, and higher steric repulsion may improve the stability of LBL systems (Benjamin, Silcock, Leus, & Everett, 2012; Gu, Decker, & McClements, 2005; Harnsilawat, Pongsawatmanit, & McClements, 2006; McClements, 1999; Moreau et al., 2003). Many studies have found that the LBL interfacial structuring can improve stability of emulsions toward environmental stresses such as heat treatment, variations in pH, aging, freeze-thaw cycles, lipid oxidation, and ionic strength (Aoki, Decker, & McClements, 2005; Gharsallaoui et al., 2010; Güzey & McClements, 2006; Moreau et al., 2003; Ogawa, Decker, & McClements, 2003) that can improve stability of encapsulated material.

Generally food solids can exist in crystalline, amorphous, and partially (e.g., semi) crystalline powders. Due to difference in structure, crystalline and amorphous materials show significantly different physicochemical properties (Bhandari, Bansal, Zhang, & Schuck, 2013). Amorphous materials are not stable compare to crystalline structure but amorphous materials are fairly stable in the glassy state (e.g., glass) (Maidannyk & Roos, 2018; Slade, Levine, & Reid, 1991). At temperatures around the onset of a calorimetric glass transition temperature (T_g), the molecules are restricted to rotation and vibrational motions, and are fixed in their location giving the solid-like features (Lim & Roos, 2018). During this process, physical properties of materials, such as viscosity, structural relaxation time, molecular mobility, etc. critically change and materials are converted to supercooled liquids (e.g., rubber) showing time-dependent flow (Angell, Ngai, McKenna, McMillan, & Martin, 2000; Maidannyk & Roos, 2018). Hence, knowing the time-dependent characteristics is practically important. Structural strength concept combine changes in temperature $(T–T_g)$ and is practically an important time factor (critical change in structural relaxation time) (Roos et al., 2015). Structural strength approach can be successfully applied for various food systems including carbohydrate-protein [trehalose-whey protein isolate (WPI); lactose-WPI], miscible carbohydrate (lactose-trehalose; trehalose-maltodextrin), partially crystalline (trehalose), encapsulant (trehalose-WPI-sunflower oil), and encapsulant with dissolved in oil phase carotenoids systems (trehalose-WPI-carotenoids dissolved in sunflowers oil and trehalose-maltodextrin-carotenoids dissolved in sunflowers oil) (Fan & Roos, 2016a, 2016b; Lim & Roos, 2018; Maidannyk, Lim, Auty, & Roos, 2018; Maidannyk, Nurhadi, & Roos, 2017; Maidannyk & Roos, 2016, 2017, 2018). These studies have confirmed that composition and water contents significantly influence structural strength parameter (S). This chapter looks at the encapsulation of carotenoids in various food matrices, loss of the encapsulated carotenoids, steps to improve stability of the encapsulated carotenoids, and prediction of carotenoids loss.

Encapsulation and delivery of carotenoids

Many technologies can be employed to protectively encapsulate and deliver carotenoids, such as liposomes, emulsions, polysaccharides complexes, nanoparticles, carbon nanotubes, and drying technology. In this section, several widely used delivery systems for carotenoids are summarized, including liposome, emulsions, polysaccharides complexes, and drying process.

Liposome

Liposome is spherical vesicles having a lipid bilayer (Fig. 2) and can be used as delivery carriers for bioactive nutrients and drugs. Liposomes usually have an aqueous solution core surrounded by a hydrophobic lipid bilayer with the hydrophobic chains of the lipids forming the bilayer and the polar head groups of the lipids oriented toward the extravesicular solution and inner cavity (Edwards & Baeumner, 2006). They have received greater attention in academic and industrial research owing to their biocompatibility and appealing ability to carry hydrophobic and hydrophilic substance. Hydrophilic solutes can be dissolved in the core, while hydrophobic chemicals associate with the bilayer. Therefore, liposome can be loaded with hydrophilic and/or hydrophobic components, delivering them to a site of action by fusing with other bilayers such as the cell membrane (Cevc & Richardsen, 1999). Liposomes can be used to encapsulate and delivery lipophilic carotenoids. It has been shown that the lipid bilayer can not

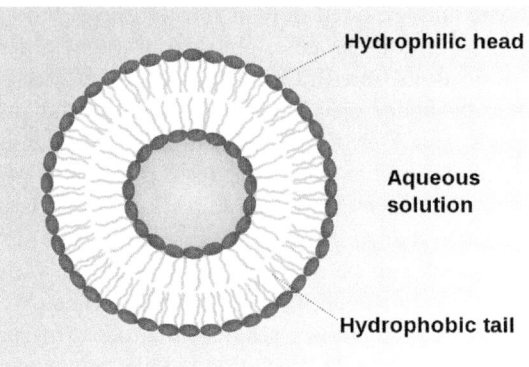

Fig. 2 Scheme of a liposome formed by phospholipids in an aqueous solution.

only provide the physiochemical barrier to incorporated carotenoids against prooxidant elements, but also make them water soluble and increase their bioavailability.

Tan et al. (2014) successfully prepared phosphatidylcholine (PTC)-based liposomes loading different carotenoids (including lutein, β-carotene, lycopene, and canthaxanthin) by thin-film evaporation method. PTC liposomes showed better different encapsulation efficiency (EE) to lutein, β-carotene, and canthaxanthin than lycopene at a high concentration. The encapsulation also significantly enhanced the antioxidant activity of these compounds, and encapsulated lutein showed the strongest antioxidant activity, followed by β-carotene, lycopene, and canthaxanthin, respectively.

Biopolymer-coated liposome as delivery carriers of carotenoids was also developed by the same group (Tan et al., 2016). The study has successfully fabricated the carotenoid nano-carriers based on the chitosan deposition through electrostatic interaction onto a negatively charged liposomal surface. The particle size of spherical liposomes was roughly in the range of 70–100 nm. The chitosan coating can restrict the motion of polar head groups of carotenoids, and slightly decrease the molecular motion of lipids in the superficial region, but did not significantly affect the fluidity of membrane hydrophobic core at the concentration of 0–1.0 mg/mL. In addition to providing the physical barrier for membrane surface, the adsorption of chitosan chains increased the condensation of liposomal structure by potential rigidification. All these contributed to a better thermal stability and dispersibility of carotenoids in liposomes. Besides, a sustained release of carotenoid from chitosan-coating liposomes in a simulated gastric-phase digestion was observed.

Emulsions

Emulsions are widely used as delivery carriers for a variety of lipophilic, hydrophilic, or amphiphilic functional ingredients, such as polyphenols, carotenoids, ω-3 unsaturated fatty acids, and vitamins (Lu, Kelly, & Miao, 2016; Mao et al., 2018; McClements, Decker, & Weiss, 2007). As delivery systems for lipophilic bioactive nutrients, for example, carotenoids, emulsions have many advantages, such as ease of preparation, maintenance of the chemical stability, potential controlled release, and improved oral bioavailability of encapsulated components. Many different emulsion-based delivery systems for lipophilic carotenoids have been developed, including single oil-in-water (O/W) emulsions, multiple-layer O/W emulsions, hydrogel-filled emulsions, or solid lipid nanoparticles (SLNs).

Conventional emulsions

Conventional O/W emulsions consist of oil droplets dispersed in an aqueous continuous phase, with the oil droplets being surrounded by a thin interfacial layer consisting of emulsifier molecules. Conventional O/W emulsions are very simple but effective way of encapsulating carotenoids. The lipophilic carotenoids, for example, β-carotene, can be easily dispersed into oil phase before mixing with water phase that contains emulsifiers. After premixing, the coarse emulsions with large droplet size are passed through a pressure homogenization, which can further rupture the large oil droplets into small ones and create final stable emulsions. The properties of final emulsions, such as droplet size, and surface charge, can be controlled by changing the pressure of homogenization, and selecting proper emulsifiers with positive, noncharged or negative charges, respectively (McClements et al., 2007).

Encapsulation in conventional emulsions can significantly improve the stability, and the bioaccessibility and cellular uptake of carotenoids by enterocytes after passing through simulated gastrointestinal tract (GIT) digestion. The bioaccessibility and cellular uptake of these encapsulated carotenoids in conventional emulsions are dependent on the initial droplet size (Salvia-Trujillo, Qian, Martin-Belloso, & McClements, 2013), composition and microstructure of the oil phase (Lu et al., 2017b; Qian, Decker, Xiao, & McClements, 2012a, 2012b), emulsifiers (Lu et al., 2017a), and the composition of water phase (Lu, Zheng, & Miao, 2018).

Structured emulsions

Generally, conventional emulsions are prone to flocculation, coalescence, or creaming when exposed to unfavorable environments, for example, extreme pH, high ion strength, or thermal processing. Hence, some novel emulsions with tailored structures in the interface, oil phase, and water phase have been developed, in order to better deliver bioactive components and enhance their stability (McClements & Li, 2010). Three types of mainly used structured emulsion-based delivery systems for lipophilic carotenoids are discussed in this section, including multilayer emulsions, SLNs, and filled hydrogels (gelled emulsions).

Multilayer emulsions

Multilayer emulsions consist of oil droplets dispersed in an aqueous phase with each oil droplets being coated with two or more interfacial layers, consisting of emulsifier and biopolymers. The multilayer interfaces can be formed by depositing oppositely charged biopolymers onto the droplets coated with emulsifiers through electrostatic attractions. Multilayer emulsions usually have better stability than conventional emulsions at acidic pH, upon heating or cooling (or freeze–thaw), or against high ionic strength (Guzey & McClements, 2006).

Hou et al. (2010) successfully prepared soybean polysaccharide-chitosan double-layer emulsions containing β-carotene. Compared with single-layer (SL) emulsion stabilized by only soybean polysaccharides, β-carotene encapsulated in double-layer emulsions showed significantly decreased degradation during storage under different temperatures, and the inhibition of the degradation is dependent on the concentration and the molecular weight of the chitosan used (Hou et al., 2012); the emulsions stabilized by chitosan of medium molecular weight at a concentration over 0.25% showed the best β-carotene stability. In addition, this double-layer interface can also significantly improve the light stability of β-carotene.

β-Carotene emulsions with lactoferrin (LF)-β-lactoglobulin (BLG) multiple layer interface by sequential electrostatic deposition of anionic (BLG) and cationic proteins (LF), was also prepared by Tokle, Mao, and McClements (2013). The formation of protein-multilayer interface could significantly improve the stability (pH and ionic strength) of emulsions containing β-carotene. However, the rate and extent of triglycerides digestion was fairly similar for lipid droplets initially coated by one, two, three, or four layers of protein when passing through a simulated GIT digestion. Multilayer interface could also improve the stability of encapsulated β-carotene in emulsions during freeze-drying process (Lim, Griffin, & Roos, 2014). Freeze-dried emulsions with WPI-gum arabic double-layer interface showed significantly slow loss of β-carotene during storage at high temperatures (45°C) compared with that with WPI SL interface.

Solid lipid nanoparticles

SLNs refer to the O/W emulsions with fully or partly solidified oil phase, and the structure, location, and packing of the crystals in the oil phase are usually controlled to obtain particular functional attributes (McClements & Li, 2010). SLC can be produced following a simple two-step thermal process:

(i) producing conventional emulsions at high temperature and.
(ii) cooling the conventional emulsions to trigger lipid solidification process (e.g., crystallization).

By control of the thermal process (temperature, heating rate, duration, cooling rate, etc.), the lipid crystallization process can be modified, and the crystals formed may have different polymorphs, leading to different emulsion properties with potentially desired functionalities. Several different SLN have been developed to encapsulate and deliver carotenoids, for example, β-carotene. The incorporation of β-carotene into the SLC can significantly slowdown the oxidation and maintain the entrapment efficiency and the chemical stability of β-carotene (Trombino et al., 2009; Zhang, Hayes, Chen, & Zhong, 2013).

The role of SLN in preventing β-carotene from degradation is significantly dependent on the emulsifiers that were used to create emulsions. Selection of emulsifiers can not only influence the interfacial properties of the SLN, but also can affect the crystallization process of the lipid phase. For example, only β-type lipid crystals were formed in Poloxamer 188 stabilized SLNs, while both β′ and β types were observed in tween 20-stabilized ones (Nik, Langmaida, & Wright, 2012), and SLN with these differently structured oil phase accordingly can influence the stability of encapsulated components. For example, the oxidative stability and the retention rates (30 days of storage at 25°C) of β-carotene in SLNs stabilized with different proteins [sodium caseinate (SC); WPI; or soy protein isolate (SPI)] decreased in the order of SC > WPI > SPI (Yi et al., 2014a, 2014b). The protein concentration could also affect the chemical stability of encapsulated β-carotene, and the stability of β-carotene increased with increasing protein concentration. In addition, the incorporation of β-carotene into these protein-stabilized SLNs could significantly improve the cellular uptake of β-carotene, and the cellular uptake of β-carotene is dependent on the emulsifiers, particle size, and surface charge of SLN, suggesting that a controlled cellular uptake of β-carotene in SLN can potentially be obtained by designing the interfacial structure and particle size of SLN. Another study also reported that SLN stabilized with lecithin showed better inhibition on the degradation of β-carotene than tween-stabilized SLN (Helgason et al., 2009). SLN can also maintain their structures when exposure to the simulated digestive conditions, decrease the lipolysis rate, and thus reduce the transferring of encapsulated carotenoids to the aqueous phase. In addition, SLN and conventional emulsions could be stable in the gastric-phase digestion, but more destabilization was observed for the conventional emulsions than SLN in the duodenal-phase digestion (Nik et al., 2012).

Filled hydrogel (gelled emulsions)

A filled hydrogel particle consists of oil droplets trapped within a hydrogel particle that is dispersed in an aqueous medium. In a filled hydrogel, a gelling agent is usually employed to form gel network in the water phase of emulsions, and turn the liquid emulsions into soft solids, and oil droplets are immobilized in the gel networks (Dickinson, 2012). Gelled emulsions are effective in encapsulating and protecting nutrients against external stresses, and they have been used to deliver polyunsaturated fatty acids, carotenoids, curcumin, etc. (McClements, 2017).

It was reported that the chemical stability of carotenoid in O/W emulsions can be improved by trapping them within calcium alginate beads (Zhang, Zhang, & McClements, 2016). Hydrogel beads may also be able to control the digestive fate of carotenoids. For example, encapsulated carotenoid in O/W emulsions had higher bioaccessibility when incorporated into starch-based hydrogels, which was attributed to the ability of the hydrogels to inhibit excessive droplet flocculation in the stomach and small intestine, thereby allowing the lipase to access the lipid droplet surfaces more easily (Mun, Kim, & McClements, 2015). In another study, carotenoid-loaded emulsion droplets were trapped inside hydrogels formed by cross-linking of starch with sodium trimetaphosphate (Wang et al., 2015). The carotenoids were retained by the hydrogel beads within the mouth and stomach, but were released once they were exposed to the small intestine conditions. This property may be useful for protecting carotenoids from chemical degradation within the highly acid conditions of the stomach, since some carotenoids are known to degrade rapidly at low pH values (Qian et al., 2012a, 2012b).

Polysaccharides complexes

Inclusion complexes are widely used in medicine to improve the solubility, stability, and oral bioavailability of insoluble drugs, and decrease their toxicity and side effects (Polyakov & Kispert, 2015). Fundamental and applied research has recently been devoted to the inclusion complexes of carotenoids, and the incorporation of carotenoids into complexes formed by natural oligosaccharides and polysaccharides is assumed to protect and increase the solubility and stability of incorporated molecules.

Tachaprutinun, Udomsup, Luadthong, and Wanichwecharungruang (2009) reported that astaxanthin encapsulated into poly (ethylene oxide)-4-methoxycinnamoyl-phthaloyl chitosan complexes showed significantly decreased heat degradation after a 2-h heating process at 70°C in an aqueous environment compared with free carotenoid molecules without encapsulation, which were almost completely destroyed, suggesting that encapsulation of astaxanthin in chitosan-based complexes can obviously improve its thermal stability. Cyclodextrins (CD, Fig. 3B) can also be used to prepare carotenoids-cyclodextrin complexes that demonstrate enhanced storage stability (Yuan, Du, Jin, & Xu, 2013). However, the poor solubility of CD greatly influences their application in encapsulation and delivery of carotenoids. Therefore, many efforts have also been done on searching proper complexes and several water-soluble natural oligosaccharides or polysaccharides-based complexes for microencapsulation of carotenoids have been developed (Apanasenko et al., 2015; Polyakov et al., 2010; Polyakov, Magyar, & Kispert, 2013).

Among these, one of the promising compounds that can be used to form carotenoids complexes is β-glycyrrhizic acid (or glycyrrhizin, GA) (Fig. 3C). GA in solution can form cyclic structures (Fig. 3D) which can accommodate various lipophilic compounds (Polyakov & Leshina, 2011). GA becomes attractive for several reasons, for example, high stability of GA complexes, enhanced functionalities of entrapped compounds, or reduced side effects of encapsulated drugs (Polyakov & Kispert, 2015). Another natural biopolymer that can be used to form carotenoid complexes is arabinogalactan (AG, Fig. 3A), a branched polysaccharides with molecular weight of 13,000–16,000 Da, consisting of arabinose and galactose. AG shows very good water solubility and produces low-viscosity solutions, and it is also a FDA-approved important source of dietary fibers with potential therapeutic benefits as an immune-stimulating agent and cancer protocol adjunct. AG also acts as a potential prebiotic and can improve the proliferation of probiotics but eliminate harmful bacteria in gut (Polyakov & Kispert, 2015).

Many GA- or AG-based carotenoids complexes have been developed and the incorporation of carotenoids into these GA- or AG-based complexes can significantly improve the solubility and chemical stability of carotenoids. However, the antioxidant activity of carotenoids in the complexes is lower than free molecules due to the partially

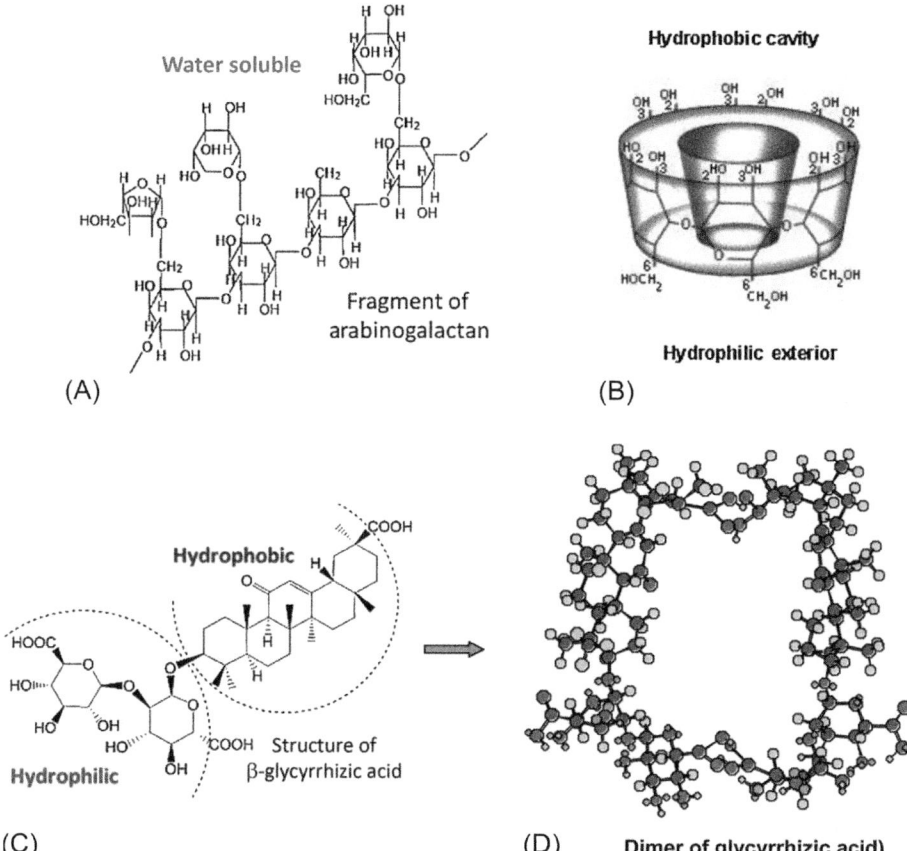

Fig. 3 The structures of arabinogalactan (A, fragment), cyclodextrin (B), β-glycyrrhizic acid (C), and schematic Chem3D Pro presentation of the suggested structures of the GA dimer (D). Arabinogalactan from the western and Siberian Larch produces low-viscosity solutions, and is approved by the US FDA as a source of dietary fiber, cancer protocol adjunct, and immune-stimulating agent. GA complexes demonstrate high stability, reduce side effects, and strengthen the therapeutic efficiency of various drugs. The GA "donut" forms a ring around the carotenoid "stick" (Polyakov and Kispert, 2015).

protection of the terminal groups from the reaction with free radicals (Polyakov & Kispert, 2015). The antioxidant of carotenoids in these complexes decreased with increasing concentration of GA or AG.

Drying process-based encapsulation

Liquid delivery systems, such as O/W emulsions, containing bioactive ingredients always have limited shelf life due to their destabilization during the storage, for example, creaming, flocculation, or coalescence. Their transportation and storage is also of high cost due to the fact that carotenoids in an aqueous dispersion are sensitive to the environmental conditions, for example, temperature, light, or heat. The dry forms of these delivery systems containing bioactive ingredients by different drying technologies (e.g., spray- or freeze-drying) were, therefore, developed with attempts of improving their self-life and lower the transportation and storage cost.

Drying process can also be used to encapsulate carotenoids and the assembly of surrounded compositions into solid particles due to the removing of water molecules during drying can be considered as an encapsulation process. Desobry et al. (1997) reported the encapsulation of β-carotene in maltodextrin (DE 25) by three drying processes, spray-, freeze-, and drum-drying. The drying method and storage temperature showed significant influence on the storage stability of β-carotene encapsulated in maltodextrin. The drum-dried powders showed the highest β-carotene preservation for all temperatures after 15 weeks storage (>47%), followed by freeze-dried, and spray-dried powders, respectively. The relative humidity (RH) of storage did not show significantly effect on the preservation of β-carotene. The slower degradation of encapsulated β-carotene in drum-dried powders is mainly attributed to their lower surface carotenoids and larger particle size as compared to the powders obtained by spray-, and freeze-drying methods.

They are also many other previous studies that produce encapsulated carotenoids by spray-drying or freeze-drying technologies, such as oleoresin, lutein, lycopene, or β-carotene (Ribeiro, Schuchmann, Engel, Walz, & Briviba, 2010). In these studies, encapsulated carotenoids were mainly prepared in two ways: (i) dissolved carotenoid molecules into a solution containing amphiphilic biopolymers, for example, proteins or polysaccharides. The mixture was then spray-dried or freeze-dried into powders; biopolymers that can be used to encapsulated carotenoids include maltodextrin, SC, soy bean proteins, pectin, or cellulose and (ii) first incorporated carotenoids into delivery carriers, for example, O/W emulsions, which was then mixed with wall materials (e.g., maltodextrin) and the mixture was applied to spray-drying or freeze-drying to obtain the final powders. Several biopolymers were usually used as wall materials in the drying process, such as gum, maltodextrin, gum arabic, cyclodextrin, native or modified starch, or gelatin. These encapsulated carotenoids in powders usually showed slow chemical degradation and thus potential extended shelf life, and the formulation of the powder and drying methods can significantly affect the properties of the powder and the storage stability of encapsulated carotenoids.

Carotenoids degradation

Bioactives such as carotenoids can undergo degradation during storage especially when exposed to elevated temperatures. The two main factors that affect reaction rates in food systems are temperature and water. Understanding the reaction kinetics is crucial to estimate stability and quality of food materials (Nelson & Labuza, 1994). Water activity was used to describe the impact of water on reaction rates and is a well-accepted approach in the prediction and control of food stability (Labuza, 1975). Glass transition was found to have an effect on the reaction rates of food systems (Meste, Champion, Roudaut, Blond, & Simatos, 2002) such as carotenoids degradation and the link between water and reaction rates can be defined using the glass transition approach (Nelson & Labuza, 1994). Storage of food below glass transition provides longer shelf life as lower diffusion rates in glassy state reduced reaction rates. Nonetheless, the consequence of glass transition on reaction rates is not well established in food processing (Roos, 2009). Changes that occur in food materials generally follow either zero- or first-order kinetics (Labuza & Riboh, 1982). The first-order reaction is described by Eq. (1) and the integrated Eq. (1) displays a linear relationship in a plot of ln C against t (2) where the change in concentration takes place exponentially with time in a first-order reaction and the rate constant, k, is defined by the slope of ln C against t plot (Roos, 1995). Temperature dependence of chemical reactions is commonly described with Arrhenius relationship (Glasstone, 1946). The Arrhenius relationship is shown as Eq. (3) and can be rewritten into the straight line form (4), where a plot of k against $1/T$ produces a straight line with a slope of E_a/R (Roos, 1995). It was established that the Arrhenius relationship is suitable to determine temperature dependence of reactions within the glassy state and 100°C above the T_g. Arrhenius kinetics, however, are not suitable to be used within the rubbery state (Slade, Levine, & Finley, 1989). Even though the Williams-Landel-Ferry (WLF) equation was deemed to be more applicable in determining temperature dependence of systems within the rubbery state, Arrhenius relationship is capable to predict changes in reaction rates within the rubbery state over a small temperature range (Nelson & Labuza, 1994). Arrhenius plot with data of up to 40°C below and above the T_g of nonenzymatic browning DMA in lactose/CMC/trehalose/xylose/lysine model system was found to be quite linear with r^2 of up to 0.999 by Karmas, Pilar Buera, and Karel (1992). Lievonen, Laaksonen, and Roos (1998) also reported r^2 of above 0.97 in the Arrhenius plots of nonenzymatic browning in various systems upon storage at temperatures approximately 15°C below and up to 35°C above the T_g.

$$-\frac{dC}{dt} = kC \tag{1}$$

$$\ln C = \ln C_0 - kt \tag{2}$$

$$k = k_0 e^{-\frac{E_a}{RT}} \tag{3}$$

$$\ln k = \ln k_0 - \frac{E_a}{RT} \tag{4}$$

Dissolving oil-soluble bioactives such as carotenoids in organic solution, for example, edible oil in the development of food products makes it less stable than naturally occurring carotenoids in tissues and these instability issues need to be addressed for successful utilization of carotenoids as nutraceutical in the food industry (Boon, McClements, Weiss, & Decker, 2010; Britton, 1995; Polyakov & Leshina, 2006). The degradation of carotenoids was found to follow first-order reaction in various studies (Achir, Randrianatoandro, Bohuon, Laffargue,

& Avallone, 2010; Desobry, Netto, & Labuza, 1999; Harnkarnsujarit et al., 2012; Henry, Catignani, & Schwartz, 1998; Hidalgo & Brandolini, 2008; Mahfoudhi & Hamdi, 2014) and the degradation rate increased with increasing storage temperature (Desobry et al., 1997; Lim et al., 2014; Spada, Noreña, Marczak, & Tessaro, 2012). Numerous factors such as temperature, type of carotenoids, physical state, reaction medium, and environmental conditions may affect degradation kinetics of carotenoids (Minguez-Mosquera & Jaren-Galan, 1995; Pesek & Warthesen, 1988). Free radicals can be found in food materials as the result of reactions such as lipid oxidation (Choe & Min, 2006) that is capable of causing degradation of the carotenoids present through electron transfer, hydrogen transfer, and formation of carotenoids-radical adducts (Britton, 1995; Mortensen, 2002; Young & Lowe, 2001). Carotenoids when exposed to heat in the presence of oxygen also showed degradation and formed volatile and larger nonvolatile compounds (Bonnie & Choo, 1999). Exposure of carotenoids to heat and light was found to cause isomerization of the unstable all-trans β-carotene to cis-isomers by Khoo, Prasad, Kong, Jiang, and Ismail (2011). Chandler and Schwartz (1988) also reported that carotenoids degradation is usually the consequence of isomerization rather than decomposition in the study on the effect of processing treatment on trans-β-carotene in sweet potatoes. Electron transfer from neutral carotenoids to radicals or metal ions produced carotenoids radical cations (Car•$^{+}$) or carotenoids radical dications (Car^{2+}) capable of isomerizing to different *cis*-species. Electron transfer plays a role in carotenoids isomerization to produce cations with lower configural transformation energy barriers than neutral carotenoids (Gao, Wei, Jeevarajan, & Kispert, 1996; Wei, Gao, & Kispert, 1997). Chandler and Schwartz (1988), Chen, Chen, and Chien (1994), and Henry et al. (1998) reported that heating of all-trans-β-carotene resulted in isomerization producing 13-cis-β-carotene, 15-cis-β-carotene, and 9-cis-β-carotene with 13-cis-β-carotene found in the largest quantity. The increase in 13-cis-β-carotene occurred simultaneously with the decrease in all-trans-β-carotene in the study by Henry et al. (1998). Carotenoids radicals too can react with other radicals to form nonradical products in low oxygen condition (Beutner et al., 2001; Burton & Ingold, 1984; Foti & Amorati, 2009).

Carotenoids stability in food systems

Nonetheless, numerous studies have found that lipid oxidation and loss of encapsulated bioactives were reduced in spray-dried system (Aberkane, Roudaut, & Saurel, 2014; Jiménez-Martín, Gharsallaoui, Pérez-Palacios, Carrascal, & Rojas, 2015; Shaw, McClements, & Decker, 2007), freeze-dried system (Klinkesorn, Sophanodora, Chinachoti, McClements, & Decker, 2005) as well as extrudates (Caliskan, Lim, & Roos, 2015) with the application of LBL interfacial structuring. LBL systems possessed multiple layers of coatings on the oil droplets through electrostatic attraction of oppositely charged secondary layer around the charged emulsifier primary layer (McClements, 2010). Fig. 4 shows the differences between conventional SL system and LBL system at the oil-water interfacial layer. Lim

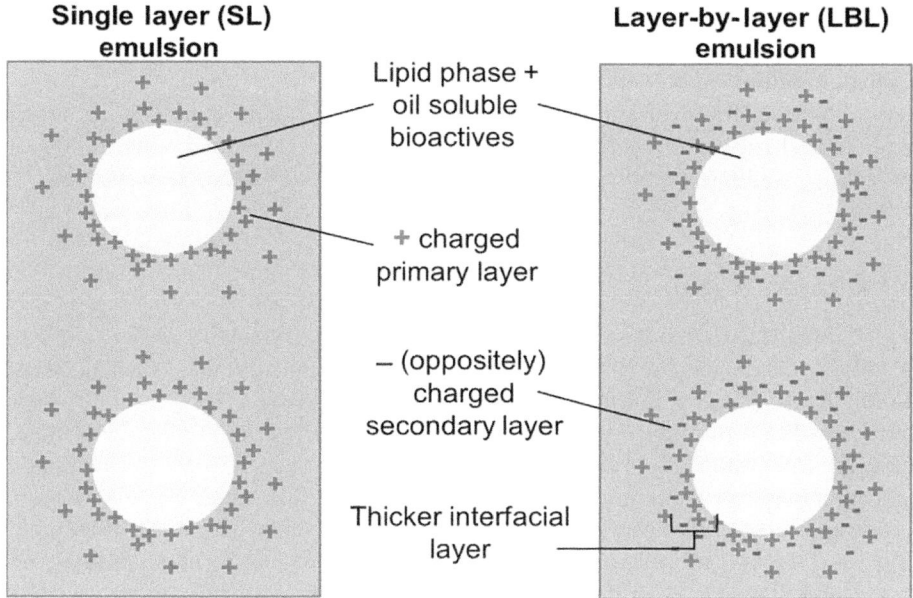

Fig. 4 Schematic diagram showing the components of oil-in-water (O/W) and the difference in interfacial layer between single-layer (SL) and layer-by-layer (LBL) emulsions.

and Roos (2016) and Lim and Roos (2017) reported in two separate studies that the degradation of lutein and all-trans-β-carotene was less rapid in LBL systems than in SL systems based on the rate constants in both freeze-dried and spray-dried materials with trehalose-maltodextrin as wall materials. Properties of the LBL interfacial layer reduced reaction rate as the thicker interfacial layer provided a better physical barrier to give an improved protection to the encapsulated lipid phase (Klinkesorn et al., 2005; Shaw et al., 2007). The thicker interfacial layer at the oil-water interface was assumed to be more efficient in minimizing diffusion of transition metal ions toward the oil phase (Aberkane et al., 2014) that can reduce the degradation of the encapsulated carotenoids.

Water activity

Water activity of dehydrated food systems may have an effect on the encapsulated carotenoids. Lipid oxidation was minimal in dehydrated systems with a_w of approximately 0.3 a_w but oxidation increased below and above 0.3 a_w in agreement with the stability map of foods (Labuza, 1971; Labuza, Cassil, & Sinskey, 1972). Labuza and Dugan Jr. (1971) proposed that the protective effect of water was due to water interaction with metal catalyst reducing their effectiveness as the result of transformation of the coordination sphere as well as bonding of water hydrogen with hydrogen peroxides to prevent initiation of decomposition reactions. Reduction in lipid oxidation of food systems was observed around a_w of the water monolayer, usually between 0.2 and $0.4a_w$ in studies of Karel, Labuza, and Maloney (1967) and Labuza

(1968). Velasco, Dobarganes, and Márquez-Ruiz (2003) attributed the role of a_w to the reduction of transition metals' prooxidant activity, higher free radicals and singlet oxygen quenching, as well as the delay in hydroperoxide decomposition. The reduction in lipid oxidation can translate to the reduced degradation of carotenoids in the oil phase at $0.3a_w$ that gives the lower degradation rate in agreement with finding of Lim and Roos (2016) that reported less rapid carotenoids degradation in systems humidified to $0.33a_w$.

Dehydrated matrix

Degradation of carotenoids was found to be more rapid in freeze-dried system than in spray-dried system in two separate studies by the same authors (Mahfoudhi & Hamdi, 2014, 2015). Lim and Roos (2016) also reported ln k value of approximately $-3\,\mathrm{day}^{-1}$ for freeze-dried emulsions with trehalose-maltodextrin at 65°C while the ln k value of spray-dried emulsion with similar a_w, glass formers, and storage temperature were much lower of about $-6\,\mathrm{day}^{-1}$. Freeze-drying gave a more porous and less dense structure than spray-drying (Fig. 5) which may allow rapid diffusion of metal ions or oxygen toward the encapsulated carotenoids that can cause faster degradation of the carotenoids. However, the formation of air vacuoles in spray-dried particles is also frequently observed (Aguilera & Stanley, 1999; Bae & Lee, 2008; Keogh et al., 2001; Klinkesorn, Sophanodora, Chinachoti, Decker, & McClements, 2006; Soottitantawat et al., 2005). Air vacuoles are formed as a result of thermal expansion of trapped air bubbles in the liquid feed and air bubbles formed during atomization in spray-drying (Duffie & Marshall, 1953; Verhey, 1972). Trapped oxygen within the spray-dried particles is capable of accelerating degradation of encapsulated bioactives. Such reactions are commonly observed as rapid initial degradation of the encapsulated oil-soluble biaoctives in spray-dried materials (Desobry et al., 1997, 1999; Jimenez, Garcia, & Beristain, 2004; Lim & Roos, 2017).

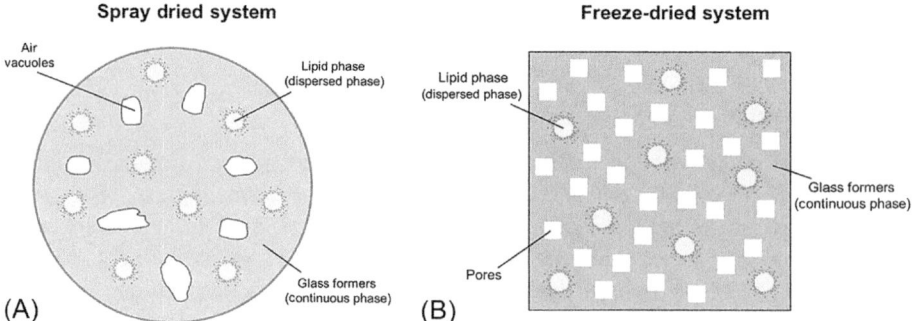

Fig. 5 Schematic diagram of a spray-dried particle (A) showing the dispersed phase and trapped air vacuoles within the continuous phase and a freeze-dried material (B) showing the dispersed phase and high amount of pores present within the continuous phase giving a more porous structure.

Wall materials

Wall materials used for encapsulation play a role in the stability of the encapsulated bioactives. The higher occluded air in system with protein as wall material than in carbohydrate only can contribute toward the higher degradation rate of carotenoids. Carneiro, Tonon, Grosso, and Hubinger (2013) reported that powders with maltodextrin-whey protein concentrate mixture as wall materials has the lowest bulk density that indicated highest amount of occluded air. The higher amount of occluded air represents a system with higher amount of trapped oxygen that can cause increased oxidation of the encapsulated carotenoids and faster degradation rate. The wall materials used will also affect particle density of the dehydrated systems as density will be higher in systems with carbohydrate wall materials than protein. Increasing the amount of lactose in WPI-lactose spray-dried systems was found to increase density and reduce porosity of powders by Moreau and Rosenberg (1999). The higher density of carbohydrate wall materials can delay migration of oxygen and metal ions toward the encapsulated carotenoids that improves encapsulation of oil-soluble bioactives. The degradation rate and retention of carotenoids was found to be less rapid and higher respectively in spray-dried emulsions with carbohydrate only (trehalose-maltodextrin) as wall materials than in emulsions with carbohydrate-protein mixture (trehalose-WPI) as wall material in several studies by Lim and Roos (2016), Lim, Burdikova, Sheehan, and Roos (2016), and Lim and Roos (2017).

The use of carbohydrate and protein as wall materials can also result in the discontinuity of the wall materials due to the presence of the surface-active protein such as whey protein. Study by Fäldt and Bergenståhl (1994) showed that the surface-active protein predominated on the surface of carbohydrate-protein particles. The surface-active protein tends to migrate to the surface (air-water interface) of the droplets during spray-drying due to its high surface activity to give a protein-rich layer (Adhikari, Howes, Bhandari, & Langrish, 2009; Wang, Jiang, & Zhou, 2013). The presence of a thin layer of WPI at the hydrophilic-hydrophobic interfaces at the surface of the powder particle and around the air vacuoles in spray-dried emulsion with trehalose-WPI mixtures as wall materials was observed by Lim et al. (2016) using Raman-focused ion beam (FIB)-scanning electron microscope (SEM) analysis. Therefore, carotenoids containing oil droplets will be encapsulated within the glass former and nonglass former in carbohydrate-protein system. The lesser amount of the denser carbohydrate glass formers to encapsulate bioactives in the carbohydrate-protein systems can result in the increased degradation rate of carotenoids.

However, carbohydrate glass formers used as wall materials can undergo dynamic process of structural collapse governed by the rate of $T - T_g$ at storage temperatures above the T_g (Levi & Karel, 1995). Storage of materials above T_g will decrease viscosity and increase molecular mobility within the solids (Roos & Karel, 1991a). Structural collapse results in the harder and denser carbohydrate glass that can improve protection of the encapsulated carotenoids. The reduced degradation of encapsulated bioactives in collapsed dehydrated systems was observed in the studies of Selim, Tsimidou, and Biliaderis (2000) and Harnkarnsujarit and Charoenrein (2011). Prado, Buera, and Elizalde (2006) and Harnkarnsujarit et al. (2012) postulated that the improved stability of encapsulated bioactives in collapsed systems was due to the reduction in oxygen permeability across the collapsed matrix with significantly reduced micropores. Besides, the presence of reducing sugar (maltodextrin, lactose) and protein amino groups (milk proteins) in dehydrated system and heat from the environment can result in Maillard reaction. Maillard reaction generates melanoidins that possesses antioxidant capacity (Wang, Qian, & Yao, 2011). Melanoidins generated thus can give protection to the encapsulated bioactives against attack from oxygen or metal ion present that will reduce degradation of the bioactives.

Carotenoids type

Carotenoids can be classified into carotenoids without oxygen, also known as carotenes, and carotenoids with oxygen as xanthophylls (McClements et al., 2007). The presence of two hydroxyl groups results in increased hydrophilicity and polarity of lutein (Farombi & Britton, 1999; Updike & Schwartz, 2003). Therefore, encapsulated lutein tends to assemble at the interface of the oil droplets, while all-trans-β-carotene is likely to remain in the bulk oil (Fig. 6). Lutein at the interface of the oil droplets can act as antioxidant to the diffusing oxygen or metal ions trapped within the wall materials resulting in rapid degradation of lutein. Degradation of lutein was predominantly more rapid than degradation of all-trans-β-carotene in both spray-dried and freeze-dried system with trehalose-maltodextrin as wall materials found in the study of Lim and Roos (2016). Lim et al. (2016) also confirmed the presence of lutein in large quantities at the interfaces that may have acted as antioxidant, while all-trans-β-carotene was dissolved within the bulk oil and only found in small quantities at the surface of a cut spray-dried particle using the combination of Raman-FIB-SEM microscopy techniques. On the

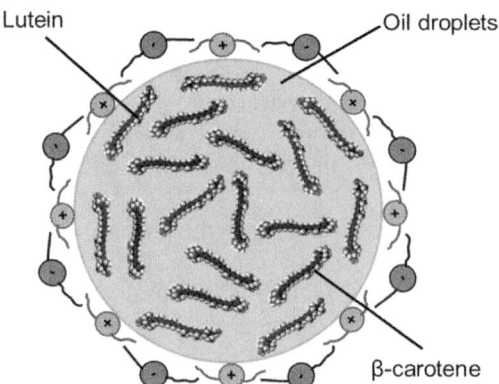

Fig. 6 Location of lutein (at in the interface) and β-carotene (in the bulk oil) dissolved and encapsulated within an oil droplet.

other hand, retention of lutein can be higher than retention of all-trans-β-carotene upon long-term storage. All-trans-β-carotene was found to readily convert into cis-isomers during thermal treatment rather than undergoing decomposition that result in total loss of β-carotene by Chandler and Schwartz (1988). Lim et al. (2014) also found higher retention of lutein than all-trans-β-carotene upon storage that was attributed to the isomerization of all-trans-β-carotene to 15-cis-β-carotene and 13-cis-β-carotene.

Glass transition, water plasticization, and α-relaxations

Physical state of a material controlling by surrounding conditions (temperature, pressure, etc.) according to its thermodynamic properties. Typically, simple one-component systems can exist as crystalline solids, liquid, and gas. The deep comprehensive studies of material properties (thermal conductivity, apparent viscosity, heat capacity, etc.) proposed the glassy state of materials as the fourth state of matter, distinct from the liquid and crystalline states (Parks & Huffman, 1927). Although such definition is not valid, any material under certain conditions (rapid condensation of vapor; quench cooling of a liquid (melt); rapid removal of solvent from solution; and removal of crystallized solvent) may enter a nonequilibrium solid in the glassy state (Maidannyk, 2017; Roos, 2008; Roos & Karel, 1991a, 1991b; Slade et al., 1991; Sperling, 2005).

Despite the fact that definition of glass transition is not clear and its characteristics are continuously discussed (Angell, 2002), it is well known that at the glassy state materials have higher thermodynamic parameters (viscosity, entropy, enthalpy, free volume, etc.) than at their equilibrium state in the same conditions. During heating to above the temperature, named the glass transition temperature (T_g), materials soften over the transition region from amorphous solids (e.g., glass) to supercooled liquid (e.g., rubber) and display dramatic change in physical properties (decrease of viscosity, increase of molecular mobility, and rapid decrease in structural relaxation time) (Angell et al., 2000; Levine & Slade, 1986; Williams, Landel, & Ferry, 1955). However, these changes are not obvious at the molecular level and materials stay topologically disordered both in the liquid and glassy state (Casalini & Roland, 2007). The glass transition usually occurs at about 100–150°C below equilibrium melting temperature (T_m) of a material (Fig. 7) (Roos, 2008). It is generally considered that liquid during cooling becomes a glass at a viscosity value 10^{12} Pa s (10^{13} P) or where relaxation time is 10^2 s (Kittel & Holcomb, 1967; Maidannyk, 2017; Ojovan & Lee, 2006).

At the liquid-glass transition (e.g., glass transition), the first derivatives of the free energy as volume, enthalpy, and entropy are continuous quantities, but the second derivatives as specific heat, compressibility, and thermal expansion coefficient manifest anomalous jumps. That means that glass transitions do not involve change in the phase but involve a change in the state of amorphous material (Roos, 2008). According to Ehrenfest (1933), glass transitions are reversible second-order (e.g., continuous) phase transitions. Mathematically, the second-order phase transition

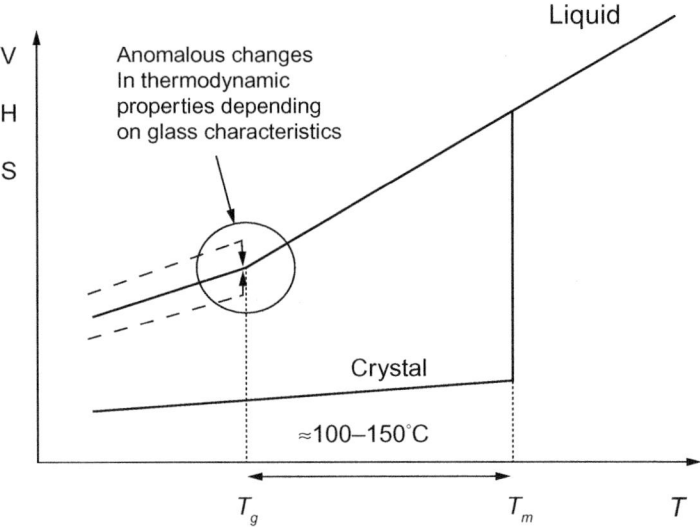

Fig. 7 Changes in physical properties (V—specific volume, H—enthalpy, and S—entropy) around glass transition and melting (Roos, 2008).

can describe the temperature behavior of the specific heat (e.g., heat capacity) (C_p) near the T_g by Landau equation (Eq. 5) in a simple form (Landau & Lifshitz, 1984; Ojovan & Lee, 2006):

$$C_p(T) \propto \frac{1}{|T - T_g|^\alpha} \tag{5}$$

where α is the universal critical exponent.

If materials exist in nonequilibrium glassy state, they exhibit thermodynamically driving force toward the equilibrium crystalline state. Materials in glassy state have time-dependent properties; thereby they cannot be described only in thermodynamic terms (Roos, 2008). Water may act as plasticizer and solvent in different amorphous materials. Water plasticization refers to the presence and interaction of water molecules within solid materials, resulting in changes of amorphous structure and significant decrease of T_g (Roos, 2008). For high water content systems (>50 g/100 g of dry solids), the determination of T_g is practically very difficult. For these aqueous systems, the Gordon-Taylor equation (Eq. 6) can predict T_g values shows the relationship between water content and T_g (Arvanitoyannis, Blanshard, Izzard, Lillford, & Ablett, 1993):

$$T_g = \frac{w_1 T_{g1} + k w_2 T_{g2}}{w_1 + k w_2} \tag{6}$$

where w_1 and w_2 are the mass fraction of amorphous material and water, T_{g1} and T_{g2} are glass transition temperatures, respectively, and k is a constant, $T_{g2} = -135°C$ (Angell, 2002) is the glass transition of water.

Due to chemical composition of carotenoids and their possibilities to dissolving in oil phase, in this work T_g of carbohydrate-protein systems contained different amount of lipids were compared. Typically, the presence of lipids very slightly increasing T_g of anhydrous carbohydrate-protein systems due to high protecting effect of trehalose on protein structures and possible proteins effect of anhydrous systems by hydrogen bonding to carbohydrate molecules (López-Díez and Bone, 2004; Maidannyk & Roos, 2016; Zhou & Roos, 2012). However, T_g are almost lipids independent with systems contained significant amount of water (Fig. 8), that were reported by many authors (Levine & Slade, 1986; Lim & Roos, 2018; Roos and Karel, 1991a, 1991b; Silalai & Roos, 2011). Fig. 8A shows that T_g occurred only in the nonfat solids components and T_g values closely followed the carbohydrate component of system at whole a_w range (Maidannyk & Roos, 2016; Maidannyk et al., 2018; Zhou & Roos, 2012).

Structural α-relaxations usually occur in amorphous systems at temperatures close to the calorimetric T_g (Champion, Le Meste, & Simatos, 2000; Roudaut, Simatos, Champion, Contreras-Lopez, & Le Meste, 2004). α-Relaxation temperatures ($T\alpha$) can be obtained from the peak temperature of dielectric loss (ε'') and dynamic tan δ [tan $\delta = E''/E'$, where E''—loss modulus (mechanical energy dissipation) and E'—storage modulus (mechanical energy storage)] of dielectric and dynamic mechanical analyses. Both DMA and DEA spectra are frequency dependent, which allows obtaining the relaxation time-temperature dependence for amorphous systems (Eq. 7) (Fan & Roos, 2016a, 2016b; Maidannyk & Roos, 2016, 2017, 2018; Potes, Kerry, & Roos, 2012; Silalai & Roos, 2011).

$$\tau = \frac{1}{2\pi f} \tag{7}$$

where τ is the structural relaxation time and f the frequency of DMA and DEA machines.

Peak of $T\alpha$ typically occurred at ~20–30°C above the onset T_g for the DMA measurements and up to ~60–70°C above the onset T_g for the DEA measurements. Systems with higher amount of lipids showed significantly broadened and less intensive DMA and DEA peaks compared to the system without lipid phase. For anhydrous samples,

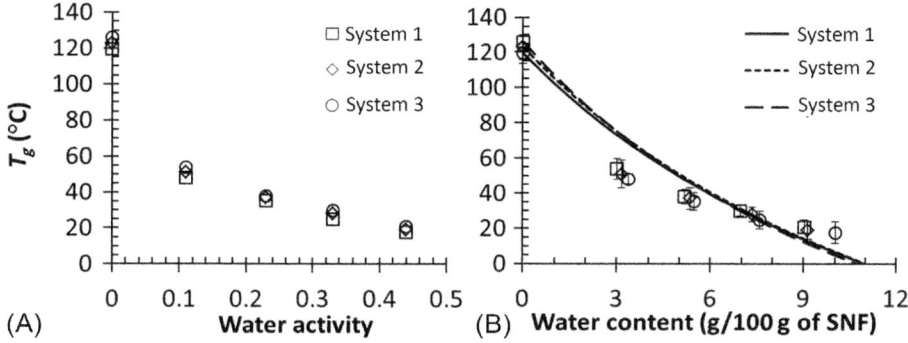

Fig. 8 Effects of water activity (A) and water content (g/100g of SNF) (B) on the onset T_g in anhydrous and humidified trehalose-WPI-SO systems 1 (0% of sunflower oil), 2 (10% of sunflower oil), and 3 (20% of sunflower oil) stored for 360h at 25±2°C. Lines correspond to the T_g predicted by Gordon-Taylor equation (Maidannyk et al., 2018).

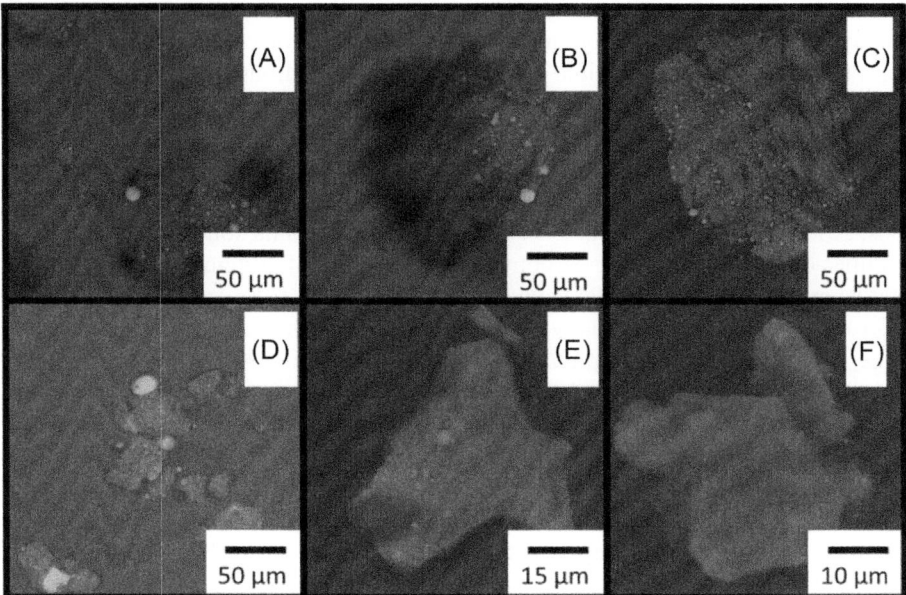

Fig. 9 Confocal scanning laser micrographs of showing internal microstructures of anhydrous trehalose-WPI-sunflower oil (10%) system (A–C) and trehalose-WPI-sunflower oil (20%) system (D–F). Figures are fluorescently labeled with Fast gray/Nile dark gray to show fat (gray) and protein (dark gray) (Maidannyk et al., 2018).

at all frequencies, $T\alpha$ slightly decreased with increasing fat content in the system, which could be caused by significant difference on powders surface composition (lubricant effect) which is in agreement with microscopies observations (Figs. 9 and 10) (Maidannyk et al., 2018). Carbohydrates may act as filler in the dry matrix which surround lipids droplets. Also, free fat and fat droplets had the lower values of diffusion coefficients than carbohydrates and protein hence they remained at the surface (Figs. 9 and 10) (Vignolles, Jeantet, Lopez, & Schuck, 2007). However, for humidified systems, the opposite effect has been observed, which is probably caused by the plasticizing effect in amorphous systems. $T\alpha$ in all systems was found to decrease with increasing water content (Maidannyk et al., 2018). Free-volume theory may explain all of these changes in systems, which shows that increasing free volume and molecular mobility significantly affected the T_g and $T\alpha$ of amorphous sugar in a complex system (Maidannyk et al., 2018; Meinders & van Vliet, 2009; Royall et al., 2005; Slade et al., 1991).

WLF modeling and strength

The WLF equation (Eq. 8) is one of the models, describing dependence of relaxation time and viscosity on the temperature. Originally, this relation showed that inorganic and organic glass materials possessed similar decreases in relaxation times and viscosity

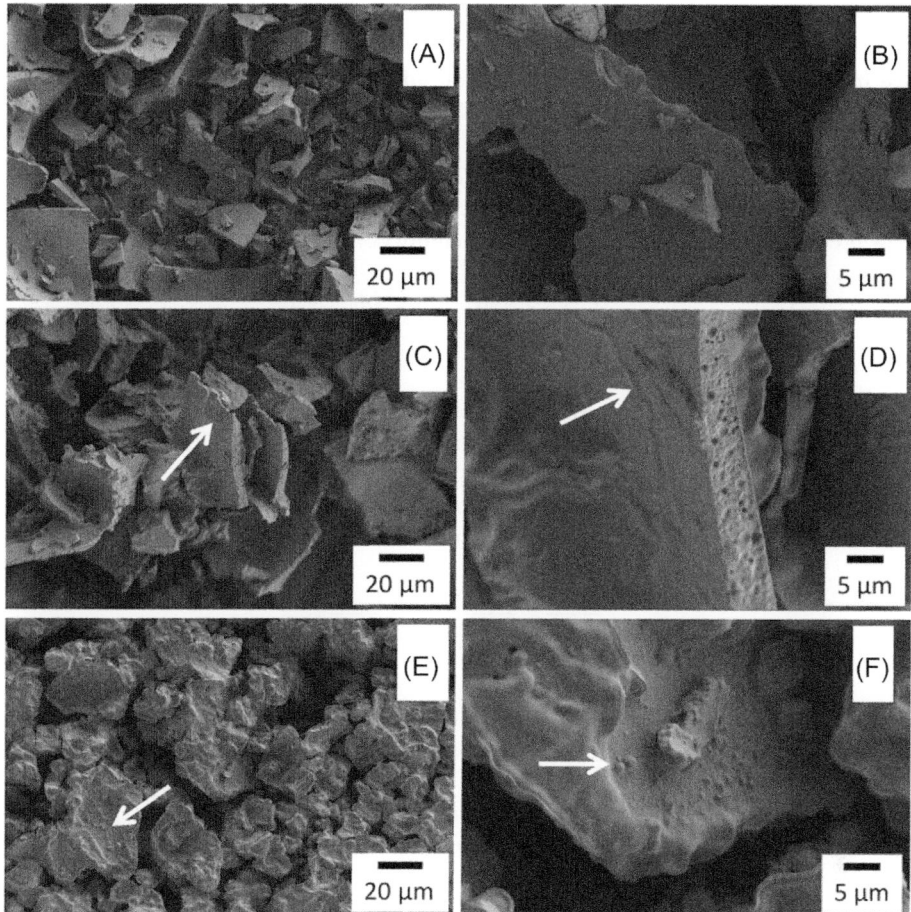

Fig. 10 Scanning electron micrographs of anhydrous trehalose-WPI-sunflower oil (0%) system (A, B), trehalose-WPI-sunflower oil (10%) system (C, D), and trehalose-WPI-sunflower oil (20%) system (E, F). Images shows powder particle surface morphology (a, c, e) and interior features of fractured particles (b, d, f). Arrows indicate fat globules and fat droplets (Maidannyk et al., 2018).

over the temperature range of T_g to $T_g + 100$ K. Williams et al. (1955) offered "universal" values for WLF constants: $C_1 = 17.44$ and $C_2 = 51.6$ and suggested their use for a wide range of materials. However, many authors (Ferry, 1980; Peleg, 1992; Roos and Drusch, 2015) advised against the use of these "universal" coefficients and suggested to determine the real constants for each system using experimental data (Eq. 5). The WLF relationship is often used to define mobility in terms of the non-Arrhenius temperature behavior of structural relaxation processes at temperatures above the T_g. WLF relationship uses structural relaxation times at a reference temperature and the corresponding relaxation time above the glass transition (T_s) (at a certain conditions: $T_s = T_g$ (Peleg, 1992; Roos and Drusch, 2015; Williams et al., 1955). Numerous studies have reported a good fit of the WLF model with unfixed constants to experimental data at temperatures above the T_g (Peleg, 1992; Peleg & Chinachoti, 1996; Slade & Levine, 1995). However, the extrapolation of the WLF equation to the range around s, proposes nonrealistic fit for systems (Peleg & Chinachoti, 1996). The use of calculated C_1 and C_2 constants gives WLF plot matching the experimental data, but does not allow predicting system behavior under changing conditions (Maidannyk, 2017).

$$\log_{10}\frac{\tau}{\tau_s} = \log_{10}\frac{\eta}{\eta_s} = -\frac{C_1\left(T - T_g\right)}{C_2 + \left(T - T_g\right)} \tag{8}$$

where τ is the relaxation time, τ_s the reference relaxation time, η the viscosity, η_s the reference viscosity, T the temperature, T_g the glass transition temperature, and C_1 and C_2 are the constants.

To fit C_1 and C_2 to experimental data, the WLF equation may be used in the form (Eq. 8). It suggests that the plot of $1/\lg(\tau/\tau_s)$ vs $1/(T - T_g)$ gives a straight line:

$$\frac{1}{\lg\dfrac{\tau}{\tau_s}} = \frac{1}{-C_1} - \frac{C_2}{C_1\left(T - T_g\right)} \tag{9}$$

Angell (1991) introduced classification of glass formers to "fragile" and "strong" structures. According to his model, viscosity or structural relaxation times of "strong" glass formers above T_g followed the Arrhenius relationship, while "fragile" materials showed non-Arrhenius characteristics near T_g. This concept allowed classifying materials according to the plot of viscosity (or structural relaxation time) vs T_g/T (Angell, 2002). However, a plot of T_g/T varies according to the differences in T_g values, while the same $T - T_g$ value often shows similar viscosity (or relaxation time). Thus, this concept applies only for materials with the same T_g and T_g/T plot cannot explain variations in structural relaxation times (or viscosities) above the T_g (Maidannyk & Roos, 2017; Roos, 2013).

Roos et al. (2015) introduced a *"strength" parameter* as a measure of variations in structural relaxation times. This parameter or *flow characteristics* of the glass formers and their interactions with other solids contribute to noncrystalline solids characteristic. Fig. 11 shows that for systems upon heating, critical and large variation in the structural relaxation time occurred between 100 and 0.01 s (between 2 and −2 in logarithmic scale).

The temperature difference, $T - T_g$, at which structural relaxation times exceed time factors critical to processing characteristics of the materials (e.g., particle stickiness in spray-drying) was defined as "strength" parameter S (Eq. 10).

$$S = \frac{dC_2}{C_1 - d} \tag{10}$$

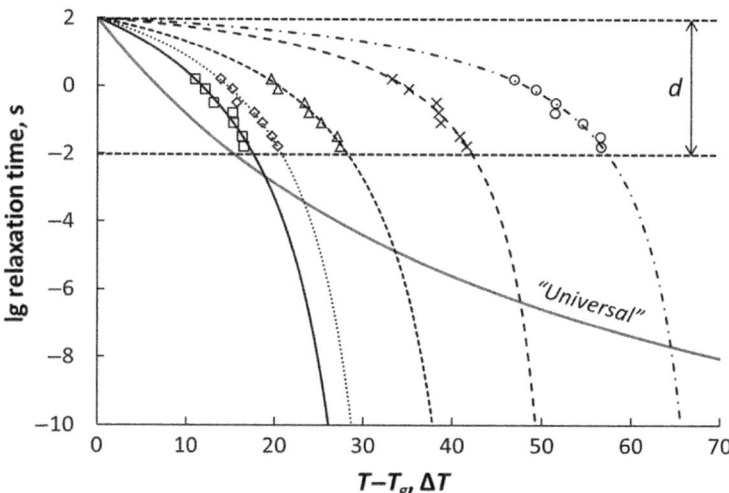

Fig. 11 "Universal" (with a fixed C_1 and C_2 constant) and calculated WLF curves (lines) and experimental data (symbols) for anhydrous trehalose-WPI mixtures (100:0, 80:20, 60:40, 40:60, 20:80) (Maidannyk & Roos, 2016).

where d is a parameter, showing the critical decrease in the number of logarithmic decades for the flow (e.g., 100–0.01 s corresponds to $d=4$; can be chosen for each system as an integer depending on the critical time for the process (Fig. 11), C_1 and C_2 are "nonuniversal" constants in the WLF equation.

Fig. 12 shows that water, as a good plasticizer, significantly decreases strength of the system. Water is one of key factor for controlling properties, processes, and storage stability for many food and pharmaceutical products (Liu, Bhandari, & Zhou, 2006). Previous studies (Fan & Roos, 2016a, 2016b; Maidannyk et al., 2017) developed an equation (Eq. 11) for interpreting the relationship between water content and strength parameters. Such relationship was also applied for describing the influence on strength and water content of each encapsulated system and achieved a very good-fitting performance (Fig. 11).

$$S = \frac{w_1 S_1 + k w_2 S_2}{w_1 + k w_2} \tag{11}$$

where w_1 is the weight fraction of dry solid; w_2 the weight fraction of water; k the coefficient; S_1 the structural strength for anhydrous system; and S_2 is the structural strength of pure water ($S_2 = 6.0$) (Maidannyk et al., 2017).

System with the low amount of lipids has more "strong" properties compared to the "weak" systems with high lipids content. Very big difference in strength values ($\sim 20°$) was observed between anhydrous (RH 0%) systems with 0% of lipid and 20% of lipids (Fig. 13), that is in agreement with microscopy observation (Figs. 9 and 10). Lipid presented on particle surface as free fat drops and fat globules may act as a lubricant

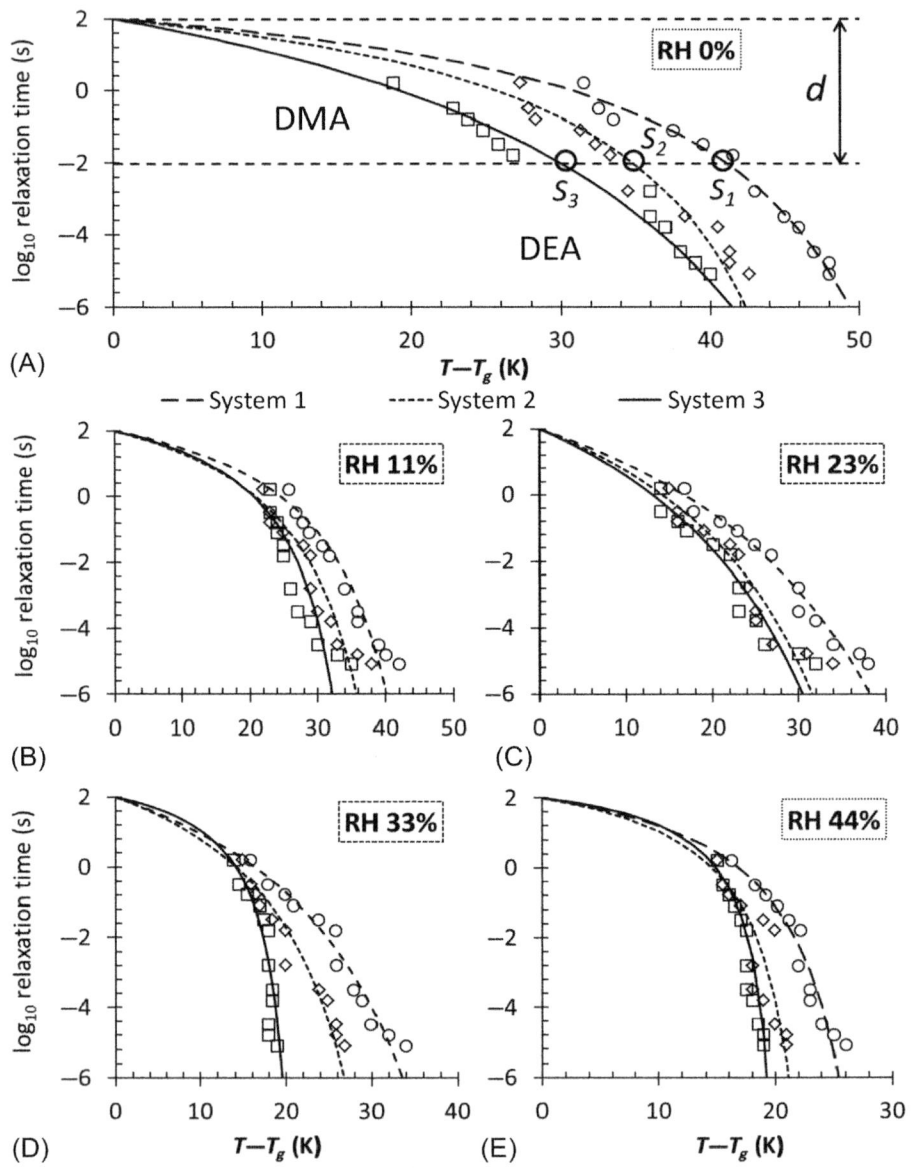

Fig. 12 Modified WLF curves (lines) and experimental data (symbols) for
(1) trehalose-WPI-sunflower oil (0%) system, (2) trehalose-WPI-sunflower oil (10%) system,
and (3) trehalose-WPI-sunflower oil (10%) system (20% of sunflower oil) stored for 360 h
at various relative humidity [0% (A), 11% (B), 23% (C), 33% (D), and 44% (E)] at $25 \pm 1°C$
(Maidannyk et al., 2018).

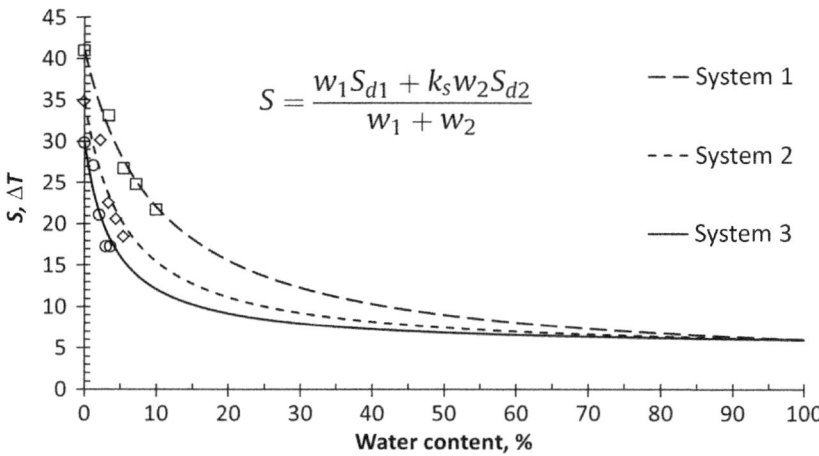

Fig. 13 Modeled by Eq. (8) (lines) and experimental (symbols) S (1) trehalose-WPI-sunflower oil (0%) system, (2) trehalose-WPI-sunflower oil (10%) system, and (3) trehalose-WPI-sunflower oil (20%) system at the different water contents (Maidannyk et al., 2018).

and affect mechanical characteristics and electrical conductivity, that reduces overall strength of the system (Maidannyk et al., 2018). It means that in systems with low amount of lipids, structural relaxation times achieved a critical level at lower temperatures than in carbohydrate-protein systems.

Strength vs degradation of carotenoids

The difference in the S of the wall materials was found to follow differences in degradation rates of carotenoids. The degradation of carotenoids was less rapid in system with a higher S (Lim & Roos, 2018). Also, in the rapid initial degradation step upon near the T_g, non-Arrhenian temperature dependence in the degradation of lutein and all-trans-β-carotene were observed (Lim & Roos, 2018). Structural collapse may occur in glass former materials during storage above or in the vicinity of the calorimetric T_g (Levi & Karel, 1995). Such collapse contributed toward the non-Arrenian temperature dependence of carotenoids degradation. The S values of carbohydrate-protein matrixes may be correlated with structural collapse of the systems. The higher S resulting from a structural collapse may be explained by oxygen diffusion delay and metal ions migration toward the carotenoid containing oil which thereby reducing carotenoids degradation rate (Lim & Roos, 2018).

Degradation of carotenoids is related to S values of the systems with different carbohydrate-protein matrixes (Fig. 14). Carbohydrates and proteins may show a phase-separated structure which can enhance migration of oxygen or metal ions toward the carotenoids containing oil phase and increasing degradation of the carotenoids. Also comparison of S and $T-T_g$ values showed that S of the systems played more important role in reducing degradation of the encapsulated carotenoids (Lim & Roos, 2018).

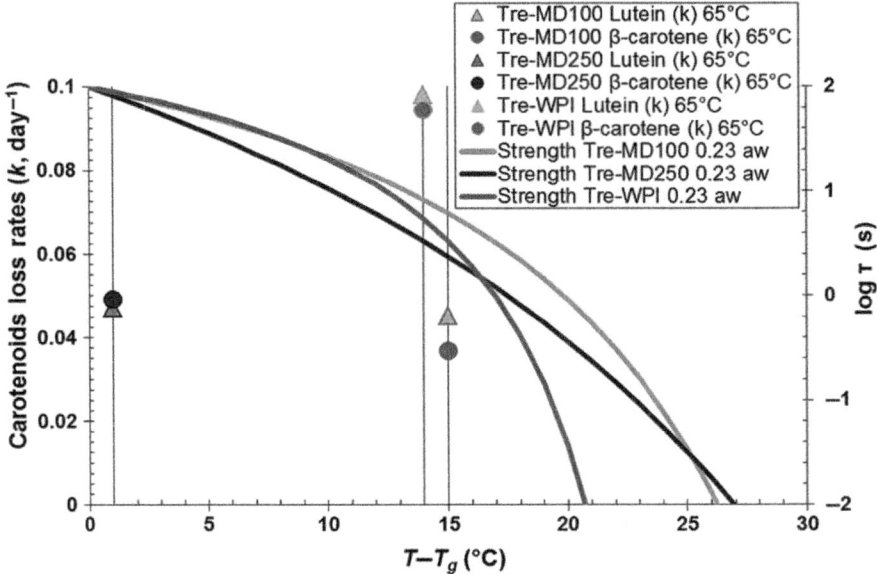

Fig. 14 Structural strength of the solids having trehalose-maltodextrin (M100), trehalose-maltodextrin (M250), and trehalose-whey protein isolate (WPI) mixtures as glass formers at 0.23 a_w and the degradation rates of lutein and all-trans-β-carotene encapsulated in layer-by-layer powders upon storage at 65°C (Lim & Roos, 2018).

Conclusion

Many food-derived bioactives such as carotenoids are water insoluble and sensitive to the environmental stresses, namely pH, temperature, heat, and light. The delivery of these molecules, therefore, needs a protective mechanism with the utilization of microencapsulation and delivery technology. Incorporation of carotenoids into different delivery carriers, such as liposomes, structured emulsions, polysaccharides complexes, or powders, can significantly improve their solubility and chemical stability and thus extend their shelf life. In addition, encapsulated carotenoids usually showed much better oral bioavailability than free molecules, and a potential controlled release of carotenoids can also be achieved by structuring the delivery carriers. The microencapsulation and delivery technologies certainly will contribute to a better and faster development of carotenoids-based functional foods. The application of LBL interfacial structuring in O/W emulsions used as delivery system may further improve stability of the encapsulated oil-soluble bioactives. Dehydration of the LBL system by either freeze-drying or spray-drying provides microencapsulation of the bioactives within glassy matrix for improved protection. Stability of the encapsulated carotenoids can be influenced by water activity of the dehydrated system, dehydration method, wall materials used, and carotenoids type. Structural changes associated with glass transition such as structural collapse also changes properties of the glass formers that can be beneficial toward the encapsulated bioactives. Strength parameter

(*S*) developed gave "strength" of amorphous food systems and can be used to predict the loss of encapsulated carotenoids. *S* was affected by numerous factors such as water content, wall materials, and encapsulated materials and can be manipulated to provide optimum protection of the encapsulated carotenoids.

References

Aberkane, L., Roudaut, G., & Saurel, R. (2014). Encapsulation and oxidative stability of PUFA-rich oil microencapsulated by spray drying using pea protein and pectin. *Food and Bioprocess Technology*, *7*(5), 1505–1517.

Achir, N., Randrianatoandro, V. A., Bohuon, P., Laffargue, A., & Avallone, S. (2010). Kinetic study of β-carotene and lutein degradation in oils during heat treatment. *European Journal of Lipid Science and Technology*, *112*(3), 349–361.

Adhikari, B., Howes, T., Bhandari, B. R., & Langrish, T. A. G. (2009). Effect of addition of proteins on the production of amorphous sucrose powder through spray drying. *Journal of Food Engineering*, *94*(2), 144–153.

Aguilera, J. M., & Stanley, D. W. (1999). Simultaneous heat and mass transfer: dehydration. In *Microstructural principles of food processing and engineering* (2nd ed., pp. 373–411). Maryland: Aspen.

Angell, C. A. (1991). Thermodynamic aspects of the glass transition in liquids and plastic crystals. *Pure and Applied Chemistry*, *63*(10), 1387–1392.

Angell, C. A. (2002). Liquid fragility and the glass transition in water and aqueous solutions. *Chemical Reviews*, *102*(8), 2627–2650.

Angell, C. A., Ngai, K. L., McKenna, G. B., McMillan, P. F., & Martin, S. W. (2000). Relaxation in glassforming liquids and amorphous solids. *Journal of Applied Physics*, *88*, 3113–3157.

Aoki, T., Decker, E. A., & McClements, D. J. (2005). Influence of environmental stresses on stability of O/W emulsions containing droplets stabilized by multi-layered membranes produced by a layer-by-layer electrostatic deposition technique. *Food Hydrocolloids*, *19*, 209–220.

Apanasenko, I. E., Selyutina, O. Y., Polyakov, N. E., Suntsova, L. P., Meteleva, E. S., Dushkin, A. V., et al. (2015). Solubilization and stabilization of macular carotenoids by water soluble oligosaccharides and polysaccharides. *Archives of Biochemistry and Biophysics*, *572*, 58–65.

Arvanitoyannis, I., Blanshard, J., Izzard, M., Lillford, P., & Ablett, S. (1993). Calorimetric study of the glass transition occurring in aqueous glucose: fructose solutions. *Journal of the Science of Food and Agriculture*, *63*, 177–188.

Bae, E. K., & Lee, S. J. (2008). Microencapsulation of avocado oil by spray drying using whey protein and maltodextrin. *Journal of Microencapsulation*, *25*(8), 549–560.

Benjamin, O., Silcock, P., Leus, M., & Everett, D. W. (2012). Multilayer emulsions as delivery systems for controlled release of volatile compounds using pH and salt triggers. *Food Hydrocolloids*, *27*, 109–118.

Beutner, S., Bloedorn, B., Frixel, S., Hernández Blanco, I., Hoffmann, T., Martin, H. D., et al. (2001). Quantitative assessment of antioxidant properties of natural colorants and phytochemicals: Carotenoids, flavonoids, phenols and indigoids. The role of β-carotene in antioxidant functions. *Journal of the Science of Food and Agriculture*, *81*(6), 559–568.

Bhandari, B., Bansal, N., Zhang, M., & Schuck, P. (2013). *Handbook of food powders: Processes and properties* (pp. 1–12). Oxford: Elsevier/Woodhead Publishing Limited.

Bonnie, T. Y. P., & Choo, Y. M. (1999). Oxidation and thermal degradation of carotenoids. *Journal of Oil Palm Research*, 2(1), 62–78.

Boon, C. S., McClements, D. J., Weiss, J., & Decker, E. A. (2010). Factors influencing the chemical stability of carotenoids in foods. *Critical Reviews in Food Science and Nutrition*, 50(6), 515–532.

Britton, G. (1995). Structure and properties of carotenoids in relation to function. *The FASEB Journal*, 9(15), 1551–1558.

Burton, G. W., & Ingold, K. U. (1984). Beta-carotene: an unusual type of lipid antioxidant. *Science*, 224(4649), 569–573.

Caliskan, G., Lim, A. S. L., & Roos, Y. H. (2015). Beta-carotene stability in extruded snacks produced using interface engineered emulsions. *International Journal of Food Properties*, 18(10), 2256–2267.

Carneiro, H. C., Tonon, R. V., Grosso, C. R., & Hubinger, M. D. (2013). Encapsulation efficiency and oxidative stability of flaxseed oil microencapsulated by spray drying using different combinations of wall materials. *Journal of Food Engineering*, 115(4), 443–451.

Casalini, R., & Roland, C. (2007). An equation for the description of volume and temperature dependences of the dynamics of supercooled liquids and polymer melts. *Journal of Non-Crystalline Solids*, 353(41), 3936–3939.

Cevc, G., & Richardsen, H. (1999). Lipid vesicles and membrane fusion. *Advanced Drug Delivery Reviews*, 38, 207–232.

Champion, D., Le Meste, M., & Simatos, D. (2000). Towards an improved understanding of glass transition and relaxations in foods: molecular mobility in the glass transition range. *Trends in Food Science and Technology*, 11(2), 41–55.

Chandler, L. A., & Schwartz, S. J. (1988). Isomerization and losses of trans-β-carotene in sweet potatoes as affected by processing treatments. *Journal of Agricultural and Food Chemistry*, 36(1), 129–133.

Chen, B. H., Chen, T. M., & Chien, J. T. (1994). Kinetic model for studying the isomerization of α- and β-carotene during heating and illumination. *Journal of Agricultural and Food Chemistry*, 42(11), 2391–2397.

Choe, E., & Min, D. B. (2006). Mechanisms and factors for edible oil oxidation. *Comprehensive Reviews in Food Science and Food Safety*, 5(4), 169–186.

Desobry, S. A., Netto, F. M., & Labuza, T. P. (1997). Comparison of spray-drying, drum-drying and freeze-drying for β-carotene encapsulation and preservation. *Journal of Food Science*, 62(6), 1158–1162.

Desobry, S. A., Netto, F. M., & Labuza, T. P. (1999). Influence of maltodextrin systems atan equivalent 25DE on encapsulated β-carotene loss during storage. *Journal of Food Processing and Preservation*, 23(1), 39–55.

Dickinson, E. (2012). Emulsion gels: the structuring of soft solids with protein-stabilized oil droplets. *Food Hydrocolloids*, 28(1), 224–241.

Duffie, J. A., & Marshall, W. R. (1953). Factors influencing the properties of spray-dried materials. *Chemical Engineering Progress*, 49(8), 417–423.

Edwards, K. A., & Baeumner, A. J. (2006). Analysis of liposomes. *Talanta*, 68(5), 1432–1441.

Ehrenfest, P. (1933). Phase changes classified according to the singularities of the thermodynamic potential. In *Proceedings of the Academy of Science, Amsterdam 36, 153; Suppl. 75b, Mitt*. Leiden: Kammerlingh Onnes Inst.

Fäldt, P., & Bergenståhl, B. (1994). The surface composition of spray-dried protein—lactose powders. *Colloids and Surfaces A: Physicochemical and Engineering Aspects*, 90(2), 183–190.

Fan, F., & Roos, Y. H. (2016a). Structural relaxations of amorphous lactose and lactose-whey protein mixtures. *Journal of Food Engineering*, 173, 106–115.

Fan, F., & Roos, Y. H. (2016b). Crystallization and structural relaxation times in structural strength analysis of amorphous sugar/whey protein systems. *Food Hydrocolloids*, *60*, 85–97.

Farombi, E. O., & Britton, G. (1999). Antioxidant activity of palm oil carotenes in organic solution: effects of structure and chemical reactivity. *Food Chemistry*, *64*, 315–321.

Ferry, J. D. (1980). *Viscoelastic properties of polymers*. New York: John Wiley & Sons.

Foti, M. C., & Amorati, R. (2009). Non-phenolic radical-trapping antioxidants. *Journal of Pharmacy and Pharmacology*, *61*(11), 1435–1448.

Gao, G., Wei, C. C., Jeevarajan, A. S., & Kispert, L. D. (1996). Geometrical isomerization of carotenoids mediated by cation radical/dication formation. *The Journal of Physical Chemistry*, *100*(13), 5362–5366.

Gharsallaoui, A., Saurel, R., Chambin, O., Cases, E., Voilley, A., & Cayot, P. (2010). Utilisation of pectin coating to enhance spray-dry stability of pea protein-stabilised oil-in –water emulsions. *Food Chemistry*, *122*, 447–454.

Glasstone, S. (1946). *Textbook of physical chemistry* (2nd ed.). Princeton, NJ, USA: Van Nostrand.

Goodwin, T. W. (1984). *Carotenoid-protein complexes the biochemistry of the carotenoids*. Dordrecht: Springer.

Gu, Y. S., Decker, E. A., & McClements, D. J. (2005). Production and characterization of oil-in-water emulsions containing droplets stabilized by multilayer membranes consisting of β-lactoglobulin, ι-carrageenan and gelatin. *Langmuir*, *21*, 5752–5760.

Güzey, D., & McClements, D. J. (2006). Influence of environmental stresses on O/W emulsions stabilized by β-lactoglobulin–pectin and β-lactoglobulin–pectin–chitosan membranes produced by the electrostatic layer-by-layer deposition technique. *Food Biophysics*, *1*(1), 30–40.

Guzey, D., & McClements, D. J. (2006). Formation, stability and properties of multilayer emulsions for application in the food industry. *Advances in Colloid and Interface Science*, *128*, 227–248.

Harnkarnsujarit, N., & Charoenrein, S. (2011). Influence of collapsed structure on stability of β-carotene in freeze-dried mangoes. *Food Research International*, *44*(10), 3188–3194.

Harnkarnsujarit, N., Charoenrein, S., & Roos, Y. H. (2012). Reversed phase HPLC analysis of stability and microstructural effects on degradation kinetics of β-carotene encapsulated in freeze-dried maltodextrin–emulsion systems. *Journal of Agricultural and Food Chemistry*, *60*(38), 9711–9718.

Harnsilawat, T., Pongsawatmanit, R., & McClements, D. J. (2006). Influence of pH and ionic strength on formation and stability of emulsions containing oil droplets coated by β-lactoglobulin–alginate interfaces. *Biomacromolecules*, *7*, 2052–2058.

Helgason, T., Awad, T. S., Kristbergsson, K., Decker, E. A., McClements, D. J., & Weiss, J. (2009). Impact of surfactant properties on oxidative stability of beta-carotene encapsulated within solid lipid nanoparticles. *Journal of Agricultural and Food Chemistry*, *57*(17), 8033–8040.

Henry, L. K., Catignani, G. L., & Schwartz, S. J. (1998). Oxidative degradation kinetics of lycopene, lutein, and 9-cis and all-trans β-carotene. *Journal of the American Oil Chemists' Society*, *75*(7), 823–829.

Hidalgo, A., & Brandolini, A. (2008). Kinetics of carotenoids degradation during the storage of einkorn (*Triticum monococcum* L. *ssp. monococcum*) and bread wheat (*Triticum aestivum* L. *ssp. aestivum*) flours. *Journal of Agricultural and Food Chemistry*, *56*(23), 11300–11305.

Hou, Z., Gao, Y., Yuan, F., Liu, Y., Li, C., & Xu, D. (2010). Investigation into the physicochemical stability and rheological properties of beta-carotene emulsion stabilized by soybean soluble polysaccharides and chitosan. *Journal of Agricultural and Food Chemistry*, *58*(15), 8604–8611.

Hou, Z., Zhang, M., Liu, B., Yan, Q., Yuan, F., Xu, D., et al. (2012). Effect of chitosan molecular weight on the stability and rheological properties of β-carotene emulsions stabilized by soybean soluble polysaccharides. *Food Hydrocolloids, 26*(1), 205–211.

Jimenez, M., Garcia, H. S., & Beristain, C. I. (2004). Spray-drying microencapsulation and oxidative stability of conjugated linoleic acid. *European Food Research and Technology, 219*(6), 588–592.

Jiménez-Martín, E., Gharsallaoui, A., Pérez-Palacios, T., Carrascal, J. R., & Rojas, T. A. (2015). Suitability of using monolayered and multilayered emulsions for microencapsulation of ω-3 fatty acids by spray drying: effect of storage at different temperatures. *Food and Bioprocess Technology, 8*(1), 100–111.

Karel, M., Labuza, T. P., & Maloney, J. F. (1967). Chemical changes in freeze-dried foods and model systems. *Cryobiology, 3*(4), 288–296.

Karmas, R., Pilar Buera, M., & Karel, M. (1992). Effect of glass transition on rates of nonenzymic browning in food systems. *Journal of Agricultural and Food Chemistry, 40*(5), 873–879.

Keogh, M. K., O'Kennedy, B. T., Kelly, J., Auty, M. A., Kelly, P. M., Fureby, A., et al. (2001). Stability to oxidation of spray-dried fish oil powder microencapsulated using milk ingredients. *Journal of Food Science, 66*(2), 217–224.

Khoo, H. E., Prasad, K. N., Kong, K. W., Jiang, Y., & Ismail, A. (2011). Carotenoids and their isomers: color pigments in fruits and vegetables. *Molecules, 16*(2), 1710–1738.

Kittel, C., & Holcomb, D. F. (1967). Introduction to solid state physics. *American Journal of Physics, 35*(6), 547–548.

Klinkesorn, U., Sophanodora, P., Chinachoti, P., Decker, E. A., & McClements, D. J. (2006). Characterization of spray-dried tuna oil emulsified in two-layered interfacial membranes prepared using electrostatic layer-by-layer deposition. *Food Research International, 39*(4), 449–457.

Klinkesorn, U., Sophanodora, P., Chinachoti, P., McClements, D. J., & Decker, E. A. (2005). Increasing the oxidative stability of liquid and dried tuna oil-in-water emulsions with electrostatic layer-by-layer deposition technology. *Journal of Agricultural and Food Chemistry, 53*, 4561–4566.

Labuza, T. P. (1968). Sorption phenomena in foods. *Food Technology, 22*, 15–24.

Labuza, T. P. (1971). Properties of water as related to the keeping quality of foods. In *Proceedings of the 3rd International Congress of Food Science and Technology.*

Labuza, T. P. (1975). Interpretation of sorption data in relation to the state of constituent water. In R. Duckworth (Ed.), *Water relation of food.* New York, USA: Academic Press.

Labuza, T. P., Cassil, S., & Sinskey, A. J. (1972). Stability of intermediate moisture foods. 2. Microbiology. *Journal of Food Science, 37*(1), 160–162.

Labuza, T. P., & Dugan, L. R., Jr. (1971). Kinetics of lipid oxidation in foods. *Critical Reviews in Food Science & Nutrition, 2*(3), 355–405.

Labuza, T. P., & Riboh, D. (1982). Theory and application of Arrhenius kinetics to the prediction of nutrient losses in foods. *Food Technology, 36*(10), 66–74.

Landau, L. D., & Lifshitz, E. M. (1984). *Physique statistique* (p. 583). Moscow: Editions Mir.

Levi, G., & Karel, M. (1995). Volumetric shrinkage (collapse) in freeze-dried carbohydrates above their glass transition temperature. *Food Research International, 28*(2), 145–151.

Levine, H., & Slade, L. (1986). A polymer physico-chemical approach to the study of commercial starch hydrolysis products (SHPs). *Carbohydrate Polymers, 6*(3), 213–244.

Lievonen, S. M., Laaksonen, T. J., & Roos, Y. H. (1998). Glass transition and reaction rates: nonenzymatic browning in glassy and liquid systems. *Journal of Agricultural and Food Chemistry, 46*(7), 2778–2784.

Lim, A. S. L., Burdikova, Z., Sheehan, J. J., & Roos, Y. H. (2016). Carotenoid stability in high total solid spray dried emulsions with gum Arabic layered interface and trehalose–WPI composites as wall materials. *Innovative Food Science & Emerging Technologies, 34,* 310–319.

Lim, A. S. L., Griffin, C., & Roos, Y. H. (2014). Stability and loss kinetics of lutein and β-carotene encapsulated in freeze-dried emulsions with layered interface and trehalose as glass former. *Food Research International, 62,* 403–409.

Lim, A. S. L., & Roos, Y. H. (2016). Spray drying of high hydrophilic solids emulsions with layered interface and trehalose–maltodextrin as glass formers for carotenoids stabilization. *Journal of Food Engineering, 171,* 174–184.

Lim, A. S. L., & Roos, Y. H. (2017). Carotenoids stability in spray dried high solids emulsions using layer-by-layer (LBL) interfacial structure and trehalose-high DE maltodextrin as glass former. *Journal of Functional Foods, 33,* 32–39.

Lim, A. S. L., & Roos, Y. H. (2018). Amorphous wall materials properties and degradation of carotenoids in spray dried formulations. *Journal of Food Engineering, 223,* 62–69.

Liu, Y., Bhandari, B., & Zhou, W. (2006). Glass transition and enthalpy relaxation of amorphous food saccharides: a review. *Journal of Agricultural and Food Chemistry, 54*(16), 5701–5717.

López-Díez, E., & Bone, S. (2004). The interaction of trypsin with trehalose: an investigation of protein preservation mechanisms. *Biochimica et Biophysica Acta (BBA)-General Subjects, 1673*(3), 139–148.

Lu, W., Kelly, A. L., & Miao, S. (2016). Emulsion-based encapsulation and delivery systems for polyphenols. *Trends in Food Science & Technology, 47,* 1–9.

Lu, W., Kelly, A. L., & Miao, S. (2017a). Bioaccessibility and cellular uptake of beta-carotene encapsulated in model O/W emulsions: influence of initial droplet size and emulsifiers. *Nanomaterials (Basel), 7*(9), 282–292.

Lu, W., Kelly, A. L., & Miao, S. (2017b). Improved bioavailability of encapsulated bioactive nutrients delivered through Monoglyceride-structured O/W emulsions. *Journal of Agricultural and Food Chemistry, 65,* 3048–3055.

Lu, W., Zheng, B., & Miao, S. (2018). Improved emulsion stability and modified nutrient release by structuring O/W emulsions using konjac glucomannan. *Food Hydrocolloids, 81,* 120–128.

Mahfoudhi, N., & Hamdi, S. (2014). Kinetic degradation and storage stability of β-carotene encapsulated by spray drying using almond gum and gum arabic as wall materials. *Journal of Polymer Engineering, 34*(8), 683–693.

Mahfoudhi, N., & Hamdi, S. (2015). Kinetic degradation and storage stability of β-carotene encapsulated by freeze-drying using almond gum and gum Arabic as wall materials. *Journal of Food Processing and Preservation, 39*(6), 896–906.

Maidannyk, V. A. (2017). *Strength analysis for understanding structural relaxations in food materials.* PhD Thesis University College Cork.

Maidannyk, V. A., Lim, A. S. L., Auty, M., & Roos, Y. H. (2018). Effects of lipids on the water sorption, glass transition and structural strength of carbohydrate-protein systems. *Food Research International Journal,* https://doi.org/10.1016/j.foodres.2018.10.008. In press.

Maidannyk, V. A., Nurhadi, B., & Roos, Y. H. (2017). Structural strength analysis of amorphous trehalose-maltodextrin systems. *Food Research International, 96,* 121–131.

Maidannyk, V. A., & Roos, Y. H. (2016). Modification of the WLF model for characterization of the relaxation time-temperature relationship in trehalose-whey protein isolate systems. *Journal of Food Engineering, 188,* 21–31.

Maidannyk, V. A., & Roos, Y. H. (2017). Water sorption, glass transition and "strength" of lactose–whey protein systems. *Food Hydrocolloids, 70,* 76–87.

Maidannyk, V. A., & Roos, Y. H. (2018). Structural strength analysis of partially crystalline trehalose. *LWT-Food Science and Technology, 88,* 9–17.

Mao, L., Wang, D., Liu, F., & Gao, Y. (2018). Emulsion design for the delivery of beta-carotene in complex food systems. *Critical Reviews in Food Science and Nutrition, 58*(5), 770–784.

McClements, D. J. (1999). *Food emulsions: Principles, practice and techniques.* Boca Raton, FL: CRC Press.

McClements, D. J. (2010). Emulsion design to improve the delivery of functional lipophilic components. *Annual Review of Food Science and Technology, 1*, 241–269.

McClements, D. J. (2017). Recent progress in hydrogel delivery systems for improving nutra-ceutical bioavailability. *Food Hydrocolloids, 68*, 238–245.

McClements, D. J., Decker, E. A., & Weiss, J. (2007). Emulsion based delivery systems for lipophilic bioactive components. *Journal of Food Science, 72*(8), R109–R124.

McClements, D. J., & Li, Y. (2010). Structured emulsion-based delivery systems: controlling the digestion and release of lipophilic food components. *Advances in Colloid and Interface Science, 159*(2), 213–228.

Meinders, M. B., & van Vliet, T. (2009). Modeling water sorption dynamics of cellular solid food systems using free volume theory. *Food Hydrocolloids, 23*(8), 2234–2242.

Meste, M. L., Champion, D., Roudaut, G., Blond, G., & Simatos, D. (2002). Glass transition and food technology: a critical appraisal. *Journal of Food Science, 67*(7), 2444–2458.

Minguez-Mosquera, M. I., & Jaren-Galan, M. (1995). Kinetics of the decolouring of carotenoid pigments. *Journal of the Science of Food and Agriculture, 67*(2), 153–161.

Moreau, L., Kim, H. J., Decker, E. A., & McClements, D. J. (2003). Production and character-ization of oil-in-water emulsions containing droplets stabilized by β-lactoglobulin-pectin membranes. *Journal of Agricultural and Food Chemistry, 51*(22), 6612–6617.

Moreau, D. L., & Rosenberg, M. (1999). Porosity of microcapsules with wall systems consist-ing of whey proteins and lactose measured by gas displacement pycnometry. *Journal of Food Science, 64*(3), 405–409.

Mortensen, A. (2002). Scavenging of benzylperoxyl radicals by carotenoids. *Free Radical Research, 36*(2), 211–216.

Mun, S., Kim, Y. R., & McClements, D. J. (2015). Control of beta-carotene bioaccessibility using starch-based filled hydrogels. *Food Chemistry, 173*, 454–461.

Nelson, K. A., & Labuza, T. P. (1994). Water activity and food polymer science: implications of state on Arrhenius and WLF models in predicting shelf life. *Journal of Food Engineering, 22*(1), 271–289.

Nik, A. M., Langmaida, S., & Wright, A. J. (2012). Digestibility and β-carotene release from lipid nanodispersions depend on dispersed phase crystallinity and interfacial properties. *Food Function, 3*, 234–245.

Ogawa, S., Decker, E. A., & McClements, D. J. (2003). Production and characterization of O/W emulsions containing cationic droplets stabilized by lecithin-chitosan membranes. *Journal of Agricultural and Food Chemistry, 51*(9), 2806–2812.

Ojovan, M. I., & Lee, W. E. (2006). Topologically disordered systems at the glass transition. *Journal of Physics: Condensed Matter, 18*(50).

Parks, G. S., & Huffman, H. (1927). Studies on glass. I. *The Journal of Physical Chemistry, 31*(12), 1842–1855.

Peleg, M. (1992). On the use of the WLF model in polymers and foods. *Critical Reviews in Food Science & Nutrition, 32*(1), 59–66.

Peleg, M., & Chinachoti, P. (1996). On modeling changes in food and biosolids at and around their glass transition temperature range. *Critical Reviews in Food Science & Nutrition, 36*(1–2), 49–67.

Pesek, C. A., & Warthesen, J. J. (1988). Characterization of the photodegradation of β-carotene in aqueous model systems. *Journal of Food Science, 53*(5), 1517–1520.

Polyakov, N. E., & Kispert, L. D. (2015). Water soluble biocompatible vesicles based on polysaccharides and oligosaccharides inclusion complexes for carotenoid delivery. *Carbohydrate Polymers*, *128*, 207–219.

Polyakov, N. E., & Leshina, T. V. (2006). Certain aspects of the reactivity of carotenoids. Redox processes and complexation. *Russian Chemical Reviews*, *75*(12), 1049.

Polyakov, N. E., & Leshina, T. V. (2011). Glycyrrhizic acid as a novel drug delivery vector synergy of drug transport and efficacy. *The Open Conference Proceedings Journal*, *2*, 64–72.

Polyakov, N. E., Leshina, T. V., Meteleva, E. S., Dushkin, A. V., Konovalova, T. A., & Kispert, L. D. (2010). Enhancement of the photocatalytic activity of TiO2 Nanoparticles by water-soluble complexes of carotenoids. *The Journal of Physical Chemistry B*, *114*, 14200–14204.

Polyakov, N. E., Magyar, A., & Kispert, L. D. (2013). Photochemical and optical properties of water-soluble xanthophyll antioxidants: aggregation vs complexation. *Journal of Physical Chemistry B*, *117*(35), 10173–10182.

Potes, N., Kerry, J. P., & Roos, Y. H. (2012). Additivity of water sorption, alpha-relaxations and crystallization inhibition in lactose–maltodextrin systems. *Carbohydrate Polymers*, *89*(4), 1050–1059.

Prado, S. M., Buera, M. P., & Elizalde, B. E. (2006). Structural collapse prevents β-carotene loss in a supercooled polymeric matrix. *Journal of Agricultural and Food Chemistry*, *54*(1), 79–85.

Qian, C., Decker, E. A., Xiao, H., & McClements, D. J. (2012a). Nanoemulsion delivery systems: influence of carrier oil on beta-carotene bioaccessibility. *Food Chemistry*, *135*(3), 1440–1447.

Qian, C., Decker, E. A., Xiao, H., & McClements, D. J. (2012b). Physical and chemical stability of β-carotene-enriched nanoemulsions: Influence of pH, ionic strength, temperature, and emulsifier type. *Food Chemistry*, *132*(3), 1221–1229.

Ré, M. I. (1998). Microencapsulation by spray drying. *Drying Technology*, *16*(6), 1195–1236.

Ribeiro, H. S., Schuchmann, H. P., Engel, R., Walz, E., & Briviba, K. (2010). Encapsulation of Carotenoids. In N. J. Zuidam (Ed.), *Encapsulation technologies for active food ingredients and food processing*. New York: Springer.

Rodriguez-Amaya, D. B. (2015). *Food carotenoids: Chemistry, biology and technology*. West Sussex, UK: Wiley Blackwell.

Roos, Y. H. (1995). *Phase transitions in foods*. San Diego, CA: Academic Press.

Roos, Y. H. (2008). *The glassy state. Food materials science* (pp. 67–81). Springer.

Roos, Y. H. (2009). Solid and liquid states of lactose. In P. L. H. McSweeeny & P. F. Fox (Eds.), *Advanced dairy chemistry. Volume 3: Lactose, water, salts and minor constituents* (pp. 17–33). New York: Springer.

Roos, Y. H. (2013). Relaxations, glass transition and engineering properties of food solids. In *Advances in food process engineering research and applications* (pp. 79–90). New York: Springer.

Roos, Y. H., & Drusch, S. (2015). *Phase transitions in foods*. Academic Press.

Roos, Y. H., Fryer, P. J., Knorr, D., Schuchmann, H. P., Schroën, K., Schutyser, M. A., et al. (2015). Food engineering at multiple scales: case studies, challenges and the future—a European perspective. *Food Engineering Reviews*, 1–25.

Roos, Y. H., & Karel, M. (1991a). Phase transitions of mixtures of amorphous polysaccharides and sugars. *Biotechnology Progress*, *7*(1), 49–53.

Roos, Y., & Karel, M. (1991b). Applying state diagrams to food processing and development. *Food Technology*, *45*(12), 66–71.

Roudaut, G., Simatos, D., Champion, D., Contreras-Lopez, E., & Le Meste, M. (2004). Molecular mobility around the glass transition temperature: a mini review. *Innovative Food Science & Emerging Technologies, 5*(2), 127–134.

Royall, P. G., Huang, C.-y., Tang, S.-w.J., Duncan, J., Van-de-Velde, G., & Brown, M. B. (2005). The development of DMA for the detection of amorphous content in pharmaceutical powdered materials. *International Journal of Pharmaceutics, 301*(1), 181–191.

Salvia-Trujillo, L., Qian, C., Martin-Belloso, O., & McClements, D. J. (2013). Influence of particle size on lipid digestion and beta-carotene bioaccessibility in emulsions and nanoemulsions. *Food Chemistry, 141*(2), 1472–1480.

Selim, K., Tsimidou, M., & Biliaderis, C. G. (2000). Kinetic studies of degradation of saffron carotenoids encapsulated in amorphous polymer matrices. *Food Chemistry, 71*(2), 199–206.

Shahidi, F., & Han, X. Q. (1993). Encapsulation of food ingredients. *Critical Reviews in Food Science & Nutrition, 33*(6), 501–547.

Shaw, L. A., McClements, D. J., & Decker, E. A. (2007). Spray-dried multilayered emulsions as a delivery method for ω-3 fatty acids into food systems. *Journal of Agricultural and Food Chemistry, 55*(8), 3112–3119.

Silalai, N., & Roos, Y. H. (2011). Mechanical relaxation times as indicators of stickiness in skim milk–maltodextrin solids systems. *Journal of Food Engineering, 106*(4), 306–317.

Slade, L., & Levine, H. (1995). Glass transitions and water-food structure interactions. *Advances in Food and Nutrition Research, 38*, 103–269.

Slade, L., Levine, H., & Finley, J. W. (1989). Protein-water interactions: water as a plasticizer of gluten and other protein polymers. In R. Phillips & J. W. Findlay (Eds.), *Protein quality and the effects of processing* (pp. 9–124). Amsterdam, New York: LAW Levier Scientific Publishing.

Slade, L., Levine, H., & Reid, D. S. (1991). Beyond water activity: recent advances based on an alternative approach to the assessment of food quality and safety. *Critical Reviews in Food Science & Nutrition, 30*(2–3), 115–360.

Soottitantawat, A., Bigeard, F., Yoshii, H., Furuta, T., Ohkawara, M., & Linko, P. (2005). Influence of emulsion and powder size on the stability of encapsulated D-limonene by spray drying. *Innovative Food Science & Emerging Technologies, 6*(1), 107–114.

Spada, J. C., Noreña, C. P. Z., Marczak, L. D. F., & Tessaro, I. C. (2012). Study on the stability of β-carotene microencapsulated with *pinhão* (*Araucaria angustifolia* seeds) starch. *Carbohydrate Polymers, 89*(4), 1166–1173.

Sperling, L. H. (2005). *Introduction to physical polymer science*. John Wiley & Sons.

Subagio, A., & Morita, N. (2001). Instability of carotenoids is a reason for their promotion on lipid oxidation. *Food Research International, 34*, 183–188.

Tachaprutinun, A., Udomsup, T., Luadthong, C., & Wanichwecharungruang, S. (2009). Preventing the thermal degradation of astaxanthin through nanoencapsulation. *International Journal of Pharmaceutics, 374*(1–2), 119–124.

Tan, C., Feng, B., Zhang, X., Xia, W., & Xia, S. (2016). Biopolymer-coated liposomes by electrostatic adsorption of chitosan (chitosomes) as novel delivery systems for carotenoids. *Food Hydrocolloids, 52*, 774–784.

Tan, C., Xue, J., Abbas, S., Feng, B., Zhang, X., & Xia, S. (2014). Liposome as a delivery system for carotenoids: comparative antioxidant activity of carotenoids as measured by ferric reducing antioxidant power, DPPH assay and lipid peroxidation. *Journal of Agricultural and Food Chemistry, 62*(28), 6726–6735.

Tokle, T., Mao, Y., & McClements, D. J. (2013). Potential biological fate of emulsion-based delivery systems: lipid particles nanolaminated with lactoferrin and beta-lactoglobulin coatings. *Pharmaceutical Research, 30*(12), 3200–3213.

Trombino, S., Cassano, R., Muzzalupo, R., Pingitore, A., Cione, E., & Picci, N. (2009). Stearyl ferulate-based solid lipid nanoparticles for the encapsulation and stabilization of beta-carotene and alpha-tocopherol. *Colloids and Surfaces B: Biointerfaces*, *72*(2), 181–187.

Updike, A. A., & Schwartz, S. J. (2003). Thermal processing of vegetables increases cis isomers of lutein and zeaxanthin. *Journal of Agricultural and Food Chemistry*, *51*, 6184–6190.

Velasco, J., Dobarganes, C., & Márquez-Ruiz, G. (2003). Variables affecting lipid oxidation in dried microencapsulated oils. *Grasas y Aceites*, *54*(3), 304–314.

Verhey, J. G. P. (1972). Vacuole formation in spray powder particles. 1. Air incorporation and bubble expansion. *Netherlands Milk and Dairy Journal*, *27*(3), 186–202.

Vignolles, M. L., Jeantet, R., Lopez, C., & Schuck, P. (2007). Free fat, surface fat and dairy powders: interactions between process and product. A review. *Le Lait*, *87*(3), 187–236.

Wang, S., Chen, X., Shi, M., Zhao, L., Li, W., Chen, Y., et al. (2015). Absorption of whey protein isolated (WPI)-stabilized β-carotene emulsions by oppositely charged oxidized starch microgels. *Food Research International*, *67*, 315–322.

Wang, W., Jiang, Y., & Zhou, W. (2013). Characteristics of soy sauce powders spray-dried using dairy whey proteins and maltodextrins as drying aids. *Journal of Food Engineering*, *119*(4), 724–730.

Wang, H., Qian, H., & Yao, W. (2011). Melanoidins produced by the Maillard reaction: Structure and biological activity. *Food Chemistry*, *128*(3), 573–584.

Wei, C. C., Gao, G., & Kispert, L. D. (1997). Selected cis/trans isomers of carotenoids formed by bulk electrolysis and iron (III) chloride oxidation. *Journal of the Chemical Society, Perkin Transactions*, *2*(4), 783–786.

Williams, M. L., Landel, R. F., & Ferry, J. D. (1955). The temperature dependence of relaxation mechanisms in amorphous polymers and other glass-forming liquids. *Journal of the American Chemical Society*, *77*(14), 3701–3707.

Yi, J., Lam, T. I., Yokoyama, W., Cheng, L. W., & Zhong, F. (2014a). Controlled release of beta-carotene in beta-lactoglobulin-dextran-conjugated nanoparticles' in vitro digestion and transport with Caco-2 monolayers. *Journal of Agricultural and Food Chemistry*, *62*(35), 8900–8907.

Yi, J., Lam, T. I., Yokoyama, W., Cheng, L. W., & Zhong, F. (2014b). Cellular uptake of β-carotene from protein stabilized solid lipid nanoparticles prepared by homogenization–evaporation method. *Journal of Agricultural and Food Chemistry*, *62*(5), 1096–1104.

Yi, J., Lam, T. I., Yokoyama, W., Cheng, L. W., & Zhong, F. (2015). Beta-carotene encapsulated in food protein nanoparticles reduces peroxyl radical oxidation in Caco-2 cells. *Food Hydrocolloids*, *43*, 31–40.

Young, A. J., & Lowe, G. M. (2001). Antioxidant and prooxidant properties of carotenoids. *Archives of Biochemistry and Biophysics*, *385*(1), 20–27.

Yuan, C., Du, L., Jin, Z., & Xu, X. (2013). Storage stability and antioxidant activity of complex of astaxanthin with hydroxypropyl-beta-cyclodextrin. *Carbohydrate Polymer*, *91*(1), 385–389.

Zhang, L., Hayes, D. G., Chen, G., & Zhong, Q. (2013). Transparent dispersions of milk-fat-based nanostructured lipid carriers for delivery of beta-carotene. *Journal of Agricultural and Food Chemistry*, *61*(39), 9435–9443.

Zhang, Z., Zhang, R., & McClements, D. J. (2016). Encapsulation of β-carotene in alginate-based hydrogel beads: impact on physicochemical stability and bioaccessibility. *Food Hydrocolloids*, *61*, 1–10.

Zhou, Y., & Roos, Y. H. (2012). Stability of α-tocopherol in freeze-dried sugar–protein–oil emulsion solids as affected by water plasticization and sugar crystallization. *Journal of Agricultural and Food Chemistry*, *60*(30), 7497–7505.

Further reading

Castelli, F., Caruso, S., & Giuffrida, N. (1999). Different effects of two structurally similar carotenoids, lutein and β-carotene, on the thermotropic behaviour of phosphatidylcholine liposomes. Calorimetric evidence of their hindered transport through biomembranes. *Thermochimica Acta, 327*(1–2), 125–131.

Cornacchia, L., & Roos, Y. H. (2011). Lipid and water crystallization in protein-stabilised oil-in-water emulsions. *Food Hydrocolloids, 25*(7), 1726–1736.

Ermolina, I., Polygalov, E., Bland, C., & Smith, G. (2007). Dielectric spectroscopy of low-loss sugar lyophiles: II. Relaxation mechanisms in freeze-dried lactose and lactose monohydrate. *Journal of Non-Crystalline Solids, 353*(47), 4485–4491.

Gearing, J., Malik, K. P., & Matejtschuk, P. (2010). Use of dynamic mechanical analysis (DMA) to determine critical transition temperatures in frozen biomaterials intended for lyophilization. *Cryobiology, 61*(1), 27–32.

Higuera-Ciapara, I., Felix-Valenzuela, L., Goycoolea, F. M., & Argüelles-Monal, W. (2004). Microencapsulation of astaxanthin in a chitosan matrix. *Carbohydrate Polymers, 56*(1), 41–45.

Kilmartin, P. A., Reid, D. S., & Samson, I. (2004). Dielectric properties of frozen maltodextrin solutions with added NaCl across the glass transition. *Journal of the Science of Food and Agriculture, 84*(11), 1277–1284.

Kokini, J., Cocero, A., Madeka, H., & De Graaf, E. (1994). The development of state diagrams for cereal proteins. *Trends in Food Science & Technology, 5*(9), 281–288.

Kostecka-Gugała, A., Latowski, D., & Strzałka, K. (2003). Thermotropic phase behaviour of α-dipalmitoylphosphatidylcholine multibilayers is influenced to various extents by carotenoids containing different structural features-evidence from differential scanning calorimetry. *Biochimica et Biophysica Acta (BBA)-Biomembranes, 1609*(2), 193–202.

Noel, T. R., Parker, R., & Ring, S. G. (2000). Effect of molecular structure and water content on the dielectric relaxation behaviour of amorphous low molecular weight carbohydrates above and below their glass transition. *Carbohydrate Research, 329*(4), 839–845.

Saini, R. K., Nile, S. H., & Park, S. W. (2015). Carotenoids from fruits and vegetables: chemistry, analysis, occurrence, bioavailability and biological activities. *Food Research International, 76*, 735–750.

Shibata, A., Kiba, Y., Akati, N., Fukuzawa, K., & Terada, H. (2001). Molecular characteristics of astaxanthin and β-carotene in the phospholipid monolayer and their distributions in the phospholipid bilayer. *Chemistry and Physics of Lipids, 113*(1), 11–22.

Socaciu, C., Jessel, R., & Diehl, H. A. (2000). Competitive carotenoid and cholesterol incorporation into liposomes: effects on membrane phase transition, fluidity, polarity and anisotropy. *Chemistry and Physics of Lipids, 106*(1), 79–88.

Vega, C., & Roos, Y. (2006). Invited review: spray-dried dairy and dairy-like emulsions—compositional considerations. *Journal of Dairy Science, 89*(2), 383–401.

Wackerbarth, H., Stoll, T., Gebken, S., Pelters, C., & Bindrich, U. (2009). Carotenoid–protein interaction as an approach for the formulation of functional food emulsions. *Food Research International, 42*(9), 1254–1258.

Williams, A. W., Boileau, T. W., & Erdman, J. W., Jr. (1998). Factors influencing the uptake and absorption of carotenoids. *Proceedings of the Society for Experimental Biology and Medicine, 218*(2), 106–108.

Zhou, P., & Labuza, T. P. (2007). Effect of water content on glass transition and protein aggregation of whey protein powders during short-term storage. *Food Biophysics, 2*(2–3), 108–116.

Extraction of carotenoids and applications

Shi-Hui Cheng*, Hock Eng Khoo†, Kin Weng Kong‡,§, Krishnamurthy Nagendra Prasad¶,‖, Charis M. Galanakis#,**
*School of Biosciences, Faculty of Science, The University of Nottingham Malaysia Campus, Semenyih, Malaysia, †Department of Nutrition and Dietetics, Faculty of Medicine and Health Sciences, Universiti Putra Malaysia, Seri Kembangan, Malaysia, ‡Department of Molecular Medicine, Faculty of Medicine, University of Malaya, Kuala Lumpur, Malaysia, §Center for Natural Products Research and Drug Discovery, University of Malaya, Kuala Lumpur, Malaysia, ¶Chemical Engineering Discipline, School of Engineering, Monash University Malaysia, Bandar Sunway, Malaysia, ‖World Pranic Healing Foundation India Research Centre, Mysore, India, #Research & Innovation Department, Galanakis Laboratories, Chania, Greece, **Food Waste Recovery Group, ISEKI Food Association, Vienna, Austria

Chapter Outline

Carotenoids: Properties, Processing and Applications. https://doi.org/10.1016/B978-0-12-817067-0.00008-7

Introduction

The consumption of a diet that rich in various essential vitamins and minerals is important for maintaining human health. One of the important food components from the human diet is carotenoid which is particularly high in fruits and vegetables. Carotenoid, also referred to as tetraterpenoid, comprises a class of natural fat-soluble pigments formed from eight molecules of five carbon isoprenoid. Carotenoid consists of a hydrocarbon containing 40 carbon atoms and two terminal rings liable for yellow, orange, and red coloration (Namitha & Negi, 2010). There are currently over 600 known carotenoids found in nature and about 40 carotenoids are regularly consumed in the human diet. Carotenoids can be divided into two groups, the hydrocarbon carotenoids, carotenes (includes lycopene, β-carotene, α-carotene) and the oxygen-containing carotenoids, xanthophylls (includes lutein, astaxanthin and zeaxanthin). Carotenoids are mainly found in yellow-orange fruits and vegetables. Indeed, the coloring properties of saffron is due to the presence of the three major apocarotenoids: crocin, crocetin, and picrocrocin. The saffron apocarotenoids are only found in the red stigmata of crocus flowers (Bouvier, Suire, Mutterer, et al., 2003). On the other hand, green leafy vegetables are rich in a number of carotenoids such as lutein, violaxanthin, β-carotene, and neoxanthin (Priyadarshani & Jansz, 2014; Saini, Nile, & Park, 2015) while β-cryptoxanthin is mainly found in peach, papaya, and citrus fruits like orange and tangerine (Sugiura, Kato, Matsumoto, Nagao, & Yano, 2002). Sweet potato, carrots, pumpkin, apricots, cantaloupe, and dark green vegetables such as spinach and broccoli are rich in α-carotene (Farre, Sanahuja, Naqvi, et al., 2010; Jaswir, Noviendri, Hasrini, & Octavianti, 2011). Most of the non-plants creatures including humans are unable to synthesize carotenoids, they need to ingest carotenoids through the daily diet and metabolize them for normal physiological functions (Berendschot & Plat, 2014). According to the literature, lycopene, α-carotene, β-carotene, lutein, zeaxanthin, and β-cryptoxanthin are the most abundant carotenoids found in human plasma (Aizawa & Inakuma, 2007).

Indeed, the medicinal properties of carotenoids have been well established. One of the most important physiological functions of carotenoids is to act as vitamin A precursors. Although not all carotenoids are served as the precursors for vitamin A but both provitamin A carotenoids (α-carotene and β-carotene) and non-provitamin A carotenoids (lutein, zeaxanthin and lycopene) at some extent play an important role in vitamin A activity which includes visual function and its protection, skin health, immunity, cell differentiation, and responsible for growth and reproduction. These compounds are also well known for their antioxidant activities due to their conjugated double bonds which allow physical quenching of many free radicals (Garrow, James, & Ralph, 2000). Epidemiological studies demonstrated that a diet rich in carotenoids was associated with a reduction of the risks of several diseases such as cancer, cataracts, and macular degradations (Ribaya-Mercado & Blumberg, 2004).

Carotenoids are also reported to reduce the risk of cardiovascular disease through reduction of oxidative stress and, hence, prevent the oxidation of low-density lipoprotein (LDL) which can further lead to a plaque formation. Cohort studies have shown that dietary carotenoids have preventive effects on cardiovascular disease in various populations such as Italy (Tavani, Gallus, Negri, Parpinel, & Vecchia, 2006), Japan (Ito et al., 2006), and Europe (Buijsse et al., 2005). In the retina, lutein and zeaxanthin are responsible for the yellow pigmentation called macular pigment and the diminished of this macular pigment is related to retinal damage and vision loss. In general, deficiency in carotenoids could result in vitamin A deficiency which can lead to keratomalacia, xerophthalmia, and night blindness (Sommer, 2008). Studies indicated that a high intake of fruits and vegetable containing carotenoids is associated with the reducing risk of getting eye disease (Johnson et al., 2000). Besides the provitamin A activity, carotenoids can also serve as the natural antioxidants to extend the shelf life of food product as well as the bioactive components in the functional foods to against oxidative stress-related diseases. On the other hand, the prominent compounds in the carotenoid groups, include lycopene and β-carotene, are natural color pigments that have been used as natural dyes and food colorants (Amr & Hussein, 2013).

In recent years, numerous studies have been carried out on the carotenoids content among the underutilized vegetables and it was reported that *Moringa oleifera* (drumstick tree), *Lactuca indica* (Indian lettuce), and *Oenanthe javanica* (water dropwort) contain rich sources of carotenoids (Andarwulan et al., 2012; Kongkachuichai, Charoensiri, Yakoh, & Kringkasemsee, 2015; Saini, Shetty, & Giridhar, 2014). Among the underutilized vegetables from Indonesia, the highest content of β-carotene (14 mg/100 g) was recorded in the leaves of *Moringa pterygosperma* (syn. *M. oleifera*) (Andarwulan et al., 2012). In another study, *L. indica* and *O. javanica* exhibited the highest β-carotene and lutein content (Kongkachuichai et al., 2015). In addition, researchers have also studied the carotenoid content in fruits. Lycopene (408 μg/g) and β-carotene (83.3 μg/g) are found to be the major constituents of carotenoids in Gac fruit (*Momordica cochinchinensis*) (Vuong, Franke, Custer, & Murphy, 2006). Among the pulps and by-products of tropical fruits, the highest content of β-carotene was recorded in the pulp of Acerola (26.23 μg/g) followed by papaya (20.24 μg/g) and Surinam Cherry pulp (15.64 μg/g) (da Silva et al., 2014). It shows that vegetables and fruits are rich in carotenoids which indicates the potential use of these vegetables and fruits species in as the materials for extracting the carotenoids.

Following the properties of carotenoids and their bioactivities, their global market demand is estimated to reach 1.8 billion USD in 2019 (Strati & Oreopoulou, 2014). Applications of carotenoids include food and feed additives, supplement, and natural colorants. The commercially available products of carotenoids are chemically synthesized, although little percentages are recovered by natural sources (Amaya Delia, 2016). The first synthetic carotenoid (β-carotene using β-ionone derived precursors like acetone and butadiene) was introduced in the market in the 1950s (Rutz, Borges, Zambiazi, Rosa, & Silva, 2016). Synthetic carotenoids are typically more stable than those derived from natural sources. They can be prepared either as colloidal suspensions, or emulsifications or dispersion colloids, whereas they are distributed in the market as water soluble and stable emulsions. Nevertheless, modern consumers show preference to natural products, as chemically synthesized compounds are known to exhibit in some cases high toxicity, carcinogenicity, and teratogenicity properties (Kirthi, Amita, Priti, Kumar, & Jyoti, 2014). This fact increases the interest of the food industry to recover carotenoids from natural sources like food processing by-products.

Extraction of carotenoids

Conventional extraction techniques

The recovery of valuable compounds from natural sources follows the principles of analytical chemistry, whereas it is well known to be conducted following the five-stages universal recovery processing: (i) macroscopic pretreatment, (ii) macro- and micro-molecules separation, (iii) extraction, (iv) purification, and (v) product formation. This methodology has been designed in order to maximize the yield of the target compounds, suite to the demands of industrial processing, clarify the valuable compounds from impurities and toxic compounds, avoid loss of functionality during processing and finally to ensure the food grade nature of the final product (Galanakis, 2012).

Specifically, macroscopic pretreatment aims at the adjustment of the water, solids and fats content, activation or deactivation of enzymes, moderation of the microbial load, and finally increase permeability of the matrix. If the substrate is fruit or vegetable by-product, a wet milling step is necessary to facilitate and improve the yield of the following separation and extraction stages (Oreopoulou & Tzia, 2007). This is conducted via swelling and tissue softening that allows the higher diffusion of extractants inside food matrix. On the other hand, if the substrate is a wastewater (i.e., of olive oil industry), concentration (thermal or vacuum) is utilized with a final purpose of removing water and increasing content of valuable components (Galanakis, 2012). With regard to the second recovery stage, alcohol precipitation is the most popular method for the separation of smaller compounds (e.g., antioxidants, acids or ions) from macromolecules (e.g., pectin, dietary fibers, or hydrocolloids), which are collected in the so-called alcohol insoluble residue (Koubala et al., 2008). Extraction, which is the next and most important stage of downstream processing, is well-documented with different methodologies employed toward the target molecules and their physicochemical characteristics (i.e., solubility or volatility). Indeed, different conventional techniques and emerging technologies have been used for this purpose (Cassano & Galanakis, 2018; Galanakis, 2013, 2015, 2016, 2017a, 2017b, 2017c, 2017d, 2017e, 2018a, 2018b, 2018c, 2019a, 2019b, 2019c, 2019d, 2019e, 2019f; Galanakis, Goulas, Tsakona, Manganaris, & Gekas, 2013; Incinur & Galanakis, 2018; Kovacevic et al., 2018; Skendi, Harasym, & Galanakis, 2018; Socaci, Fărcaş, & Galanakis, 2019; Ucak, Gokoglu, Kiessling, Toepfl, & Galanakis, 2019; Ucak, Gokoglu, Toepfl, & Galanakis, 2018; Zinoviadou & Galanakis, 2017) depending on the nature of the initial substrate and the target compounds.

Solvent extraction is the most typical and widely used method. This is happening because it is very convenient, since the solvent provides a physical carrier to transfer the valuable compounds between different phases (e.g., solid, liquid and vapor), following their physicochemical characteristics (e.g., solubility or volatility). One of the essential criteria in the process of extraction is the solvent used for extraction (Arvayo-Enríquez, Mondaca-Fernández, Gortárez-Moroyoqui, López-Cervantes, & Rodríguez-Ramírez, 2013). For instance, antioxidants like polyphenols are easily solubilized in polar protic mediums such as hydroalcoholic mixtures, and respective fractions can be obtained on the basis of polarity by varying alcohol concentration (Galanakis et al., 2013; Tsakona, Galanakis, & Gekas, 2012). In addition, among the several alcohols, ethanol is most preferable because it is rather cheap and is generally recognized as safe in the food industry (Galanakis, 2012). Due to their hydrophobic nature, carotenoids are conventionally extracted using the organic solvents such as dichloromethane, hexane, methanol, ethanol, dimethyl ether, diethyl ether, toluene, 2-propanol, n-butanol, heptane, acetonitrile, tetradecane, dodecane, hexadecane, and tetrahydrofuran. Nonpolar solvents such as hexane or petroleum ether, are commonly used to extract the nonpolar carotenes like β-carotene. Hexane is one of the most widely used solvents in the industry to extract β-carotene, due to its high affinity for carotenoids. Semipolar solvents such as acetone, ethanol, and ethyl acetate are used to extract those semipolar carotenoids like lutein (Saini & Keum, 2018).

A review on the methods of carotenoid extraction has shown that the most common solvents used for plant samples are hexane, acetone, and ethanol/hexane (4:3) (Amorim-Carrilho, Cepeda, Fente, & Regal, 2014). However, most of the solvents used in the conventional extraction methods possess environmental health and safety hazards (Saini & Keum, 2018). In view of the environmental and health issues, ethanol and acetone are the two preferred solvents for food application over other common solvents used to extract carotenoids such as hexane, diethyl ether, and dichloromethane (Alfonsi et al., 2008; Capello, Fischer, & Hungerbu, 2007).

The carotenoids content in the plant is influenced by several factors, including genetic, climate condition, and cultivation method used to grow the plant. However, postharvest processes can also influence the bioavailability of the carotenoids (Kopsell & Kopsell, 2006). Different part of the same plant may also contain different amounts of carotenoids. Packaging and processing methods such as heat drying or ultrasound drying are also able to provide a great influence to the carotenoids content in the food products (Saini, Shetty, Prakash, & Giridhar, 2014). Another problem is the low efficiency in the extraction process of carotenoids. Owing to numerous physical and chemical barriers present in food matrices, it is difficult for the solvent molecule to penetrate the plant matrices to solubilize the carotenoids during extraction. It ended up with a low level of recovery for carotenoids when extracting them through a complex matrix (Lavecchia & Zuorro, 2008). In addition, various factors found in the process of carotenoid extraction such as overexposure to heat, light, acids, and long extraction times could also reduce the recovery of carotenoids (Arvayo-Enríquez et al., 2013). All these factors led to increased efforts in recent years for improving the extraction methods.

The fat-soluble properties of carotenoids make them suitable to be used in food and cosmetic products. Carotenoids have been reported to have high market potential, with β-carotene has the highest market value followed by lutein, capsanthin, and zeaxanthin. In the market, the sales for β-carotene have been reported to surpass USD 280 million in 2015 (Arvayo-Enríquez et al., 2013). The applications of carotenoids as food additives, ingredients for cosmetics, healthy foods, and pharmaceutical products are the main reason that carotenoids are of interest among the researchers. However, the existing extraction technologies have some shortcomings to overcome. With the increase of energy cost and the drive to reduce the greenhouse gas emissions, there have been continuous efforts in the development of new extraction methods for carotenoids over the past decades to shorten the extraction time, reduce solvent consumption, reduce the processing cost, and increased the functionality (Saini & Keum, 2018).

Disadvantages of conventional methods in extraction of carotenoids

Extraction of carotenoids from fruits and vegetables for commercial application needs a simple, rapid, and inexpensive method. However, the use of conventional extraction methods not only threatened the environment and human health but the extraction techniques also required a long extraction time and a huge volume of solvent. In addition, conventional technologies have other problems that often restrict their utilization in practice. For instance, membrane technologies (e.g., ultrafiltration) require increased energy consumption, whereas others like show high-operational cost. Besides, thermal processes (e.g., concentration, spray drying) may cause detrimental effects on antioxidants or loss of their functionality due to overheating of the substrate's matrix (Mujumdar & Law, 2010). Finally, additional problems like the generation of unstable products (that are difficult to preserve in the shelf) may arise during encapsulation or emulsification of the final product (Galanakis, 2013). Regarding carotenoids extraction, Soxhlet is one of the conventional techniques used. It utilizes solvents at their boiling temperatures and low pressure to selectively extract the targeted compounds (Luque de Castro & Garcia-Ayuso, 1998). The cost of the extraction for Soxhlet method is higher as compared to other methods because this method requires a long extraction time and uses significant amounts of solvents.

As explained earlier, selection of an appropriate solvent is considered the most important factor for the conventional technique because different solvents provide a different amount of extraction yield and extract compositions (Arvayo-Enríquez et al., 2013). The extraction of carotenoids with an organic solvent is usually carried out under a high temperature to demonstrate the interaction between the solvent and compound. Hence, increase the mass transfer rate. When an organic solvent is used along with the high temperature, the solvent surface becomes tension, and thus the solvent can easily reach the solute in the matrix, solubilizing a variety of solutes (Mezzomo & Ferreira, 2016).

Carotenoids are susceptible to enzymatic and nonenzymatic oxidation, oxygen availability, the high temperature, and light exposure. Thus the extraction of carotenoids should be carried out in the shortest possible time. However, many of the conventional extraction methods introduce temperature to the sample. The high temperature during the extraction can cause rapid degradation of carotenoids and leads to isomerization of trans-carotenoids which is the most stable form in nature, to form cis-form, promoting the slight loss of color and a reduction in the provitamin activity (Aman, Schieber, & Carle, 2005). Besides the possible thermal degradation of the extract, the other major disadvantage is the incomplete solvent removal from the final product. Normally, the final product may have a trace amount of solvent and thus reduces the use of the resulted extract in food products (Babu, Chakrabarti, & Sambasivarao, 2008). The use of organic solvents in the industry often requires expensive disposal measures

(Craft & Soares, 1992). In addition, the solvent removal step also leads to environmental and safety problems. A huge amount (20 million tons) of organic solvent is released to the atmosphere every year, leading to severe environmental pollution (Jutz, Andanson, & Baiker, 2011).

These disadvantages together with increased ecological concern and economic considerations have called for the development of other extraction solvents. In the past few decades, the term "green chemistry" becomes a major focus of research in academia and industry to minimize the environment and health impacts. A green solvent must fulfill some basic requirements such as low toxicity, easily available, ability to recycle, and high efficiency in the extraction (Song & Han, 2015). By using a green solvent, the extraction process can be optimized, solvent usage can be reduced, and this helps to achieve a sustainable environment. Extraction using ionic liquid is termed as green extraction, and this method of carotenoids extraction has been discussed in the subsequent section.

Emerging extraction techniques

The disadvantages of conventional techniques could be overcome using new (typically nonthermal) technologies, so-called emerging ones. These technologies are nowadays investigated in research level and in some cases applied in the food industry, promising shortening of processing and residence times, accelerated heat and mass transfer, control of Maillard reactions, improvement of product quality, enhancement of functionality, protection from environmental stresses, and extended preservation. The most popular emerging or reconsidered technologies examined in the broad field of food science are radio-frequency drying, electro-osmotic dewatering, cold plasma treatment, high-pressure processing and homogenization, ultrasound-assisted extraction (UAE), laser ablation, high-voltage electrical discharge, pulsed electric field, pulsed fluid-bed agglomeration, and nanoencapsulation (Galanakis, 2013). For instance, high hydrostatic pressure improves the mass transfer rate of carotenoids during their extraction by increasing the plant cell permeability, allowing diffusion of the molecules in phase transition (Oroian & Escriche, 2015). In particular, elevated pressures ranging from 100 to 1000 Mpa are employed to induce pressure stress on the plant matrix for a short period of time from few seconds to over 20 min. The applied pressure acts uniformly in all directions of the reaction medium, providing equal pressure distribution to the sample (Nagarajan, Ramanan, Raghunandan, Galanakis, & Prasad, 2017). Pulsed electric field is another nonthermal technology that enhances carotenoids' transfer rate by softening plant tissues and reducing cell's membrane integrity, as well as influencing the texture and electroporation of the plant (Oroian & Escriche, 2015). It involves the application of high-voltage pulses ($20–80 \text{kVcm}^{-1}$) in liquid or semisolid food between two electrodes for short period of time. Carotenoid accessibility has been reported to be high in treated samples with pulsed electric field, for example, in the case of carrot pomace in sunflower oil using a field strength of 0.6kV cm^{-1} and 5 Hz (Roohinejad, Everett, & Oey, 2014).

Irradiation process is another technology that involves exposure of a sample to ionizing or nonionizing energy known as cold pasteurization. Its main goal is to destroy and inactivate microorganism activity in the food that reduces the shelf life of the food. Ionizing radiation is generated by electron beams, gamma-rays (Cobalt-60), and X-rays. Nonionizing radiations include ultraviolet rays (UV), microwaves, and visible lights that do not carry energy to ionize atoms (Nagarajan et al., 2017). The effect of radiation treatment (0, 2.5, 5, 7.5, and 10 kGy) has been compared with thermal treatment on strawberry and papaya blended nectar. As the radiation dosage increases, the content of carotenoids (particularly β-cryptoxanthin) in the nectar blend reduced and increases 7.4% at 10 kGy. It was concluded that the increased radiation dosage up to 7.5 kGy negatively affects β-cryptoxanthin, β-carotene, and lycopene content in the sample in all ratio composition. However at 10 kGy, the carotenoids content increased significantly compared to sample radiated at 7.5 kGy. At higher radiation, the polygalacturonase enzyme in the plant cell, hydrolyses the glycosidic bonds and degrades the pectin. Therefore, the nectar sample become much susceptible to release carotenoid, hence more bioavailable (Swada, Keeley, Ghane, & Engeseth, 2016).

Ionic liquids as solvents for extraction

In addition to nonthermal technologies, innovative approaches have been proposed to address the use of safer and cleaner alternatives for solvent extraction. The use of greener solvents as an extraction solvent has recently become a priority and gained significant attention worldwide. In the advancement of extraction technology, green solvents are more favorable due to their harmlessness to the environment and health impacts. Ionic liquids are termed as a green solvent for carotenoids extraction in achieving the goal of a sustainable environment. Further, we highlight the recent development of extraction methods particularly ionic liquids which would open a new alternative to the pharmaceutical or food industry for carotenoids extractions.

Ionic liquid is defined as ionic salt with a low melting point (<100 °C) in its liquid state (Dietz, 2006). Ionic solutions are the promising media for separation and extraction of a wide array of analytes from diverse plant origins (Passos, Freire, & Coutinho, 2014). The nature of the ionic liquid components has been reported by Saini and Keum (2018), where these ionic liquids are typically in the range from dipolar to polar. Ionic liquids consist of anions (such as imidazolium, ammonium and pyridinium) and cations including Br^-, Cl^- tetrafluoroborate ($BF4^-$), and methylsulfate (MS^-). In the extraction of bioactive compounds from an oily sample, an ionic liquid is diluted either in the water or organic solvents. On the other hand, the ionic liquid is classified as a new class of cationic hydrotrope. It shows that ionic liquids are the good candidates to dissolve compounds with different polarities (Seddon, 1997).

The use of ionic liquids as an extracting solvent could provide a good alternative to overcome the limitations found in the traditional extraction methods. These ionic liquids exhibit several properties that make them a potential solvent for improved extraction processes, among them are a wide liquid range, nonflammable, low vapor pressure, good thermal stability, and nonvolatile versatile salts composed of loosely held anions and cations which has the ability to solubilize a wide range of solutes (García, Larriba, García, Torrecilla, & Rodríguez, 2012; Saini & Keum, 2018).

The low vapor pressure of ionic liquids facilitates the isolation of the organic compounds which is slightly soluble. Another advantage of ionic liquids is these liquids that are reusable, and this would reduce the material required and waste generated. In addition, ionic solutions can increase the solubility and stability of a solute in a given solvent (Sivapragasam, Moniruzzaman, & Goto, 2016). Ionic liquids are also categorized as thermally stable solvents. These high thermal and chemical stability properties enable ionic liquid to be used as a solvent to extract carotenoids at high temperature (Ibrahim, Moniruzzaman, Yusup, & Uemura, 2015).

It is noteworthy that ionic liquid generally exhibits a low surface tension even at the condition above the room temperature (Tariq et al., 2012). Surface tension is a measure of the cohesive forces between the liquid molecules present at the surface. Low surface tension is essential for the solvent to better dissolve to the plant matrix. The low vapor pressure, hydrophilic property, nontoxic, and reusability of the ionic liquids are seen as their strength to be employed in food processing (Martins, Braga, & de Rosso, 2017). Ionic liquids are used as the green solvent for carotenoids in a pretreatment step to improve the extraction yield (Rajabi, Moniruzzaman, Mahmood, Sivapragasam, & Bustam, 2017). A previous study also showed that addition of ionic liquid (1-methyl-3-octyloxymethylimidazolium tetrafluoroborate) in the extraction solvent (n-hexane) elevated the extraction yield of all-trans β-carotene which was 100 times higher than in the extraction solvent alone (Bialek-Bylka, Pawlak, Jazurek, Skrzypczak, & Koyama, 2007). The study also revealed that the extraction yield of 15-cis β-carotene was >100 times higher than the yield obtained from n-hexane.

Besides the physicochemical properties of ionic liquids, ionic liquids are gaining increasing interest as an eco-friendly solvent to replace volatile organic solvents for the extraction of bioactive compounds, especially carotenoids. In contrast, traditional extraction methods that are usually involved with highly toxic, volatile, and flammable organic solvents can lead to many environmental issues (Huddleston, Willauer, Swatloski, Visser, & Rogers, 1998). Corrosive and inflammable solvents also increase the cost of pre and posttreatment of the waste products. In addition, only nontoxic solvents should be taken into consideration when it comes to food and pharmaceutical processing.

Ionic liquids have also been used for extraction of carotenoids from seaweeds. For instance, Vieira et al. (2018) revealed that fucoxanthin was extracted from brown seaweeds using aqueous solutions of different ionic states. The study showed that surface-active ionic liquids and anionic surfactants were first screened for their effectiveness in extracting fucoxanthin from the seaweed sample. The used of sodium dodecyl sulfate yielded the highest concentration of the carotenoid, whereas some of the ionic liquids and surfactants failed to recover fucoxanthin from the sample. As one of the ionic solution, sodium dodecyl sulfate has a great potential in extracting carotenoids from plants without utilizing n-hexane as the extraction solvent. Another study also revealed that antioxidant activity value of the carotenoids extracted from tomatoes using the ionic solvent containing 1-butyl-3-methylimidazolium (0.1 M) was 7.4 which was lower than the antioxidant activity value (12.4) reported for the acetone extracted carotenoids. The extraction was done by the using an ultrasound probe in the range of 65% for 30 min. The values were relative to the α-tocopherol

Table 1   Advantages and disadvantages of different methods of extraction

Extraction methods	Advantages	Disadvantages
Soxhlet extraction	• Conventional method providing the highest recovery of carotenoids • Simple, no sophisticated instruments needed • Continuously contact with the fresh solvent	• Longer extraction time • Consume a large amount of solvents which increases the cost of extraction • Can cause thermal degradation and cis-trans isomerization of carotenoids
Microwave-assisted extraction	• Simple • Shorter extraction time • Economic method	• Can cause thermal degradation and cis-trans isomerization of carotenoids
Ultrasound-assisted extraction	• Simple • shorter extraction time • Efficient extraction	• Aging of the ultrasound probe surface can change the extraction efficiency
Enzyme-assisted extraction	• Shorter extraction time • Efficient extraction • Minimal consumption of solvents	• High cost of the enzymes
Accelerated solvent extraction	• Shorter extraction time • Efficient extraction • Minimal consumption of solvents	• Difficult to apply to large volumes due to clogging caused by sugars and pectins of plant matrices.

standard (Martins & de Rosso, 2016). The study also reported the interaction between ionic liquids and carotenoids was complex. It could be due to the variation of both anion and cation in the ionic solvent. Besides the extraction of carotenoids from tomatoes, 1-butyl-3-methylimidazolium (0.50 M) has been used to extract astaxanthin from shrimp waste (Saini, Moon, & Keum, 2018). The use of ionic liquid in UAE of astaxanthin from shrimp waste contributed to higher astaxanthin yield than the conventional UAE (Bi, Tian, Zhou, & Row, 2010). It was suggested that the length of alkyl chain of the ionic liquid affects the extraction yield of astaxanthin from shrimp waste. The possible reasons are hydrogen bonding occurred between astaxanthin and the ionic liquid, as well as π-effects (Ventura et al., 2017).

The extraction of carotenoids using ionic solutions can be accelerated using non-thermal and other extraction techniques. The most extensively applied techniques include microwave-assisted extraction (MAE), UAE, accelerated solvent extraction (ASE), supercritical fluid extraction, and enzyme-assisted extraction (EAE). The following section describes the ionic liquid-assisted extraction by means of different extraction methods. Advantages and disadvantages of different assisted methods of extraction are listed in Table 1.

Microwave-assisted extraction

MAE is a simple, rapid, and inexpensive method for carotenoid extraction. MAE works by increasing pressure on the cell wall from the evaporation of moisture inside the cells using heat generated by microwaves (Hiranvarachat & Devahastin, 2014). Waves transmitted by the microwave penetrate biomaterials, then interact with the polar molecules like water to create heat. The increased pressure disrupts the physical properties of the sample tissues/matrix, and the increased porosity of its matrix allows the extracting solvent for better penetration and improves the recovery of carotenoids (Wang & Weller, 2006). The effect of the microwave is dependent on the dielectric susceptibility of the ionic solvent used and the solid plant matrix. Moistening plant samples with water can improve carotenoid recovery, as water has a comparatively high dielectric constant. The rehydrated biomaterial is also able to interact better with microwave energy to create heat, expand in the cell wall, and eventually causing them to rupture and releasing carotenoids into the solvent.

Choosing an appropriate ionic solvent is critical for its optimal use. Three main parameters for selecting an appropriate solvent are solubility, dielectric constant, and dissipation factors (Routray & Orsat, 2012). Solvents like water, ethanol, and methanol with a high dielectric constant can strongly absorb microwave energy compared to nonpolar solvents like hexane which has a low dielectric constant. The mixtures of solvents can be used to modulate the interaction between the solvent and the microwave. Dissipation factor represents the efficiency of a solvent heated up under a microwave. Even though water has a high dielectric constant, it has a low dissipation factor in which it is inefficient in heating up the moisture inside the sample. Therefore, microwave helps in the extraction of carotenoids even without the use of water as the ionic solvent (Chemat, Fabiano-tixier, Abert, Allaf, & Vorobiev, 2015). As reported in the literature, extraction efficiency is affected by the type of solvent; extraction yield increased when the ethanol concentration increased to 50% (Zhang, Yang, Su, & Guo, 2009). Using ethyl acetate as an MAE solvent is also reported to have a higher recovery for lycopene compared to hexane. Using MAE can result in a great yield of carotenoids with the reduced extraction time as compared to the Soxhlet extraction technique (Poojary et al., 2016). MAE require a very short extraction time with a low amount of solvents, making it comparable to other extraction methods like supercritical fluid extraction. Previous studies also showed that the application of MAE enhanced the efficiency, reduced the extraction time and amount of solvent used for carotenoid extraction from plants compared to those conventional extraction methods (Hiranvarachat, Devahastin, Chiewchan, & Vijaya Raghavan, 2013; Pasquet et al., 2011). However, MAE requires additional filtration or centrifugation to remove the solid residues.

Ultrasound-assisted extraction

UAE is an inexpensive, quick, and efficient method for extraction of carotenoids from food and environmental samples. The effectiveness of this method compared to the other conventional methods is mainly due to the acoustic cavitation.

Apart from food processing ultrasound applications are also versatile in extraction, emulsification, and homogenization. Acoustic cavitation occurs when liquids are exposed to ultrasounds in the frequency range of 20 kHz to >1 MHz. Low-pressure voids or vacuum bubbles are formed in the liquid and continues to grow and oscillate briefly after which they implode with great intensity, causing the cell wall to rupture (Chemat, Huma, & Khan, 2011). The disruption to the cell wall facilitates the mass-transfer of extractants, allows the diffusion of the of the solvent to extract the bioactive compounds. UAE increases the yield of carotenoids at low temperature as acoustic cavitation is very efficient in enhancing the diffusion through cell membranes (Tzanakis, Lebon, Eskin, & Pericleous, 2017). In addition, UAE is a green extraction method that uses a lesser quantity of solvent as compared to Soxhlet (Chemat, Rombaut, Sicaire, Meullemiestre, & Abert-vian, 2017). UAE enables the extraction to be carried out within a shorter period with high reproducibility, reducing the consumption of solvent, and thus eliminating the posttreatment of waste solvent. Compounds from the plant have been extracted efficiently by using UAE. Studies showed that β-carotene and other carotenoids are extracted from carrot peels using UAE via intermittent radiation without thermal degradation (Hiranvarachat & Devahastin, 2014; Li, Fabiano-tixier, Tomao, Cravotto, & Chemat, 2013).

UAE allows processing conditions to be changed such as a decrease in temperature and pressure which makes it suitable for thermolabile compounds, particularly carotenoids that are vulnerable to decomposition or alter in their molecular structures when exposed to heat (Poojary et al., 2016). It is also reasonably easier to operate compared to other sophisticated extraction methods; it can be used with any solvent to extract numerous compounds. However, the extraction yield and mechanical effects of ultrasound are dependent on the nature of the carotenoids to be extracted. As an example, ultrasound increases the yield of extracted pyrethrins from Pyrethrum flowers but has weak effects on the yield of extracted oil from woad seeds (Wang & Weller, 2006). UAE also has been proved to be a promising technology to extract carotenoids from tomato by-products (skin, seeds, and pulp) as it significantly increased the extraction yield by 43% as compared to traditional extraction without causing any degradation of carotenoids (Luengo, Condón-abanto, Condón, Álvarez, & Raso, 2014). On the other hand, ultrasonic processing has been proven to reduce the in vitro bioaccessibility of lycopene compared to untreated sample. Specifically, the sonication energy is able to cause a rapid compression and expansion of plant cells, resulting in bubble formation around the sample. Subsequently, tomato pulp is partially de-esterified and pectin molecules (in integral part of plant) are released. This fact leads to the formation of gelling substances due to hydrogen and hydrophobic interactions (Anese et al., 2015). An interesting finding was observed when pasteurized carrot juice was subjected for sonication at different time intervals. In particular, β-carotene concentration was increased up to 95 µg/g, resulting in oxidation and increasing peroxide content of the sample. This was due to the prooxidant effect shown by β-carotene at higher concentration (Shanmugam & Ashokkumar, 2015). These studies indicate that the optimization of extraction conditions is always important, as the effect of nonthermal technologies like ultrasounds for the recovery of carotenoids may not always be beneficial.

Enzyme-assisted extraction

Enzymatic treatment is usually done prior to conventional solvent extraction as a pretreatment. EAE normally uses hydrolytic enzymes in plant extraction such as pectinase and cellulase. These enzymes are used to break down the structure of the cell wall for allowing efficient extraction and the release of bioactive compounds (Saini & Keum, 2018). The use of raw enzymes has been shown to obtain a high carotene content with a reduction in processing time as compared to the commercial enzyme (Navarrete-bolan, Rangel-cruz, Jime, Botello-alvarez, & Rico-martı, 2005). The disintegration of the cell wall structure usually accelerates metabolic transformation resulting in undesirable colors and changes in flavor. However, these changes have not been observed in the enzymatically treated plant matrices. It is because the extractants such as carotenoids, released by pectinase and cellulase are still bound to proteins keeping the highly unsaturated pigment structure stable (Arvayo-Enríquez et al., 2013). The concentrations of enzymes used for pretreatment of plant range from 0.01% to 0.1% (w/w) (Delgado-vargas & Paredes-lpez, 1997). Water is crucial to allow the enzymatic hydrolysis to take place. However, excessive water leads to the formation of an aqueous phase and prevent the solvent in contact with the carotenoids and hence slow down the extraction process. Agitation plays an important role in enzymatic treatment to facilitate the diffusion of enzyme from the aqueous phase (supernatant) into the solid phase (plant); this will enhance the lysis of the cell wall and will increase the extraction yield (Arvayo-Enríquez et al., 2013).

Pectinase and cellulase are the two common enzymes used in enzyme-assisted extraction. The primary cell wall consists of cellulose, pectin compounds, hemicellulose, and glycoproteins (Choudhari & Ananthanarayan, 2007). Pectinase breaks down the pectin found in the plant primary cell walls and the middle lamella. Cellulase hydrolyses the 1,4-β-d-glycosidic linkages of cellulose that also found in the primary cell wall. The breakdown of pectin and cellulose increases cell wall permeability, thus increasing the extraction yield of the compounds. These enzymes, although normally functioning at their optimal temperature, can be used over a range of temperatures which provide flexibility on the adjustment of production cost and product quality (Choudhari & Ananthanarayan, 2007). Treating carotenoid-containing samples with enzymes cellulase and pectinase before extraction has been shown to improve the yield of carotenoids. In the extraction of total carotenoids and lycopene from tomatoes, there was an increase in the extraction yield of the treated samples compared to untreated samples (Strati & Oreopoulou, 2014). Cellulase is reported to be more efficient to attain a higher lycopene yield compared to pectinase, probably due to the high content of cellulose and hemicellulose in the tomato. Extraction by using ethyl lactate in the samples after enzyme treatment is also reported to achieve a higher yield of total carotenoids and lycopene as compared to acetone, ethanol, and ethyl acetate/hexane (Saini & Keum, 2018). Using enzymes are cost effective and can reduce the processing time while achieving a high yield of carotenoids. However, on an industrial-scale, enzyme-assisted extraction is not feasible because enzymes are expensive for processing of large quantity of raw material and they behave differently in different environmental conditions.

Accelerated solvent extraction

ASE or pressurized liquid extraction, acknowledged as a green and alternative technique due to the use of ionic solvents involves extraction at a constant high pressure to increase the extraction rate of carotenoids. The constant high pressure improves cell permeability and intermolecular physical interactions, facilitates penetration of extracting solvent, and enhances mass transfer of carotenoids (Saini & Keum, 2018). The pressures are usually between 10 and 15 MPa and the temperatures are between 50 °C and 200 °C. This extraction method is similar to supercritical fluid extraction. The high temperature positively improves the carotenoid extraction and applying high temperature ensures that the carotenoid-binding protein is denatured. The high pressure speeds up the extraction process while reducing the amount of solvent consumption (Mendiola, Herrero, Cifuentes, & Iba, 2007). Laboratory scale equipment for ASE has been invented to allow perfect control of temperature, pressure, time of extraction, and solvent together with a program to allow the extraction to run a maximum of 24 samples placed in the high-pressure stainless steel vessels where they are protected from oxygen and light. ASE has been used previously for extraction of carotenoids from carrot by-products (Mustafa, Trevino, & Turner, 2012), peppers (Barbero, Palma, & Barroso, 2006), microalgae (Koo, Cha, Song, Chung, & Pan, 2012), and various food such as pudding mixes, breakfast cereals, cookies, sausages, and commercial beverages (Breithaupt, 2004).

ASE is a good alternative for supercritical fluid extraction because this method uses the nontoxic extracting solvent such as water which has economic and environmental advantages. ASE is an ideal method for the recovery of carotenoids. As temperature rises, the dielectric constant of solvents decreases which lower the polarity of the solvent. Therefore, the temperature can match the solvent polarity to the compounds (Strati & Oreopoulou, 2014). In addition, higher temperature also helps to facilitate the diffusion of solvent into the solid matrix which in turn shortening the extraction time. It has been previously reported that high recovery of nonpolar carotenoids such as β-carotene (101%) and β-cryptoxanthin (84%) was obtained within a short duration of extraction (5 min) by using ASE (Zaghdoudi, Pontvianne, Framboisier, & Achard, 2015). Another study also revealed that a higher extraction yields from tomato waste are achieved in a relatively short time (10 min) compared to conventional solvent extraction process of 30 min (Strati, Gogou, & Oreopoulou, 2015). Moreover, ASE utilizes a lower amount of solvents (6 mL/g) as compared to conventional solvent extraction (10 mL/g), with an increased in the extraction yield (Strati et al., 2015).

Hydrotropes

A hydrotrope is an amphiphilic compound that possesses hydrophilic and hydrophobic chains within the molecule (Hodgdon & Kaler, 2007). They are usually composed of an aromatic ring which is substituted by a sulfate, sulfonate, or carboxylate group. The compound can be solubilized in both oil and water because it has both hydrophilic and hydrophobic ends (Dhapte & Mehta, 2015). It also increases the solubility of compounds which are poorly soluble in water. Hydrotropes are able to increase the solubility of the organic solvents up to 200 times in water. Hydrotropes consist of hydrotropic salts and esterified mineral. Hydrotropic agents are ionic organic salts which help to increase the solubility of the solute in a given solvent. Hydrotropic agents can be anionic, cationic, or neutral. The hydrotropic salts such as sodium, potassium, and

Table 2 Examples of hydrotropic agents

Type	Examples
Aromatic anionics	Sodium benzoate, sodium salicylate, sodium benzene sulfonate, sodium benzene di-sulfonate, sodium cinnamate, sodium 3-hydroxy-2-naphthoate, sodium para toluene sulfonate, sodium cumene sulfonate, nicotinamide, N,N-diethylnicotinamide and *N,N*-dimethyl benzamide
Aromatic cationics	Para-aminobenzoic acid hydrochloride, procaine hydrochloride and caffeine
Aliphatics and linear compounds	Para-aminobenzoic acid hydrochloride, procaine hydrochloride and caffeine

ammonium, are the typical hydrotropes used by industries. Most of the ingredients used in detergents consist of hydrotropic salts such as sodium alkane sulfonate, sodium xylene, xylene sulfonates, toluene sulfonates, sodium xylene sulfonate, ammonium xylene sulfonate, sodium cumene sulfonate, sodium toluene sulfonate, potassium toluene sulfonate, and others. Besides these sulfonates, cationic compounds and neutral molecule such as pyrogallol also have hydrotropic properties (Saleh & El-Khordagui, 1985). Some of the examples of hydrotropic agents are provided in Table 2.

The term "hydrotropy" is first discovered by the scientist named Carl A. Neuberg. Hydrotropy is the situation that occurs when the hydrotrope salt promotes the solubility of insoluble solutes in water. The efficiency of the hydrotrope depends on the balance between hydrophobic and hydrophilic part of the hydrotrope (Kim, Kim, Papp, Park, & Pinal, 2010). The larger the hydrophobic part of hydrotrope, the better the hydrotropic efficiency. Various efforts have been made by researchers to clarify the mechanisms of hydrotropes. There are three main ways on the mechanisms behind hydrotropy (Dhapte & Mehta, 2015). The first mechanism proposes that hydrotrope molecules have self-aggregation potential and the interaction between hydrotropes and solutes results in the formation of hydrotrope-solute complexes. The second mechanism is that hydrotropes change the structure of the solvent and they are known as structure breaker and structure maker. The final mechanism proposes that hydrotropes are able to form aggregates to act as micelles above a concentration, known as the minimum hydrotrope concentration (Subbarao, Kalyan, Sai Bharadwaj, & Krishna, 2012).

There are many advantages in applying hydrotropes for the extraction of carotenoids over the conventional extraction methods. Hydrotropes are cheap, nontoxic, and environmentally friendly. In addition to being a green solvent, hydrotropes also possess other properties such as the pH-independent solvent character, nonflammability, easy availability, and inexpensive aqueous phase (Gaikar & Sharma, 1993). Another characteristic of the hydrotropes is the simple recovery from the reaction, and they are recyclability. Hydrotrope solutions tend to separate the dissolved compound, leaving the hydrotrope in the aqueous solution to be used anew for extraction purposes. In addition, hydrotropes offer other advantages such as trouble-free handling, efficient, and cleaner extraction process as well as short extraction time making it superior compared with the other extraction methods (Dhapte & Mehta, 2015).

The use of hydrotropes

Hydrotropes enable hydrophobic compounds to solubilize in a hydrophilic solution. These compounds significantly increase the solubility of hydrophobic or organic compounds and solutes in water. Hydrotrope works with the molecule adsorbs onto the surface of the cell walls of the plant matrix. The penetration of hydrotropes into the cell walls alters the permeability of the cell membrane, and the hydrotropic solution can then easily access the desired phytochemical compound (Raman & Gaikar, 2002). Hydrotropes are the ingredients used for a wide range of applications, including food, cosmetic, pharmaceutical, and laundry industries. In food processing, hydrotropes are used to recover the valuable components from the processing wastes.

A hydrotropic solution is another type of green solvent for extraction of bioactive compounds from plants and wastes of food processing. Literature shows that bioactive limonin (0.65 mg/g seed) has been extracted from the seeds of sour orange using a hydrotropic solution of sodium salicylate and sodium cumene sulfonate mixture at concentrations of 0.65 and 0.1 M, respectively (Dandekar, Jayaprakasha, & Patil, 2008). Another study also reported that sodium alkyl benzene sulfonates and sodium butyl monoglycol sulfate are used to extract piperine from black pepper, where a high recovery rate of about 90% found (Raman & Gaikar, 2002). In the pulp and paper industry, hydrotropes successfully recovered a huge amount of plant components in papermaking. A previous study reported that sodium xylene sulfonate, sodium cumene sulfonate, and sodium n-butyl benzene sulfonate were effectively recovered lignin from sugarcane bagasse of up to 99% of the recovery rate (Ansari & Gaikar, 2014).

Hydrotropic extraction of carotenoids

Since a few decades ago, hydrotropes had been applied in the extraction and recovery of carotenoids from plants. There are a few United States's patents on the recoveries of carotenoids from plants using hydrotropic agents. The first patent on this technique has been filed by Burdick in 1966. He patented the method on separation of carotenoids from papaya leaves using an aqueous solution of a mixture of sodium benzene sulfonate and sodium paracymene sulfonate (Burdick, 1966). The plant material is also digested with enzymes and saponificated before the separation of carotenoid-containing fraction. Xylene sulfonate and cumene sulfonate have also been patented as the hydrotropes used in the extraction of carotenoids from brown algae gametophytes (Cattuzzato, Dumont, Le Gelebart, & Loeuil, 2018). The literature reported that hydrotropic solvents are extensively used to extract several compounds from plants such as piperine from pepper (Raman & Gaikar, 2002), curcumin from turmeric (Dandekar & Gaikar, 2003), and limonin from sour orange seeds (Dandekar et al., 2008). However, to the best of our knowledge, research on the extraction of carotenoids using hydrotropic solution are still scarce. Only a few studies reported their findings in this area. In addition, Yara-Varón et al. (2016) revealed that cyclopentyl methyl ether and 2-methyltetrahydrofuran were the green solvents for the extraction of carotenoids from dehydrated carrots which gave the highest yield.

Application of hydrotropes in the extraction of carotenoids from several types of samples has been compiled and reported by Amorim-Carrilho et al. (2014).

Hydrotrope such as sodium dodecyl sulfate has been used to extract carotenoids from the red blood cells. Pyrogallol is also applied in the extraction of carotenoids from red blood cells, fruits, and processed foods. The aqueous solution of sodium dodecyl sulfate has been selected as the best hydrotropic solution to extract fucoxanthin from brown seaweeds (Vieira et al., 2018). Another study also supports the fact that solutions of higher than 0.2% sodium dodecyl sulfate help in increasing the solubility of lycopene extracted from watermelon in water (Fish, 2006). The application of hydrotropes in the food industry is further discussed in the following section.

Final product formation

After the extraction process, the final product does not have to be present in pure form. In addition, the extracted carotenoids may be masked by other subextracted plant components such as chlorophyll, lipids, fatty acids, and esters. Due to the presence of hydroxyl groups, carotenoids like xanthophylls are often present in esterified form (Sarkar et al., 2012). Retrieving carotenoids is conducted with saponification to eliminate chlorophylls or undesired lipids that might cause intercalation during spectrophotometric analysis. Saponification process can be directly performed during sample homogenization before extraction or even after extraction (Nagarajan et al., 2017). During this stage, solvents such as methanolic sodium or potassium hydroxide are added and stirred under atmosphere of nitrogen to remove the lipid or chlorophyll phase from the extract (Larsen & Christensen, 2005). In any case, saponification step can be omitted to non-chlorophyll plant species such as carrot or tomato as the defatting process shows only negligible differences in the total carotenoid content. Unnecessary process of saponification can also lead to structural alteration or degradation of carotenoids (Singh, Ahmad, & Ahmad, 2015). Carotenoids in raw food are usually added in crystalline form that has to be effectively released from the matrix, solubilized and absorbed in the intestine in order to increase its bioaccessibility (Zhang et al., 2015). Their bioaccessibility can be increased through excipient emulsions. These emulsions are not bioactive, but when they are co-ingested with other pharmaceutical preparations, their efficacy is increased (Mcclements & Xiao, 2014). Basically, emulsions are thermodynamically unstable, whereas their stability is affected by different processes, namely creaming, flocculation, coalescence, and Ostwald ripening. Carotenoid incorporated excipient food has been prepared using any of them to enhance food's bioavailability (Gerding et al., 2016).

Applications of carotenoids

Carotenoids containing at least one unsubstituted β-ionone ring, (e.g., β-carotene, α-carotene, γ-carotene, and β-cryptoxanthin) are classified as provitamin A carotenoids and can be converted into retinal by humans and animals (Bai, Twyman, Farre, et al., 2011). Compounds like lutein and zeaxanthin accumulate in the macula of the eye; thus are able to protect the retina from damaging from blue and near ultraviolet light (Landrum & Bone, 2001). To this point, individuals having a rich diet in carotenoids diet may be protected against age-related macular degeneration (Fraser & Bramley, 2004; Hammond Jr, Johnson, Russel, et al., 1997); a disease affecting almost one-third of people over 75 years old (Berman et al., 2015; Mozaffarieh, Sacu, & Wedrich, 2003). Lycopene and astaxanthin are effective scavengers of reactive oxygen species that can be compared to other dietary antioxidants, such as α-tocopherol and ascorbic acid. They are also potent inhibitors of lipid peroxidation in foods, as well as lipopolysaccharide-induced superoxide production, peroxide-induced cytotoxicity, and LDL oxidation In addition, the antiinflammatory and immunomodulatory activities of carotenoids have received significant attention for their potential role in preventing oxidative stress, cancer, and CVD disease (Kim et al., 2011; Visioli & Artaria, 2017). To this line, they have been proposed as potential food antioxidants and bioactive compounds to fortify foods. For example, ketocarotenoids like astaxanthin have important applications in the nutraceutical, cosmetics, and feed industries (Fassett & Coombes, 2005; Zhu, Naqvi, Capell, et al., 2009), reflecting their antiinflammatory properties, ability to inhibit the oxidation of LDL and to produce animal pigmentation (Iwamoto, Hosoda, Hirano, et al., 2000).

In the food industry, carotenoids are mainly extracted to be used as colorants in fruit juices, pasta, beverages, candies, margarine, cheeses, and sausages. The demands for natural colorants have been growing recently due to the increase of awareness of consumer toward more natural food products. Carotenoids are often fortified to foods because of their coloring properties as well as due to their potent antioxidant and biological functions to human health. For example, the yellow color of many fruits and vegetables may be attributed to carotenoids like β-carotene and α-carotene, whereas orange fruits such as mandarin, papaya, and orange are also rich in cryptoxanthin and zeaxanthin. The red color of tomato, watermelon, pink grapefruit, guava, and gac fruits is due to the presence of lycopene (Aoki, Kieu, Kuze, et al., 2002; Bramley, 2000) that today is commercially important as a natural dark red pigment.. On the other hand, zeaxanthin is preferred over other carotenoids (e.g., it is at least 1.5-fold as potent as lutein) for enhancing pigmentation in several products (e.g., poultry and fish) due to its potency to provide a true color. When administered to poultry in high doses, carotenoid or carotenoid-containing compounds such as canthaxanthin, alfalfa, and cayenne pepper cause abnormal red or purple colors in the flesh and color striations in yolks (Orndorff, Campbell, & Medwid, 1994; Sajilata, Singhal, & Kamat, 2008).

Applications of ionic liquids in the food industry and toxicity issues

As referred earlier, carotenoids may be recovered using ionic liquids. The latest are used in the food industry as solvents for synthesizing food ingredients. Traces of ionic liquid residual can be found in the marketed food products (Martins et al., 2017). However, Larangeira, de Rosso, da Silva, de Moura, and Ribeiro (2016) recommended that a low dose of 1-butyl-3-methyl-imidazolium at 10 mg/kg body weight per day that used in the extraction of carotenoids from tomatoes is unable to exhibit toxicological effects.

These nontoxicological effects were indicated by the genotoxicity, mutagenicity, and cytotoxicity analyses using multiple organs of the experimental rats treated with the ionic liquid. Although ionic liquids have been extensively studied for its potential use in food industry, a recent metaanalysis revealed that there is a need to fill in the knowledge gap in terms of the effect on human health and the environment safety (Heckenbach, Romero, Green, & Halden, 2016). Considering the benefits of ionic liquids, therefore, further studies are required to address the safety of ionic liquids on human consumption.

In particular, the toxicity of ionic liquids is a major health issue since the dramatic growth of the use of ionic liquid in food research and development. Ionic liquids which known as environment-friendly chemicals are toxic to aquatic organisms (Pham, Cho, & Yun, 2010). Although ionic liquids are considered as the green solvents, the cations of these liquids are able to be oxidized in various position on the alkyl side chain (Zhao, Liao, & Zhang, 2007). In many cases, the ionic liquids are used together with toxic organic solvents such as acetone and 2-propanol (Eckstein, Villela Filho, Liese, & Kragl, 2004). The addition of organic solvent to ionic liquid during extraction of carotenoid contributes to the increase ecotoxicological risk. Thus it is another issue for ionic liquid application. A previous study also reported that imidazolium salt with longer alkyl chain length showed a higher inhibition of marine algae growth (Cho et al., 2007).

Ionic liquids are not only toxic to aquatic organisms (Pretti et al., 2009), but the anionic and cationic compounds also cytotoxic (Frade & Afonso, 2010) to human body. Literature shows that ionic liquids are more toxic than water-soluble organic solvents which include acetone, acetonitrile, ethanol, dimethylformamide, and dimethyl sulfoxide (Wang et al., 2007). The study found that 1-ethyl-3-methylimidazolium tetrafluoroborate ($[C_2MIM][BF_4]$) induced apoptosis in HeLa cells. Another study also determined the cytotoxic effect of 27 anions with addition of imidazolium cation using promyelocytic leukemia rat cell line IPC-81 and WST-1 assay (Stolte et al., 2006). The results show mixed toxicity effects of these anionic liquids, and 10 of 27 tested anions had the anionic effect. A review paper also reported the toxic effect of ionic liquids, where it covers aquatic system, microbiological approach, cytotoxicity, and animal studies (Zhao et al., 2007). The in vivo toxicity studies used experimental animals such as nematode (Swatloski et al., 2004), snails (Bernot, Kennedy, & Lamberti, 2005), zebrafish (Pretti et al., 2006), and rats (Landry, Brooks, Poche, & Woolhiser, 2005). All these studies show that ionic liquids are toxic. Due to the toxic effect of ionic liquids has been reported in the literature, the use of ionic liquids in the extraction of carotenoids for food colorant and as nutraceutical is not recommended.

Conclusion

Carotenoid extraction has been under intensive research efforts during the past few years since carotenoids have been reported to exhibit antioxidative and anticarcinogenic effects as well as reducing the risk of getting other chronic diseases. Natural carotenoids are more stable and have the desired biological active compounds as compared to the synthetic carotenoids. Conventional extraction of carotenoids is known to require long extraction time, consume large amounts of solvents, and require several extraction steps. Owing to the drawbacks on the conventional extraction methods and the concerns about the health and safety issues, this has led to the search of the alternative extraction methods using ionic liquids as well as the hydrotropic solutions, for reducing the use of organic solvent and protect against environmental pollution. Regardless of the techniques employed, ionic liquids have proved to be a better solvent for extraction and separation of carotenoids from plants. The cation and anion in the ionic liquids increase the extraction efficiency, significantly reduce the extraction time and reduce the amount of solvent consumption. In conclusion, ionic liquids appear to be an excellent alternative as a promising green extraction solvent, with potential applications within the food industry. The limited information of its toxicity, bioactivity and stability in food application warrants further studies in these areas.

References

Aizawa, K., & Inakuma, T. (2007). Quantitation of carotenoids in commonly consumed vegetables in Japan. *Food Science and Technology Research, 13*(3), 247–252. https://doi.org/10.3136/fstr.13.247.

Alfonsi, K., Colberg, J., Dunn, P. J., Fevig, T., Jennings, S., Johnson, T. A., et al. (2008). Green chemistry tools to influence a medicinal chemistry and research chemistry based organisation. *Green Chemistry, 10*(1), 31–36. https://doi.org/10.1039/b711717e.

Aman, R., Schieber, A., & Carle, R. (2005). Effects of heating and illumination on trans–cis isomerization and degradation of β-carotene and lutein in isolated spinach chloroplasts. *Journal of Agricultural and Food Chemistry, 53*, 9512–9518. https://doi.org/10.1021/jf050926w.

Amaya Delia, B. R. (2016). Natural food pigments and colorants. *Current Opinion in Food Science, 7*, 20–26. https://doi.org/10.1016/j.cofs.2015.08.004.

Amorim-Carrilho, K. T., Cepeda, A., Fente, C., & Regal, P. (2014). Review of methods for analysis of carotenoids. *Trends in Analytical Chemistry, 56*, 49–73. https://doi.org/10.1016/j.trac.2013.12.011.

Amr, A. S., & Hussein, D. S. (2013). Tomato pomace pigment: extraction and use as food colorant. *Jordan Journal of Agricultural Sciences, 9*(1), 72–85. Retrieved from https://journals.ju.edu.jo/JJAS/article/view/3646.

Andarwulan, N., Kurniasih, D., Aris, R., Rahmat, H., Roto, A. V., & Bolling, B. W. (2012). Polyphenols, carotenoids, and ascorbic acid in underutilized medicinal vegetables. *Journal of Functional Foods, 4*(1), 339–347. https://doi.org/10.1016/j.jff.2012.01.003.

Anese, M., et al. (2015). Effect of ultrasound treatment, oil addition and storage time on lycopene stability and in vitro bioaccessibility of tomato pulp. *Food Chemistry, 172*, 685–691. https://doi.org/10.1016/j.foodchem.2014.09.140.

Ansari, K. B., & Gaikar, V. G. (2014). Green hydrotropic extraction technology for deligni fi cation of sugarcane bagasse by using alkybenzene sulfonates as hydrotropes. *Chemical Engineering Science, 115*, 157–166. https://doi.org/10.1016/j.ces.2013.10.042.

Aoki, H., Kieu, N. T., Kuze, N., et al. (2002). Carotenoid pigments in GAC fruit (*Momordica cochinchinensis* SPRENG). *Bioscience, Biotechnology, and Biochemistry, 66*, 2479–2482. https://doi.org/10.1271/bbb.66.2479.

Arvayo-Enríquez, H., Mondaca-Fernández, I., Gortárez-Moroyoqui, P., López-Cervantes, J., & Rodríguez-Ramírez, R. (2013). Carotenoids extraction and quantification: a review. *Analytical Methods, 5*(12), 2916. https://doi.org/10.1039/c3ay26295b.

Babu, C. M., Chakrabarti, R., & Sambasivarao, K. R. S. (2008). Enzymatic isolation of carotenoid-protein complex from shrimp head waste and its use as a source of carotenoids. *LWT—Food Science and Technology, 41*(2), 227–235. https://doi.org/10.1016/j.lwt.2007.03.006.

Bai, C., Twyman, R. M., Farre, G., et al. (2011). A golden era—provitamin A enhancement in diverse crops. *In Vitro Cellular & Developmental Biology Plant, 47,* 205–221. https://doi.org/10.1007/s11627-011-9363-6.

Barbero, G. F., Palma, M., & Barroso, C. G. (2006). Pressurized liquid extraction of capsaicinoids from peppers. *Journal of Agricultural and Food Chemistry, 54,* 3231–3236. https://doi.org/10.1021/jf060021y.

Berendschot, T.T.J.M., & Plat, J. (2014). Plant stanol and sterol esters and macular pigment optical density. In *Handbook of nutrition, diet and the eye.* Elsevier. https://doi.org/10.1016/B978-0-12-401717-7.00044-7.

Berman, J., Zorrilla-Lopez, U., Farre, G., Zhu, C., Sandmann, G., Twyman, R. M., et al. (2015). Nutritionally important carotenoids as consumer products. *Phytochemistry Reviews, 14,* 727–743. https://doi.org/10.1007/s11101-014-9373-1.

Bernot, R. J., Kennedy, E. E., & Lamberti, G. A. (2005). Effects of ionic liquids on the survival, movement, and feeding behavior of the freshwater snail, *Physa acuta. Environmental Toxicology and Chemistry, 24*(7), 1759–1765. https://doi.org/10.1897/04-614R.1.

Bi, W., Tian, M., Zhou, J., & Row, K. H. (2010). Task-specific ionic liquid-assisted extraction and separation of astaxanthin from shrimp waste. *Journal of Chromatography B, 878*(24), 2243–2248. https://doi.org/10.1016/j.jchromb.2010.06.034.

Bialek-Bylka, G. E., Pawlak, K., Jazurek, B., Skrzypczak, A., & Koyama, Y. (2007). Spectroscopic properties and temperature induced electronic configuration changes of all-trans and 15-cis β-carotenes in ionic liquids. *Photosynthetica, 45*(2), 161–166. https://doi.org/10.1007/s11099-007-0027-z.

Bouvier, F., Suire, C., Mutterer, J., et al. (2003). Oxidative remodeling of chromoplast carotenoids: identification of the carotenoid dioxygenase CsCCD and CsZCD genes involved in crocus secondary metabolite biogenesis. *Plant Cell, 15,* 47–62. https://doi.org/10.1105/tpc.006536.

Bramley, P. M. (2000). Is lycopene beneficial to human health? *Phytochemistry, 54,* 233–236.

Breithaupt, D. E. (2004). Simultaneous HPLC determination of carotenoids used as food coloring additives: applicability of accelerated solvent extraction. *Food Chemistry, 86,* 449–456. https://doi.org/10.1016/j.foodchem.2003.10.027.

Buijsse, B., Feskens, E. J. M., Schlettwein-gsell, D., Ferry, M., Kok, F. J., & Kromhout, D. (2005). Plasma carotene and α-tocopherol in relation to 10-y all-cause and cause-specific mortality in European elderly: the survey in europe on nutrition and the elderly, a concerted action (SENECA). *American Journal of Clinical Nutrition, 82,* 879–886. https://doi.org/10.1093/ajcn/82.4.879.

Burdick, E. M. (1966). U.S. Patent No. 3,248,301. Washington, DC: U.S. Patent and Trademark Office. Retrieved from https://patents.google.com/patent/US3248301A/en.

Capello, C., Fischer, U., & Hungerbu, K. (2007). What is a green solvent? A comprehensive framework for the environmental assessment of solvents. *Green Chemistry, 9*(9), 927–934. https://doi.org/10.1039/b617536h.

Cassano, A., & Galanakis, C. M. (2018). Membrane technologies for the fractionation of compounds recovered from cereal processing by-products. In C. M. Galanakis (Ed.), *Sustainable recovery and reutilization of cereal processing by-products.* Waltham: Elsevier Inc. [chapter 6].

Cattuzzato, L., Dumont, S., Le Gelebart, E., & Loeuil, J. (2018). *Obtaining an extract from brown algae gametophytes, and use of said extract as a cosmetic anti-aging active principle.* U.S. Patent Application No. 15/553,018. Retrieved from https://patents.google.com/patent/US20180028437A1/en.

Chemat, F., Fabiano-tixier, A. S., Abert, M., Allaf, T., & Vorobiev, E. (2015). Solvent-free extraction of food and natural products. *Trends in Analytical Chemistry, 71*, 157–168. https://doi.org/10.1016/j.trac.2015.02.021.

Chemat, F., Huma, Z., & Khan, M. K. (2011). Applications of ultrasound in food technology: processing, preservation and extraction. *Ultrasonics Sonochemistry, 18*, 813–835. https://doi.org/10.1016/j.ultsonch.2010.11.023.

Chemat, F., Rombaut, N., Sicaire, A., Meullemiestre, A., & Abert-vian, M. (2017). Ultrasonics assisted extraction of food and natural products. Mechanisms, techniques, combinations, protocols and applications. A review. *Ultrasonics Sonochemistry, 34*, 540–560. https://doi.org/10.1016/j.ultsonch.2016.06.035.

Cho, C. W., Pham, T. P. T., Jeon, Y. C., Vijayaraghavan, K., Choe, W. S., & Yun, Y. S. (2007). Toxicity of imidazolium salt with anion bromide to a phytoplankton *Selenastrum capricornutum*: effect of alkyl-chain length. *Chemosphere, 69*(6), 1003–1007. https://doi.org/10.1016/j.chemosphere.2007.06.023.

Choudhari, S. M., & Ananthanarayan, L. (2007). Enzyme aided extraction of lycopene from tomato tissues. *Food Chemistry, 102*, 77–81. https://doi.org/10.1016/j.foodchem.2006.04.031.

Craft, N. E., & Soares, J. H. (1992). Relative solubility, stability, and absorptivity of lutein and β-carotene in organic solvents. *Journal of Agricultural and Food Chemistry, 40*(3), 431–434. https://doi.org/10.1021/jf00015a013.

da Silva, L. M. R., De Figueiredo, E. A. T., Ricardo, N.M.P.S., Vieira, I. G. P., De Figueiredo, R. W., Brasil, I. M., et al. (2014). Quantification of bioactive compounds in pulps and by-products of tropical fruits from Brazil. *Food Chemistry, 143*, 398–404. https://doi.org/10.1016/j.foodchem.2013.08.001.

Dandekar, D. V., & Gaikar, V. G. (2003). Separation science and technology hydrotropic extraction of curcuminoids from turmeric hydrotropic extraction of curcuminoids. *Separation Science and Technology, 38*(5), 1185–1215. https://doi.org/10.1081/SS-120018130.

Dandekar, D. V., Jayaprakasha, G. K., & Patil, B. S. (2008). Hydrotropic extraction of bioactive limonin from sour orange (*Citrus aurantium* L.) seeds. *Food Chemistry, 109*, 515–520. https://doi.org/10.1016/j.foodchem.2007.12.071.

Delgado-vargas, F., & Paredes-lpez, O. (1997). Effects of enzymatic treatments on carotenoid extraction from marigold flowers (*Tagetes erecta*). *Food Chemistry, 58*(3), 255–258. https://doi.org/10.1016/S0308-8146(96)00163-X.

Dhapte, V., & Mehta, P. (2015). Advances in hydrotropic solutions: an updated review. *St. Petersburg Polytechnical University Journal: Physics and Mathematics, 1*(4), 424–435. https://doi.org/10.1016/j.spjpm.2015.12.006.

Dietz, M. L. (2006). Ionic liquids as extraction solvents: where do we stand? *Separation Science and Technology, 41*(10), 2047–2063. https://doi.org/10.1080/01496390600743144.

Eckstein, M., Villela Filho, M., Liese, A., & Kragl, U. (2004). Use of an ionic liquid in a two-phase system to improve an alcohol dehydrogenase catalysed reduction. *Chemical Communications, 2004*, 1084–1085. https://doi.org/10.1039/B401065E.

Farre, G., Sanahuja, G., Naqvi, S., et al. (2010). Travel advice on the road to carotenoids in plants. *Plant Science, 179*(28), 48. https://doi.org/10.1016/j.plantsci.2010.03.009.

Fassett, R. G., & Coombes, J. S. (2005). Astaxanthin: a potential therapeutic agent in cardiovascular disease. *Marine Drugs, 9*, 447–465. https://doi.org/10.3390/md9030447.

Fish, W. W. (2006). Interaction of sodium dodecyl sulfate with watermelon chromoplasts and examination of the organization of lycopene within the chromoplasts. *Journal of Agricultural and Food Chemistry*, *54*, 8294–8300. https://doi.org/10.1021/jf061468+.

Frade, R. F., & Afonso, C. A. (2010). Impact of ionic liquids in environment and humans: an overview. *Human & Experimental Toxicology*, *29*(12), 1038–1054. https://doi.org/10.1177/0960327110371259.

Fraser, P. D., & Bramley, P. M. (2004). The biosynthesis and nutritional uses of carotenoids. *Progress in Lipid Research*, *43*, 228–265. https://doi.org/10.1016/j.plipres.2003.10.002.

Gaikar, V. G., & Sharma, M. M. (1993). Separations with hydrotropes. *Separations Technology*, *3*(1), 2–11. https://doi.org/10.1080/07366298608917896.

Galanakis, C. M. (2012). Recovery of high added-value components from food wastes: conventional, emerging technologies and commercialized applications. *Trends in Food Science & Technology*, *26*, 68–87. https://doi.org/10.1016/j.tifs.2012.03.003.

Galanakis, C. M. (2013). Emerging technologies for the production of nutraceuticals from agricultural by-products: a viewpoint of opportunities and challenges. *Food and Bioproducts Processing*, *91*, 575–579. https://doi.org/10.1016/j.fbp.2013.01.004.

Galanakis, C. M. (2015). Preface. In C. M. Galanakis (Ed.), *Food waste recovery: Processing technologies and industrial techniques*.

Galanakis, C. M. (2016). *Innovation strategies for the food industry: Tools for implementation*. Elsevier-Academic Press, ISBN: 9780128037515.

Galanakis, C. M. (2017a). *Handbook of coffee processing by-products: Sustainable applications*. Elsevier-Academic Press.

Galanakis, C. M. (2017b). *Handbook of grape processing by-products: Sustainable solutions*. Elsevier-Academic Press, ISBN: 9780128098707.

Galanakis, C. M. (2017c). *Olive mill waste: Recent advances for the sustainable management*. Elsevier-Academic Press, ISBN: 9780128053140.

Galanakis, C. M. (2017d). *Nutraceutical and functional food components: Effects of innovative processing techniques*. Elsevier-Academic Press, ISBN: 9780128052570.

Galanakis, C. M. (2017e). Membrane technologies for the separation of compounds recovered from grape processing by-products. In C. M. Galanakis (Ed.), *Handbook of grape processing by-products: Sustainable solutions*. Waltham: Elsevier Inc. [chapter 6].

Galanakis, C. M. (2018a). *Polyphenols: Properties, recovery and applications*. Elsevier-Academic Press.

Galanakis, C. M. (2018b). *Sustainable recovery and reutilization of cereal processing by-products*. Elsevier-Woodprint.

Galanakis, C. M. (2018c). *Sustainable food systems from agriculture to industry: Improving production and processing*. Elsevier-Academic Press.

Galanakis, C. M. (2019a). *Dietary fiber: Properties, recovery & applications*. Elsevier Inc.

Galanakis, C. M. (2019b). *Proteins: Sustainable source, processing and applications*. Elsevier Inc.

Galanakis, C. M. (2019c). *The role of alternative and innovative food ingredients and products in consumer wellness*. Elsevier Inc..

Galanakis, C. M. (2019d). *Saving food: Production, supply chain, food waste and food consumption*. Elsevier-Academic Press.

Galanakis, C. M. (2019e). *Separation of functional molecules in food by membrane technology (2019)*. Elsevier-Academic Press.

Galanakis, C. M. (2019f). In C. M. Galanakis (Ed.), *Sustainable meat production and processing (2018)*. Elsevier-Academic Press. ISBN: 9780128148747.

Galanakis, C. M., Goulas, V., Tsakona, S., Manganaris, G. A., & Gekas, V. (2013). A knowledge
base for the recovery of natural phenols with different solvents. *International Journal of
Food Properties*, *16*, 382–396. https://doi.org/10.1080/10942912.2010.522750.

García, S., Larriba, M., García, J., Torrecilla, J. S., & Rodríguez, F. (2012). Liquid-liquid extraction of toluene from n-heptane using binary mixtures of N-butylpyridinium tetrafluoroborate and N-butylpyridinium bis(trifluoromethylsulfonyl)imide ionic liquids. *Chemical
Engineering Journal*, *180*, 210–215. https://doi.org/10.1016/j.cej.2011.11.069.

Garrow, J. S., James, W. P. T., & Ralph, A. (2000). *Human nutrition and dietetics* (10th ed.).
London: Churchill Livingstone Press.

Gerding, D. S., et al. (2016). High carotenoid bioaccessibility through linseed oil nanoemulsions with enhanced physical and oxidative stability. *Food Chemistry*, *199*(2016), 463–
470. https://doi.org/10.1016/j.foodchem.2015.12.004.

Hammond, B. R., Jr., Johnson, E. J., Russel, R. M., et al. (1997). Dietary modification of
human macular pigment density. *Investigative Ophthalmology & Visual Science*, *38*,
1795–1801.

Heckenbach, M. E., Romero, F. N., Green, M. D., & Halden, R. U. (2016). Meta-analysis of ionic
liquid literature and toxicology. *Chemosphere*, *150*, 266–274. https://doi.org/10.1016/j.
chemosphere.2016.02.029.

Hiranvarachat, B., & Devahastin, S. (2014). Enhancement of microwave-assisted extraction
via intermittent radiation: extraction of carotenoids from carrot peels. *Journal of Food
Engineering*, *126*, 17–26. https://doi.org/10.1016/j.jfoodeng.2013.10.024.

Hiranvarachat, B., Devahastin, S., Chiewchan, N., & Vijaya Raghavan, G. S. (2013). Structural
modification by different pretreatment methods to enhance microwave-assisted extraction
of β-carotene from carrots. *Journal of Food Engineering*, *115*(2), 190–197. https://doi.
org/10.1016/j.jfoodeng.2012.10.012.

Hodgdon, T. K., & Kaler, E. W. (2007). Hydrotropic solutions. *Current Opinion in Colloid and
Interface Science*, *12*(3), 121–128. https://doi.org/10.1016/j.cocis.2007.06.004.

Huddleston, J. G., Willauer, H. D., Swatloski, R. P., Visser, A. E., & Rogers, R. D. (1998). Room
temperature ionic liquids as novel media for 'clean' liquid—liquid extraction. *Chemical
Communications*, 1765–1766. https://doi.org/10.1039/A803999B.

Ibrahim, F., Moniruzzaman, M., Yusup, S., & Uemura, Y. (2015). Dissolution of cellulose with
ionic liquid in pressurized cell. *Journal of Molecular Liquids*, *211*, 370–372. https://doi.
org/10.1016/j.molliq.2015.07.041.

Incinur, H., & Galanakis, C. M. (2018). Recovery technologies and encapsulation techniques.
In C. M. Galanakis (Ed.), *Polyphenols: Properties, recovery and applications*. Waltham:
Elsevier Inc. [chapter 7].

Ito, Y., Suzuki, K., Ishii, J., Hishida, H., Tamakoshi, A., Hamajima, N., et al. (2006). A
population-based follow-up study on mortality from cancer or cardiovascular disease and
serum carotenoids, retinol and tocopherols in Japanese inhabitants. *Asian Pacific Journal of
Cancer Prevention*, *7*, 533–546. Retrieved from http://journal.waocp.org/article_24522.html.

Iwamoto, T., Hosoda, K., Hirano, R., et al. (2000). Inhibition of lowdensity lipoprotein oxidation by astaxanthin. *Journal of Atherosclerosis and Thrombosis*, *7*, 216–222.

Jaswir, I., Noviendri, D., Hasrini, R. F., & Octavianti, F. (2011). Carotenoids: sources, medicinal
properties and their application in food and nutraceutical industry. *Journal of Medicinal
Plant Research*, *5*(33), 7119–7131. https://doi.org/10.5897/JMPRX11.011.

Johnson, E. J., Hammond, B. R., Yeum, K., Qin, J., Wang, X. D., Castaneda, C., et al. (2000).
Relation among serum and tissue concentrations of lutein and zeaxanthin and macular
pigment density. *American Journal of Clinical Nutrition*, *71*, 1555–1562. https://doi.
org/10.1093/ajcn/71.6.1555.

Jutz, F., Andanson, J. M., & Baiker, A. (2011). Ionic liquids and dense carbon dioxide: a beneficial biphasic system for catalysis. *Chemical Reviews*, *111*(2), 322–353. https://doi. org/10.1021/cr100194q.

Kim, J. Y., Kim, S., Papp, M., Park, K., & Pinal, R. (2010). Hydrotropic solubilization of poorly water-soluble drugs. *Journal of Pharmaceutical Sciences*, *99*(9), 3953–3965. https://doi. org/10.1002/jps.22241.

Kim, J. Y., Paik, J. K., Kim, O. Y., Park, H. W., Lee, J. H., Jang, Y., et al. (2011). Effects of lycopene supplementation on oxidative stress and markers of endothelial function in healthy men. *Atherosclerosis*, *215*(1), 189–195. https://doi.org/10.1016/j. atherosclerosis.2010.11.036.

Kirthi, K., Amita, S., Priti, S., Kumar, A. M., & Jyoti, S. (2014). Colourful world of microbes: carotenoids and their applications. *Advances in Biology*, *2014*, 1–13. https://doi. org/10.1155/2014/837891.

Kongkachuichai, R., Charoensiri, R., Yakoh, K., & Kringkasemsee, A. (2015). Nutrients value and antioxidant content of indigenous vegetables from Southern Thailand. *Food Chemistry*, *173*, 838–846. https://doi.org/10.1016/j.foodchem.2014.10.123.

Koo, S. Y., Cha, K. H., Song, D., Chung, D., & Pan, C. H. (2012). Optimization of pressurized liquid extraction of zeaxanthin from *Chlorella ellipsoidea*. *Journal of Applied Phycology*, *24*(4), 725–730. https://doi.org/10.1007/s10811-011-9691-2.

Kopsell, D. A., & Kopsell, D. E. (2006). Accumulation and bioavailability of dietary carotenoids in vegetable crops. *Trends in Plant Science*, *11*(10), 1360–1385. https://doi.org/10.1016/j. tplants.2006.08.006.

Koubala, B. B., Mbome, L. I., Kansci, G., Tchouanguep Mbiapo, F., Crepeau, M.–J., Thibault, J.–.F., et al. (2008). Physicochemical properties of pectins from ambarella peels (*Spondias cytherea*) obtained using different extraction conditions. *Food Chemistry*, *106*, 1202–1207. https://doi.org/10.1016/j.foodchem.2007.07.065.

Kovacevic, D. B., Barba, F. J., Granato, D., Galanakis, C. M., Herceg, Z., Dragovic-Uzelac, V., et al. (2018). Pressurized hot water extraction (PHWE) for the green recovery of bioactive compounds from steviol glycosides from stevis rebaudiana bertoni Leaves. *Food Chemistry*, *254*, 150–157. https://doi.org/10.1016/j.foodchem.2018.01.192.

Landrum, J. T., & Bone, R. A. (2001). Lutein, zeaxanthin, and the macular pigment. *Archives of Biochemistry and Biophysics*, *385*, 28–40. https://doi.org/10.1006/abbi.2000.2171.

Landry, T. D., Brooks, K., Poche, D., & Woolhiser, M. (2005). Acute toxicity profile of 1-butyl-3-methylimidazolium chloride. *Bulletin of Environmental Contamination and Toxicology*, *74*(3), 559–565. https://doi.org/10.1007/s00128-005-0620-4.

Larangeira, P. M., de Rosso, V. V., da Silva, V. H. P., de Moura, C. F. G., & Ribeiro, D. A. (2016). Genotoxicity, mutagenicity and cytotoxicity of carotenoids extracted from ionic liquid in multiples organs of wistar rats. *Experimental and Toxicologic Pathology*, *68*(10), 571–578. https://doi.org/10.1016/j.etp.2016.09.003.

Larsen, E., & Christensen, L. (2005). Simple Saponification method for the quantitative determination of carotenoids in green vegetables. *Journal of Agricultural and Food Chemistry*, *53*, 6598–6602. https://doi.org/10.1021/jf050622+.

Lavecchia, R., & Zuorro, A. (2008). Improved lycopene extraction from tomato peels using cellwall degrading enzymes. *European Food Research and Technology*, *228*, 153–158. https:// doi.org/10.1007/s00217-008-0897-8.

Li, Y., Fabiano-tixier, A. S., Tomao, V., Cravotto, G., & Chemat, F. (2013). Ultrasonics sonochemistry green ultrasound-assisted extraction of carotenoids based on the biorefinery concept using sunflower oil as an alternative solvent. *Ultrasonics Sonochemistry*, *20*, 12–18. https://doi.org/10.1016/j.ultsonch.2012.07.005.

Luengo, E., Condón-abanto, S., Condón, S., Álvarez, I., & Raso, J. (2014). Improving the extraction of carotenoids from tomato waste by application of ultrasound under pressure. *Separation and Purification Technology*, *136*, 130–136. https://doi.org/10.1016/j.seppur.2014.09.008.

Luque de Castro, M. D., & Garcia-Ayuso, L. E. (1998). Soxhlet extraction of solid materials: an outdated technique with a promising innovative future. *Analytica Chimica Acta*, *369*, 1–10. https://doi.org/10.1016/S0003-2670(98)00233-5.

Martins, P. L. G., Braga, A. R., & de Rosso, V. V. (2017). Can ionic liquid solvents be applied in the food industry? *Trends in Food Science and Technology*, *66*, 117–124. https://doi.org/10.1016/j.tifs.2017.06.002.

Martins, P. L. G., & de Rosso, V. V. (2016). Thermal and light stabilities and antioxidant activity of carotenoids from tomatoes extracted using an ultrasound-assisted completely solvent-free method. *Food Research International*, *82*, 156–164. https://doi.org/10.1016/j.foodres.2016.01.015.

Mcclements, D. J., & Xiao, H. (2014). Excipient foods: designing food matrices that improve the oral bioavailability of pharmaceuticals and nutraceuticals. *Food & Function*, *5*(7), 1320–1333. https://doi.org/10.1039/C4FO00100A.

Mendiola, J. A., Herrero, M., Cifuentes, A., & Iba, E. (2007). Use of compressed fluids for sample preparation: food applications. *Journal of Chromatography A*, *1152*, 234–246. https://doi.org/10.1016/j.chroma.2007.02.046.

Mezzomo, N., & Ferreira, S. R. S. (2016). Carotenoids functionality, sources, and processing by supercritical technology: a review. *Journal of Chemistry*, *2016*, 3164312. https://doi.org/10.1155/2016/3164312.

Mozaffarieh, M., Sacu, S., & Wedrich, A. (2003). The role of the carotenoids, lutein and zeaxanthin, in protecting against age-related macular degeneration: a review based on controversial evidence. *Nutrition Journal*, *11*, 20–28. https://doi.org/10.1186/1475-2891-2-20.

Mujumdar, A. S., & Law, C. L. (2010). Drying technology: trends and applications in postharvest processing. *Food and Bioprocess Technology*, *3*(6), 843–852. https://doi.org/10.1007/s11947-010-0353-1.

Mustafa, A., Trevino, L. M., & Turner, C. (2012). Pressurized hot ethanol extraction of carotenoids from carrot by-products. *Molecules*, *17*, 1809–1818. https://doi.org/10.3390/molecules17021809.

Nagarajan, J., Ramanan, R. N., Raghunandan, Galanakis, C. M., & Prasad, N. K. (2017). Carotenoids. In C. M. Galanakis (Ed.), *Nutraceutical and functional food components: Effect of innovative processing techniques*. Waltham: Elsevier Inc.

Namitha, K. K., & Negi, P. S. (2010). Chemistry and biotechnology of carotenoids. *Critical Reviews in Food Science and Nutrition*, *50*(8), 1040–8398. https://doi.org/10.1080/10408398.2010.499811.

Navarrete-bolan, L., Rangel-cruz, C. L., Jime, H., Botello-alvarez, E., & Rico-marti, R. (2005). Pre-treatment effects on the extraction efficiency of xanthophylls from marigold flower (*Tagetes erecta*) using hexane. *Food Research International*, *38*(2), 159–165. https://doi.org/10.1016/j.foodres.2004.09.007.

Oreopoulou, V., & Tzia, C. (2007). Utilization of plant by-products for the recovery of proteins, dietary fibers, antioxidants, and colorants. In V. Oreopoulou & W. Russ (Eds.), *Utilization of by-products and treatment of waste in the food industry* (pp. 209–232). New York: Springer Science+Business Media.

Orndorff, S. A., Campbell, E. A., & Medwid, R. D. (1994). inventors *Zeaxanthin producing strains of neospongiococcum excentricum*. U.S. patent 5,360,730.

Oroian, M., & Escriche, I. (2015). Antioxidants: characterization, natural sources, extraction and analysis. *Food Research International*, *74*, 10–36. https://doi.org/10.1016/j.foodres.2015.04.018.

Pasquet, V., Chérouvrier, J. R., Farhat, F., Thiéry, V., Piot, J. M., Bérard, J. B., et al. (2011). Study on the microalgal pigments extraction process: performance of microwave assisted extraction. *Process Biochemistry*, *46*(1), 59–67. https://doi.org/10.1016/j.procbio.2010.07.009.

Passos, H., Freire, M. G., & Coutinho, J. A. P. (2014). Ionic liquid solutions as extractive solvents for value-added compounds from biomass. *Green Chemistry*, *16*(12), 4786–4815. https://doi.org/10.1039/c4gc00236a.

Pham, T. P. T., Cho, C. W., & Yun, Y. S. (2010). Environmental fate and toxicity of ionic liquids: a review. *Water Research*, *44*(2), 352–372. https://doi.org/10.1016/j.watres.2009.09.030.

Poojary, M. M., Barba, F. J., Aliakbarian, B., Donsì, F., Pataro, G., Dias, D. A., et al. (2016). Innovative alternative technologies to extract carotenoids from microalgae and seaweeds. *Marine Drugs*, *14*(11), 1–34. https://doi.org/10.3390/md14110214.

Pretti, C., Chiappe, C., Baldetti, I., Brunini, S., Monni, G., & Intorre, L. (2009). Acute toxicity of ionic liquids for three freshwater organisms: *Pseudokirchneriella subcapitata*, *Daphnia magna* and *Danio rerio*. *Ecotoxicology and Environmental Safety*, *72*(4), 1170–1176. https://doi.org/10.1016/j.ecoenv.2008.09.010.

Pretti, C., Chiappe, C., Pieraccini, D., Gregori, M., Abramo, F., Monnia, G., et al. (2006). Acute toxicity of ionic liquids to the zebrafish (*Danio rerio*). *Green Chemistry*, *8*, 238–240. https://doi.org/10.1039/B511554J.

Priyadarshani, A. M. B., & Jansz, E. R. (2014). A critical review on carotenoid research in Sri Lankan context and its outcomes. *Critical Reviews in Food Science and Nutrition*, *54*(5), 561–571. https://doi.org/10.1080/10408398.2011.595019.

Rajabi, M. S., Moniruzzaman, M., Mahmood, H., Sivapragasam, M., & Bustam, M. A. (2017). Extraction of β-carotene from organic phase using ammonium based ionic liquids. *Journal of Molecular Liquids*, *227*, 15–20. https://doi.org/10.1016/j.molliq.2016.12.008.

Raman, G., & Gaikar, V. G. (2002). Extraction of piperine from *Piper nigrum* (black pepper) by hydrotropic solubilization. *Industrial & Engineering Chemistry Research*, *41*(12), 2966–2976. https://doi.org/10.1021/ie0107845.

Ribaya-Mercado, J.D.., & Blumberg, J.B..b. (2004). Lutein and zeaxanthin and their potential roles in disease prevention. *Journal of the American College of Nutrition*, *23*(6 Suppl), 567S–587S.

Roohinejad, S., Everett, D. W., & Oey, I. (2014). Effect of pulsed electric field processing on carotenoid extractability of carrot puree. *International Journal of Food Science and Technology*, *49*, 2120–2127. https://doi.org/10.1111/ijfs.12510.

Routray, W., & Orsat, V. (2012). Microwave-assisted extraction of flavonoids: a review. *Food and Bioprocess Technology*, *5*(2), 409–424. https://doi.org/10.1007/s11947-011-0573-z.

Rutz, J. K., Borges, C. D., Zambiazi, R. C., Rosa, C. G., & Silva, M. M. (2016). Elaboration of microparticles of carotenoids from natural and synthetic sources for applications in food. *Food Chemistry*, *202*(2016), 324–333. https://doi.org/10.1016/j.foodchem.2016.01.140.

Saini, R. K., & Keum, Y. S. (2018). Carotenoid extraction methods: a review of recent developments. *Food Chemistry*, *240*, 90–103. https://doi.org/10.1016/j.foodchem.2017.07.099. April 2017.

Saini, R. K., Moon, S. H., & Keum, Y. (2018). An updated review on use of tomato pomace and crustacean processing waste to recover commercially vital carotenoids. *Food Research International*, *108*, 516–529. https://doi.org/10.1016/j.foodres.2018.04.003.

Saini, R. K., Nile, S. H., & Park, S. W. (2015). Carotenoids from fruits and vegetables: chemistry, analysis, occurrence, bioavailability and biological activities. *Food Research International, 76*, 735–750. https://doi.org/10.1016/j.foodres.2015.07.047.

Saini, R. K., Shetty, N., & Giridhar, P. (2014). Carotenoid content in vegetative and reproductive parts of commercially grown *Moringa oleifera* Lam. cultivars from India by LC–APCI–MS. *European Food Research and Technology, 238*, 971–978. https://doi.org/10.1007/s00217-014-2174-3.

Saini, R. K., Shetty, N. P., Prakash, M., & Giridhar, P. (2014). Effect of dehydration methods on retention of carotenoids, tocopherols, ascorbic acid and antioxidant activity in *Moringa oleifera* leaves and preparation of a RTE product. *Journal of Food Science and Technology, 51*(9), 2176–2182. https://doi.org/10.1007/s13197-014-1264-3.

Sajilata, M. G., Singhal, R. S., & Kamat, M. Y. (2008). The carotenoid pigment, zeaxanthin-a review. *Comprehensive Reviews in Food Science and Food Safety, 7*, 29–49. https://doi.org/10.1111/j.1541-4337.2007.00028.x.

Saleh, A. M., & El-Khordagui, L. K. (1985). Hydrotropic agents: a new definition. *International Journal of Pharmaceutics, 24*, 231–238. https://doi.org/10.1016/0378-5173(85)90023-7.

Sarkar, C., et al. (2012). An efficient condition of Saponification of lutein ester from marigold flower. *Annals of Biological Research, 3*(3), 1461–1466.

Seddon, K. R. (1997). Ionic liquids for clean technology. *Journal of Chemical Technology & Biotechnology, 68*, 351–356. https://doi.org/10.1002/(SICI)1097-4660(199704)68:4<351::AID-JCTB613>3.0.CO;2-4.

Shanmugam, A., & Ashokkumar, M. (2015). Characterization of ultrasonically prepared flaxseed oil enriched beverage/carrot juice emulsion and process-induced changes to the functional properties of carrot juice. *Food and Bioprocess Technology, 8*, 1258–1266. https://doi.org/10.1007/s11947-015-1492-1.

Singh, A., Ahmad, S., & Ahmad, A. (2015). Green extraction methods and environmental applications of carotenoids-a review. *RSC Advances, 5*(77), 62358–62393. https://doi.org/10.1039/C5RA10243J.

Sivapragasam, M., Moniruzzaman, M., & Goto, M. (2016). Recent advances in exploiting ionic liquids for biomolecules: solubility, stability and applications. *Biotechnology Journal, 11*, 1000–1013. https://doi.org/10.1002/biot.201500603.

Skendi, A., Harasym, J., & Galanakis, C. M. (2018). Recovery of high added value compounds from brewing and distillate processing by-products. In C. M. Galanakis (Ed.), *Sustainable recovery and reutilization of cereal processing by-products*. Waltham: Elsevier Inc. [chapter 7].

Socaci, S. A., Fǎrcaş, A. C., & Galanakis, C. M. (2019). Introduction in functional components for membrane separations. In C. M. Galanakis (Ed.), *Separation of functional molecules in food by membrane technology*. Waltham: Elsevier Inc. [chapter 2].

Sommer, A. (2008). Vitamin a deficiency and clinical disease: an historical overview. *The Journal of Nutrition, 138*(10), 1835–1839. https://doi.org/10.1016/B978-0-7506-8816-1.50021-5.

Song, J., & Han, B. (2015). Green chemistry: a tool for the sustainable development of the chemical industry. *National Science Review, 2*(3), 255–256. https://doi.org/10.1093/nsr/nwu076.

Stolte, S., Arning, J., Bottin-Weber, U., Matzke, M., Stock, F., Thiele, K., et al. (2006). Anion effects on the cytotoxicity of ionic liquids. *Green Chemistry, 8*(7), 621–629. https://doi.org/10.1039/B602161A.

Strati, I. F., Gogou, E., & Oreopoulou, V. (2015). Enzyme and high pressure assisted extraction of carotenoids from tomato waste. *Food and Bioproducts Processing, 94*, 668–674. https://doi.org/10.1016/j.fbp.2014.09.012.

Strati, I. F., & Oreopoulou, V. (2014). Recovery of carotenoids from tomato processing by-products—a review. *Food Research International*, *65*, 311–321. https://doi.org/10.1016/j.foodres.2014.09.032. PC.

Subbarao, C. V., Kalyan, I. P., Sai Bharadwaj, A.V.S.L., & Krishna, K. M. M. (2012). Functions of hydrotropes in solutions. *Chemical Engineering and Technology*, *35*(2), 225–237. https://doi.org/10.1002/ceat.201100484.

Sugiura, M., Kato, M., Matsumoto, H., Nagao, A., & Yano, M. (2002). Serum concentration of β-cryptoxanthin in Japan reflects the frequency of satsuma mandarin (*Citrus unshiu* Marc.) consumption. *Journal of Health Science*, *48*(4), 350–353. https://doi.org/10.1248/jhs.48.350.

Swada, J. G., Keeley, C. J., Ghane, M. A., & Engeseth, N. J. (2016). Synergistic potential of papaya and strawberry nectar blends focus on specific nutrients and antioxidants using alternative thermal and non thermal processing techniques. *Food Chemistry*, *199*(2016), 87–95. https://doi.org/10.1016/j.foodchem.2015.11.087.

Swatloski, R. P., Holbrey, J. D., Memon, S. B., Caldwell, G. A., Caldwell, K. A., & Rogers, R. D. (2004). Using *Caenorhabditis elegans* to probe toxicity of 1-alkyl-3-methylimidazolium chloride based ionic liquids. *Chemical Communications*, (6), 668–669. https://doi.org/10.1039/B316491H.

Tariq, M., Freire, M. G., Saramago, B., Coutinho, J. A. P., Lopes, J. N. C., & Rebelo, L. P. N. (2012). Surface tension of ionic liquids and ionic liquid solutions. *Chemical Society Reviews*, *41*, 829–868. https://doi.org/10.1039/c1cs15146k.

Tavani, A., Gallus, S., Negri, E. V. A., Parpinel, M., & Vecchia, C. L. A. (2006). Dietary intake of carotenoids and retinol and the risk of acute myocardial infarction in Italy. *Free Radical Biology and Medicine*, *40*(6), 659–664. https://doi.org/10.1080/10715760600615649.

Tsakona, S., Galanakis, C. M., & Gekas, V. (2012). Hydro-ethanolic mixtures for the recovery of phenols from mediterranean plant materials. *Food and Bioprocess Technology*, *5*(4), 1384–1393. https://doi.org/10.1007/s11947-010-0419-0.

Tzanakis, I., Lebon, G. S. B., Eskin, D. G., & Pericleous, K. A. (2017). Characterizing the cavitation development and acoustic spectrum in various liquids. *Ultrasonics Sonochemistry*, *34*, 651–662. https://doi.org/10.1016/j.ultsonch.2016.06.034.

Ucak, I., Gokoglu, N., Kiessling, M., Toepfl, S., & Galanakis, C. M. (2019). Inhibitory effects of high pressure treatment on microbial growth and biogenic amine formation in marinated herring (clupea harengus) inoculated with morganella psychrotolerans. *LWT—Food Science and Technology*, *99*, 50–56. https://doi.org/10.1016/j.lwt.2018.09.058.

Ucak, I., Gokoglu, N., Toepfl, S., & Galanakis, C. M. (2018). Inhibitory effects of high pressure processing on photobacterium phosphoreum and morganella psychrotolerans in vacuum packed herring (clupea harengus). *Journal of Food Safety*, https://doi.org/10.1111/jfs.12519. [in press].

Ventura, S. P., e Silva, F. A., Quental, M. V., Mondal, D., Freire, M. G., & Coutinho, J. A. (2017). Ionic-liquid-mediated extraction and separation processes for bioactive compounds: past, present, and future trends. *Chemical Reviews*, *117*(10), 6984–7052. https://doi.org/10.1021/acs.chemrev.6b00550.

Vieira, F. A., Guilherme, R. J. R., Neves, M. C., Rego, A., Abreu, M. H., Coutinho, J. A. P., et al. (2018). Recovery of carotenoids from brown seaweeds using aqueous solutions of surface-active ionic liquids and anionic surfactants. *Separation and Purification Technology*, *196*, 300–308. https://doi.org/10.1016/j.seppur.2017.05.006.

Visioli, F., & Artaria, C. (2017). Astaxanthin in cardiovascular health and disease: mechanisms of action, therapeutic merits, and knowledge gaps. *Food & Function*, *8*(1), 39–63. https://doi.org/10.1039/C6FO01721E.

Vuong, L. T., Franke, A. A., Custer, L. J., & Murphy, S. P. (2006). *Momordica cochinchinensis* Spreng. (gac) fruit carotenoids reevaluated. *Journal of Food Composition and Analysis*, *19*, 664–668. https://doi.org/10.1016/j.jfca.2005.02.001.

Wang, X., Ohlin, C. A., Lu, Q., Fei, Z., Hu, J., & Dyson, P. J. (2007). Cytotoxicity of ionic liquids and precursor compounds towards human cell line HeLa. *Green Chemistry*, *9*(11), 1191–1197. https://doi.org/10.1039/B704503D.

Wang, L., & Weller, C. L. (2006). Recent advances in extraction of nutraceuticals from plants. *Trends in Food Science and Technology*, *17*(6), 300–312. https://doi.org/10.1016/j. tifs.2005.12.004.

Yara-Varón, E., Fabiano-Tixier, A. S., Balcells, M., Canela-Garayoa, R., Bily, A., & Chemat, F. (2016). Is it possible to substitute hexane with green solvents for extraction of carotenoids ? A theoretical versus experimental solubility study. *RSC Advances*, *6*, 27750–27759. https://doi.org/10.1039/c6ra03016e.

Zaghdoudi, K., Pontvianne, S., Framboisier, X., & Achard, M. (2015). Accelerated solvent extraction of carotenoids from: tunisian kaki (*Diospyros kaki* L.), peach (*Prunus persica* L.) and apricot (*Prunus armeniaca* L.). *Food Chemistry*, *184*, 131–139. https://doi. org/10.1016/j.foodchem.2015.03.072.

Zhang, F., Yang, Y., Su, P., & Guo, Z. (2009). Microwave-assisted extraction of rutin and quercetin from the stalks of *Euonymus alatus* (Thunb.) sieb. *Phytochemical Analysis*, *20*(1), 33–37. https://doi.org/10.1002/pca.1088.

Zhang, R., et al. (2015). Enhancing nutraceutical bioavailability from raw and cooked vegetables using excipient emulsions: influence of lipid type on carotenoid bioaccessibility from carrots. *Journal of Agricultural and Food Chemistry*, *63*(48), 10508–10517. https://doi. org/10.1021/acs.jafc.5b04691.

Zhao, D., Liao, Y., & Zhang, Z. (2007). Toxicity of ionic liquids. *Clean: Soil, Air, Water*, *35*(1), 42–48. https://doi.org/10.1002/clen.200600015.

Zhu, C., Naqvi, S., Capell, T., et al. (2009). Metabolic engineering of ketocarotenoid biosynthesis in higher plants. *Archives of Biochemistry and Biophysics*, *483*, 182–190. https://doi. org/10.1016/j.abb.2008.10.029.

Zinoviadou, K. G., & Galanakis, C. M. (2017). Glucosinolates and respective derivatives. In M. Puri (Ed.), *Food bioactives: Extraction and biotechnology applications*. New York: Springer.

Further reading

Galanakis, C. M. (2019g). *Innovations in traditional foods*. Elsevier-Woodhead Publishing, ISBN: 9780128148877.

Carotenoids as potential biocolorants: A case study of astaxanthin recovered from shrimp waste

Farah Ayuni Mohd Hatta, Rashidi Othman
International Institute for Halal Research and Training (INHART), Herbarium Unit, Department of Landscape Architecture, Kulliyyah of Architecture and Environmental Design, International Islamic University Malaysia, Kuala Lumpur, Malaysia

Chapter outline

Carotenoids: Properties, Processing and Applications. https://doi.org/10.1016/B978-0-12-817067-0.00009-9

Introduction

Colorant

Colorant is defined as chemical compounds that absorb light within the range of wavelengths of the visible region (Delgado-vargas & Paredes-Lopez, 2000; Jiménez, 2000). Historically, the art of natural colorant was established alongside the development of *Homo sapiens* civilization (Gulrajani, 1992). This is attributable to the nature of man and their ever-present attraction to colorful and beautiful elements. In the second half of the nineteenth century, the coloring using natural colorant evolved with the invention of synthetic colorant, which provided numerous attractive spectra (Ul-Islam, 2017). Aberoumand (2011) and Mortensen (2006) have stated that colors can be classified into different types of natural, synthetic, nature-identical, and inorganic colorants, respectively. Natural colors are found in renewable resources, oftentimes extracted from plant sources, but also from other sources such as insects, algae, cyanobacteria, and fungi. Meanwhile, synthetic colors are formulated colors that do not originate from nature, such as azo dyes, whereas nature-identical colors are defined as synthesized colors that can also be found in nature, such as carotene, canthaxanthin, and riboflavin. Finally, inorganic colors are derived from metals, such as titanium dioxide, gold, and silver.

Perceptible visual aesthetics in terms of color is one of the most important aspects for product marketability and acceptability, as color itself is ubiquitous and is capable of conveying valuable messages regarding products. A study titled "Impact of Color in Marketing" has revealed the tendency for the average people to make a judgment within 90 seconds of their first impression of a product, where up to 90% of the judgment is influenced solely by the colors (Singh, 2006). The addition of colorants to products is needed because of things such as color replacement for those colors that have vanished during product processing, enhancement of the existing color, and ensuring minimal dissimilarity in the same batch of products (Aberoumand, 2011). Furthermore, the effectiveness and economic factors offered by synthetic colorants have resulted in wide use in various industries, including the food industry. Unfortunately, the application of synthetic colorants or color additives has been reported to negatively contribute toward human development and health, as their toxicity can cause health problems (Bridle & Timberlake, 1997; Samanta & Agarwal, 2009).

Controversial issues regarding the safety of synthetic colorants have drawn great attention among consumers. The European Union (EU) has enforced all food manufacturers to label their products with cautionary clarifications in case of the presence of "Southampton six colorant." These are tartrazine, quinoline yellow, sunset yellow, carmoisine, ponceau red, and allura red (Munawar, Makiah, & Jamil, 2014). Research by Buchweitz, Nagel, Crle, and Kammerer (2012) has shown that children who consume drinks containing azo dyes and benzoic acid may potentially trigger the attention deficit hyperactivity disorder (ADHD). The International Agency for Research on Cancer (IARC, 1975) has previously classified azo dyes of Sudan I, Sudan II, Sudan III, and Sudan IV as human carcinogens. Therefore, the EU has banned the use of azo dye as a food additive or colorant, but the practice of using this dye is still present in some countries, including Malaysia.

Carotenoids as biocolorants

Natural colors produced by living organisms can be categorized into three major groups, which include flavonoids, tetrapyrroles, and tetraterpenoids (Aberoumand, 2011). An example of a flavonoid is anthocyanin, which is responsible for colors, ranging from red to purple, of many fruits such as berries. Meanwhile, chlorophyll is considered as the most important element of the tetrapyrroles that can be found in higher plants. Similar to chlorophyll, tetraterpenoids like carotenoids are widely found as they absorb light as energy during photosynthesis and protect the chlorophyll from photodegradation.

Carotenoids are pigments naturally occurring in several fruits, vegetables, algae, and crustaceans, whereas they are synthesized by all photosynthetic organisms and many nonphotosynthetic bacteria and fungi (Sajilata, Singhal, & Kamat, 2008). Epidemiological studies have shown an inverse relationship between the risk of laryngeal, lung, and colon cancers and the consumption of carotenoid-rich foods (Block, Patterson, & Subar, 1992; Steinmetz & Potter, 1993). Approximately 700 carotenoids have been found, contributing to the different colors of yellow, orange, and red (Fortes, 2006; Mezzomo & Ferreira, 2016; Polyakov et al., 2009; Rodriguez-Amaya, Rodriguez, & Amaya-Farfan, 2006). Carotenoids are liposoluble tetraterpenes originating from the condensation of isoprenyl units that form a series of conjugated double bonds constituting a chromophoric system (Britton, 1995).

Carotenoids are typically categorized according to their functional groups, specifically carotenes and xanthophylls. There are two main classes of naturally occurring carotenoids: β-carotene, α-carotene and lycopene that are hydrocarbons (linear or cyclized at one or both ends of the molecule), and xanthophylls (lutein, zeaxanthin, β-cryptoxanthin and astaxanthin), which are oxygenated derivatives of carotenes (Fortes, 2006; Rivera, Vilaró, & Canela, 2011; Rodriguez-Amaya, 2001). All xanthophylls produced by higher plants, such as violaxanthin, antheraxanthin, zeaxanthin, neoxanthin, and lutein, are also synthesized by green algae (Eonseon, Polle, Lee, Hyun, & Chang, 2003).

β-Carotene is one of the best-known food carotenoids, and it is sometimes found together with α-carotene in certain foods. It can be detected in carrots, mangoes, and apricots, whereas α-carotene is typically found in carrots and pumpkins. Lutein, the dihydroxy derivative of β-carotene is commonly detected in yellow or orange fruits and flowers as well as green vegetables. Lutein is isomeric with zeaxanthin. Specifically, the two carotene alcohols differ from one another just by the shift of a single double bond so that in zeaxanthin, all double bonds are conjugated. Both zeaxanthin and lutein are important in the prevention of age-related macular degeneration (AMD), the leading cause of blindness (Moeller, Jacques, & Blumberg, 2000; Snodderly, 1995). Zeaxanthin is yellow and is naturally found in corn, egg yolks, as well as some of the orange and yellow vegetables and fruits like alfalfa and marigold flowers (Handelman, Nightingale, Lichtenstein, Schaefer, & Blumberg, 1999; Humphries & Khachik, 2003; Nelis & DeLeenheer, 1991; Sajilata et al., 2008). Zeaxanthin is used as a feed additive and colorant in the food industry for birds, swine, and fish (Hadden et al., 1999). The pigment imparts a yellow coloration to the skin and egg yolks of birds, whereas in pigs and fish it is used for skin pigmentation (Nelis & DeLeenheer, 1991). Meanwhile, lycopene is a typical food carotenoid found in many red fruits and vegetables, such as watermelon, pink guava, grapes, and tomatoes (Fortes, 2006; Rodriguez-Amaya, 2001).

Unique carotenoids like bixin may be sourced in annatto, whereas crocin is present in saffron (Rodriguez-Amaya, 2001). The red pigment from bixin is widely and typically used in the food, pharmaceutical, cosmetic, and textiles industries accordingly (Santos, Albuquerque, & Meireles, 2011). In contrast, astaxanthin is the major form of carotenoid detected in marine animals like salmon, shrimp, lobster, and crab, as well as other microorganisms (Ushakumari & Ramanujan, 2012). Astaxanthin (3,3′-dihydroxy-β,β-carotene-4,4′-dione) is classified as one of the lipophilic carotenoids (C_{40}) and is categorized under the xanthophyll group (Rodrigo-Baños, Garbayo, Vílchez, Bonete, & Martínez-Espinosa, 2015). However, the primary carotenoids in a type of food may differ depending on the genetics, locality, seasonality, and handling techniques (Arvayo-Enríquez, Mondaca-Fernández, Gortáres-Moroyoqui, Lopez-Cervantes, & Rodríguez-Ramírez, 2013; Fortes, 2006; Manzi, Flood, Webb, & Mitchell, 2002; Othman, 2009).

Chemical structure of carotenoids

Carotenoids are developed from acyclic C_{40} isoprenoid lycopene, which is also categorized as a tetraterpene (Arvayo-Enríquez et al., 2013). Generally, most of them are lipophilic in nature, which means they are soluble in organic solvents like alcohol, chloroform, ethyl ether, ethyl acetate, and acetone, and they are insoluble in water. Therefore, the best organic solvent to dissolve carotenes is either petroleum ether, hexane, or toluene, whereas methanol and ethanol are the best options for xanthophylls (Rodriguez-Amaya, 2001). Regardless, food carotenoids are mostly found as polytenes in all-*trans* forms made from eight 5-carbon isoprenoid units. However, during processing especially involving thermal conditions, a nonnegligible proportion of *cis*-isomers can be formed (Arvayo-Enríquez et al., 2013; Borel, 2003).

Generally, one double bond is added to the molecule during the process of conversion from phytoene to lycopene, which is made up of 3 to 13 conjugated double bonds accordingly. After lycopene, the biosynthetic process will result in enzymatic cyclization of the end groups, which would next create γ-carotene (one beta ring) and β-carotene (two beta rings). The limit of the biosynthetic step is determined by the concentration of carotenoids available in the sources (Fortes, 2006). For example, red tomatoes containing lycopene at a very high concentration are not capable of converting them to β-carotene due to inadequate enzyme activity. According to McClements, Decker, Park, and Weiss (2009), certain cases display the formation of six carbon ring structures at one or both ends of the molecules. Some carotenoid structures are shown in Fig. 1.

Bioactive compound properties in carotenoids

According to Farre et al. (2015), all carotenoids comprise a polyisoprenoid structure containing long, conjugated double bonds at the center of the compound. The acyclic structure is capable of transforming and yielding a large family of more than 800 compounds via cyclization of the end of groups or the introduction of oxygen-rich

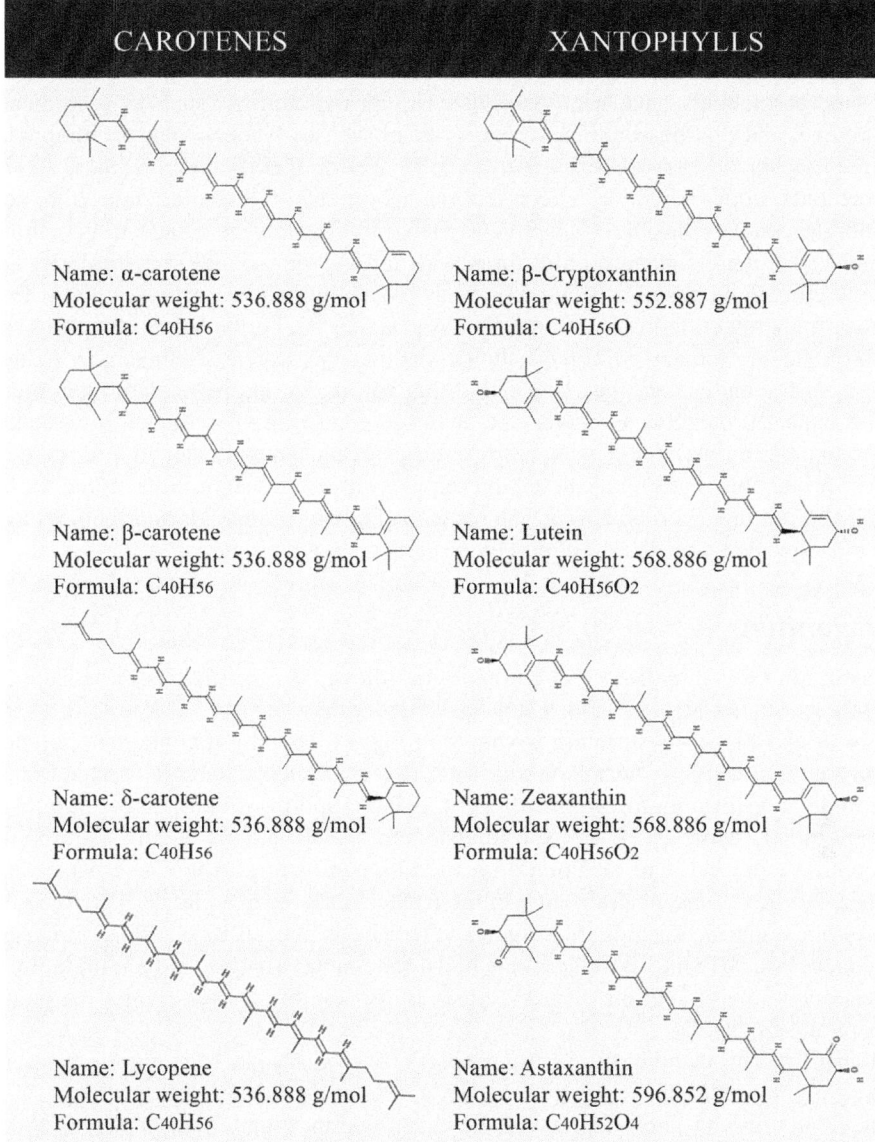

Fig. 1 Examples of carotenoid structure (National Center for Biotechnology Information, 2018).

functional groups (Britton, Liaaen-Jensen, & Pfander, 2004). Therefore, their polyene structure has rendered carotenoids to be recognized as excellent free-radical scavengers with singlet-oxygen quenching properties and the ability to trap peroxyl radicals. In principle, the presence of greater conjugated chains causes greater antioxidant activity in the compound. Besides, the higher polarity of end groups (such as carbonyl and hydroxyl groups) due to β-ionone rings also greatly contribute to such antioxidant function. In fact, extracts from natural sources commonly contain bioactive compounds with antiinflammatory, antitumor, antiobesity, antimicrobial, antibacterial, antiviral, antifungal, and antioxidant properties (da Silva, Rocha-Santos, & Duarte, 2016).

Some carotenoids have been recognized as pro-vitamin A, such as β-carotene, γ-carotene, and β-cryptoxanthin, whereas others such as lycopene and xanthophylls are not recognized (Arvayo-Enríquez et al., 2013; Borel, 2003; Stahl & Sies, 2005). Carotenoids, in particular, have been reported as capable of lessening damage to cell membranes and are linked to receptors triggered by free radicals, controlling cellular immune reactions, and preventing tumor-cell growth (Fortes, 2006). Similarly, the annatto carotenoid has also been reported as having antioxidant activity against free radicals and protecting from sunlight (Santos et al., 2011). Furthermore, numerous epidemiological research studies have shown that dietary carotenoid intake may reduce the risks of some cancer, thus suggesting that antioxidant properties are instrumental for cancer protection. However, the evidence concerning β-carotene, α-carotene, β-cryptoxanthin, lutein, and zeaxanthin in terms of ideal supplementation dosage as cancer protection is still inadequate and requires further research in the context of a well-balanced diet (Fortes, 2006). The sources of some carotenoids and their respective bioactive compounds as reported by researchers are presented in Table 1.

Astaxanthin

Astaxanthin (3,3′-dihydroxy-β,β-carotene-4,4′-dione) is classified as one of the lipophilic carotenoids (C_{40}) and is categorized under the xanthophyll group (Rodrigo-Baños et al., 2015). Its structure is shown in Fig. 1, whereby it contains a polyene chain that connects two terminal rings and two asymmetric carbons situated at 3. The molecular formula for astaxanthin is $C_{40}H_{52}O_4$ and the molar mass is 596.85 g/mol (Ambati, Moi, Ravi, & Aswathanarayana, 2014). This reddish lipophilic carotenoid can be found accumulating predominantly in seafood or crustaceans, such as shrimp, lobster, crab, and salmon (Mezzomo & Ferreira, 2016; Radzali, Masturah, Baharin, Rashidi, & Rahman, 2016; Rodriguez-Amaya, 2001; Sui, Yue, Wang, & Han, 2015). Its buildup in the body of some microalgae and phytoplankton is also due to their being the primary source of astaxanthin consumption (Senthamil & Kumaresan, 2015).

Regardless, astaxanthin from shrimp wastes (byproduct) has been reported as containing highly antioxidant activities, which can improve human health through UV-light protection and antiinflammatory activity (Guerin, Huntley, & Olaizola, 2003; Kidd, 2011; Sui et al., 2015; Ushakumari & Ramanujan, 2012; Yamashita, 2013; Yang, Kim, & Lee, 2013). Despite not being a vitamin A precursor, several studies have reported that its biological activity is more potent than other carotenoids (Ambati et al., 2014; Lin, Chen, Chen, Chen, & Ho, 2016; Mezzomo & Ferreira, 2016; Naguib, 2000). According to Miki (1991), astaxanthin's antioxidant activity is 10 times greater than zeaxanthin, lutein, canthaxanthin, β-carotene, and is 100-fold better than α-tocopherol. This is attributable to its unique molecular structure that contains hydroxyl and keto moieties on each ionone ring (Hussein, Sankawa, Goto, Matsumoto, & Watanabe, 2006; Liu & Osawa, 2007), as well as long, conjugated double bonds at the center

Table 1 Carotenoids and their bioactive compounds

Sources	Carotenoids	Bioactivities	References
Algae (*Haematococcus pluvialis*)	Astaxanthin	Antioxidant	Wang, Yang, Yan, and Yao (2012)
Arabian red shrimp (*Aristeus alcocki*)	Astaxanthin	Antioxidant, antiinflammatory	Sindhu and Sherief (2011)
Aztec marigold (*Tagetes erecta*)	Lutein	Antimutagenicity	González-de-Mejía, Loarca-Piña, and Ramos- Gómez (1997)
Crabs (*Portunus sanguinolentus, Callinectes sapidus*, and *Paralithodes brevipes*)	Astaxanthin	Antioxidant, antimicrobial	Suganya and Asheeba (2015)
Green and dark green, leafy vegetables, e.g., spinach, parsley, kale, broccoli, corn, avocado, Brussels sprouts, beans	Lutein	Prevention against age-related Macular Degeneration (AMD), anticancer	Jaswir, Noviendri, Hasrini, and Octavianti (2011)
Green leafy vegetables	α-Carotene	Antioxidants, anticarcinogenic	Jaswir et al. (2011)
Peaches, oranges, tangerines, mangoes, papayas	β-Cryptoxanthin	Antioxidants, anticancer	Jaswir et al. (2011)
Seaweed (*Undaria pinnatifida*)	Fucoxanthin	Anticancer	Liu, Huang, Hosokawa, Miyashita, and Hu (2009)
Seaweed (*Undaria pinnatifida*)	Fucoxanthin	Antiobesity	Maeda, Hosokawa, Sahima, Funayama, & Miyashita (2005)
Shrimps (*Penaeus brasiliensis* and *Penaeus paulensis*)	Astaxanthin	Antiobesity and hypolipidemic	Mezzomo et al. (2015)
Tomato	Lycopene	Anticancer	Kim, Rao, and Rao (2002)
Tomato	Lycopene	Antioxidant	Erge and Karadeniz (2011)
Tomato and carrot	Carotenoids	Antioxidant	Patras, Brunton, Da, Butler, and Downey (2009)
Tomatoes, pink-red grapefruit, red-fleshed papayas, watermelon	Lycopene	Antioxidant, anticancer, anticholesterol	Jaswir et al. (2011)
Yellow-orange fruit and vegetables, e.g., carrot, broccoli, spinach, parsley, celery, tomatoes	β-Carotene	Antioxidants	Jaswir et al. (2011)

of the compound (13 conjugated double bonds) (Delgado-vargas & Paredes-Lopez, 2000). Therefore, their nutritional benefits have caused the United States Food and Drug Administration (USFDA) to approve astaxanthin as a color additive (pigment) in animal feeds (Pashkow, Watumull, & Campbell, 2008). Other than that, it is also used widely as a nutritious supplement in food, pharmaceutical products, and nutraceutical products (Ambati et al., 2014).

Astaxanthin production from shrimp waste

Malaysia's fishery sector has contributed extensively to the country's economic growth, with the marine-capture fishery serving as the main supplier for the sector. The aquaculture industry has also expanded significantly to cater to both local and international demands for fish products (*Investment Opportunities in the Aquaculture Industry in Sabah, Malaysia*, 2010). For example, the incentives offered by the National Key Economic Areas (NKEA) have spurred the Northern Corridor Implementation Authority (NCIA) and Hannan Corporation Sdn. Bhd. (HCSB) to invest in developing two phases of shrimp aquaculture complexes located in Perak Darul Ridzuan (Economic Transformation Programme). Both complexes are projected to produce 14,000 tons of white shrimp per year. In 2002, the global aquaculture industry has contributed more than 50 million Metric ton valued at US$60 billion, whereby more than 90% of the amount has been contributed from Asia (Primavera, 2005).

However, the shrimp aquaculture industry specifically has led to serious ecological impacts, one of which is a result of the tremendous amount of shrimp waste produced (Famino, Oduguwa, Onifade, & Olotunde, 2000). Shrimp waste usually consists of the head part from a processed shrimp, called the cephalothorax and the exoskeleton, which generates up to 70% of the raw material (Simpson & Haard, 1985; Quan & Turner, 2009; Mezzomo, Martínez, Maraschin, & Ferreira, 2013). Therefore, researchers have advocated various alternatives to overcome this issue, as well as to attain sustainability in aquacultural practices. For example, shrimp waste has been reported to contain valuable carotenoid compounds that are usable in the food, nutraceuticals, and pharmaceutical industries alike (Ambati et al., 2014; Mezzomo et al., 2013; Sui et al., 2015).

Furthermore, the aquaculture industry typically makes use of synthetic carotenoid as an animal-feed supplement, which constitutes up to 20% of the feed expenses (Quan & Turner, 2009). In particular, astaxanthin is added to the feed to enhance the pigmentation of cultured animals. Thus, this component that is produced from shrimp waste may be used as a colorant in salmonid and crustacean feed (Mezzomo & Ferreira, 2016). These opportunities have increased the demand for colorants or pigments from natural sources, drawing the attention of many researchers to explore the potential natural sources as colorants for various products. In this current work, the raw material of white shrimp waste, *Litopenaeus vannamei* (Fig. 2), has been specially chosen because the cephalothorax and exoskeleton parts are known to potentially generate other by-products.

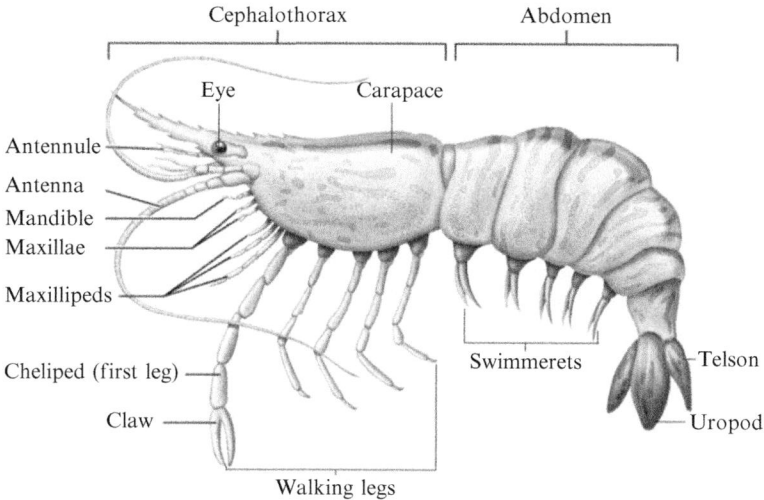

Fig. 2 Anatomy of *L. vannamei*.

Extraction technologies for astaxanthin production

Astaxanthin can be produced through various extraction methods, such as chemical extraction, the alkaline method, soxhlet, ultrasound, oil extraction, or supercritical fluid extraction (Gildberg & Stenberg, 2001; Macías-sanchez et al., 2009; Meyers & Chen, 1985; Mezzomo, Maestri, Dos Santos, Maraschin, & Ferreira, 2011; Sui et al., 2015; Sun, Sangkatumvong, & Shung, 2006). However, the applicability of the extraction methods used is a monumental factor in ensuring product quality (Mezzomo et al., 2013). A large volume of alkaline and acid chemicals are typically utilized in the conventional methods, which not only lead to environmental pollution but may also decrease the quality of the astaxanthin generated (Sui et al., 2015). Furthermore, the toxic organic solvent used during the process may leave traces in the final product that can cause further harm to human health (Mezzomo & Ferreira, 2016). Moreover, the conventional extraction method normally consumes more time and a higher amount of solvent, and it also causes compound degradation (Herrero, Cifuentes, & Iban, 2006). Further investigation on green technologies for carotenoid extraction has steadily amassed scholarly attention with surging demand in the global market trending toward products generated from natural compounds.

Hence, such weaknesses have been addressed and progress toward improvement achieved by the introduction of supercritical fluid extraction (SFE), which allowed a high extraction yield within a shorter time while maintaining the extract compound concomitantly (Santos et al., 2011; Arapitsas & Turner, 2008; Silva, Gamarra, Oliveira & Cabral, 2008). Some research has been done on extracting carotenoids from shrimp waste using vegetable oils as cosolvent via supercritical carbon dioxide extraction, such as sunflower oil, soybean oil, palm oil, and flaxseed oil (Sachindra & Mahendrakar, 2005; Handayani, Sutrisno, Indraswati, & Ismadji, 2008; Pu, Bechtel,

& Sathivel, 2010). Regardless, SFE technology is well known for its numerous advantages over the conventional extraction methods (Cadoni, De Giorgi, Medda, & Poma, 2000; da Silva et al., 2016; Mezzomo et al., 2013). The use of cheaper, nontoxic, and inflammable gas (i.e., carbon dioxide) has rendered it a paramount element in various industrial applications. Moreover, the high consumption of carbon dioxide on an industrial scale can be controlled by recycling efforts, thus minimizing the operating costs and preventing an environmental carbon footprint. Although the low polarity of the gas complicates the process of extracting compounds with high polarity, cosolvent use coupled with high polarity has made the process more efficient (Herrero et al., 2006).

The low critical temperature and pressure of carbon dioxide at 31.3°C and 72.9 atm, respectively, have allowed the compounds to maintain and preserve their thermally labile samples (Durante, Lenucci, & Mita, 2014). SFE, in particular, can have a shorter extraction time due to high diffusivity and low viscosity of the supercritical fluid, allowing easy diffusion of the fluid through the samples (Herrero et al., 2006). Moreover, manipulation of the pressure and temperature used has allowed the fluid density to be modified and has improved its solubility. Additionally, selective extraction of the compound via SFE is undertaken using a systematic experimental design approach, where response variables of samples can be optimized through modification of parameters such as temperature, pressure, and time. It can also be ensured that the sample output is of high purity. Therefore, the green technology is an efficient alternative for implementation in a wide range of industries, such as dye, food and beverage, pharmaceutical, cosmetic, and others (Cadoni et al., 2000).

Another emerging method of extraction is high-pressure processing (HPP), which is a new and safe technology in research and development that is capable of reducing the loss of bioactive compounds during processing (Tadapaneni, Daryaei, Krishnamurthy, Edirisinghe, & Burton-freeman, 2014). HPP is also widely recognized in the food industry due to its capability to preserve food nutrients, quality, sensory properties, as well as offering a longer shelf life. These properties are attributable to its very minimal effect on the covalent bonds of low molecular-mass compounds (Patras et al., 2009). Furthermore, nonthermal technology has allowed for the quality of thermo-labile compounds to be preserved (Ahmed & Ramaswamy, 2006), whereby the pressure during the process can increase the mass transfer rate, thus enhancing the sample permeability (Xi, 2006). A few studies have reviewed the use of HPP as an extraction method, and one study (Xi, 2013) has used it to extract active compounds from plants. Moreover, Sánchez, Baranda, and Martínez de Marañón (2014) and McInerney, Seccafien, Stewart, and Bird (2007) have also studied the total carotenoid content in several plants extracted using HPP. When HPP has initiated its operation, the different pressures between the internal and external cell membranes have resulted in continuous penetration until the concentration between them reaches the equilibrium state (Xi, 2006). This process is attainable in a short time. Like SFE, extraction via HPP can also produce high extraction yield despite not being a time-consuming process.

Future prospects of biocolorant for polymer products

When selecting colorant materials used especially for polymer products in contact with food, toys, and graphic-arts tools, the toxicology and environmental aspects should be taken into consideration. Some synthetic colorants contain toxic heavy metals like cadmium and lead, which are illegal for use in these products as per quality-assurance and safety standards outlined by European Union (BS EN 71-3:1995) and International Standards (International Organization for Standardization, ISO 8124-3:1997 Migration of Certain Elements) (Kumar & Pastore, 2006). However, the rising consumer awareness regarding the negative impacts of synthetic-colorant consumption has also increased the demand for natural products, spurring product manufacturers to opt for natural colorants (Samanta & Agarwal, 2009; Santos et al., 2011). This is evident in the various works done on biocolorant application in mitigating environmental pollution caused by industries associated with synthetic colorant (Ali, El-Khatib, El-Mohamedy, & Ramadan, 2014).

Incorporating colorants as an additive in polymers is synonymous with altering the optical properties so as to attract consumers in purchasing the products (Christie, 1994). The technique of colorant incorporation has been selected in accordance with the desired finish and quality in product application. The dispersion process involves the dispersion of colorants into the liquid phase of a polymer, whereby physical retainment is seen in the polymer matrix after solidification concludes. Meanwhile, it may also be retained in the polymer matrix by completely dissolving in a polymeric medium to create an affinity between the colorant and the polymer molecules (Christie, 1994). Incorporating biocolorants from carotenoids with biodegradable polymers has been reported to show a protective element against the oxidation process (Martín, Mattea, Gutiérrez, Miguel, & Cocero, 2007). The application of biocolorant to polymer is a promising invention in various applied sectors, starting from the production of colorant materials in the agrotechnology sector until the final product is manufactured by the polymer industry. Thus, these biocolored polymers may accordingly be applied as safe food-contact items (e.g., packaging, kitchen utensils), baby and kids' items (e.g., toys, polymer clay), medical devices (e.g., implants, gloves, bandages), cosmetics, and pharmaceutical products. Therefore, further research is encouraged to discover the use, challenges, and technologies of carotenoids production and its development as a potential biocolorant for polymer products.

Current research

This chapter aims at exploring the application of carotenoids as biocolorants, focusing on a case study of astaxanthin recovered from shrimp waste. It assesses its chromaticity stability across various environmental factors involving UV irradiation, heat, salinity, and pH stability tests throughout 4 weeks. The color analysis was performed using the CIELAB system. According to Sant'Anna, Gurak, Ferreira Marczak, and Tessaro (2013) and Torskangerpoll and Andersen (2005), CIELAB is a useful system to describe colors, as it involves the complete visible spectrum of the eye. When a visual assessment is performed on an object, three factors can determine the color output: namely, light source, light-receptor mechanism, and the object itself. Although there are various standards of light source, standard daylight illuminant, D65, is the commonly used option in food color measurement by CIE (Vidal Zaragoza, 2012).

The CIELAB system can measure the index of lightness (L^*) and two color coordinates (a^* and b^*). The luminosity or lightness is described by the L^* index at the vertical axis, whereby every color is associated with vividness or dullness in the range of black ($L^* = 0$) and white ($L^* = 100$). The positive coordinates of the a* index refer to the reddish colors, whereas its negative coordinates refer to the greenish colors. In contrast, the positive coordinates of the b^*index denote the yellowish colors, whereas its negative coordinates represent the bluish colors. Moreover, important information can be gathered from the values of the chroma (C^*_{ab}) (quantitatively) and the hue (h_{ab}) (qualitatively) (Sant'Anna et al., 2013). Boonsong, Laohakunjit, and Kerdchoechuen (2012) have defined hue angle ($h°$) as an angle ranging from $0°$ to $360°$. Red, orange, and yellow are indicated by angles that range from $0°$ to $90°$, whereas yellow to green is displayed by the angle between $90°$ and $180°$. Meanwhile, green, cyan, and blue ranges between $180°$ and $270°$, whereas blue, purple, magenta, and red are indicated by angles from $270°$ to $360°$.

Experimental design

Raw materials preparation

The raw material of *Litopenaeus vannamei* consists of white shrimp waste made up of the cephalothorax and supplied by the shrimp aquaculture company, Hannan Corporation Sdn. Bhd. The materials are transported to the laboratory in a container filled with ice at a temperature of 4°C. On arrival, the sample is stored in the freezer at a temperature of –20°C prior to further processing, before approximately 30 kg of them are dried using a freeze dryer (FDU-1100, EYELA, Tokyo Rikakikai Co., Japan). This has been done at a temperature of –50°C and vacuum level at 6.5 Pa for three days. At the same time, approximately 30 kg of shrimp waste is dried at 60°C for 1 week in an oven with air circulation (UF55, Memmert) for HPP extraction. Then, the sample is ground into fine powder using a heavy-duty blender (LB20E, Laboratory Blender). The ground sample is conveniently stored under appropriate conditions at a temperature of –20°C to minimize enzymatic reactions (Othman, 2009).

Extraction of astaxanthin by chemical extraction

One g of ground shrimp waste has been added into 50 mL tubes and was rehydrated via the addition of 1 mL distilled water. Then, 5 mL of different solvents [i.e., acetone:methanol mixture (9:1, v/v), acetone, methanol, ethanol] prepared with 0.1% butylated hydroxytoluene (BHT) was added into each tube. BHT is used to avoid any oxidation and isomerization from occurring during the extraction (Arvayo-Enríquez et al., 2013). The samples are then stored overnight in a dark condition at room temperature, and each has been prepared in triplicate. The next day, the samples were vortexed and centrifuged for 2 minutes at $13,500 \times g$ (NU-C200R-E, Nuaire, United States), with the resulting supernatant being transferred into 50 mL graduated polypropylene centrifuge tubes. This step is then repeated by adding 5 mL of the same solvent until the supernatant of the sample become colorless (normally 2 or 3 times). Then, an equal volume of hexane and distilled water (5 mL) is added to extract the carotenoid from the combined supernatants. The solution is then allowed to separate, with the upper hexane layer containing the carotenoids being collected. This procedure is repeated with hexane alone until it becomes colorless. After that, the combined upper layer is dried to completion under a gentle stream of oxygen-free nitrogen. Tubes are then capped and sealed with parafilm to exclude oxygen, and they are immediately stored at −20°C before further analysis. Fig. 3 shows the collected astaxanthin and nitrogen-dried astaxanthin.

High-performance liquid chromatography (HPLC) analysis

One mg of dried astaxanthin extract was dissolved in 1 mL ethyl acetate. Then, 450 μL of the sample was added into Whatman Mini-UniPrep Syringeless Filters vials, with the prepared sample being inserted into HPLC for analysis. HPLC employing diode-array detection (DAD) is the most common analytical method in determining the qualitative and quantitative carotenoid profiles. The HPLC analysis was done following the procedure described by previous authors (Othman, 2009; Radzali et al., 2016), with the HPLC Agilent 1200 series (Agilent Technologies, United States) being used to analyze the carotenoid content extracted from *L. vannamei* waste. It is equipped with a binary pump with autosampler injector, microvacuum degassers, and a thermostatic column compartment, whereas the reverse-phase column is a ZORBAX Eclipse XDB-C_{18} end capped (5 μm) and sized at 4.6×150 mm. An HPLC grade of acetonitrile:water (9:1, v/v) has been prepared as eluent A, whereas the HPLC grade of ethyl acetate is designated as eluent B. Meanwhile, Ultrapure water 18.0 MΩ is prepared using a Milipore S.A.S water purification system.

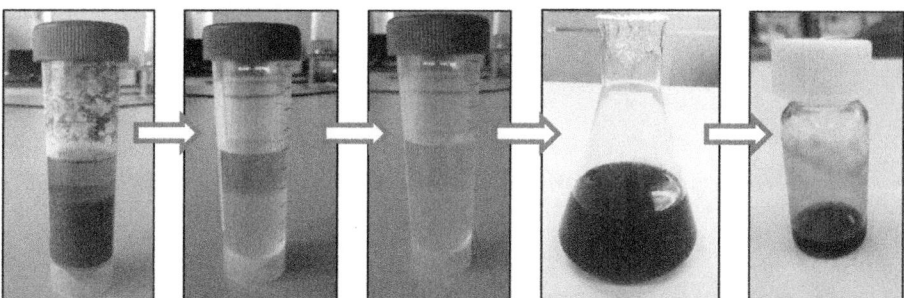

Fig. 3 Astaxanthin extracted using chemical extraction.

The solvent gradient used has been established as follows: 0%–40% solvent B (0–20 min), 40%–60% solvent B (20–25 min), 60%–100% solvent B (25–25.1 min), 100% solvent B (25.1–35 min), and 100%–0% solvent B (35–35.1 min). The flow rate is set at $1.0 \, mL \, min^{-1}$ and the injection volume is $10 \, \mu L$. The column was thermostatic at 25°C, with carotenoid peak identification performed in the range of 350–550 nm. The stop time was set at 40 min, with astaxanthin detection done at the maximum absorption wavelength (480 nm). Triplicate samples were prepared, with three injections being performed for each vial. The concentration of the astaxanthin was determined using the standard curve in regard to its structure and properties. The chromatographic peak is then identified by comparing the retention time and spectra against the astaxanthin standard. The carotenoids concentration has been quantified in terms of microgram per 1.0 g dry weight of sample ($\mu g/g$ DW).

Astaxanthin pigment preparation for stability test

Astaxanthin extract stored at –20°C have been used for color-stability tests. Three concentrations comprised of 1, 2, and 3 g/L of astaxanthin (Fig. 4) have been prepared by dissolving in ethanol. The chromaticity of the sample without any treatment has been measured as a blank.

UV irradiation test

All glass tubes containing samples of three different concentrations were placed in a laminar hood and exposed under UVA (long wavelength = 365 nm, intensity 5500 lux) and UVB (middle wavelength = 312 nm, intensity 2900 lux) perpendicularly 10 cm below the light source for 8 hours at room temperature (Fig. 5). The samples were prepared in triplicate and were analyzed hourly to monitor their chromaticity. Any changes in color before and after the experiment have been measured accordingly.

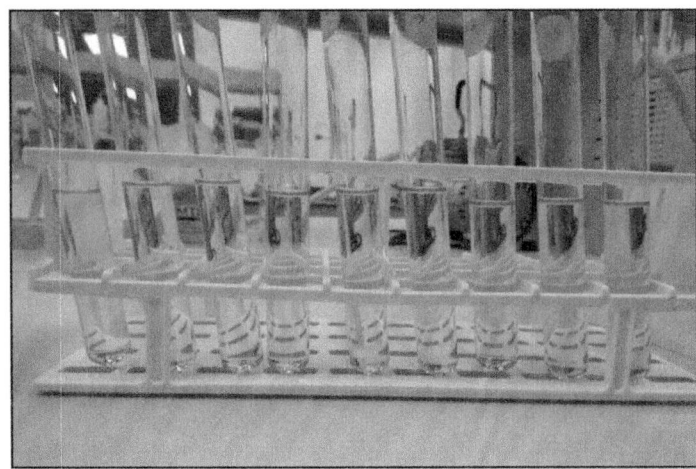

Fig. 4 Prepared 1, 2, and 3 g/L of astaxanthin pigment.

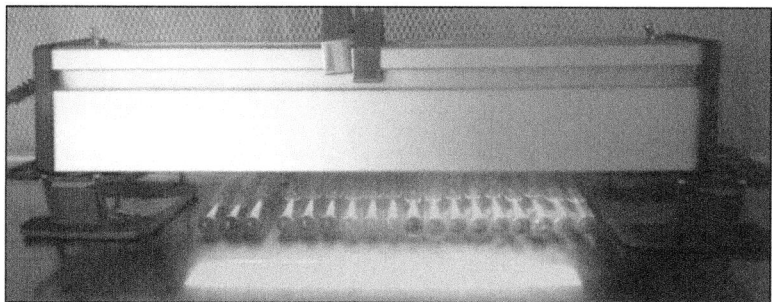

Fig. 5 Samples exposed under UV irradiation.

pH test

The pH of samples was adjusted to 3, 5, 7, 9, and 11 using acid hydrochloric (HCl) and sodium hydroxide (NaOH). They were prepared at three concentrations and were exposed under dark and light conditions (cool light of a fluorescent lamp with light intensity, 3100 lux, perpendicularly 30 cm below) at room temperature for 4 weeks. The samples were prepared in triplicate and were analyzed hourly to monitor their chromaticity. The chromaticity of a sample for day 1 was also measured.

Salinity test

Sodium chloride (NaCl) was added into each sample at three concentrations, making the final concentration of the NaCl of 1, 3, and 5 g/L, respectively. Samples were incubated in dark and light conditions at room temperature for 4 weeks. The samples were prepared in triplicate and were analyzed hourly to monitor their chromaticity. The chromaticity of the sample for day 1 was also measured.

Heat test

An astaxanthin sample at concentration 1, 3, and 5 g/L was prepared accordingly. All samples were incubated in the oven at eight points of temperature (i.e., 25°C, 35°C, 45°C, 55°C, 65°C, 75°C, 85°C, and 95°C) for 3 hours. The samples were prepared in triplicate and were analyzed hourly to monitor their chromaticity. The changes in color before the experiment were also measured.

Analysis of chromaticity

A total of 1 mL of carotenoid pigment was pipetted into a glass cuvette and was introduced into the CIELab colorimeter (Cary Win UV Color Application, Agilent Technologies). The CIELab system is then used to analyze L^* (lightness), a^* (red-green), and b^* (yellow-blue) values of the samples' colors. Meanwhile, the three measured color parameters are calculated into C^* (Chroma) representing color saturation, h (hue angle) indicating color intensity, and ΔE (total color change) using the following equations (Eq. 1) (Licón, Carmona, Rubio, Molina, & Berruga, 2012; Yawadio & Morita, 2007).

$$\Delta E = \left[\left(\Delta L^* \right)^2 + \left(\Delta a^* \right)^2 + \left(\Delta b^* \right)^2 \right]^{1/2} \tag{1}$$

Statistical analysis

One-way analysis of variance (ANOVA) has been conducted using SPSS (version 20) to compare CIELAB parameters in different treatments, and the resulting values have been given as a mean. Significant ($P < .0001$) differences between means of three replicates are subsequently identified using Tukey's test.

Result and discussion

Analysis of total astaxanthin content

HPLC analysis has been performed to characterize the total astaxanthin content extracted from *L. vannamei* waste using a reference calibration curve. Fig. 6 shows the HPLC chromatogram for astaxanthin obtained via chemical extraction. Astaxanthin has been detected at the retention time of 15.674 minutes with a purity greater than 85%, and the amount of total astaxanthin has been calculated on a dry weight (DW) basis. The results obtained have been presented as an average of the three replicates (mean ± standard deviation) and they are demonstrated in Fig. 7. The highest amount of astaxanthin content has been obtained from extraction using 100% acetone, which is $5701.99 \pm 261.15 \, \mu g/g$ DW, followed by acetone:methanol (7,3, v/v), ethanol, and methanol (4184.14 ± 312.14, 3100.62 ± 136.66, and $2294.57 \pm 165.18 \, \mu g/g$ DW, respectively).

The extraction using solvent typically involves the interaction resulting in an affinity between the sample and the solvent. The low polarity of carotenoid compounds normally makes the extraction more efficient, with solvents, such as petroleum ether and hexane, having low polarities. However, some carotenoids also contain a polar part, thereby rendering a proper selection of solvent to assist in increasing the

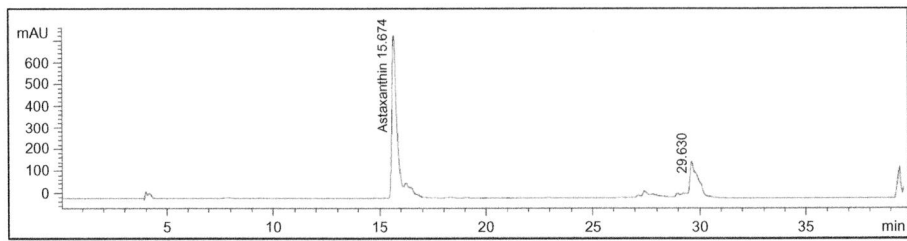

Fig. 6 Chromatogram of total astaxanthin obtained by chemical extraction.

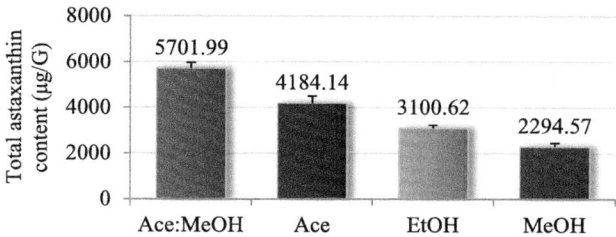

Fig. 7 Total astaxanthin content obtained by the different solvent used.

extraction yield (Arvayo-Enríquez et al., 2013). The result of the chemical extraction has shown that the use of an acetone:methanol mixture (7:3, v/v) and acetone as a solvent has produced a significant amount of total astaxanthin. This result is supported by those obtained by Mezzomo et al. (2011), Sachindra, Bhaskar, and Mahendrakar (2005), Sindhu and Sherief (2011), and Vimala and Paul (2009), whereby astaxanthin is effectively extracted by acetone. The high polarity of acetone renders it the best solvent for the extraction of carotenoids from shrimp waste. This is due to the higher molecular chain in etherified astaxanthin and the presence of a hydrophobic mass surrounding the pigments of xanthophylls, which requires more polar solvents. This will assist the penetration in the sample matrix, which increases the concentration of extraction yield.

However, the result of previous authors has also shown that the use of polar solvent has caused low selectivity, in which other compounds aside from carotenoids are also extracted. This has resulted in an increased yield of extract. In the food and pharmaceutical industries, the use of acetone is intolerable, as its traces found in the final product can consequently cause harm to human health (Arvayo-Enríquez et al., 2013). Hence, there are numerous studies done using environmentally friendly solvents like ethyl acetate and ethanol for carotenoid extraction.

Color analysis of astaxanthin pigment stability

Salinity test

Color stability is demonstrated by the chromaticity and color saturation graphs of astaxanthin pigment, once added with 1, 3, and 5 g/L NaCl and stored in dark and light conditions. Undertaken across 4 weeks, the results are shown in Figs. 8 and 9, respectively. Color intensity and brightness are responsible for the chromaticity (C^*) values of the pigment, whereas the saturation (s) is defined as the vividness of an area visualized, which is given by the ratio of chromaticity to lightness (Nor, Aziz, Mohd-adnan, Taha, & Arof, 2016). From the results, it can be seen that the values for astaxanthin pigment chromaticity and saturation increase linearly with the concentration of the pigments. Furthermore, the pigments stored in light conditions have shown higher degradation rates than those stored in a dark condition. The graphs have also confirmed that pigment without salt treatment (blank) has shown the least degradation effect, followed by the pigment treated with the sodium chloride (NaCl) concentration of 1, 3, and 5 g/L, respectively, both in dark and light conditions.

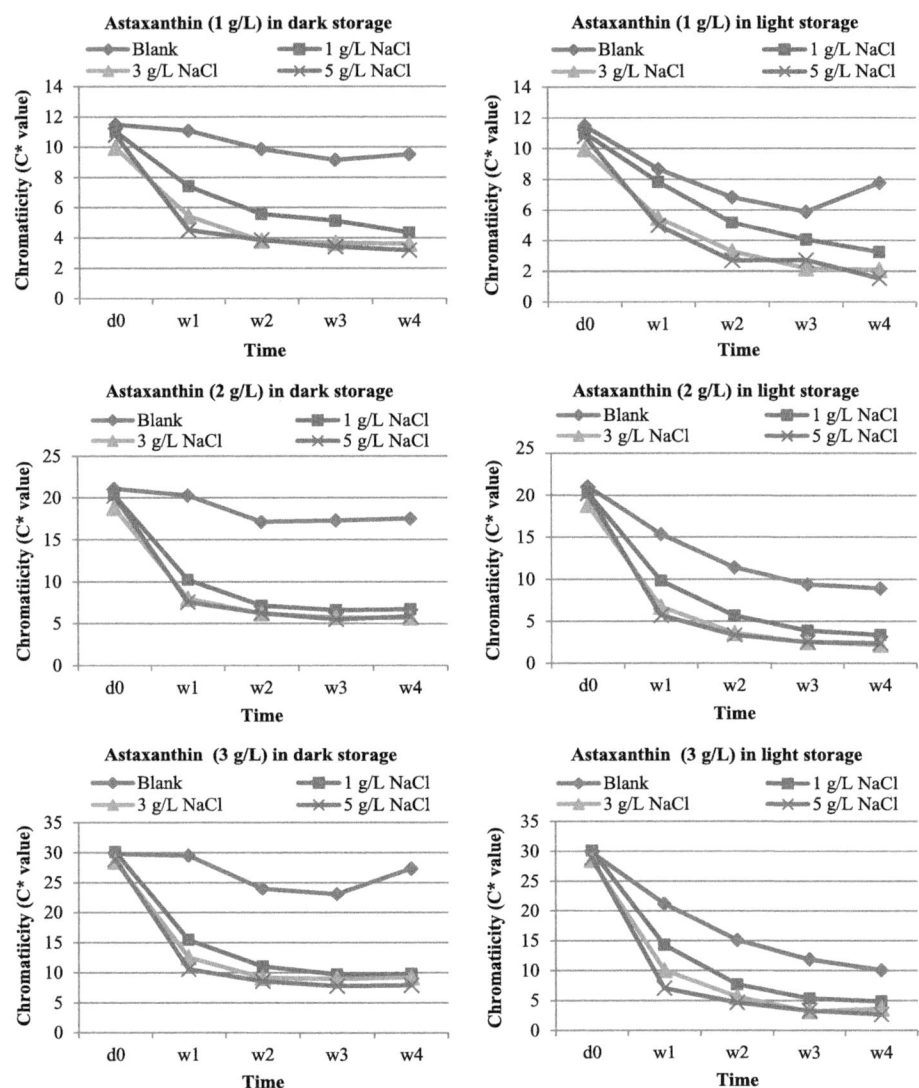

Fig. 8 Chromaticity of astaxanthin pigments at different concentrations 1, 2, 3 g/L and different salinities, stored in dark and light conditions, measured initially and every 1, 2, 3, and 4 weeks.

By the end of the treatment in a dark condition, the lowest concentration of a pigment treated with 0, 1, 3, and 5 g/L NaCl was obtained as 17.01%, 60.57%, 63.92%, and 70.52% of chromaticity degradation. Meanwhile, the medium concentration of astaxanthin pigments (2 g/L) show 16.80%, 66.87%, 69.71%, and 70.88% degradation, whereas the highest concentration of pigments (3 g/L) show 8.2, 67.49, 67.77, and 72.65% degradation correspondingly. In contrast, the end of the treatment in a light condition resulted in a chromaticity degradation of 32.45, 70.64, 79.14, and 85.90% for the lowest concentration pigments, 57.72, 83.28, 88.33, and 88.07% for

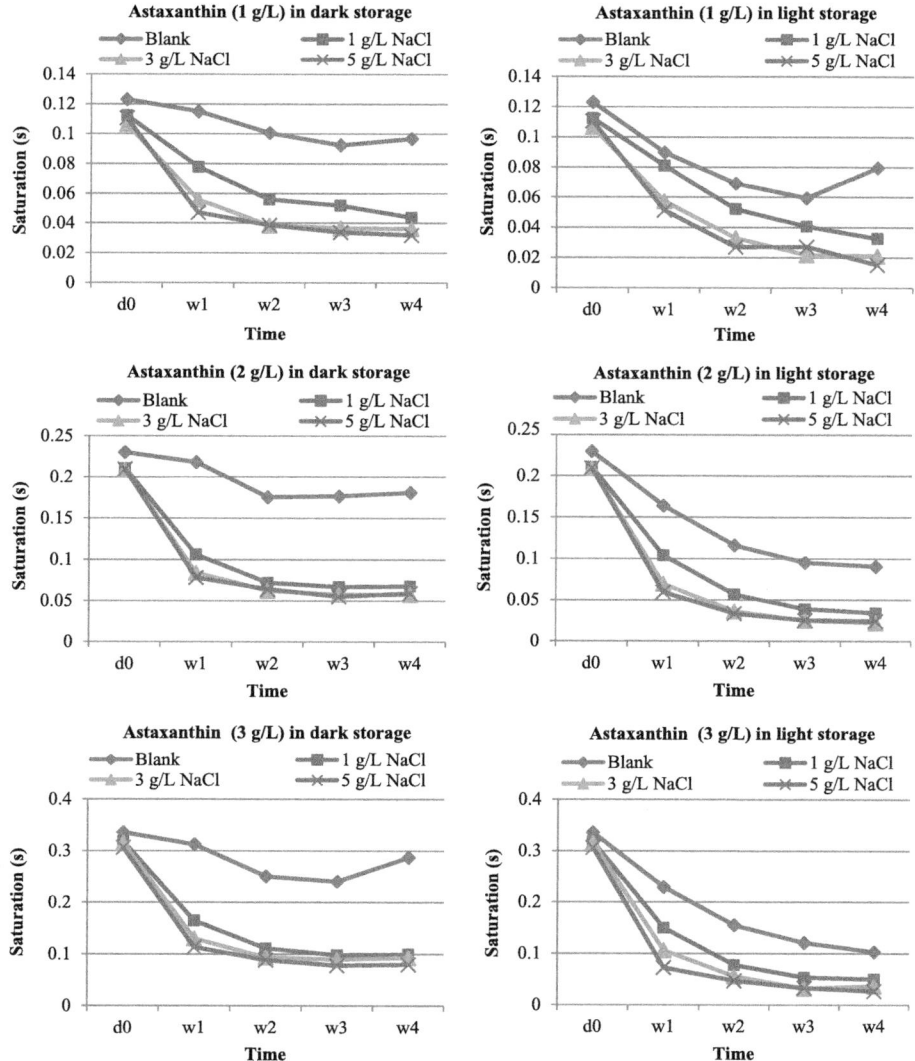

Fig. 9 Color saturation of astaxanthin pigments at different concentrations 1, 2, 3 g/L and different salinities, stored at room temperature, in dark and light conditions, measured initially and every 1, 2, 3, and 4 weeks.

medium concentration pigments, and 66.18, 83.94, 87.34, and, 90.76% for the highest concentration pigments, respectively. This corresponded with the concentrations of NaCl across each class. Therefore, the color-difference values (ΔE^*) shown in Fig. 10 support the result of salinity stability tests, where it shows significant changes affected by different pigment concentrations, the presence of NaCl, and the storage condition. Almost consistent increments have also been seen throughout the 4 weeks of experiment duration, despite the smallest differences from 1 week to another.

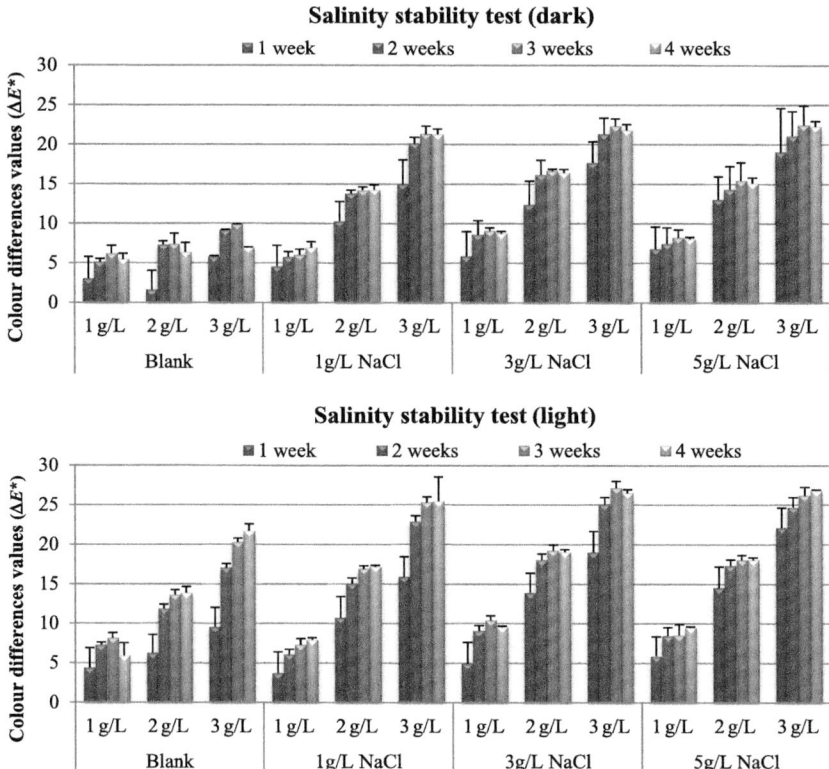

Fig. 10 Color difference values (ΔE^*) of astaxanthin pigments at different concentrations 1, 2, 3 g/L and different salinities, stored at room temperature, in dark and light conditions, measured initially and every 1, 2, 3, and 4 weeks.

The statistical analysis is performed via One-Way ANOVA for color changes difference value, indicating any statistically significant differences between pigment concentrations, NaCl concentrations, time, and storage conditions. The output indicated by the P value confirmed a statistically significant difference in the mean of the color difference value between different pigment concentrations, NaCl concentrations, time, and storage conditions, respectively, with a P value less than .0001. Then, a Tukey post hoc test was performed to show how each group differs from one another, revealing statistically significant differences in color values between each group of pigment concentrations of 1, 2, and 3 g/L ($P < .0001$). The test also revealed a statistically significant difference in color value between the 1-week group with other groups of 2, 3, and 4 weeks, as well as between the blank with other groups of 1, 3, and 5 g/L NaCl.

From the results, it can be deduced that the pigment degradation is increased in higher concentrations of salt treatment. This is due to salinity being one of the environmental stresses that can destabilize the molecular structure of the pigment (Mohajer, Taha, & Azmi, 2016). Besides, it can be concluded that the presence of light induces the photodegradation process. Therefore, during processing and storage of the carotenoid products, light exposure should be avoided to minimize quality deterioration.

pH test

Color stability is demonstrated by the chromaticity and color saturation graphs of the astaxanthin pigment, which is treated with pH 3, 5, 7, 9, and 11 and is stored in dark and light conditions accordingly throughout 4 weeks. The graphs are shown in Figs. 11 and 12, respectively. The values of astaxanthin pigment chromaticity and saturation have increased linearly with the concentration of the pigments, with those

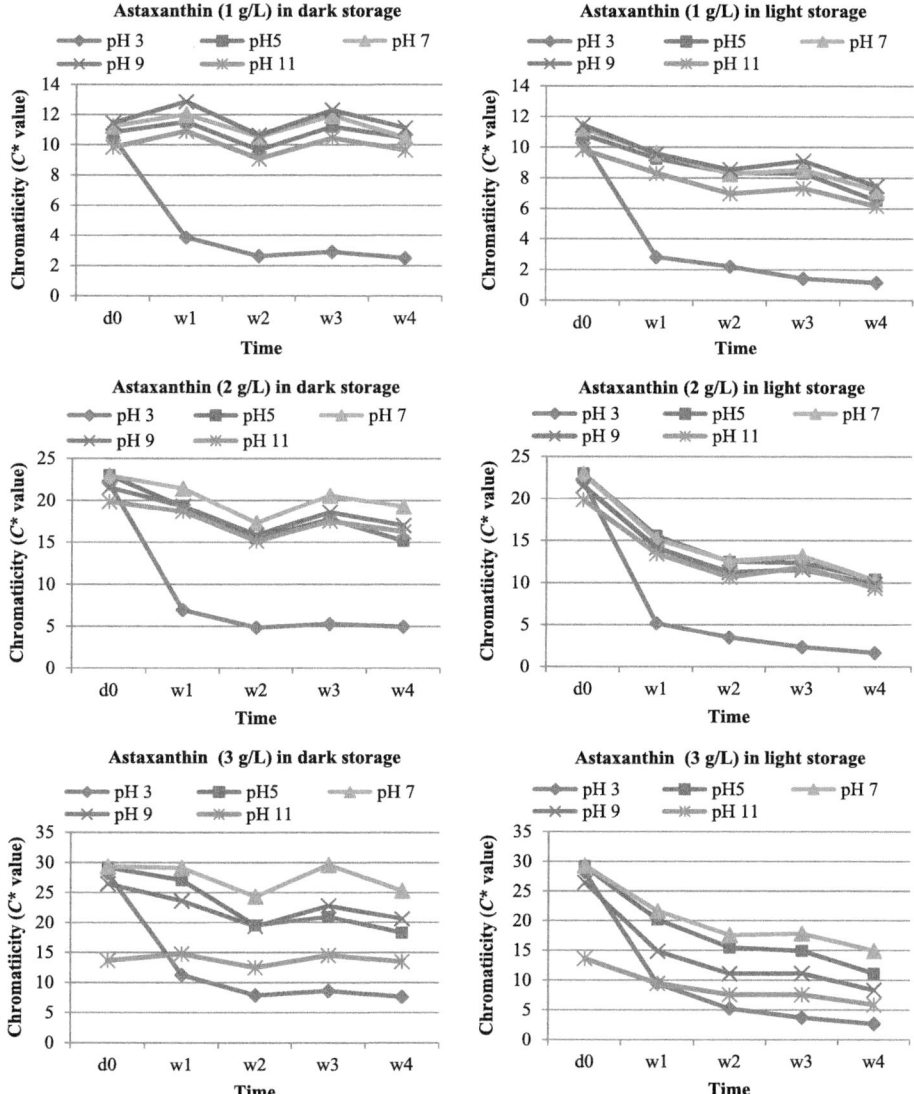

Fig. 11 Chromaticity of astaxanthin pigments at different concentrations 1, 2, 3 g/L and different pH values, stored at room temperature, in dark conditions, measured initially and every 1, 2, 3, and 4 weeks.

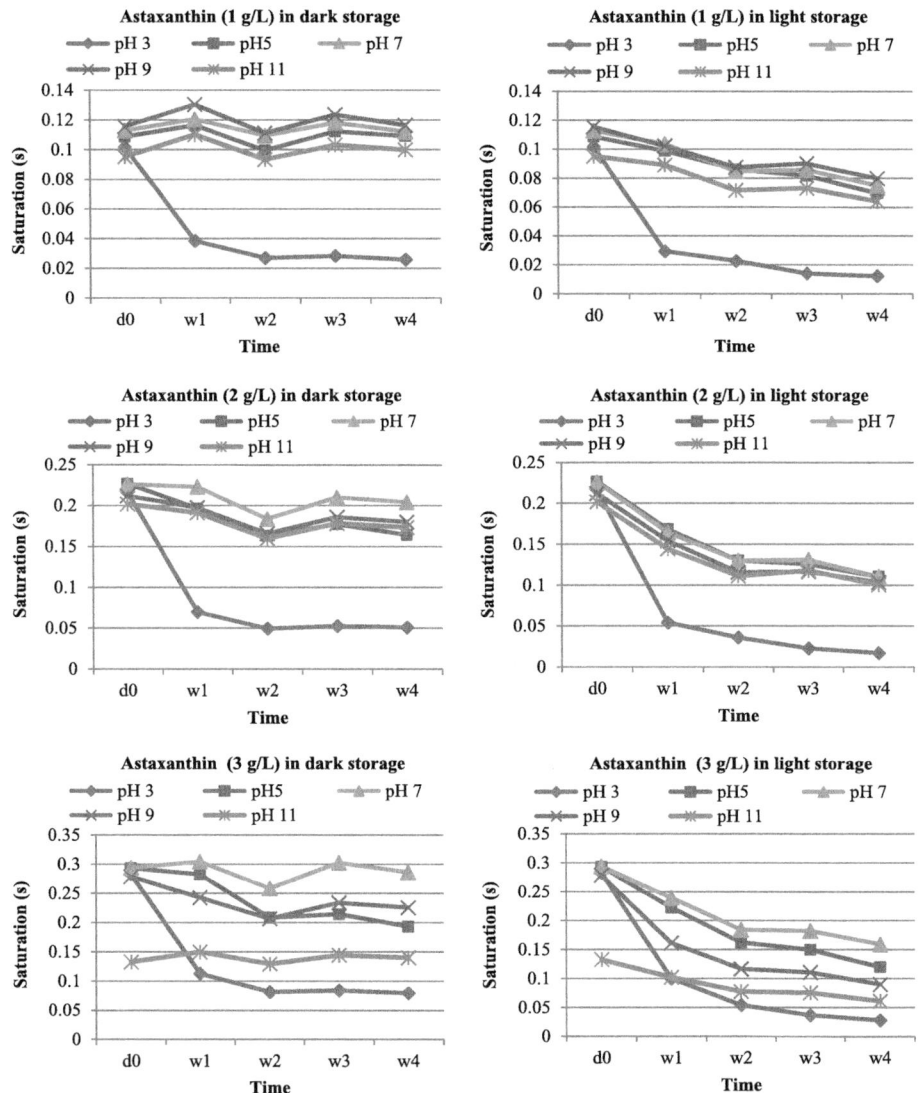

Fig. 12 Color saturation of astaxanthin pigments at different concentrations 1, 2, 3 g/L and different pH values, stored at room temperature, in dark and light conditions, measured initially and every 1, 2, 3, and 4 weeks.

stored in light conditions showing a higher degradation rate than the pigments stored in dark conditions. The graphs also demonstrate that the pigment with pH 3 has shown the highest degradation effect compared to those treated with other pHs for both dark and light conditions.

By the end of the treatment in a dark condition, the lowest concentration of pigment treated with pH 3, 5, 7, 9, and 11 has shown 76.19%, 3.45%, 6.69%, 2.87%, and 1.92% of chromaticity changes. Then, the medium concentration of astaxanthin pigments (2 g/L) showed 77.41%, 34.00%, 16.11%, 21.04%, and 18.09% changes, whereas the highest concentration of pigments (3 g/L) showed 72.94%, 37.37%, 13.69%, 21.96%, and 1.16% changes correspondingly. In contrast, the end of the treatment in light conditions resulted in chromaticity changes of 88.92%, 39.70%, 36.05%, 34.76%, and 37.45% for the lowest concentration pigments. This is followed by 92.55%, 54.79%, 55.28%, 54.39%, and 52.85% for the medium concentration pigments, and 90.51%, 61.94%, 49.16%, 68.56%, and 56.92% for the highest concentration pigments. This corresponded with pH 3, 5, 7, 9, and 11, respectively. The color difference values (ΔE^*) shown in Fig. 13 have supported the result of the pH stability test, whereby the pigment has shown significant changes when adjusted to very acidic conditions, and it showed fluctuation throughout the treatment period.

The statistical analysis performed via One-Way ANOVA for color-change difference value displayed the presence of any statistically significant difference between astaxanthin pigment concentrations, pHs, time, and storage conditions. The output indicated by the P value showed that there is a statistically significant difference ($P < .0001$) in the mean of the color difference value between different pigment concentrations, pHs, time, and storage conditions. The Tukey post hoc test was done showing which groups differing for each other, revealing a statistically significant variance ($P < .0001$) in color difference value between the 1 g/L concentration group

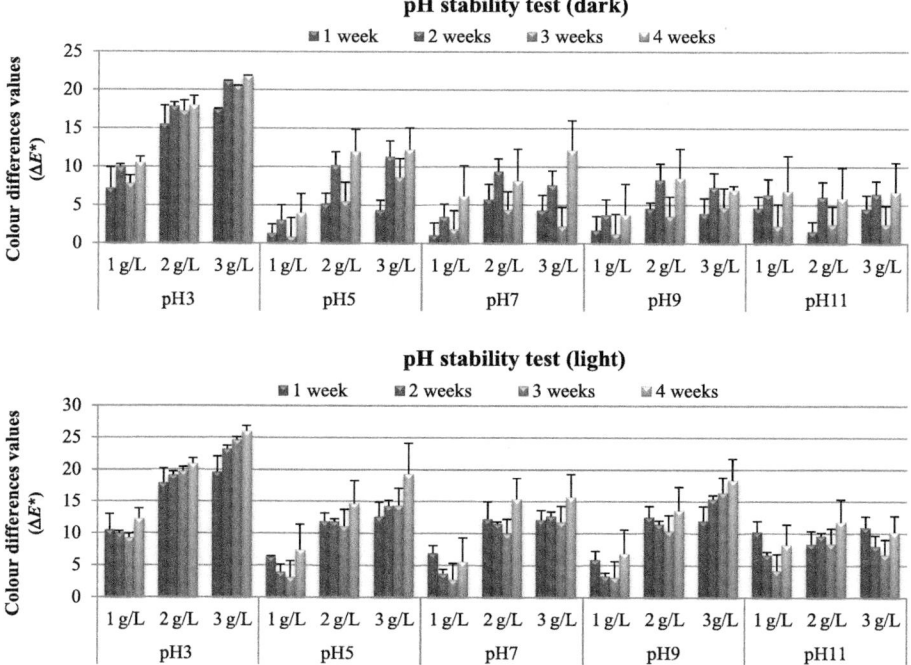

Fig. 13 Color difference values (ΔE^*) of astaxanthin pigment at different concentrations 1, 2, 3 g/L and different pH values, stored at room temperature, in dark and light conditions, measured initially and every 1, 2, 3, and 4 weeks.

with 2 and 3 g/L groups. In terms of time, there are statistically significant differences ($P < .0001$) between the 4-week group and the 1-week and 3-week groups. There are also statistically significant differences ($P < .0001$), between pH 3 with each of the other pH groups.

The observed color degradation suggested that the pigment is unstable in highly acidic conditions. This might be due to trans-cis isomerization occurring with the presence of acid (Gliemmo, Latorre, Gerschenson, & Campos, 2009; Rodriguez-Amaya, 2001; Ye & Eitenmiller, 2006; Yip, Joe, Mustapha, Maskat, & Said, 2014). The result of the pH stability test is also in agreement with the studies done by Rodriguez-Amaya (2001), Ye and Eitenmiller (2006), and Chen, Peng, and Chen (1996), where carotenoids in an alkaline condition are commonly more stable than in acidic conditions. An acidic pH is also believed to create ion pairs that form a carotenoid carbocation [e.g., $Car + AH \leftrightarrow (CarH^{+\cdots}A^-) \leftrightarrow CarH^+ + A^-$] (Boon, Mcclements, Weiss, & Decker, 2010). Besides, it can be concluded that the presence of light has a strong effect on astaxanthin stability, causing photodegradation of the pigment.

Heat test

Color stability is presented by the chromaticity and color saturation graphs of astaxanthin pigment, which are incubated in various temperatures (i.e., 4°C, 25°C, 35°C, 45°C, 65°C, 75°C, 85°C, and 95°C) for 3 hours as shown in Figs. 14 and 15. The values of astaxanthin pigment chromaticity and saturation fluctuated over 3 hours of incubation, but the changes observed are at a very minimal range. The color difference values (ΔE^*) shown in Fig. 16 supported the results of the heat stability test, where the pigment showed insignificant changes across different temperatures and periods of experiments.

The statistical analysis performed by One-Way ANOVA for the color difference value has indicated the presence of a statistically significant difference between astaxanthin pigment concentrations, temperatures, and time. The output indicated by the P value showed that there is no statistically significant difference by means of color difference value across different pigment concentrations, temperatures, and time. The Tukey post hoc test is performed afterward, confirming that no groups are statistically different from each other.

The minimal fluctuation trend over 3 hours at all temperatures applied showed the resistance of astaxanthin pigment toward heat. The results of this study are also supported by other research, where the pigment is found stable at 70–90°C in various carriers and is reported to degrade only at 120–150°C (Ambati et al., 2014). This may be due to esterified astaxanthin, which is more stable in nature than free astaxanthin, which has lower stability against light, oxygen, acidity, and heat. This subsequently causes oxidation, degradation, and isomerization processes (Mezzomo et al., 2013; Mezzomo & Ferreira, 2016).

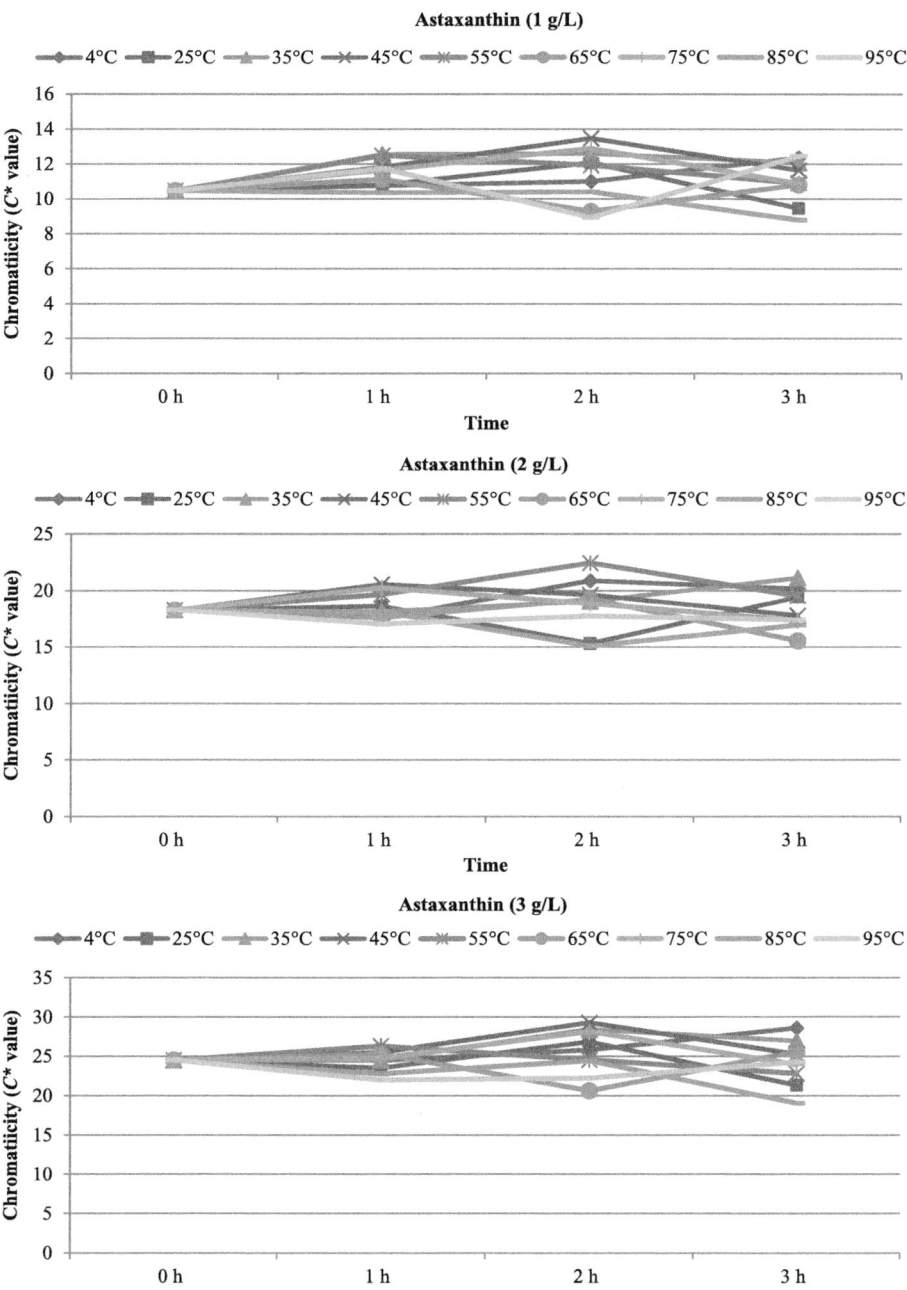

Fig. 14 Chromaticity of astaxanthin pigments at different concentrations 1, 2, 3 g/L incubated in different temperatures measured initially and every 1, 2, and 3 hours.

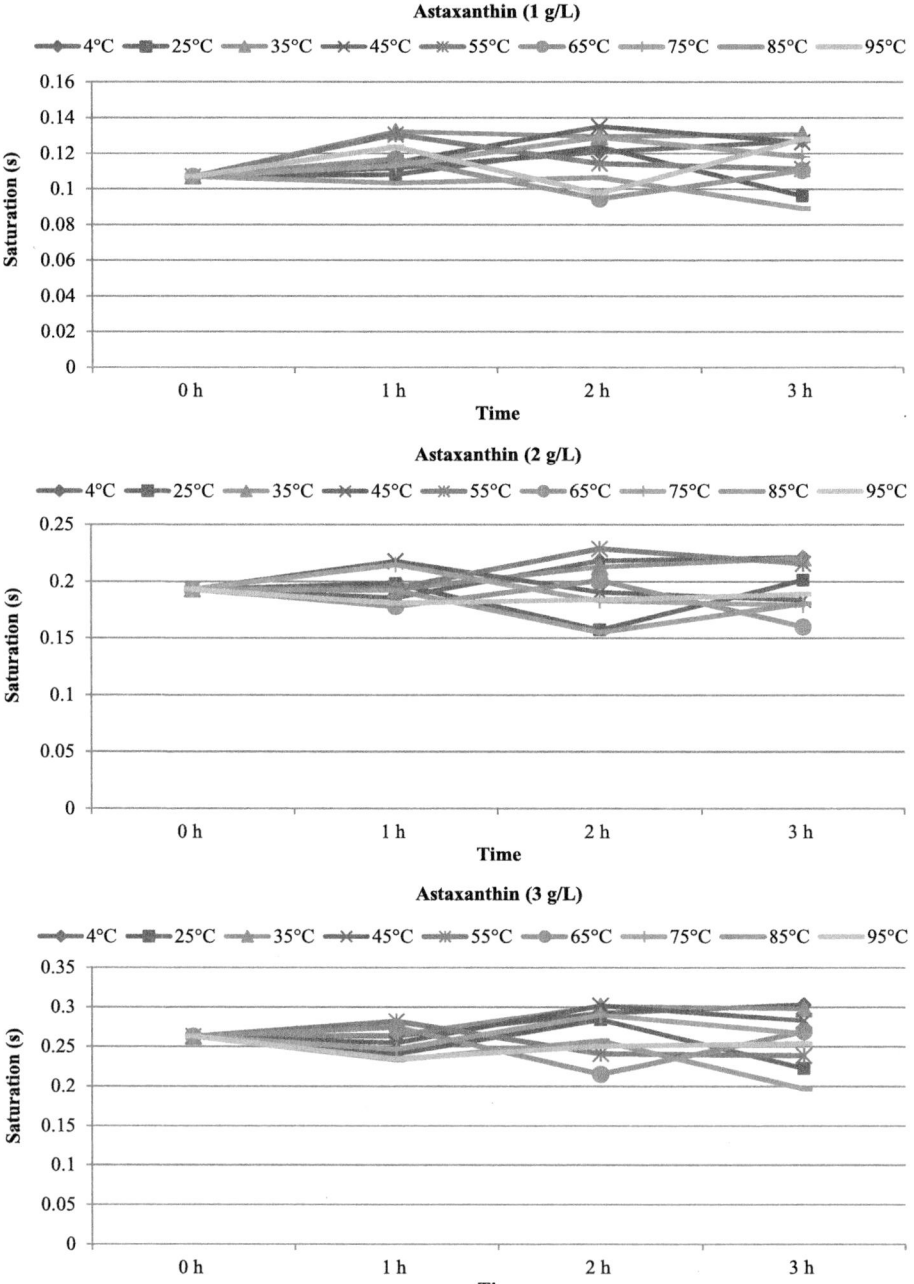

Fig. 15 Color saturation of astaxanthin pigments at different concentrations 1, 2, 3 g/L incubated in different temperatures measured initially and every 1, 2, and 3 hours.

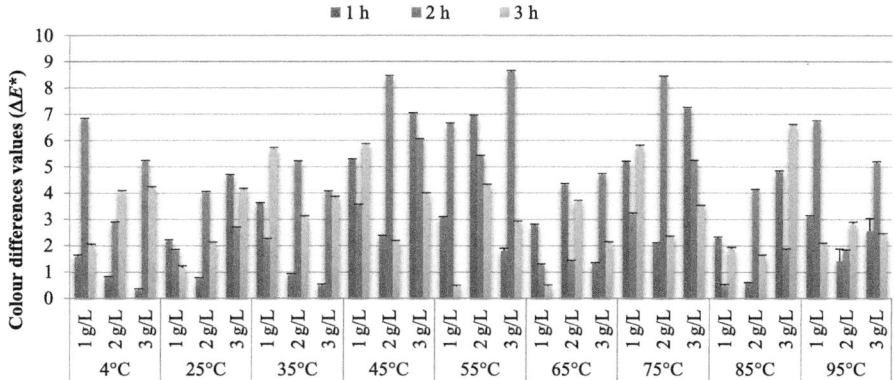

Fig. 16 Color difference values (ΔE^*) of astaxanthin pigment at different concentrations 1, 2, 3 g/L temperatures, measured initially and every 1, 2, and 3 hours.

UV irradiation test

The color stability of the astaxanthin pigment that is irradiated under UVA (365 nm) and UVB (312 nm) for 8 hours is exhibited by the chromaticity and color saturation graphs as shown in Figs. 17 and 18. After 8 hours of irradiation under UVA light, the chromaticity of 1, 2, and 3 g/L astaxanthin pigments show 14.54%, 38.71%, and 31.61% of degradation, respectively. Meanwhile, after being irradiated under UVB light, the chromaticity of 1, 2, and 3 g/L astaxanthin pigments shows 39.81%, 30.69%, and 52.67% of degradation, respectively. Therefore, the color difference values (ΔE^*) shown in Fig. 19 have supported the results of the UV stability test, where the highest pigment concentration irradiated under UVB light shows significant changes over 8 hours of experimentation.

The statistical analysis performed using One-Way ANOVA for color-difference value showed whether there is a statistically significant difference between astaxanthin pigment concentrations, UVs, and time. The output indicated by the P value shows that there is a statistically significant difference ($P < .0001$), by means of the color-difference value between different pigment concentrations. Then, the Tukey post hoc test is done to show whether different groups differ from each other, revealing a statistically significant difference ($P < .0001$) in color difference value between the 1 g/L concentration group with 2 and 3 g/L groups.

Light exposure can affect the stability of carotenoids (Boon et al., 2010; Rodriguez-Amaya, 2001), as trans-cis photoisomerization may occur (Rodriguez-Amaya, 2001; Yip et al., 2014). The light absorption may also lead to the single oxygen formation resulting in the excited state of the carotenoid molecule. This may subsequently involve a chemical-degradation pathway (Boon et al., 2010; Meléndez-Martínez, Britton, Vicario, & Heredia, 2006).

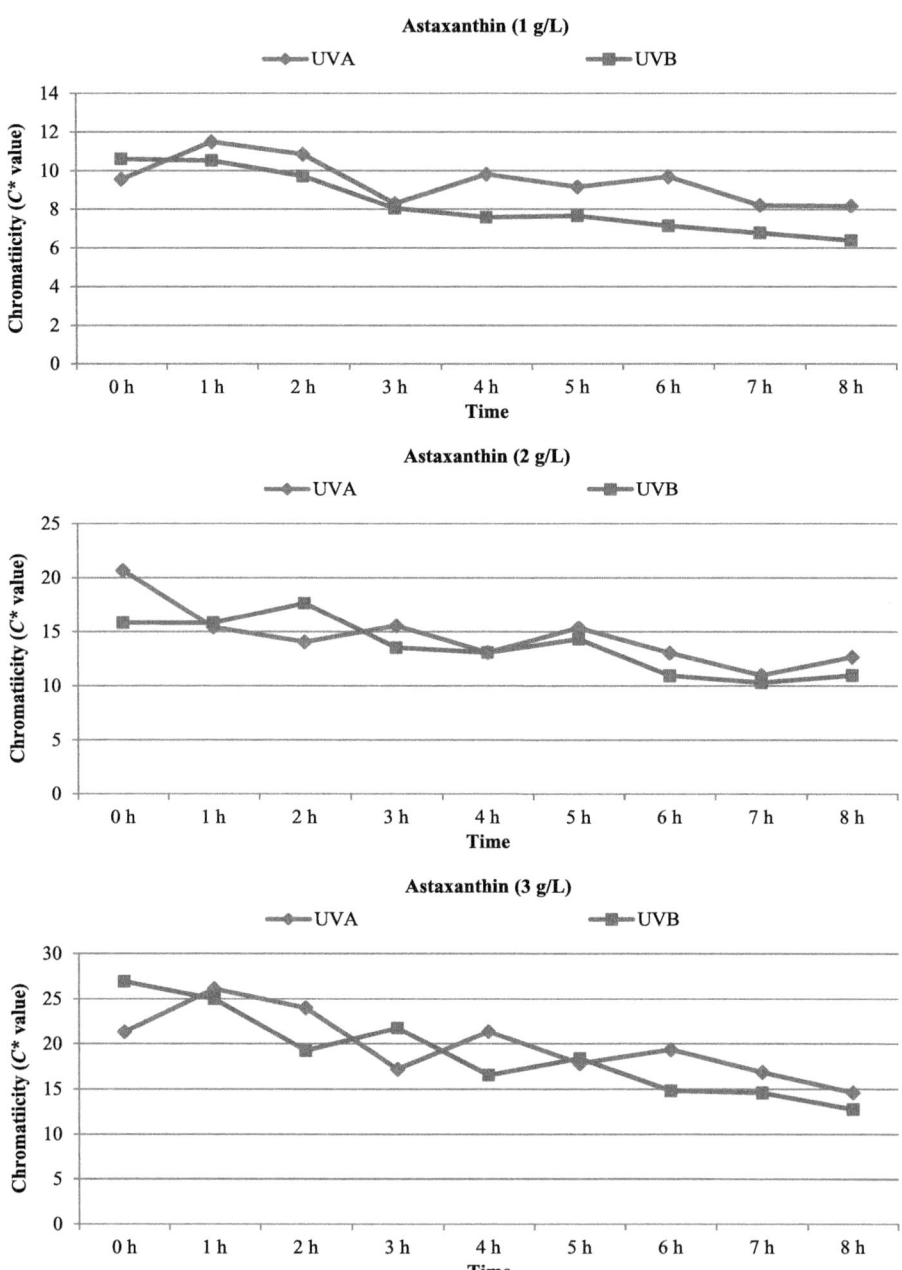

Fig. 17 Chromaticity of astaxanthin pigments at different concentrations 1, 2, 3 g/L exposed under UVA (365 nm) and UVB (312 nm) light, at room temperature, measured every hour for 8 hours.

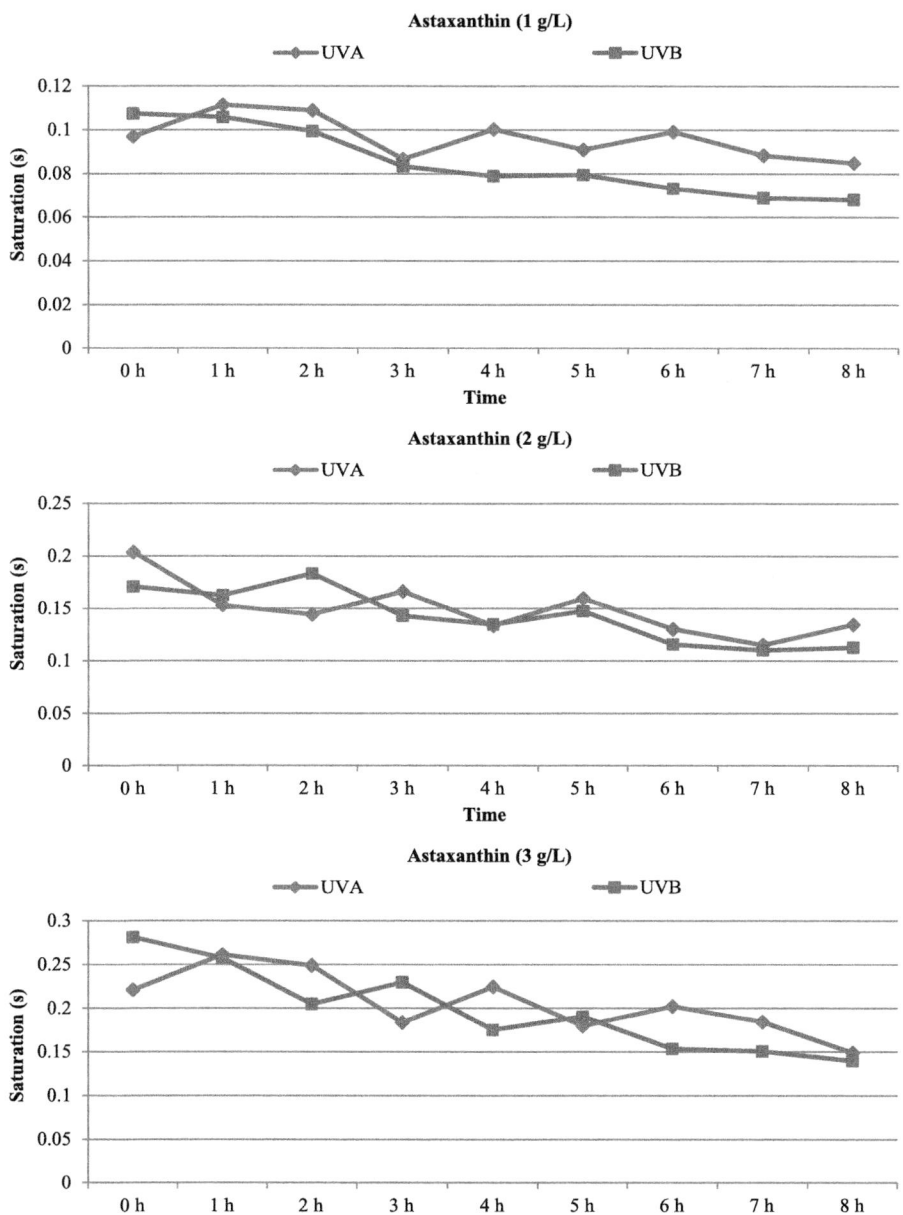

Fig. 18 Color saturation of astaxanthin pigments at different concentrations 1, 2, 3 g/L exposed under UVA (365 nm) and UVB (312 nm) light, at room temperature, measured every hour for 8 hours.

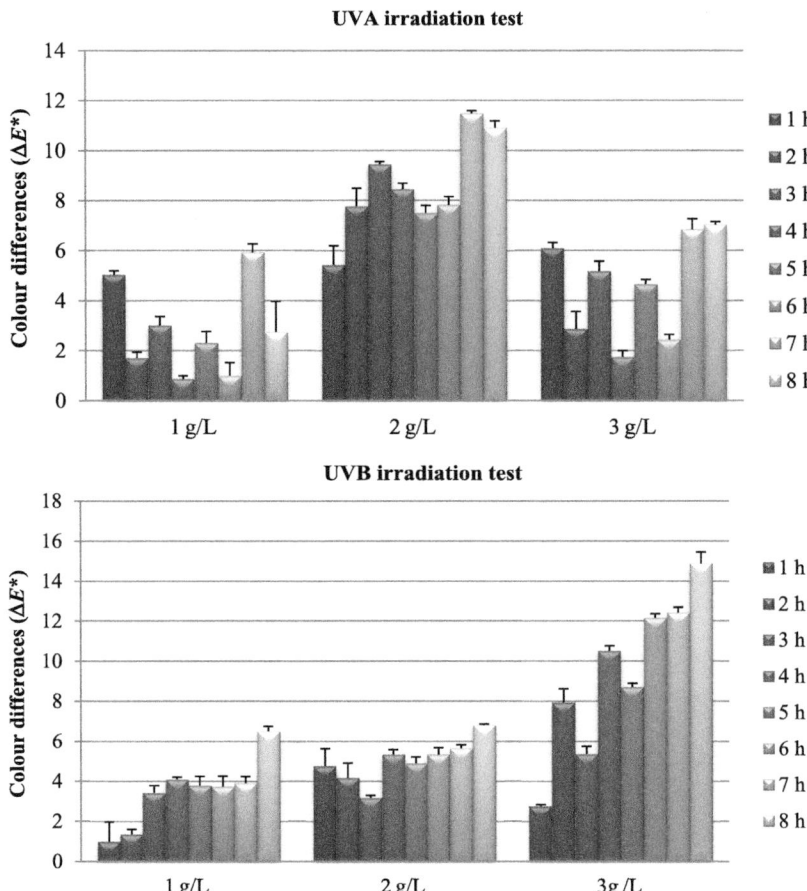

Fig. 19 Color difference values of astaxanthin pigment exposed under UVA (365 nm) and UVB (312 nm).

Conclusion

There are several outcomes of the chromaticity-stability assessment of astaxanthin throughout different periods of exposure to pH, salinity, UV, and heat. Salinity treatment has displayed a significant effect on astaxanthin where the highest degradation rate has been observed at higher concentrations of NaCl given that they are stored in light storage, displaying 91% degradation. NaCl, as one of the known environmental stresses, can destabilize the molecular structure. The highest degradation rate has also been found in pigments stored in light conditions; at an acidic condition, astaxanthin has resulted in chromaticity changes greater than 89%. This is explained by the occurrence of tran-cis isomerization that contributes to the decoloration of the pigment. The astaxanthin pigment has shown fluctuation over 3 hours of incubation but within a minimal range, indicating its resistance against high temperature. UVA and

UVB irradiation can also cause photodegradation of carotenoids. In the UV irradiation stability test, astaxanthin has shown a low degradation rate of only 40%.

Therefore, the properties of carotenoids in terms of color appearance have been correlated with various environmental factors, such as heat, light, oxygen, pH, and others. Color is also attributed to the conjugated double bonds system within their structure, which develops the light-absorbing chromophore that substantiates the carotenoid characterization and quantification. During the production, storage, delivery, and consumption of carotenoid products, various environmental stresses will be encountered and will influence the stability of the pigments. Therefore, this study has successfully provided a basic understanding regarding the carotenoid pigment stability related to these factors.

References

Aberoumand, A. (2011). A review article on edible pigments properties and sources as natural biocolorants in foodstuff and food industry. *World Journal of Dairy & Food Sciences*, *6*(1), 71–78.

Ali, N. F., El-Khatib, E. M., El-Mohamedy, R. S. S., & Ramadan, M. A. (2014). Antimicrobial activity of silk fabrics dyed with saffron dye using microwave heating. *International Journal of Current Microbiology and Applied Sciences*, *3*(12), 140–146.

Ahmed, J., & Ramaswamy, H. S. (2006). Changes in color during high-pressure processing of fruits and vegetables. *Stewart Postharvest Review*, *5*(9), 1–8. http://doi.org/10.2212/spr.2006.5.9.

Ambati, R. R., Moi, P. S., Ravi, S., & Aswathanarayana, R. G. (2014). Astaxanthin: Sources, extraction, stability, biological activities and its commercial applications—A review. *Marine Drugs*, *12*(1), 128–152. https://doi.org/10.3390/md12010128.

Arapitsas, P., & Turner, C. (2008). Pressurized solvent extraction and monolithic column-HPLC/DAD analysis of anthocyanins in redmcabbage. *Talanta*, *74*, 1218–1223.

Arvayo-Enríquez, H., Mondaca-Fernández, I., Gortáres-Moroyoqui, P., Lopez-Cervantes, J., & Rodríguez-Ramírez, R. (2013). Carotenoids extraction and quantification: a review. *Analytical Methods*, *5*(12), 2916–2924. https://doi.org/10.1039/c3ay26295b.

Block, G., Patterson, B., & Subar, A. (1992). Fruit, vegetables, and cancer prevention: a review of epidemiological evidence. *Nutrition and Cancer*, *18*, 1–29.

Boon, C. S., Mcclements, D. J., Weiss, J., & Decker, E. A. (2010). Factors influencing the chemical stability of carotenoids in foods factors influencing the chemical stability of carotenoids in foods. *Critical Reviews in Food Science and Nutrition*, *50*(November), 515–532. https://doi.org/10.1080/10408390802565889.

Boonsong, P., Laohakunjit, N., & Kerdchoechuen, O. (2012). Natural pigments from six species of Thai plants extracted by water for hair dyeing product application. *Journal of Cleaner Production*, *37*, 93–106. https://doi.org/10.1016/j.jclepro.2012.06.013.

Bridle, P., & Timberlake, C. F. (1997). Anthocyanins as natural food colour selected aspects. *Food Chemistry*, *58*, 103–109.

Borel, P. (2003). Factors affecting intestinal absorption of highly lipophilic food microconstituents (fat-soluble vitamins, carotenoids, and phytosterols). *Clinical Chemistry and Laboratory Medicine*, *41*, 979.

Britton, G. (1995). Structure and properties of carotenoids in relation to function. *The FASEB Journal*, *9*, 1551–1558.

Britton, G., Liaaen-Jensen, S., & Pfander, H. (Eds.), (2004). *Carotenoids: Handbook*. Birkhäuser.

Buchweitz, M., Nagel, A., Crle, R., & Kammerer, D. R. (2012). Characterisation of sugar beet pectin fractions providing enhanced stability of anthocyanin-based natural blue food colourants. *Food Chemistry, 12*(4), 1971–1979.

Chen, H. E., Peng, H. Y., & Chen, B. H. (1996). Stability of carotenoids and vitamin A during storage of carrot juice. *Food Chemistry, 57*(4), 497–503.

Cadoni, E., De Giorgi, M. R., Medda, E., & Poma, G. (2000). Supercritical CO<ce:inf>2</ce:inf> extraction of lycopene and beta-carotene from ripe tomatoes. *Dyes and Pigments, 44*(1), 27–32.

Delgado-vargas, F., & Paredes-Lopez, O. (2000). Natural pigments: Carotenoids, anthocyanins, and betalains—characteristics, biosynthesis, processing, and stability. *Critical Reviews in Food Science and Nutrition, 40*(3), 173–289. https://doi.org/10.1080/10408690091189257.

Christie, R. M. (1994). Pigments, dyes and fluorescent brightening agents for plastics: an overview. *Polymer International, 34*(4), 351–361. https://doi.org/10.1002/pi.1994.210340401.

da Silva, R.P.F.F., Rocha-Santos, T. A. P., & Duarte, A. C. (2016). Supercritical fluid extraction of bioactive compounds. *Trends in Analytical Chemistry, 76*, 40–51. https://doi.org/10.1016/j.trac.2015.11.013.

Eonseon, J., Polle, J. W., Lee, H. K., Hyun, S. M., & Chang, M. J. (2003). Xanthophylls in microalgae: from biosynthesis to biotechnological mass production and application. *Microbial Biotechnology, 13*(2), 165–174.

Durante, M., Lenucci, M. S., & Mita, G. (2014). Supercritical carbon dioxide extraction of carotenoids from Pumpkin (Cucurbita spp.): a review. *International Journal of Molecular Sciences, 15*(1), 6725–6740.

Famino, A. O., Oduguwa, O. O., Onifade, A. O., & Olotunde, T. O. (2000). Protein quality of shrimp-waste meal. *Bioresource Technology, 72*(1), 185.

Erge, H. S., & Karadeniz, F. (2011). Bioactive compounds and antioxidant activity of tomato cultivars. *International Journal of Food Properties, 14*(5), 968–977. https://doi.org/10.1080/10942910903506210.

Fortes, C. (2006). Carotenoids in Cancer Prevention. In W. Baer-Dubowska, A. Bartoszek, & D. Malejka-Giganti (Eds.), *Carcinogenic and Anticarcinogenic Food Components* (pp. 283–302). United States of America: CRC Press.

Farre, G., Zhu, C., Sandmann, G., Twyman, R. M., Capell, T., & Christou, P. (2015). Nutritionally important carotenoids as consumer products. *Phytochemistry Reviews, 14*, 727–743. https://doi.org/10.1007/s11101-014-9373-1.

Gildberg, A., & Stenberg, E. (2001). A new process for advanced utilization of shrimp waste. *Process Biochemistry, 36*(8), 809–812.

Gliemmo, M. F., Latorre, M. E., Gerschenson, L. N., & Campos, C. A. (2009). Color stability of pumpkin (Cucurbita moschata, Duchesne ex Poiret) puree during storage at room temperature: Effect of pH, potassium sorbate, ascorbic acid and packaging material. *LWT—Food Science and Technology, 42*, 196–201.

González-de-Mejía, E., Loarca-Piña, G., & Ramos- Gómez, M. (1997). Antimutagenicity of xanthophylls present in Aztec marigold (*Tagetes erecta*) against 1-nitropyrene. *Mutation Research, 389*, 219–226.

Guerin, M., Huntley, M. E., & Olaizola, M. (2003). Haematococcus astaxanthin: applications for human health and nutrition. *Trends on Biotechnology, 21*(5), 210–216.

Gulrajani, M. L. (1992). *Introduction to Natural Dyes*. New Delhi: Indian Institute of Technology.

Hadden, W. L., Watkins, R. H., Levy, L. W., Regalado, E., Rivadeneira, D. M., van Breemen, R. B., et al. (1999). Carotenoid composition of marigold (*Tagetes erecta*) flower extract used as nutritional supplement. *Journal of Agricultural and Food Chemistry, 47*, 4189–4194.

Handayani, A. D., Sutrisno, Indraswati, N., & Ismadji, S. (2008). Extraction of astaxanthin from giant tiger (Penaeus monodon) shrimp waste using palm oil: Studies of extraction kinetics and thermodynamic. *Bioresource Technology, 99*, 4414–4419.

Handelman, G. J., Nightingale, Z. D., Lichtenstein, A. H., Schaefer, E. J., & Blumberg, J. B. (1999). Lutein and zeaxanthin concentrations in plasma after dietary supplementation with egg yolk. *The American Journal of Clinical Nutrition, 70*, 247–251.

Humphries, J. M., & Khachik, F. (2003). Distribution of lutein, zeaxanthin, and related geometrical isomers in fruit, vegetables, wheat, and pasta products. *Journal of Agricultural and Food Chemistry, 51*, 1322–1327.

Herrero, M., Cifuentes, A., & Iban, E. (2006). Sub- and supercritical fluid extraction of functional ingredients from different natural sources: plants, food-by-products, algae and microalgae. A review. *Food Chemistry, 98*, 136–148.

Hussein, G., Sankawa, U., Goto, H., Matsumoto, K., & Watanabe, H. (2006). Astaxanthin, a carotenoid with potential in human health and nutrition. *Journal of Natural Products, 69*, 443–449.

IARC. (1975). *World Health Organisation. International Agency for Research on Cancer. IARC Monographs on the evaluation of the carcinogenic risk of chemicals to man: Some aromatic azo compounds. 8*. Lyon.

Jiménez, A. R. (2000). Natural pigments: carotenoids, anthocyanins, and betalains—Characteristics, biosynthesis, processing, and stability. *Critical Reviews in Food Science and Nutrition, 40*(3), 173–289.

Jaswir, I., Noviendri, D., Hasrini, R. F., & Octavianti, F. (2011). Carotenoids: sources, medicinal properties and their application in food and nutraceutical industry. *Journal of Medicinal Plants Research, 5*(33), 7119–7131. https://doi.org/10.5897/JMPRx11.011.

Kidd, P. (2011). Astaxanthin, cell membrane nutrient with diverse clinical benefits and anti-aging potential. *Alternative Medicine Review, 16*, 355–364.

Kim, L., Rao, A. V., & Rao, I. G. (2002). Effect of lycopene on prostate LNCaP cancer cells in culture. *Journal of Medicinal Food, 5*, 181–187.

Kumar, A., & Pastore, P. (2006). *Toying with toxics*. . Retrieved from www.toxicslink.org.

Licón, C. C., Carmona, M., Rubio, R., Molina, A., & Berruga, M. I. (2012). Preliminary study of saffron (Crocus sativus L. stigmas) color extraction in a dairy matrix. *Dyes and Pigments, 92*(3), 1355–1360. https://doi.org/10.1016/j.dyepig.2011.09.022.

Lin, S., Chen, Y., Chen, R., Chen, L., & Ho, H. (2016). Improving the stability of astaxanthin by microencapsulation in calcium alginate beads. *PLoS ONE, 11*(4), 1–10. https://doi.org/10.1371/journal.pone.0153685.

Liu, C. L., Huang, Y. S., Hosokawa, M., Miyashita, K., & Hu, M. L. (2009). Inhibition of proliferation of hepatoma cell line by fucoxanthin in relation to cell cycle arrest and enhanced gap junctional intercellular communication. *Chemico-Biological Interactions, 182*, 165–172.

Liu, X., & Osawa, T. (2007). *Cis* astaxanthin and especially 9-cis astaxanthin exhibits a higher antioxidant activity in vitro compared to the all trans isomer. *Biochemical and Biophysical Research Communications, 357*, 187–193.

Macías-sanchez, M. D., Mantell, C., Rodríguez, M., La ossa, E. M., Lubian, L. M., & Montero, O. (2009). Comparison of supercritical fluid and ultrasound-assisted extraction of carotenoids and chlorophyll from *Dunaliella salina*. *Talanta, 77*(3), 948.

Maeda, H., Hosokawa, M., Sahima, T., Funayama, K., & Miyashita, K. (2005). Fucoxanthin from edible seaweed, *Undaria pinnatifida*, shows antiobesity effect through UCP1 expression in white adipose tissue. *Biochemical and Biophysical Research Communications, 332*, 392–397.

Manzi, F., Flood, V., Webb, K., & Mitchell, P. (2002). The intake of carotenoids in an older Australian population: the Blue Mountains Eye Study. *Public Health Nutrition, 5*, 347.

McClements, D. J., Decker, E. A., Park, Y., & Weiss, J. (2009). Structural design principles for delivery of bioactive components in nutraceuticals and functional foods. *Critical Reviews in Food Science and Nutrition, 49*, 577–606.

Martín, A., Mattea, F., Gutiérrez, L., Miguel, F., & Cocero, M. J. (2007). Co-precipitation of carotenoids and bio-polymers with the supercritical anti-solvent process. *Journal of Supercritical Fluids, 41*(1), 138–147.

McInerney, J. K., Seccafien, C. A., Stewart, C. M., & Bird, A. R. (2007). Effects of high pressure processing on antioxidant activity, and total carotenoid content and availability, in vegetables. *Innovative Food Science & Emerging Technologies, 8*(4), 543–548.

Meléndez-Martínez, A. J., Britton, G., Vicario, I. M., & Heredia, F. J. (2006). Relationship between the colour and the chemical structure of carotenoid pigments. *Food Chemistry, 101*(3), 1145–1150. https://doi.org/10.1016/j.foodchem.2006.03.015.

Meyers, S. P., & Chen, H. M. (1985). Process for utilization of shellfish waste. US Patent 4,505,936.

Mezzomo, N., & Ferreira, S. R. S. (2016). Carotenoids functionality, sources, and processing by supercritical technology: A review. *Journal of Chemistry, 2016*, 1–17.

Mezzomo, N., Maestri, B., Dos Santos, R. L., Maraschin, M., & Ferreira, S. R. S. (2011). Pink shrimp (P. brasiliensis and P. paulensis) residue: Influence of extraction method on carotenoid concentration. *Talanta, 85*(3), 1383–1391. https://doi.org/10.1016/j.talanta.2011.06.018.

Mezzomo, N., Martínez, J., Maraschin, M., & Ferreira, S. R. S. (2013). Pink shrimp (P. brasiliensis and P. paulensis) residue: Supercritical fluid extraction of carotenoid fraction. *Journal of Supercritical Fluids, 74*, 22–33. https://doi.org/10.1016/j.supflu.2012.11.020.

Mezzomo, N., Tenfen, L., Farias, M. S., Friedrich, M. T., Pedrosa, R. C. S., & Ferreira, R. S. (2015). Evidence of anti-obesity and mixed hypolipidemic effects of extracts from pink shrimp (*Penaeus brasiliensis* and *Penaeus paulensis*) processing residue. *Journal of Supercritical Fluids, 96*, 252–261.

Miki, W. (1991). Biological functions and activities of animal carotenoids. *Pure and Applied Chemistry, 63*, 141–146.

Moeller, S. M., Jacques, P. F., & Blumberg, J. B. (2000). The potential role of dietary xanthophylls in cataract and age-related macular degeneration. *Journal of the American College of Nutrition, 5*, 522–527.

Mohajer, S., Taha, R. M., & Azmi, S. Z. (2016). Phytochemical screening and potential of natural dye colourant from pomegranate (*Punica granatum* L.). *Pigment & Resin Technology, 45*(1), 38–44. https://doi.org/10.1108/PRT-10-2014-0100.

Mortensen, A. (2006). Carotenoids and other pigments as natural colorants. *Pure and Applied Chemistry, 78*(8), 1477–1491. https://doi.org/10.1351/pac200678081477.

Munawar, N., Makiah, H., & Jamil, H. (2014). The islamic perspective approach on plant pigments as natural food colourants. *Procedia-Social and Behavioral Sciences, 121*, 193–203. https://doi.org/10.1016/j.sbspro.2014.01.1120.

Naguib, Y. M. A. (2000). Antioxidant activities of astaxanthin and related carotenoids. *Journal of Agricultural and Food Chemistry, 48*, 1150–1154.

Nelis, J. H., & DeLeenheer, P. A. (1991). Microbial sources of carotenoid pigments used in foods and feeds. *The Journal of Applied Bacteriology, 70*, 181–191.

Nor, N. A. M., Aziz, N., Mohd-adnan, A. F., Taha, R. M., & Arof, A. K. (2016). Chromaticity and color saturation of ultraviolet irradiated poly (vinyl alcohol)-anthocyanin coatings. *Optical Materials, 56*(1), 18–21. https://doi.org/10.1016/j.optmat.2015.12.031.

Othman, R. (2009). *Biochemistry and Genetics of Carotenoid Composition in Potato Tubers*. Lincoln University.

Pashkow, F. J., Watumull, D. G., & Campbell, C. L. (2008). Astaxanthin: A novel potential treatment for oxidative stress and inflammation in cardiovascular disease. *The American Journal of Cardiology*, *101*, 58D–68D.

Patras, A., Brunton, N., Da, S., Butler, F., & Downey, G. (2009). Effect of thermal and high pressure processing on antioxidant activity and instrumental colour of tomato and carrot purées. *Innovative Food Science and Emerging Technologies*, *10*(1), 16–22. https://doi.org/10.1016/j.ifset.2008.09.008.

Polyakov, N. E., Leshina, T. V., Meteleva, E. S., Dushkin, A. V., Konovalova, T. A., & Kispert, L. D. (2009). Water Soluble Complexes of Carotenoids with Arabinogalactan. *The Journal of Physical Chemistry B*, *113*, 275–282. https://doi.org/10.1021/jp805531q.

Radzali, S. A., Masturah, M., Baharin, B. S., Rashidi, O., & Rahman, R. A. (2016). Optimisation of supercritical fluid extraction of astaxanthin from Penaeus monodon waste using ethanol-modified carbon dioxide. *Journal of Engineering Science and Technology*, *11*(5), 722–736.

Primavera, J. H. (2005). *Mangroves and aquaculture in Southeast Asia. In Regional technical consultation for the development of code of practice for responsible aquaculture in mangrove ecosystem*. 25–37.

Tigbauan, Iloilo, Philippines: SEAFDEC Aquaculture Department. Quan, C., & Turner, C. (2009). Extraction of astaxanthin from shrimp waste using pressurized hot ethanol. *Chromatographia*, *70*(1–2), 247–251. http://doi.org/10.1365/s10337-009-1113-0.

Pu, J., Bechtel, P. J., & Sathivel, S. (2010). Extraction of shrimp astaxanthin with flaxseed oil: effects on lipid oxidation and astaxanthin degradation rates. *Biosystems Engineering*, *107*(4), 364–371.

Rivera, S., Vilaró, F., & Canela, R. (2011). Determination of carotenoids by liquid chromatography/mass spectrometry: Effect of several dopants. *Analytical and Bioanalytical Chemistry*, *400*(5), 1339–1346. https://doi.org/10.1007/s00216-011-4825-6.

Rodrigo-Baños, M., Garbayo, I., Vílchez, C., Bonete, M. J., & Martínez-Espinosa, R. M. (2015). Carotenoids from Haloarchaea and their potential in biotechnology. *Marine Drugs*, *13*, 5508–5532. https://doi.org/10.3390/md13095508.

Rodriguez-Amaya, D. B. (2001). *A Guide to Carotenoid Analysis in Foods*. Washington, DC: OMNI Research.

Rodriguez-Amaya, D. B., Rodriguez, E. B., & Amaya-Farfan, J. (2006). Advances in Food Carotenoid Research: Chemical and Technological Aspects, Implications in Human Health. *Malaysian Journal of Nutrition*, *12*(1), 101–121.

Sachindra, N. M., Bhaskar, N., & Mahendrakar, N. S. (2005). Carotenoids in different body components of Indian shrimps. *Journal of the Science of Food and Agriculture*, *5*, 167–172.

Sachindra, N. M., & Mahendrakar, N. S. (2005). Process optimization for extraction of carotenoids from shrimp waste with vegetable oils. *Bioresource Technology*, *96*, 1195–1200.

Sajilata, M., Singhal, R., & Kamat, M. (2008). The Carotenoid Pigment Zeaxanthin—A Review. *Comprehensive Reviews in Food Science and Food Safety*, *7*, 29–49. https://doi.org/10.1111/j.1541-4337.2007.00028.x.

Samanta, A. K., & Agarwal, P. (2009). Application of natural dyes on textiles. *Indian Journal of Fibre & Textile Research*, *34*(December), 384–399.

Sánchez, C., Baranda, A. B., & Martínez de Marañón, I. (2014). The effect of High Pressure and High Temperature processing on carotenoids and chlorophylls content in some vegetables. *Food Chemistry*, *163*, 37–45.

Sant'Anna, V., Gurak, P. D., Ferreira Marczak, L. D., & Tessaro, I. C. (2013). Tracking bioactive compounds with colour changes in foods—A review. *Dyes and Pigments*, *98*(3), 601–608. https://doi.org/10.1016/j.dyepig.2013.04.011.

Santos, D. T., Albuquerque, C. L. C., & Meireles, M. A. A. (2011). Antioxidant dye and pigment extraction using a homemade pressurized solvent extraction system. *Procedia Food Science, 1*, 1581–1588. https://doi.org/10.1016/j.profoo.2011.09.234.

Senthamil, L., & Kumaresan, R. (2015). Extraction and identification of astaxanthin from shrimp waste. *Indian Journal of Research in Pharmacy and Biotechnology, 3*(3), 192–195.

Simpson, B. K., & Haard, N. F. (1985). The use of proteolytic enzymes to extract caroteno- proteins from shrimp wastes. *Journal of Applied Biochemistry, 7*, 212.

Silva, G. F., Gamarra, F. M. C., Oliveira, A. L., & Cabral, F. A. (2008). Extraction of bixin from annatto seeds using supercritical carbon dioxide. *Brazilian Journal of Chemical Engineering, 25*, 419–426.

Sindhu, S., & Sherief, P. M. (2011). Extraction, characterization, antioxidant and anti-inflammatory properties of carotenoids from the shell waste of Arabian Red Shrimp Aristeus alcocki, Ramadan 1938. *The Open Conference Proceedings Journal, 2*, 95–103.

Singh, S. (2006). Impact of color on marketing. *Management Decision, 44*(6), 783–789. https://doi.org/10.1108/00251740610673332.

Snodderly, D. M. (1995). Evidence for protection against age-related macular degeneration by carotenoids and antioxidant vitamins. *The American Journal of Clinical Nutrition, 62*, 1448S–1461S. Suppl.

Stahl, W., & Sies, H. (2005). Bioactivity and protective effects of natural carotenoids. *Biochimica et Biophysica Acta, 1740*, 101–107.

Steinmetz, K. A., & Potter, J. D. (1993). Food-group consumption and colon cancer in the Adelaide case-control study. *International Journal of Cancer, 53*, 711–719.

Sui, X., Yue, R., Wang, L., & Han, Y. (2015). *Process optimization of astaxanthin extraction from antarctic kill (Euphausia superba) by subcritical R134a*. In: *3rd International Conference on Material, Mechanical and Manufacturing Engineering (IC3ME 2015)* (pp. 47–53). Qingdao, China: Atlantis Press.

Suganya, V., & Asheeba, S. T. (2015). Antioxidant and antimicrobial activity of astaxanthin isolated from three varieties of crabs. *International Journal of Recent Scientific, 6*(10), 6753–6758.

Sun, L., Sangkatumvong, S., & Shung, K. K. (2006). *A high resolution digital ultrasound system for imaging of zebrafish*. 2202–2205.

Torskangerpoll, K., & Andersen, Ø.M. (2005). Colour stability of anthocyanins in aqueous solutions at various pH values. *Food Chemistry, 89*(3), 427–440. https://doi.org/10.1016/j.foodchem.2004.03.002.

Tadapaneni, R. K., Daryaei, H., Krishnamurthy, K., Edirisinghe, I., & Burton-freeman, B. M. (2014). High-pressure processing of berry and other fruit products: implications for bioactive compounds and food safety. *Journal of Agricultural and Food Chemistry, 62*, 3877–3885.

Ul-Islam, S. (2017). Plant-Based Natural Products: Derivatives and Applications. In *Scrivener Publishing*. Hoboken, NJ.

Ushakumari, U. N., & Ramanujan, R. (2012). Astaxanthin from shrimp shell waste. *International Journal of Pharmaceutical Chemistry Research, 1*(3), 1–6.

Vidal Zaragoza, A. (2012). *Measurement of colour of citrus fruits using an automatic computer vision system*. Universidad Politécnica de Valencia. http://hdl.handle.net/10251/27912.

Vimala, S., & Paul, V. I. (2009). Utilization of crustacean fishery waste as a source of carotenoids. *Journal of Experimental Zoology India, 12*(2), 377–380.

Wang, L., Yang, B., Yan, B., & Yao, X. (2012). Supercritical fluid extraction of astaxanthin from *Haematococcus pluvialis* and its antioxidant potential in sunflower oil. *Innovative Food Science and Emerging Technologies, 13*, 120–127.

Yamashita, E. (2013). Astaxanthin as a medical food. *Functional Foods in Health and Disease, 3*, 254–258.

Xi, J. (2006). Effect of high-pressure processing on the extraction of lycopene in tomato paste waste. *Chemical Engineering & Technology*, *29*(6), 736–739. https://doi.org/10.1002/ceat.200600024.

Xi, J. (2013). High-pressure processing as emergent technology for the extraction of bioactive ingredients from plant materials. *Critical Reviews in Food Science and Nutrition*, *53*(8), 837–852. https://doi.org/10.1080/10408398.2011.561380.

Yang, Y., Kim, B., & Lee, J. Y. (2013). Astaxanthin structure, metabolism, and health benefits. *Journal of Human Nutrition & Food Science*, *1*, 1003–1011.

Yawadio, R., & Morita, N. (2007). Color enhancing effect of carboxylic acids on anthocyanins. *Food Chemistry*, *105*(1), 421–427. https://doi.org/10.1016/j.foodchem.2006.12.066.

Ye, L., & Eitenmiller, R. R. (2006). Fat-soluble vitamins. In Y. H. Hui (Ed.), *Handbook of Food Science, Technology, and Engineering* (pp. 212–241). USA: CRC Press.

Yip, W. H., Joe, L. S., Mustapha, W. A. W., Maskat, M. Y., & Said, M. (2014). Characterisation and Stability of Pigments Extracted from Sargassum binderi Obtained from Semporna, Sabah. *Sains Malaysiana*, *43*(9), 1345–1354.

Commercialization aspects of carotenoids

Ludmila Bogacz-Radomska*, Joanna Harasym*, Arkadiusz Piwowar[†]
*Adaptive Food Systems Accelerator, Department of Biotechnology and Food Analysis, Wroclaw University of Economics, Wroclaw, Poland, [†]Department of Management and Food Economy, Wroclaw University of Economics, Wroclaw, Poland

Chapter Outline

Carotenoids are part of a large group of natural and synthetic pigments, but only a few have met with industrial exploitation. The carotenoid market shares are divided into astaxanthin, beta-carotene, lycopene, lutein, and zeaxanthin. Due to their bioactive and color properties, they can be included in the food matrix, cosmetics, and pharmaceutical products. The main factors of carotenoid application are the color and the protective functions.

Capsanthin is widely used in the food and cosmetic industry as a natural colorant. The carotenoid is regarded as a functional material owing to its antioxidant activity (Kim, Ha, & Hwang, 2009; Matsufuji, Nakamura, Chino, & Takeda, 1998). Capsanthin is also added to chicken feed to make the color of the egg yolk more intense (Lokaewmanee, Yamauchi, & Okuda, 2013). Astaxanthin is mainly used in the animal feed industry

Carotenoids: Properties, Processing and Applications. https://doi.org/10.1016/B978-0-12-817067-0.00010-5

(feed for salmon and trout, for chicken, and for cattle). Multidirectional biological action of astaxanthin makes it a good ingredient of diet supplements and functional food (Pogorzelska, Hamułka, & Wawrzyniak, 2016; Sieradzka & Kołodziejczyk-Czepas, 2016). Astaxanthin is also used in the nutraceutical and pharmaceutical sector, and it has become popular in the cosmetic industry. Beta-carotene, owing to its characteristics, finds a number of applications in the food, pharmaceutical, and cosmetic sector (Saini, Nile, & Park, 2015). β-Carotene is an active vitamin A precursor. Lutein, similar to most carotenoids, has strong antioxidant characteristics, which contributes to its potential health-promoting properties. The unique feature characteristic of lutein (and zeaxanthin) is its ability to accumulate in the eyeball (in the macula and retina). Owing to the aforementioned properties, lutein and zeaxanthin reduce the risk of age-related macular degeneration (AMD) (Mozaffarieh, Sacu, & Wedrich, 2003). The literature mentions a number of potential benefits of using lutein as a nutrient or cosmetic agent (Shegokar & Mitri, 2012). Annatto is used in the food sector to add yellow or orange color in a wide range of food products (e.g., processed meat, smoked fish, beverages) (Scotter, 2009). Lycopene is also used as a coloring agent in the food sector. Antioxidant properties of lycopene make it a good active ingredient of cosmetics (Chiu et al., 2007). As emphasized by Igielska-Kalwat et al., the interest in carotenoids (lycopene in particular) as natural active ingredients of cosmetics is growing (Igielska-Kalwat, Gościańska, & Nowak, 2014). Cantaxanthin in the food sector is used as a colorant. Moreover, it finds application in the animal feed, pharmaceutical, and cosmetic sector. The literature emphasized the anticancer properties of lycopene (Mein, Lian, & Wang, 2008; Story, Kopec, Schwartz, & Harris, 2010).

Production methods

The production of natural carotenoids is expensive, which is why these compounds are produced mainly by chemical synthesis. The extraction process is a basic physicochemical method used for the production of natural carotenoids. These are extracted from flowers, fruits, seeds, roots, tubers, and the green parts of plants (Dasgupta & Klein, 2014). They occur in great quantities in carrots, pumpkins, and tomatoes, and also in fruits such as watermelons or raspberries. The production procedure is divided into several steps that are shown in Fig. 1.

The critical step is the extraction method. Until now, many extraction procedures have been developed. They are classified by Saini and Keum into five groups, as follows (Saini & Keum, 2018):

1. maceration, extraction in Soxhlet apparatus, microwave- or ultrasound-assisted extraction,
2. accelerated solvent extraction,
3. pulsed electric-field assisted extraction,
4. supercritical fluid extraction,
5. enzyme-assisted extraction.

The extraction process influences the efficiency of carotenoid production based on plant material. Hexane is a nonpolar organic solvent that is authorized for carotenoid

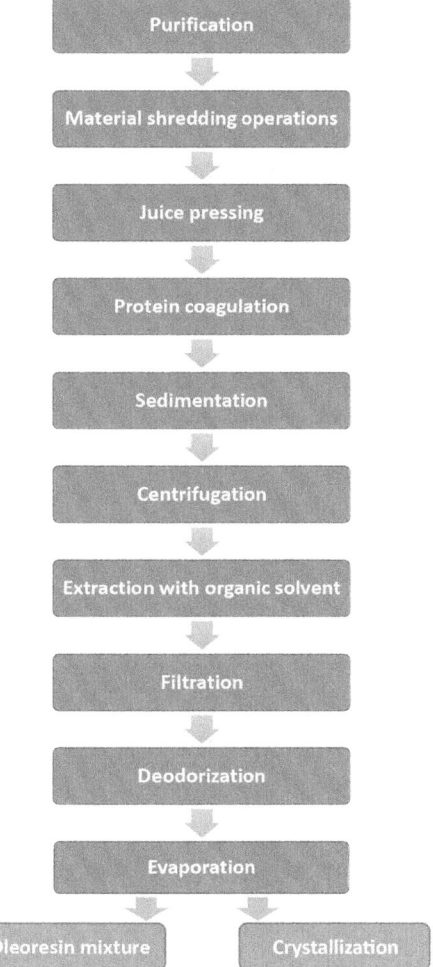

Fig. 1 Industrial production of natural carotenoids from plants.
Source: authors' own study.

extraction in commercial production. The presented production procedure is sometimes completed with fermentation and drying, whereupon the material is refermented. These additional processes increase the efficiency of carotenoid extraction. There are many carotenoid additives that are applied in different food products. Some examples of carotenoid products of plant origin are presented in Table 1.

The marigold flower (*Tagetes erecta L.*), because of its high lutein content (up to 0.2% of dry matter) is applied at the production of that carotenoid. This plant is cultivated primarily in China, Ecuador, India, Mexico, Peru, and Spain.

The lutein production from marigold flower first includes the drying of the plant material, and grinding is next. Thereafter, as a result of the extraction process, a nonpolar oleoresin extract is obtained. Then follows the conversion from trans-lutein into

Table 1 Examples of natural carotenoid formulations with plant origin

Carotenoid formulation		Plant material	Extraction method	Solvent	Carotenoids formula	Application
Carotene mixture CI Food Orange 5	**Carotenes**	Palm oil unrefined Carrot Alfa alfa	Solvent extraction	Oil Fat Hexane	Mainly ß-carotene (85%) and carotene (15%) i trace amount of γ-carotene $C_{40}H_{56}$	**Pigment** Nonalcoholic drinks, nonfiltered, with citrus taste; Edible fats; Processed cheese; Pastry: ice cream
Oleoresins Natural Yellow 27		Grass Urtica Tomatoes *Lycopersicon esculentum*	Solvent extraction	Fat	Lycopene $C_{40}H_{56}$	**Pigment** Tomato products; Jam, Marmalade
Annato CI Natural Orange 4	**Xanthophylls**	Annato—Bixa orleana,annatto seed extract	Solvent extraction Water alkali hydrolyze of extracted bixin Extraction of the external seed cover with NaOH and KOH Extraction of the external seed cover with edible plant oil	Oil Water Oil	Bixin $C_{26}H_{33}O_3$ Norbixin $C_{24}H_{28}O_4$ Norbixin $C_{24}H_{28}O_4$ Mainly bixin	**Pigment:** Fruit drink; Juice; Tomato products; Butter; Margarine; Ice cream; Nuddles; Instant soup
Oleoresisn-form paprika		Annual paprika, (mixed lemmas *Capsicum annuum* L. without seeds)	Solvent extraction	Fat	Kapsanthin $C_{40}H_{56}O_3$ Capsorubin $C_{40}H_{56}O_4$	**Pigment and taste additive:** Cold meat; Delicatessen food; Cheese; Canned vegetables; Canned meat; Canned fish
Lutein Mixture of carotenes and xanthophylls		Leavey *Tagetes erecta* Alfa alfa	Solvent extraction	Oil Ethanol	Lutein $C_{40}H_{54}(OH)_2$	**Pigment:** Muzzy citrus drinks; Dips; Ice creams; Dairy products; Confectionary

cis-lutein, which is catalyzed by several factors, for example, light, oxygen, heat, or acid. Finally, the nonpolar extract needs to be purified. To achieve a free lutein, it is necessary to apply a saponification process. The final products are in the form of capsules, oil, or powder, and as such they are implemented in the food matrix (Šivel, Kráčmar, Fišera, Klejdus, & Kubáň, 2014).

The main disadvantages of the production of carotenoids from plant material are the high cost, geographic determinants, and the seasonality of the raw material. To counter these drawbacks, synthetic methods have been developed. The first methods to synthesize carotenoids chemically were developed in the 1950s. Until now, they have served as the major source of carotenoid pigments in the market. The chemical synthesis of carotenoids used Wittig reactions or Grignard compounds. Lycopene, canthaxanthin, astaxanthin, β,β-carotene, β-apo-8′-carotenal, β-apo-8′-carotene, and cytranaxanthin are synthesized using these methods (Alvarez, Vaz, Gronemever, & de Lera, 2014).

Because of consumer demand for these natural pigments, the biotechnological production of carotenoids has garnered a lot of interest (Torregrosa-Crespo et al., 2018). There are many microorganisms that produce carotenoids, but only the alga *Dunaliella salina* and mold *Blakeslea trispora* are commercially applied (Fazeli, Tofighi, Samadi, & Jamalifar, 2006; Marchal, Mojaat-Guemir, Foucault, & Prevost, 2013; Mogedas, Casal, Forjan, & Vilchez, 2009). Cultures are created in three main stages, involving inoculum multiplication, biomass biosynthesis, and centrifugation.

The final commercial form influences the next steps of biomass treatment. In the case of the powder form, the biomass is spray dried. In the case of oleoresin with carotenoids or the crystalline form, it is necessary to squeeze the biomass and then to proceed as with the plant material (Pawłowska, 2009; Perez et al., 2003; Xinde, Mingqing, Dong, Bin, & Leming, 2012). The crystallization process requires alcohols (containing 1–6 carbon atoms), for example, n-propanol at 60°C. On mixing with gelatin, sucrose, starch, or vegetable oils, carotenoids can be applied as food additives (Joseph & Anandane, 2011; Perez et al., 2001; Xinde et al., 2012).

The alga *Dunaliella salina* is the main commercial source of natural β-carotene of microbiological origin. Its cultivation needs special conditions such as intense sunlight and relatively saline water. To assure efficient β-carotene biosynthesis, it is necessary to provide sodium chloride content in the range of 24% w/w. Cultivations of *D. salina* are mainly conducted in open tanks. The biomass productivity totals up to 40 g of dry mass per day per m^2. The β-carotene productivity depends on the tank's volumetric size and decreases with capacity extension. The β-carotene isolation process is determined by the product's commercial form. To obtain an alga powder containing 3% β-carotene, the biomass is centrifuged and dried. In contrast, to obtain a carotenoid emulsion, the algae dye is subjected to extraction, purification, and color separation. Thereafter, β-carotene is dissolved in vegetable oils (Mykolaiovych et al., 2008; Pisal & Lele, 2005).

Because of the healthy properties of lutein, especially the prevention of age-related macular degeneration, new technologies are developed that involve algae cultivations. Some reports claim higher lutein content in microalgae. Moreover the high growth rate of microalgae influences the yield productivity, which significantly exceeds the marigold crops on a per-square-meter basis (Fernández-Sevilla, Acién Fernández, & Molina Grima, 2010; Lin, Lee, & Chang, 2015).

Algae are cultivated in open ponds. The advantages of that process are simplicity and low production costs. There are, however, several disadvantages to this mode of production, for example, the poor use of light, evaporation losses, the requirement of a large area, bacterial infections, and variable weather.

Therefore, the cultivation of algae in photobioreactors is preferred. The use of photobioreactors enables full control of the cultivation, high efficiency of light use, higher biomass concretion, the control of gas emissions, the reduction of substrate evaporation, keeping the optimal temperature, protection against infections, and better use of space. On the downside, the costs of photo-bioreactors are high. Moreover, there are technical problems related to sterilization.

Algae-containing carotenoids have gained the trust of consumers. The main risk of their production, however, is the accumulation of heavy metals. Only clean production with clean oxygen input can assure healthy products. That is the reason why a clean label has such great importance.

Legal regulations

Carotenoid applications in the European Union are underlined in regulation (EC) No. 1333/2008 on food additives of the European Parliament and the Council of 16 December, 2008.

Food additive is any substance not normally consumed as a food in itself and not normally used as a characteristic ingredient of food, whether or not it has nutritive value, the intentional addition of which to food for a technological purpose in the manufacture, processing, preparation, treatment, packaging, transport or storage of such food results, or may be reasonably expected to result, in it or its by-products becoming directly or indirectly a component of such foods.

A list of approved carotenoid food additives have *E*-numbers E160 and E161. They are applied as colors. Only a few—carotenes E160a, paprika extract, capsanthin, and capsorubin E160c—are authorized at *quantum satis.* As such, these carotenoids are authorized to be used in the following food products:

- ripened orange, yellow, and broken-white cheese,
- processed cheese,
- ripened orange, yellow, and broken-white products,
- fats,
- butter and concentrated butter and butter oil and anhydrous milkfat, except butter from sheep and goats' milk,
- other fat and oil emulsions including spreads as defined by Council Regulation (EC) No 1234/2007 and liquid emulsions,
- preserves of red fruit,
- only vegetables (excluding olives),
- fruit and vegetable preparations excluding compote, preserves of red fruit, and seaweed-based fish roe analogues,

- jam, jellies, and marmalades and sweetened chestnut purée as defined by Directive 2001/113/EC, except chestnut purée,
- processed potato products, only dried potato granules and flakes,
- extruded puffed and or fruit-flavored breakfast cereals,
- fish paste and crustacean paste,
- precooked crustacean,
- smoked fish.

In some food products, for example, cheese or sausages, pâtés, and terrines, the aforementioned additives have limits of application up to 20 mg/L or mg/kg as appropriate. These specific application limits are set for carotenoids that depend on food products (mg/L or mg/kg as appropriate):

- lycopene 5–500,
- lutein 100–200,
- annatto, bixin, and norbixin 10–50,
- beta-apo-8′-carotenal 100–250.

In the food industry, lycopene is authorized for the commercial production of:

- flavored fermented milk products including heat-treated products,
- edible cheese rind,
- flavored processed cheese,
- edible ices,
- jam, jellies, and marmalades and sweetened chestnut purée as defined by Directive 2001/113/EC, except chestnut purée,
- fruit or vegetable spreads, except crème de pruneaux,
- breath-freshening microsweets,
- chewing gum,
- decorations, coatings, and fillings, except fruit-based fillings, except red coating of hard-sugar–coated chocolate confectionery,
- red coating of hard-sugar–coated chocolate confectionery,
- batters for coating,
- fine bakery wares,
- decorations and coatings except edible external coating of pasturmas,
- edible casings,
- salmon substitute,
- fish and crustacean paste, precooked crustaceans, surimi, smoked fish,
- fish roe, except sturgeons' eggs (caviar),
- seasonings and condiments,
- soups and broths,
- sauces, excluding tomato-based sauces,
- meat and fish analogues based on vegetable proteins,
- dietary foods for special medical purposes defined in Directive 1999/21/EC,
- dietary foods for weight control diets intended to replace total daily food intake or an individual meal (the whole or part of the total daily diet),
- flavored drinks, excluding dilutable drinks,
- fruit wine and made wine, excluding wino owocowe markowe,
- aromatized wine-product cocktails,
- other alcoholic drinks including mixtures of alcoholic drinks with nonalcoholic drinks and

spirits with less than 15% alcohol,
- ready-to-eat savories and snacks,
- processed nuts,
- desserts,
- food supplements supplied in a solid form, excluding food supplements for infants and young children,
- food supplements supplied in a liquid form, excluding food supplements for infants and young children,
- food supplements supplied in a syrup-type or chewable form.

The application of lutein at a food market is very low. Only a few food products are commercially pigmented with lutein:

- flavored processed cheese,
- jam, jellies, and marmalades and sweetened chestnut purée as defined by Directive 2001/113/EC, except chestnut purée,
- fruit or vegetable spreads, except crème de pruneaux,
- fish paste and crustacean paste,
- precooked crustacean.

Annatto, bixin, and norbixin are widely used in the production of:

- flavored fermented milk products including heat-treated products,
- ripened orange, yellow, and broken-white cheese and red and green pesto cheese,
- red Leicester cheese,
- Mimolette cheese,
- edible cheese rind,
- processed cheese,
- ripened orange, yellow and broken-white products,
- fats and oils essentially free from water (excluding anhydrous milk fat),
- other fat and oil emulsions including spreads as defined by Council Regulation (EC) No. 1234/2007 and liquid emulsions, excluding reduced fat butter,
- edible ices,
- decorations and coatings except fruit-based fillings,
- extruded puffed and or fruit-flavored breakfast cereals,
- batters for coating,
- fine bakery wares,
- casings and coatings and decorations for meat,
- smoked fish,
- liqueurs,
- alcoholic drinks with less than 15% alcohol,
- potato-, cereal-, flour-, or starch-based snacks, excluding extruded or expanded savory snack products,
- savory-coated nuts,
- desserts.

Beta-apo-8′-carotenal, similar to lutein, is used only in the production of four products:

- flavored processed cheese,
- fish paste and crustacean paste,

- precooked crustacean,
- smoked fish.

All carotenoids are added at dimethyl polysiloxane (PDMS) that is commonly referred to as silicones. PDMS is nontoxic and nonflammable.

Canthaxanthin is not authorized in the food categories listed in Parts D and E. The substance is in list B1 because it is used in medicinal products in accordance with Directive 2009/35/EC of the European Parliament and the Council, 2009 (OJ L 109, 30.4.2009, p. 10).

The following are sources of E160a carotenes:

E160a (i)—chemical synthesis.
E160a (ii)—palm carotenes (natural).
E160a (iii)—biosynthesis by *Blakeslea trispora* (called fungal or fermented beta carotene).
E160a (iv)—algal carotenes, extracted from *Dunaliella salina.*

The application of carotenoids in food depends on regulations, which can differ. Similar regulations are applied in the European Union, United States, Canada, Colombia, Venezuela, Chile, South Korea, and Japan, where carotenoids are used mainly according to *Good Manufacturing Practice*. Limited values are set in Mexico, Central America, GCC, India, China, the Philippines, Vietnam, and Thailand. Limited application amounts concern, in particular, synthetic, natural and fungal beta-carotene, lycopene, and lutein.

Many companies in the European Union replaced synthetic colors with natural. This resulted from changes in consumers' behavior. Civilization diseases are associated with processed food and synthetic additives.

Many consumers associate the E number with an ingredient that is "not natural"; therefore, this term that describes natural pigments was replaced with a full description of the added pigment or with the term "clean label." Food products achieve "clean-label" status if they are coloring food. Coloring food is a food ingredient derived from a food source or a characteristic ingredient of food processed in such a way so as not to extract the pigment selectively, even when used principally for the purpose of coloration of the final application. There are guidance notes on the classification of food extracts with coloring properties, published in November 2013. These notes serve to differentiate food-color additives (*E*-number) from extracts/concentrates with coloring properties (coloring foodstuffs). To consider a foodstuff as an ingredient and not as an additive, the extract must be obtained by nonselective extraction and from a source that is typically consumed as food in the European Union. Moreover, an Enrichment factor (*Fn*) is in force, which is calculated as follows:

$$Fn = \frac{Cp \, / \, Np}{Cs \, / \, Ns}$$

where:

Cp—% pigment in the primary extract.
Np—% nutrients in the primary extract.
Cs—% pigment in the source.
Ns—% nutrients in the source.

The *Fn* must be less than 6. If the food product fulfils all conditions, then it will be labeled as an ingredient, even when added principally for coloring purposes. In the guidance notes, an Annex III was scheduled to present reference values for the source materials. Since 2013, however, it has not been published. Therefore, the Joint Research Center (JRC) determines these values. Until Annex III is published, producers are obligated to file evidence of coloring foodstuffs used. There is a list of source materials (e.g., fruits, vegetables) that have been presented in the JRC Technical Report. That report is not an EU regulation, but until Annex III is published, the JRC Technical Report serves as guidance and awards penalties.

Carotenoids market

The rising knowledge about carotenoids importance resulted in a multiplicity of attempts to create, protect, and implement those compounds into different branches of the market, mainly connected with the just-assessed properties of carotenoids. Additionally, the observed global megatrend toward natural carotenoid-use amplification resulted in the important reconstruction of market players and suppliers. Based on the actual application, the carotenoid market is divided into feed, food, supplements, cosmetics, and pharmaceuticals. The feed segment, because of less restricted regulations, is estimated to constitute the majority of the carotenoids market in 2023 [Global Carotenoids Market, n.d.]. Additionally the increase in meat, poultry, and dairy-product consumption, mainly connected with protein diet trends and the appearance and fitness culture, drive the growth of carotenoid feed-market development.

Moreover, the growing concern about the animal-diseases outbreak, growing domestic and international quick-service restaurants in developing countries, and the demand for quality meat products create a demand for carotenoids in the feed market. In 2016, Europe had the largest share of the world carotenoid market in terms of value due to the presence of leading producers in the region. Strict EU rules for the use of synthetic carotenoids also drive the natural carotenoids market in the region.

The main carotenoid markets in Europe are Germany, France, Italy, the Netherlands, and Spain. The carotenoid market in the Asia-Pacific region is expected to grow thanks to investments by several international producers. In addition, extensive research and development initiatives have been undertaken in the region to investigate the use of carotenoids.

Associated health risks and high doses, as well as strict regulatory and approval standards, are the main factors hindering the development of the carotenoid market in emerging countries. In addition, another major challenge related to the use of carotenoids is their harmful effects on animals, humans, and the environment.

The main companies identified in the global carotenoid market are BASF SE (Germany), Royal DSM N.V. (The Netherlands), Chr. Hansen A/S (Denmark), FMC Corporation (USA), Kemin Industries, Inc. (USA), and Cyanotech Corporation (USA).

According to reports published by BCC Research, the value of the global market of carotenoids in 2017 was estimated to amount to 1.5 billion USD, whereas according to the forecasts the value will increase to 2.0 billion USD in 2022. For comparison, the value of the global market of carotenoids in 2007 was estimated at 766 million USD, which means that its value in the global scale increased almost twice in the period between 2007 and 2017 (BCC Research, 2018).

World carotenoids consumption

The volume of world carotenoids consumption in 2007 was equal to 4193 metric tons and has increased within 10 years by about 1500 metric tons, thereby it was equal to 5693.6 metric tons. That growing trend will remain constant, and in 2022, the world consumption of carotenoids will achieve 6222.6 metric tons (Euromonitor International).

Between 2007 and 2017, the highest year-on-year growth of the world carotenoids market was observed between 2008 and 2009 and totaled 5.8%. Recently the year-on-year growth was very low and achieved the lowest value in 2015–16, equal to 0.1%. The years 2016 and 2017 observed a slow increase of year-on-year growth up to 1.1%. That trend will be stable, and the 2019-on-2022 growth will achieve 1.9%. During 2007–17, the volume of carotenoids consumption increased 35.1% and achieved 3.1% CAGR. The forecast for 2019–22 shows a slow growth of carotenoids consumption up to 5.7% and 1.9% CAGR (Euromonitor International).

Carotenoids added to food totaled 4020.8 metric tons in 2017. In that year, the market shares of carotenoids applied to food products were estimated as follows (Euromonitor International):

- frozen pizza—2297.9 metric tons,
- margarine and spreads—740.1 metric tons,
- frozen desserts—296.4 metric tons,
- salad dressings—251.7 metric tons,
- staple foods—178.3 metric tons,
- cooking sauces—89.8 metric tons,
- processed cheese—10.1 metric tons.

The market of beverages with carotenoids added totaled 1609.8 metric tons. The highest consumption volume of carotenoids in that market were in sectors mentioned below (Euromonitor International):

- functional bottled water—1186.1 metric tons,
- orange carbonates—409.4 metric tons,
- nectars (25%–99% juice)—12.8 metric tons,
- sports drinks—1.5 metric tons.

Nonfood market consumed 63.0 metric tons of carotenoids in 2017. The particular market shares are as follows (Euromonitor International):

- pet care—62.9 metric tons, especially premium dry dog and cat food,
- beauty and personal care—0.1 metric tons.

The value of these markets are forecasted in 2022 to achieve (Euromonitor International):

- frozen pizza—2528.0 metric tons,
- functional bottled water—1372.1 metric tons,
- margarine and spreads—745.7 metric tons,
- orange carbonates—457.3 metric tons,
- frozen desserts—307.2 metric tons,
- salad dressings—266.0 metric tons,
- staple foods—188.6 metric tons,
- cooking sauces—96.3 metric tons,
- pet care—70.9 metric tons,
- nectars (25–99% juice)—12.4 metric tons,
- processed cheese—10.8 metric tons,
- sports drinks—1.7 metric tons.

CAGR of listed products within the period from 2019 and 2022 is estimated as follows [%] (Euromonitor International):

- frozen pizza—1.7,
- functional bottled water—3.5,
- margarine and spreads—0.6,
- orange carbonates—2.4,
- frozen desserts—0.7,
- salad dressings—0.9,
- staple foods—1.1,
- cooking sauces—1.5,
- pet care—2.4,
- nectars (25%–99% juice)—minus 0.4,
- processed cheese—1.8,
- sports drinks—1.5.

Western Europe

The largest market of carotenoids consumption is Western Europe. Based on Euromonitor statistics, the volume of carotenoids consumption in 2017 totaled 1689.5 metric tons and will come to 2010.2 metric tons in 2022. Over the years 2007 to 2017, the year-on-year growth achieved the highest value (4.6%) in 2009–10. This growth slowed in 2016 and 2017 and totaled 1.4%. The forecast shows a slight increase up to 1.6% in 2022. The growth in period 2007–17 was equal to 25% and the CAGR 2.3%. The anticipations show that the index of period growth will achieve 4.8% between 2019 and 2022 and CAGR will total 1.6% (Euromonitor International).

In 2017, the significant market size of carotenoids consumption in Western Europe by country is listed below (Euromonitor International):

- France—142.5 metric tons,
- Italy—101.2 metric tons,
- Netherlands—97.4 metric tons,
- Spain—70.9 metric tons,

- Turkey—57.9 metric tons,
- Norway—55.8 metric tons,
- Belgium—43.5 metric tons,
- Sweden—39.7 metric tons,
- Austria—37.7 metric tons.

In some countries, the volume of carotenoids consumption will decline in 2022, as the analytics project (Euromonitor International):

- France—137.8 metric tons,
- Spain—69.5 metric tons,
- Netherlands—96.8 metric tons.

In the other countries, the market for carotenoids will continue to grow. In 2022, these markets will total the estimates listed below (Euromonitor International):

- Italy—112.8 metric tons,
- Turkey—80.1 metric tons,
- Norway—64.5 metric tons,
- Belgium—43.9 metric tons,
- Sweden—42.7 metric tons,
- Austria—42.2 metric tons.

Middle and Eastern Europe

The carotenoids market in Eastern Europe achieved 448.4 metric tons in 2017. Within the years 2009–10, the highest year-on-year index was achieved, which was equal to 9.9%. That index dropped, and in 2016–17 it totaled 3.7%. The analytics anticipate a slight decrease to 3.5% in 2021–22. The period growth within 2007 and 2017 of total carotenoids consumption was 44.2% and CAGR 3.7%. The forecast for the years 2019–22 predicts 11.2% of period growth and CAGR 3.6%. Comparing these data with the world forecast, the market of carotenoids in Eastern Europe will develop fast. The growth rate of Eastern Europe is higher than of Western Europe, because the eastern region consists of developing countries, and the market is still not replete (Euromonitor International).

The biggest carotenoids markets in Eastern Europe are Russia, Poland, Slovakia, and the Czech Republic. In 2017, the volume of carotenoid consumption totaled the following (Euromonitor International):

- Russia—137.2 metric tons,
- Poland—79.3 metric tons,
- Slovakia—53.1 metric tons,
- Czech Republic—48.5 metric tons,
- Ukraine—24.7 metric tons,
- Hungary—18.5 metric tons,
- Romania—13.3 metric tons,
- Belarus—13.2 metric tons,
- Bulgaria—11.7 metric tons,
- Croatia—10.4 metric tons,
- Other countries with a volume of carotenoid consumption below 10 metric tons.

The forecast for 2022 shows an increase of carotenoid consumption in the following countries (Euromonitor International):

- Russia—162.5 metric tons,
- Poland—101.8 metric tons,
- Slovakia—63.7 metric tons,
- Czech Republic—52.1 metric tons,
- Ukraine—27.0 metric tons,
- Hungary—25.1 metric tons,
- Romania—13.9 metric tons,
- Belarus—13.5 metric tons,
- Bulgaria—15.1 metric tons,
- Croatia—11.9 metric tons.

Asia and Pacific

The Asia and Pacific region was the second-largest market of carotenoid consumption. In 2017, that market totaled 1505.8 metric tons. The forecast for that region is 1535.6 metric tons in 2019 and 1632.8 metric tons in 2022. That market develops very quickly. The year-on-year index in 2017 achieved a value of 1.3% and is estimated to reach 1.9% in 2022. The period growth is predicted on 6.3% and CAGR 2.1% within 2019 and 2022 (Euromonitor International).

The biggest carotenoids markets in Asia and the Pacific are China and Japan. In 2017, particular country markets achieved the following volume of carotenoid consumption (Euromonitor International):

- China—939.7 metric tons,
- Japan—168.0 metric tons,
- Philippines—72.7 metric tons,
- Indonesia—55.9 metric tons,
- Thailand—53.8 metric tons,
- India—50.0 metric tons,
- Taiwan—35.5 metric tons,
- South Korea—24.4 metric tons,
- Malaysia—11.6 metric tons,
- Other countries had the volume of carotenoid consumption under 10 metric tons.

The forecast for 2022 shows an increase of carotenoid consumption in the following countries (Euromonitor International):

- China—982.5 metric tons,
- Japan—171.2 metric tons,
- Philippines—92.8 metric tons,
- India—74.6 metric tons,
- Taiwan—45.5 metric tons,
- South Korea—31.3 metric tons,
- Malaysia—13.1 metric tons.

In Indonesia, the carotenoids consumption should remain at the same level of 55.9 metric tons, and in Thailand, consumption will decrease to 48.1 metric tons (Euromonitor International).

Australasia

Australasia is composed of two countries: Australia and New Zealand. That region is the smallest market of carotenoids consumption and totaled 88.3 metric tons in 2017 and CAGR 4.1%. The forecast in 2022 is estimated at 111.9 metric tons. Within 2019 and 2022, analytics forecasted CAGR 5.0% and the period growth 15.8% (Euromonitor International).

Latin America

The market for carotenoid consumption in Latin America was estimated at 362.0 metric tons in 2017. The analytics forecasted the small market growth up to 379.7 in 2022. The CAGR for 2016 and 2017 was equal to −3.8%. The estimate for period growth was 5.2% and CAGR 1.7% within 2019 and 2022 (Euromonitor International).

The biggest carotenoid markets in Latin America are Brazil and Mexico. In 2017, market shares were divided between Latin American countries as listed below (Euromonitor International):

- Brazil—161.8 metric tons,
- Mexico—76.5 metric tons,
- Chile—20.2 metric tons,
- Venezuela—17.7 metric tons,
- Colombia—14.6 metric tons,
- Peru—10.6 metric tons,
- Argentina—10.4 metric tons,
- Other countries with a consumption value below 10 metric tons.

The forecast for 2022 shows the following volume of carotenoid consumption in Latin America (Euromonitor International):

- Brazil—175.8 metric tons,
- Mexico—81.7 metric tons,
- Chile—20.3 metric tons,
- Venezuela—10.9 metric tons,
- Colombia—15.1 metric tons,
- Peru—11.8 metric tons,
- Argentina—11.0 metric tons.

North America

The market's data of North America concern Canada and the United States. The volume of carotenoid consumption totaled in North America 1321.1 metric tons in 2017.

The US share was equal to 1180.6 metric tons, and Canada consumed 140.5 metric tons. The forecast for 2022 estimates an increase of market volume in the United States up to 1278.5 metric tons and a decrease in the carotenoid application in Canada to 130.2 metric tons. The CAGR for North America was 0.6% in 2017, however CAGR achieved by the United States totaled 0.9%, and by Canada −1.8%. The CAGR for North America as forecasted by analytics will grow up to 0.9% and the period growth to 2.8% within 2019 and 2022. The CAGR (2019–22) for Canada will still have minus value (−1.4%) and for the United States will slightly increase to 1.2% (Euromonitor International].

Carotenoids market division

The carotenoid market is divided into areas related to the use of particular compounds such as astaxanthin, beta-carotene, lutein, lycopene, zeaxanthin, canthaxanthin, and others (annatto, capsanthin, fucoxanthin, rhodoxanthin and trans-β-apo-8′-carotenal). The astaxanthin segment dominated the carotenoid market by value in 2016. Europe is a key market for astaxanthin; the various health benefits of astaxanthin and its increasing use in animal feed are driving the market in these regions. The Asia-Pacific region is expected to grow to the highest level of CAGR. In addition, rising per capita income and increased consumption of healthy food in the Asia-Pacific region are other factors driving the growth of the astaxanthin market in the area.

The market of carotenoids can be divided into segments according to the kind of products, the origins of resources, and the application areas. Fig. 2 presents the structure of the global market of carotenoids (in a value-based approach) according to the types of products in 2016.

Taking into account the structure of the market of carotenoids in 2016 (in a value-based approach), seven main product types can be distinguished. Capsanthin

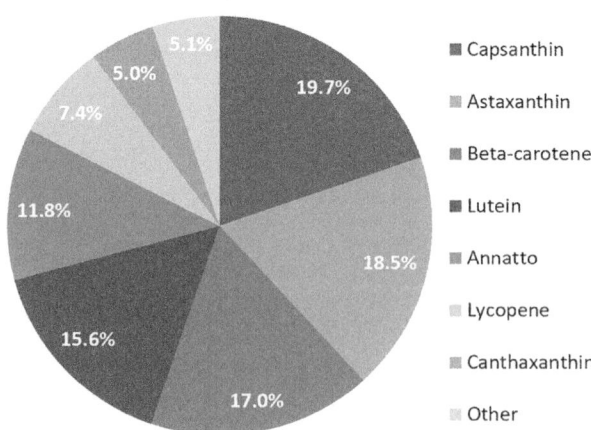

Fig. 2 Structure of the global market of carotenoids (value-based approach) according to the type of products in 2016.
Source: BCC Research Report Overview.

constituted the largest segment of the market (285 million USD, i.e., 19.7% in the structure of the carotenoid market). The following products also held a significant share in the value and structure of the reference market: astaxanthin (267.5 million USD, i.e., 18.5% of the market value), beta-carotene (246.2 million USD, i.e., 17%), lutein (225 million USD, i.e., 15.6%), annatto (170 million USD, i.e., 11.8%), and lycopene (107 million USD, i.e., 7.4%). The aforementioned carotenoids constituted of almost 90% of the total value of the market of carotenoids in 2016. According to market forecasts published by BCC Research, the value of the market of astaxanthin in 2022 will reach 426.9 million USD. This way, the segment of astaxanthin will reach the greatest share in the structure of the global market of carotenoids (in a value-based approach) according to the product types.

There are several factors that determine the growth of the market of carotenoids. The factors include changes in consumer behavior, including greater consumer awareness on the impact of food on our health. Numerous studies revealed a beneficial health impact of carotenoids owing to their antioxidant and antiinflammation characteristics, which is used in the production of food and animal feed. Carotenoids are mainly used as colorants—natural coloring agents have been gaining popularity in the food sector (e.g., to standardize the colors of food products). The development of the market of carotenoid-containing products results from a number of economic, demographic and sociocultural factors. Balanced consumption (conscious, responsible consumption) can be observed among contemporary consumer behaviors, which also fosters the demand for diet supplements (including the ones with carotenoids). Strong antioxidant action enables the use of carotenoids in the cosmetic and pharmaceutical sector. Moreover, carotenoid decomposition products are used as aromas.

The structure of the market of carotenoids is oligopolistic, dominated by two manufacturers: BASF SE (Germany) and Koninklijke DSM NV (The Netherlands). The entities dominate on the markets of beta-carotene, astaxanthin, and cantaxanthin. The range of products offered by BASF includes, for example, Lucantin Pink (Astaxanthin), a popular product for pigmentation in aquaculture. DSM produces, for example, ROVIMIX ß-Carotene. Other major entities operating on the market of carotenoids include: Chr. Hansen Holding A/S (Denmark), Sensient Technologies Corporation (USA), Novus International, Inc. (USA), FMC Corporation (USA), Kemin Industries, Inc. (USA), Cyanotech Corporation (USA) and Lycored Ltd. (Israel). Recent years have seen an increase in the competitiveness of business entities from Asia (mainly from China) and India on the global market of carotenoids.

Carotenoids commercialization

Investigating the scope of carotenoid commercialization by manufacturing, when processing an application using patent databases several trends can be observed. The most abundant inventions, which are related to human needs and are worthy of intellectual property protection, are located in the following International Patent Classification categories—A61K, A23L, and A23K, and are related to: preparations for medical, dental, or toilet purposes; foods, foodstuffs, or nonalcoholic beverages;

and feeding-stuffs especially adapted for animals; methods especially adapted for the production thereof, respectively.

The last 10 years have provided the evidence that astaxanthin and also lutein are two boosting market carotenoids, whereas beta-carotene solution rose in 2009 and now maintains their average innovation level (Fig. 3). The group of other carotenoids is also gaining increased attention (Fig. 4).

The strong distribution of carotenoid interest is especially visible when comparing the particular compounds within the six carotenoids of most industrial interest (Figs. 5–10).

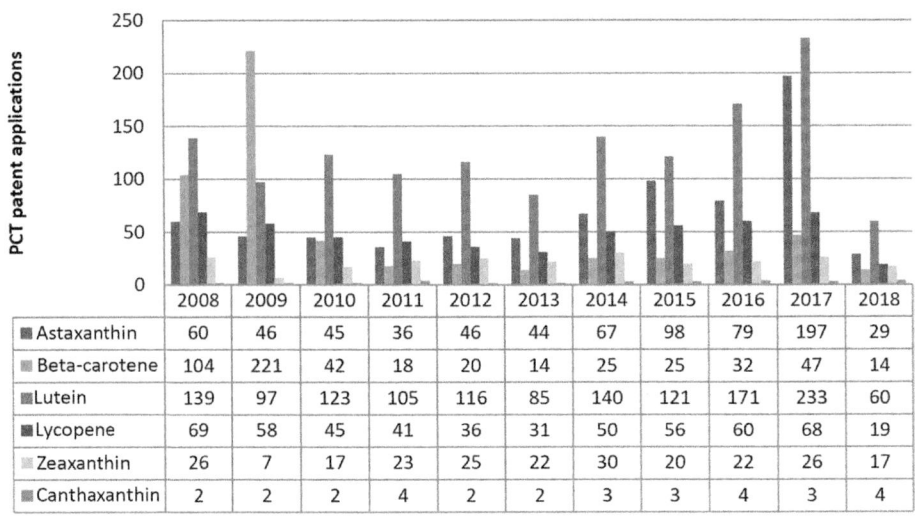

	2008	2009	2010	2011	2012	2013	2014	2015	2016	2017	2018
Astaxanthin	60	46	45	36	46	44	67	98	79	197	29
Beta-carotene	104	221	42	18	20	14	25	25	32	47	14
Lutein	139	97	123	105	116	85	140	121	171	233	60
Lycopene	69	58	45	41	36	31	50	56	60	68	19
Zeaxanthin	26	7	17	23	25	22	30	20	22	26	17
Canthaxanthin	2	2	2	4	2	2	3	3	4	3	4

Fig. 3 Main carotenoids patent applications within the 10-year period of 2008–18 (https:// patentscope.wipo.int/search/en/structuredSearch.jsf).

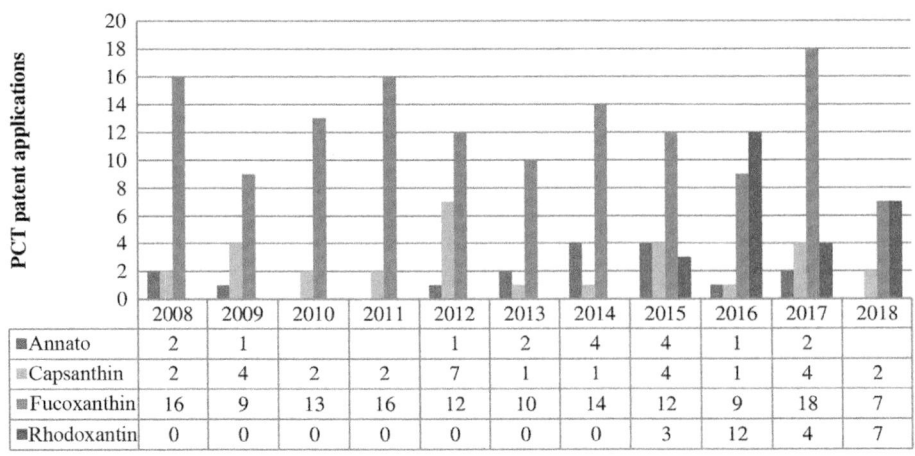

	2008	2009	2010	2011	2012	2013	2014	2015	2016	2017	2018
Annato	2	1			1	2	4	4	1	2	
Capsanthin	2	4	2	2	7	1	1	4	1	4	2
Fucoxanthin	16	9	13	16	12	10	14	12	9	18	7
Rhodoxantin	0	0	0	0	0	0	0	3	12	4	7

Fig. 4 Minor carotenoids patent applications within the 10-year period of 2008–18 (https:// patentscope.wipo.int/search/en/structuredSearch.jsf).

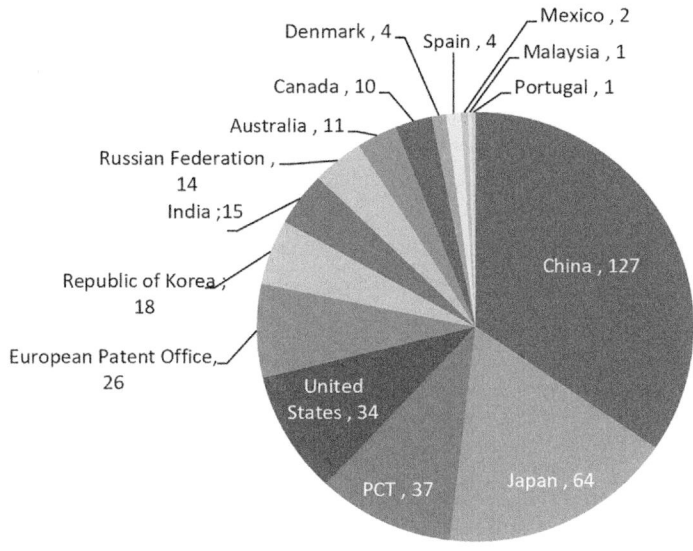

Astaxanthin

Fig. 5 Astaxanthin-related patent applications related to country, or patent-procedure type involved, within the period of 2008–18 (https://patentscope.wipo.int/search/en/structuredSearch.jsf).

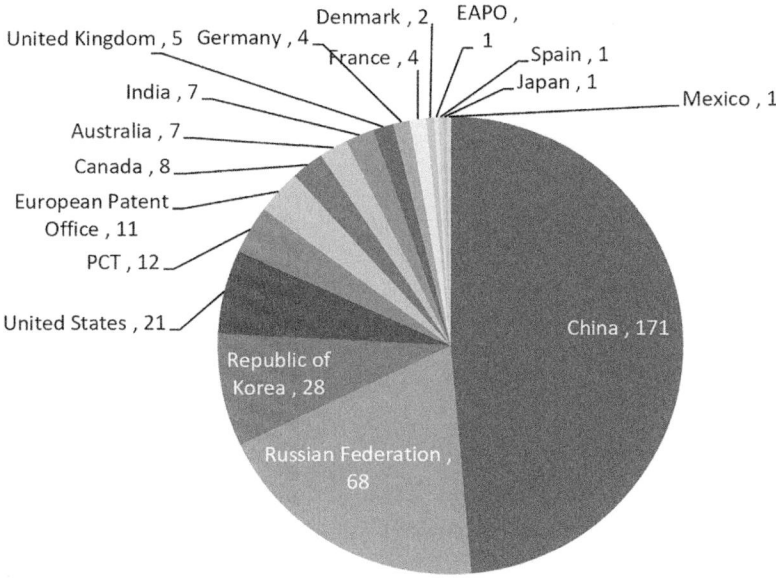

Beta-carotene

Fig. 6 Beta-carotene–related patent applications related to country or patent-procedure type involved within the period of 2008–18 (https://patentscope.wipo.int/search/en/structuredSearch.jsf).

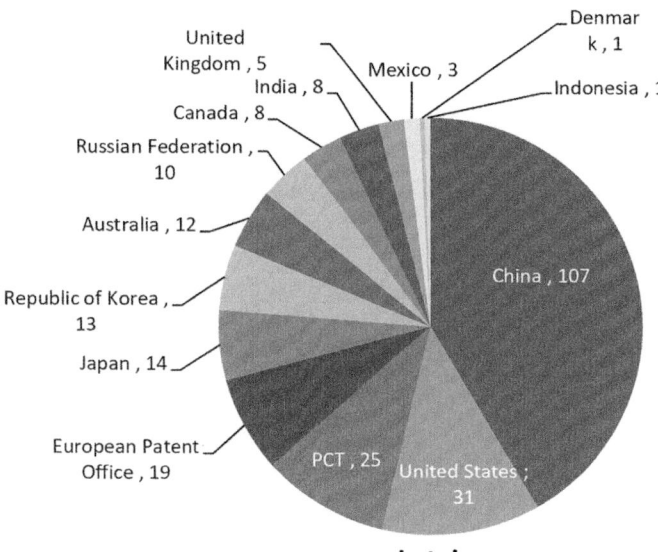

Lutein

Fig. 7 Lutein-related patent applications related to country or patent-procedure type involved within the period of 2008–18 (https://patentscope.wipo.int/search/en/structuredSearch.jsf).

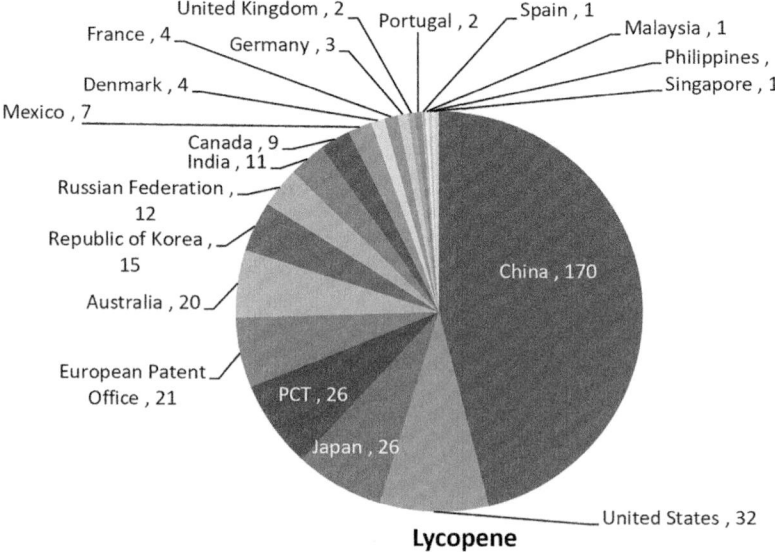

Lycopene

Fig. 8 Lycopene-related patent applications related to country or patent-procedure type involved within the period of 2008–18 (https://patentscope.wipo.int/search/en/structuredSearch.jsf).

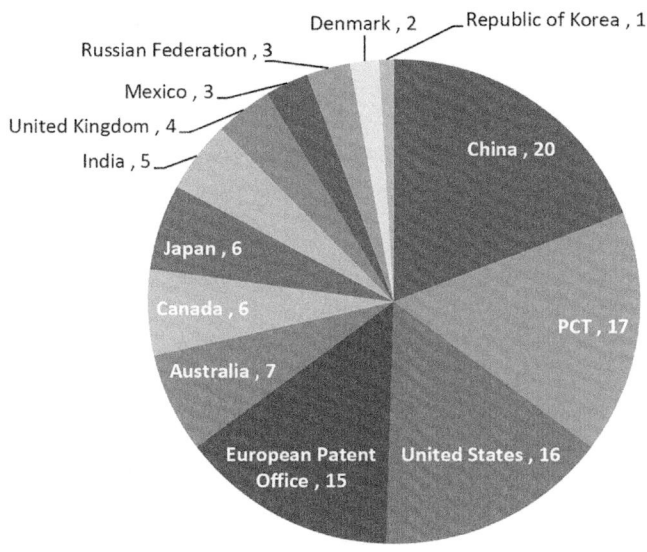

Zeaxanthin

Fig. 9 Zeaxanthin-related patent applications related to country or patent-procedure type involved within the period of 2008–18 (https://patentscope.wipo.int/search/en/structuredSearch.jsf).

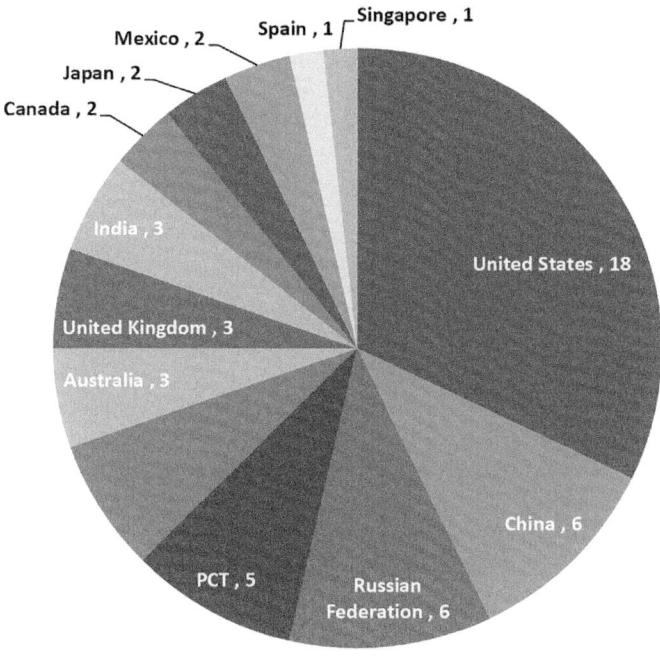

Canthaxanthin

Fig. 10 Canthaxanthin-related patent applications related to country or patent procedure type involved within the period of 2008–18 (https://patentscope.wipo.int/search/en/structuredSearch.jsf).

The specific food application of particular carotenoids of high market importance are presented in Fig. 11.

The main industrial players in the feed application of carotenoids are Tianjin Chenhui Feed Co., Ltd., Norsk Hydro AS, BASF SE, DSM, and Astacarotene. Chinese producer focuses mainly on fish food application, providing a feed mixture both for ornamental pet and meat fish, mainly for guppies (CN107183333, 2017), *Astronotus ocellatus* (CN106213049, 2016), *Trichogaster microlepis* (CN107223805, 2017), red lion head goldfish (CN106213043, 2016), tropic ornamental fishes (CN106213045, 2016), butterfly tail golden fish (CN106173547, 2016), *Scleropages formosus* (CN104397381, 2014), rainbow trout (CN103549205, 2013), kohaku (CN104621403, 2015), goldfish (CN104664145, 2015), *Pseudorabora parva* (CN104397386, 2014), *Oncorhynchus mykiss* (CN106173540, 2016), yellow-head catfish (CN107183412, 2017), dragonfish (CN106173543, 2016), *Cyprinus carpio* (CN107173636, 2017), and red crucian carps (CN107173635, 2017). Norsk Hydro applications focus on salmonids group feed and different modifications of astaxanthin for their better utilization as feed (CA2336272, 1999; CN1589296, 2002; US6709688, 2000); BASF concern applications are more general, as they have dedicated their astaxanthin-containing mixtures as medicament for feed, food, and food supplement incorporation (CN107404905, 2016; CN107427029, 2016). DSM Company dominates the method for astaxanthin biosynthesis using *Phaffia rhodozyma* as well as marigold extract exploitation as a source for semisynthesis and astaxanthin esters manufacturing for functionality improvement (CN1628097, 2003; US20060037543, 2003; US20060134734, 2003). Meanwhile, the ASTACAROTENE Company protects the astaxanthin application both for mammals and poultry breeding and improved production (US6054491, 1997). Several feed applications related to astaxanthin also cover the food and food supplements area being mainly formulated as additives.

Astaxanthin

Food market of astaxanthin application is dominated by Fuji Chem Ind Co. Ltd., which protects solutions containing astaxanthin as: a medicament for therapy and/ or prevention of failure of eye accommodation and food/drink containing the same (EP1396264, 2002), composition having an ameliorating and preventing effect on metabolic syndrome (EP1938810, 2006), preparation for improving muscle atrophy by gene expression regulation (EP2653157, 2005), food/drink preventing effect for cerebral dysfunction (JP2007126455, 2006), compositions for body fat reduction (EP1829537, 2005), improving agent with ability for organisms to use oxygen under a low-oxygen condition (JP2002159279, 2000), active oxygen inhibitor inhibiting active oxygen for preventing easily oxidizable components of food and cosmetics (JP2014019660, 2012), an inhibitor against oxidative damage to erythrocytes (JP2002226368, 2001), a peripheral blood circulation ameliorative composition (JP2008239619, 2008), a life-extending and fatigue-improving agent (JP2006347927, 2005; JP2012072132, 2011), a vascular endothelial cell-protecting agent and a food having the effect of protecting vascular endothelial cells (EP1864658, 2006), prophylactics for diabetes-combined diseases and prophylactic foods and drinks for diabetes

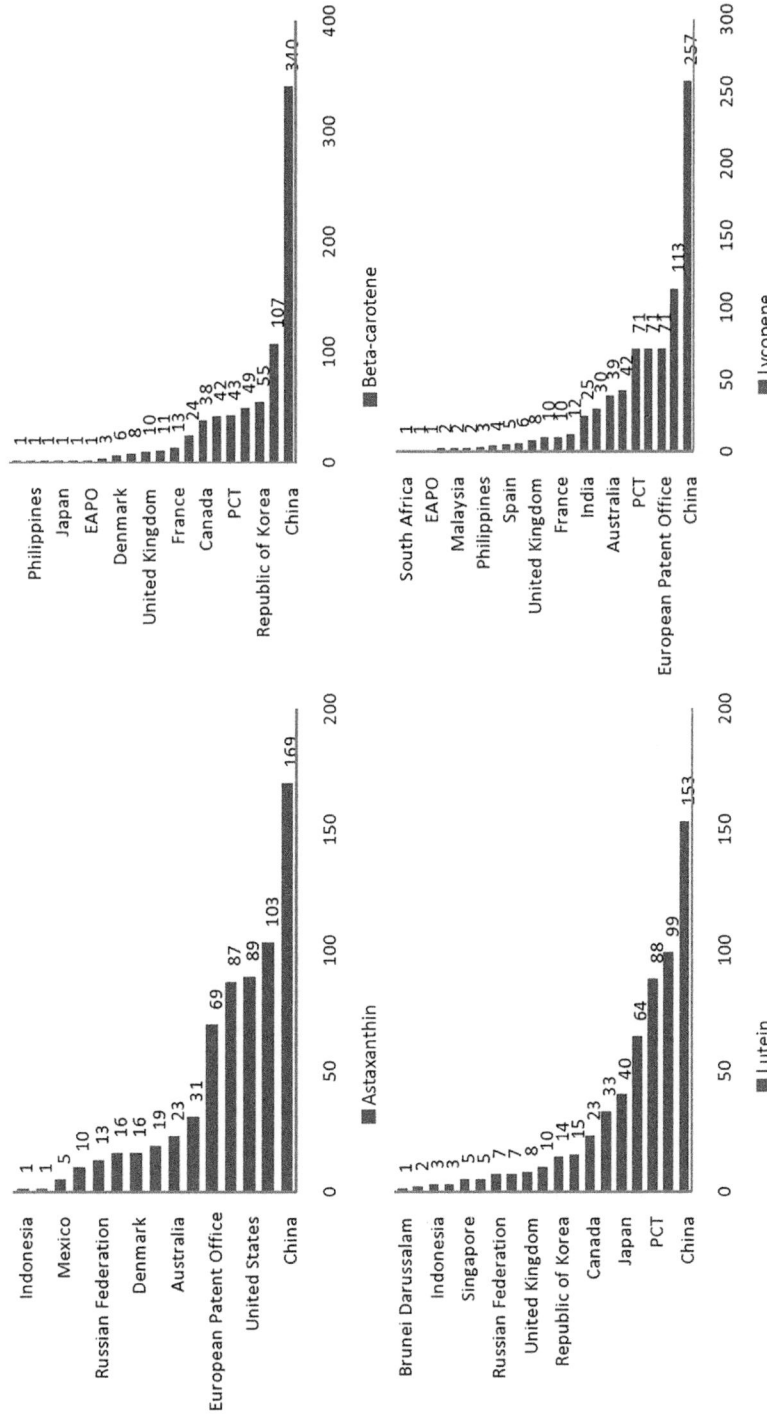

Fig. 11 Food application of astaxanthin, beta-carotene, lutein, and lycopene within the period of 2008–2018 (https://patentscope.wipo.int/search/en/structuredSearch.jsf).

(JP2009007346, 2008), an oral formulation for the prevention and/or treatment of inflammation of mucosa of mammals' digestive tracts (especially the human belly) caused by infection of Helicobacter (especially, *H. pylori*) (JP2010111689, 2010), and an emulsion containing a stable carotenoid that can be used as an aqueous solution of a colorant for food products (JP 2001316601, 2001).

BASF company patent applications and patents focus on: astaxanthin-containing compositions of multiple use (CN107404905, 2016; CN107427029, 2016; WO/2016/146802, 2016; WO/2016/146803, 2016; WO/2016/146804, 2016), astaxanthin derivatives obtaining (7163/CHENP/2011, 2012), and astaxanthin coloring properties exploitation as a pigment source (JP 10327801, 1998). DSM properties are dedicated to purification methods of astaxanthin (CN105705039, 2014; CN105705041, 2014), as well as encapsulation methods for further incorporation into products (JP2014097999, 2014) whereas AstaCarotene mainly provides solutions dedicated for the prevention and treatment of Helicobacter pylori infections (; AU1998062951, 1998; US6262316, 1998).

Suntory Company protects food or drink having the action or preventing cataracts or the action of suppressing the progress of the cataract (JP10276721, 1998), antistress composition (US6265450, 2001), a circadian rhythm normalizing composition (US20030091614, 2003), the agent for ameliorating the functional disorder of the exocrine gland, and the food and drink (JP2008127303, 2008) as well as an astaxanthin medium-chain fatty acid ester and its production method (WO/2003/093229, 2003).

Beta-carotene

Beta-carotene is one of best-known carotenoids and the application is widespread in any possible fat-containing and color-needing food or feed product. The natural beta-carotene market is dominated by the DSM and BASF Companies as suppliers, but looking into natural beta-carotene production methods, Abbott Laboratories, LycoRed, and PAN Quian appear as innovative product manufactures.

An enteral nutritional product has been formulated for persons who are currently undergoing radiation therapy and/or chemotherapy (US5547927A, 1996), persons having a neurological injury (US5308832, 1994), as well as therapeutic composition comprising one or more polyphenols and two or more carotenoids selected from the group consisting of lutein, lycopene, and beta-carotene (EP2381935, 2016).

Lycopene

The addition of lycopene to food intends to exploit its health potential by protecting the method for producing healthcare foods of lycopene soft capsule by using tomato peel and dregs as raw materials (CN107259562, 2017), a lycopene food and a preparation method (CN107411076, 2017), an anticancer combined healthcare food (CN107361356, 2017), health foods containing a nutrient for protecting and improving male prostate functions (CN107518398, 2017), special diet tomato nutrition powder (CN107467573, 2017), oxidation-preventing functional food (CN107136504, 2017), radiation protection composition containing tea polysaccharide (CN107519195,

2017), tomato-derived thickening agent (US20160029671, 2016), nutritional powder as a specifically developed nutritional food, which is highly matched with a low-sugar diet and moderate exercise in a solution for treating obesity and high blood pressure (US20160324204, 2016), or the preparation of lycopene containing oleoresin and lycopene crystals for human consumption (EP2757904, 2017).

Lutein

Lutein commercialization on the market is also widespread. In 2017, 22 patent applications appeared providing a lutein ester aqueous suspension and a production process (CN107625126, 2018), a dietary supplement or food additive that improves contrast sensitivity (EP 3372280, 2018a, 2018b), a water-dispersible colorant composition and a process for its preparation (RU0002664579, 2018), an application of lutein extracted from marigold (CN107625126, 2018), a lutein ester solid beverage (CN107712537, 2018), a method of treating photoinduced ocular fatigue and associated reduction in speed of ocular focus (US 20180042978, 2018a, 2018b), solid beverage with hygroscopicity resistance and efficient absorption and utilization capability (CN107647237, 2018), a polymer capsule having a double-layered structure and stabilizing lutein (WO/2018/030579, 2018), a lutein ester microcapsule drink (CN107616399, 2018), liquid nutritional compositions that include functional ingredients such as beta-hydroxy-beta-methylbutyrate, docosahexaenoic acid, and lutein (EP3349596, 2018) or brain-nourishing walnut oil capsules based on phosphatidylserine containing lutein (CN107616506, 2018).

Zeaxanthin

The application of zeaxanthin is mainly explored for visual impairment, and the condition is improved by: (1) improving the visual performance of a human subject without age-related macular degeneration by administering an effective amount of a composition comprising mesozeaxanthin, lutein, and zeaxanthin as a dietary supplement or food additive (EP 3372280, 2018a, 2018b), (2) a photoinduced ocular fatigue and associated reduction in speed of ocular focus in humans by administering a therapeutic amount of a dietary supplement (US 20180042978, 2018a, 2018b), (3) a method of enhancing a subject's macular pigment optical density by administering an effective amount of one or more xanthophyll carotenoids (CN107410811, 2017), (4) an agent, food, and beverage for improving a carotenoid balance in the blood (WO/2017/195504, 2017) or the use of granules in beverages, wherein the granules comprise a milled carotenoid selected from the group consisting of lutein and zeaxanthin (WO/2017/168006, 2017).

Canthaxanthin

Canthaxanthin usage is gradually expanding and is looking for its own niche in the market. There are several applications including: (1) the use of canthaxanthin and at least one vitamin-D metabolite for improving internal egg quality (US20160128359, 2017),

(2) a salmon-flesh color-improving method and a salmon-flesh color-improving feed (US20100319077, 2015), (3) a process for preparing a soybean protein material having a red color, which, when combined with uncured meat, makes a product that has a uniform red color in the raw state and which when cooked has a uniform gray-brown color that is similar to cooked natural meat (US3958019, 1976), (4) water-dispersible carotenoid formulation that contains a mixture of canthaxanthine and marigold soap, which has a pigmenting potential on eggs and animal tissues much greater than that obtained when these xanthophylls are applied separately (WO/2009/022034, 2009), (5) a method for coloring a ham (JP2015029442, 2017) or powdery or encapsulated compositions containing fat-soluble materials to be blended into food products, beverages, animal feeds, cosmetics, or pharmaceuticals as additives (JP2014097999, 2014).

Summary

Carotenoids form a group of socially and economically valuable compounds. Beneficial characteristics of carotenoids contribute to a growing interest in the development of methods and techniques for acquiring them and for using them to enrich food, pharmaceutical, and cosmetic products. The global market of carotenoids has grown significantly in the last several years because of an increasing number of end uses in food, beverages, animal feed, diet supplements, pharmaceuticals, and cosmetics.

References

7163/CHENP/2011. (2012). *Formulation of astaxanthin derivatives and use.* 16.11.2012.

Alvarez, R., Vaz, B., Gronemeyer, H., & de Lera, A. R. (2014). Functions, therapeutic applications, and synthesis of retinoids and carotenoids. *Chemical Reviews, 114*(1), 1–125.

AU1998062951. (1998). *Oral preparation for the prophylactic and therapeutic treatment of helicobacter.* 03.09.1998.

BCC Research https://www.bccresearch.com/market-research/food-and-beverage/the-global-market-for-carotenoids-fod025f.html (11.07.2018) 2018.

CA2336272. (1999). *Stabilisation of pigments and polyunsaturated oils.* 25.06.1999.

Chiu, Y. T., Chiu, C. P., Chien, J. T., Ho, G. H., Yang, J., & Chen, B. H. (2007). Encapsulation of lycopene extract from tomato pulp waste with gelatin and poly(γ-glutamic acid) as carrier. *Journal of Agricultural and Food Chemistry, 55*, 5123–5130.

CN103549205. (2013). *Compound feed for enhancing color of rainbow trout.* 07.11.2013.

CN104397381. (2014). *Body strengthening and redness increasing Scleropages formosus compound feed and preparation method thereof.* 06.11.2014.

CN104397386. (2014). *Compound feed capable of enabling Pseudorabora parva to quickly produce head, brightening body color and promoting growth and preparation method thereof.* 06.11.2014.

CN104621403. (2015). *Feed for kohaku.* 05.02.2015.

CN104664145. (2015). *Goldfish head developing feed.* 05.02.2015.

CN105705039. (2014). *Process for the purification of astaxanthin.* 06.11.2014.

CN105705041. (2014). *Process for the purification of astaxanthin.* 06.11.2014.

CN106173540. (2016). *Low-nitrogen high-energy compound feed for growing Oncorhynchus mykiss and preparation method thereof.* 22.07.2016.

CN106173543. (2016). *Dragonfish puffed mixed feed and preparation method thereof.* 22.07.2016.

CN106173547. (2016). *Butterfly tail golden fish head swelling feed and preparation method thereof.* 22.07.2016.

CN106213043. (2016). *Feed for red lion head goldfish caruncle formation and preparation method thereof.* 22.07.2016.

CN106213045. (2016). *Formula feed for tropic ornamental fishes and preparation method thereof.* 22.07.2016.

CN106213049. (2016). *Astronotus ocellatus brightening feed and preparation method thereof.* 22.07.2016.

CN107136504. (2017). *Oxidation preventing functional food.* 08.09.2017.

CN107173635. (2017). *Color increasing feed for red crucian carps and preparation method thereof.* 07.06.2017.

CN107173636. (2017). *Feed for cyprinus carpio and preparation method thereof.* 07.06.2017.

CN107183333. (2017). *Color enhancing feed for guppies, and preparation method of color enhancing feed.* 07.06.2017.

CN107183412. (2017). *Feed for improving meat quality of yellow-head catfish and preparation method thereof.* 07.06.2017.

CN107223805. (2017). *Feed for rapidly increasing color of trichogaster microlepis and preparation method thereof.* 07.06.2017.

CN107259562. (2017). *Method for producing health care food of lycopene soft capsule by using tomato peel and dregs as raw materials.* 20.10.2017.

CN107361356. (2017). *Anticancer health-care food.* 21.11.2017.

CN107404905. (2016). *Astaxanthin Compositions.* 18.03.2016.

CN107410811. (2017). *Preparation method of lutein microcapsules and lutein microcapsule instant beverage.* 01.12.2017.

CN107411076. (2017). *Method for producing health care food of lycopene soft capsule by using tomato peel and dregs as raw materials.* 20.10.2017.

CN107427029. (2016). *Astaxanthin compositions.* 18.03.2016.

CN107467573. (2017). *Extraction method of lycopene and special diet tomato nutrition powder.* 15.12.2017.

CN107518398. (2017). *Nutrient for protecting and improving male prostate functions.* 29.12.2017.

CN107519195. (2017). *Radiation protection composition containing tea polysaccharide.* 29.12.2017.

CN107616399. (2018). *Lutein ester microcapsule drink and preparation method thereof.* 23.01.2018.

CN107616506. (2018). *Brain nourishing walnut oil capsules based on phosphatidylserine and preparation method thereof.* 23.01.2018.

CN107625126. (2018). *Lutein ester aqueous suspension and a production process thereof.* 26.01.2018.

CN107647237. (2018). *Solid beverage with hygroscopicity resistance and efficient absorption and utilization capability and preparation method thereof.* 02.02.2018.

CN107712537. (2018). *Lutein ester solid beverage.* 23.02.2018.

CN1589296. (2002). *Pigment.* 15.10.2002.

CN1628097. (2003). *Astaxanthin esters.* 29.01.2003.

Dasgupta, A., & Klein, K. (2014). *Antioxidants in food, vitamins and supplements*(pp. 209–235).

EP1396264. (2002). *Linderung von fehlern in der augenkontrollfunktion*. 23.05.2002.

EP1829537. (2005). *Zusammensetzung zur reduzierung von körperfett*. 02.12.2005.

EP1864658. (2006). *Mittel zur linderung von gefässinsuffizienz*. 31.03.2006.

EP1938810. (2006). *Agent d'amelioration pour le syndrome metabolique*. 29.09.2006.

EP2381935. (2016). *Synergistische kombinationen aus carotenoiden und polyphenolen*. 01.06.2016.

EP2653157. (2005). *Astaxanthin zur Verbesserung der Muskelatrophie*. 04.02.2005.

EP2757904. (2017). *Effizientes verfahren zur herstellung von lycopinhaltigem ölharz und lycopin kristalle für menschlichen verzehr*. 11.01.2017.

EP3349596. (2018). *Reduced fat, shelf stable liquid nutritional composition*. 25.07.2018.

EP3372280. (2018a). *Improvements in or relating to visual performance*. 12.09.2018.

EP3372280. (2018b). *Verbesserungen an oder im zusammenhang mit der sehleistung*. 12.09.2018.

European Parliament and the Council. (2008). *Regulation (EC) No 1333/2008 of the European Parliament and of the Council of 16 December 2008 on food additives*.

European Parliament and the Council. (2009). *Directive 2009/35/EC of the European Parliament and of the Council of 23 April 2009 on the colouring matters which may be added to medicinal products (recast)*.

Fazeli, M. R., Tofighi, H., Samadi, N., & Jamalifar, H. (2006). Effects of salinity on β-carotene production by Dunaliella tertiolecta DCCBC26 isolated from the Urmia salt lake, north of Iran. *Bioresource Technology*, 97(18), 2453–2456.

Fernández-Sevilla, J., Acién Fernández, F. G., & Molina Grima, E. (2010). Biotechnological production of lutein and its applications. *Applied Microbiology and Biotechnology*, 86(1), 27–40.

Global Carotenoids Market Global carotenoids market research report and industry analysis 2016–2023 n.d. published by: QYRESEARCH.

Igielska-Kalwat, J., Gościańska, J., & Nowak, I. (2014). Zastosowanie likopenu w dermokosmetykach. *Przemysl Chemiczny*, 93(7), 1110–1113.

Joseph, S., & Anandane, A. (2011). *Process for production of high purity beta-carotene and lycopene crystals from fungal biomass*. [Patent PCT/IN2011/000343].

JP 10327801. (1998). *Use of carotenoid as color stabilizer, food pigment mixture and color stabilized food*. 15.12.1998.

JP 2001316601. (2001). *Stable emulsion for coloring and method for preparing the same*. 16.11.2001.

JP10276721. (1998). *Astaxanthin containing food or drink*. 20.10.1998.

JP2002159279. (2000). *Improving agent with ability to utilize oxygen*. 27.11.2000.

JP2002226368. (2001). *Inhibitor against oxidative damage to erythrocyte*. 02.02.2001.

JP2006347927. (2005). *Fatigue-improving agent*. 14.06.2005.

JP2007126455. (2006). *Cerebral dysfunction improving agent*. 06.10.2006.

JP2008127303. (2008). *A—Agent for ameliorating functional disorder of exocrine gland, and food and drink for ameliorating functional disorder*. 23.10.2008.

JP2008239619. (2008). *Peripheral blood circulation ameliorative composition*. 28.02.2008.

JP2009007346. (2008). *Prophylactic for diabetes.combined disease*. 30.05.2008.

JP2010111689. (2010). *Oral formulation for prevention and treatment of infection by helicobacter*. 20.05.2010.

JP2012072132. (2011). *Life-extending agent*. 31.08.2011.

JP2014019660. (2012). *Active oxygen inhibitor*. 13.07.2012.

JP2014097999. (2014). *Reparation method of compositions containing fat soluble physiologically active components*. 29.05.2014.

JP2015029442. (2017). *Method for coloring ham.* 29.11.2017.

Kim, S., Ha, T. Y., & Hwang, I. K. (2009). Analysis, bioavailability, and potential healthy effects of capsanthin, natural red pigment from Capsicum spp. *Food Reviews International*, *25*(3), 198–213.

Lin, J.-H., Lee, D.-J., & Chang, J.-S. (2015). Lutein production from biomass: marigold flowers versus microalgae. *Bioresource Technology*, *184*, 421–428.

Lokaewmanee, K., Yamauchi, K., & Okuda, N. (2013). Effects of dietary red pepper on egg yolk colour and histological intestinal morphology in laying hens. *Journal of Animal Physiology and Animal Nutrition*, *97*(5), 986–995.

Marchal, L., Mojaat-Guemir, M., Foucault, A., & Prevost, J. (2013). *Prevost Centrifugal partition extraction of β-carotene from Dunaliella* salina *for efficient and biocompatible recovery of metabolites. Bioresource Technology*, *134*, 396–400.

Matsufuji, H., Nakamura, H., Chino, M., & Takeda, M. (1998). Antioxidant activity of capsanthin and the fatty acid esters in paprika (Capsicum annuum). *Journal of Agricultural and Food Chemistry*, *46*(9), 3468–3472.

Mein, J. R., Lian, F., & Wang, X. D. (2008). Biological activity of lycopene metabolites: implications for cancer prevention. *Nutrition Reviews*, *66*(12), 667–683.

Mogedas, B., Casal, C., Forjan, E., & Vilchez, C. (2009). β-Carotene production enhancement by UV-A radiation in Dunaliella bardawil cultivated in laboratory reactors. *Journal of Bioscience and Bioengineering*, *108*(1), 47–51.

Mozaffarieh, M., Sacu, S., & Wedrich, A. (2003). The role of the carotenoids, lutein and zeaxanthin, in protecting against age-related macular degeneration: a review based on controversial evidence. *Nutrition Journal*, *2*(1), 20.

Mykolaiovych, R. O., Volodymyrovyc, T. Y., Ivanovyvh, C. S., Hryhorovyc, T. V., Viktorovych, D. S., & Pavlivna, K. V. (2008). *Device for concentration of carotene-containing biomass of micro-alga Dunaliella salina.* [Patent UA20070008450U 20070723].

Pawłowska, B. (2009). Biotechnologiczne zrodla barwnikow spozywczych. *Inzynieria I Aparatura Chemiczna*, *48*, 79–80.

Perez, C. J., Castro, E. A., Rodriguez, M. A. T., de Prado, G. J. E., Cezon, P. E. R., Collados De La, V. A., et al. (2001). *Method for the production of beta-carotene.* Patent PCT/ES2001/000284.

Perez, C. J., Rodriguez, M. A. T., De la Fuente Moreno, J. L., Saiz, R. M., Garcia, D. B., Cezon, P. E., et al. (2003). *Method of producing β-carotene by means of mixed culture fermentation using (+) and (−) strains of Blakeslea trispora.* Patent PCT/ES2003/000047.

Pisal, D. S., & Lele, S. S. (2005). Carotenoid production from microalga Dunaliella salina. *Indian Journal of Biotechnology*, *4*, 476–483.

Pogorzelska, E., Hamułka, J., & Wawrzyniak, A. (2016). Astaksantyna—budowa, właściwości i możliwości zastosowania w żywności funkcjonalnej. *Żywność Nauka Technologia Jakość*, *1*(104), 5–16.

RU0002664579. (2018). *Hue controlled β-carotene compositions.* 08.21.

Saini, R. K., & Keum, Y.-S. (2018). Carotenoid extraction methods: a review of recent developments. *Food Chemistry*, *240*, 90–103.

Saini, R. K., Nile, S. H., & Park, S. W. (2015). Carotenoids from fruits and vegetables: chemistry, analysis, occurrence, bioavailability and biological activities. *Food Research International*, *76*, 735–750.

Scotter, M. (2009). The chemistry and analysis of annatto food colouring: a review. *Food Additives and Contaminants*, *26*(8), 1123–1145.

Shegokar, R., & Mitri, K. (2012). Carotenoid lutein: a promising candidate for pharmaceutical and nutraceutical applications. *Journal of Dietary Supplements*, *9*(3), 183–210.

Sieradzka, M., & Kołodziejczyk-Czepas, J. (2016). Astaksantyna–karotenoidowy przeciwutleniacz o właściwościach kardioprotekcyjnych. *Problemy Higieny i Epidemiologii, 97*(3), 197–206.

Šivel, M., Kráčmar, S., Fišera M., Klejdus, B., & Kubáň, V. (2014). Lutein content in marigold flower (Tagetes erecta L.) concentrates used for production of food supplements. *Czech Journal of Food Sciences, 32*(6), 521–525.

Story, E. N., Kopec, R. E., Schwartz, S. J., & Harris, G. K. (2010). An update on the health effects of tomato lycopene. *Annual Review of Food Science and Technology, 1*, 189–210.

Torregrosa-Crespo, J., Montero, Z., Fuentes, J. F., García-Galbis, M. R., Garbayo, I., Vílchez, C., et al. (2018). Exploring the valuable carotenoids for the large-scale production. *Marine Drugs*.

US20030091614. (2003). *Compositions normalizing circadian rhythm.* 15.05.2003.

US20060037543. (2003). *Enhanced feeding and growth rates of aquatic animals fed an astaxanthin product derived from marigold extract.* 11.03.2003.

US20060134734. (2003). *Astaxanthin production using fed-batch fermentation process by Phaffia rhodozyma.* 16.09.2003.

US20100319077. (2015). *Method of improving salmon meat color.* 07.04.2015.

US20160029671. (2016). *Tomato derived thickening agent.* 04.02.2016.

US20160128359. (2017). *Novel use of canthaxanthin.* 21.03.2017.

US20160324204. (2016). *Complete nutritional powder and preparation method thereof.* 10.11.2016.

US20180042978. (2018a). *Method of treating photoinduced ocular fatigue and associated reduction in speed of ocular focus.* 15.02.2018a.

US20180042978. (2018b). *Method of treating photo.Induced ocular fatigue and associated reduction in speed of ocular focus.* 15.02.2018b.

US3958019. (1976). *Color treatment for soybean food products.* 18.05.1976.

US5308832. (1994). *Nutritional product for persons having a neurological injury.* 03.05.1994.

US5547927A. (1996). *Enteral nutritional product for patients undergoing radiation therapy and/or chemotherapy.* 20.08.1996.

US6054491. (1997). *Agent for increasing the production of/in breeding and production mammals.* 21.03.1997.

US6262316. (1998). *Oral preparation for the prophylactic and therapeutic treatment of helicobacter sp. Infection.* 05.02.1998.

US6265450. (2001). *Anti-stress composition.* 24.07.2001.

US6709688. (2000). *Pigment.* 17.04.2000.

WO/2003/093229. (2003). *Astaxanthin medium-chain fatty acid ester, process for producing the same and composition containing the ester.* 13.11.2003.

WO/2009/022034. (2009). *Water dispersable carotenoid formulation.* 19.02.2009.

WO/2016/146802. (2016). *Astaxanthinzusammensetzungen (ii).* 18.03.2016.

WO/2016/146803. (2016). *Astaxanthinzusammensetzungen (iii).* 18.03.2016.

WO/2016/146804. (2016). *Astaxanthinzusammensetzungen (iv).* 18.03.2016.

WO/2017/168006. (2017). *Beverages comprising stable granules of milled lutein.* 05.10.2017.

WO/2017/195504. (2017). *Agent for improving carotenoid balance in blood.* 16.11.2017.

WO/2018/030579. (2018). *Polymer capsule having double layered structure and improved elution rate and stability of lutein, preparation method there for, and pharmaceutical composition for preventing or treating ophthalmologic diseases, containing same.* 15.02.2018.

Xinde, X., Mingqing, J., Dong, S., Bin, S., & Leming, Y. (2012). *Method of producing natural β-carotene by fermentation and use thereof.* [Patent PCT/CN2012/000655].

Further reading

Bogacz-Radomska, L., & Harasym, J. (2016). Vegetables as a source of carotenoids. *Nauki Inzynierskie i Technologie*, *4*(23), 26–39.

CA2280715. (1998). *Oral preparation for the prophylactic and therapeutic treatment of helicobacter sp.infection.* 03.09.2019.

Euromonitor database https://go.euromonitor.com/passport.html (10.12.2018) 2018.

Patentscope https://patentscope.wipo.int/search/en/structuredSearch.jsf (18.11.2018) 2018.

Index

Note: Page numbers followed by *f* indicate figures and *t* indicate tables.

X

Z